# Current Radiation Oncology

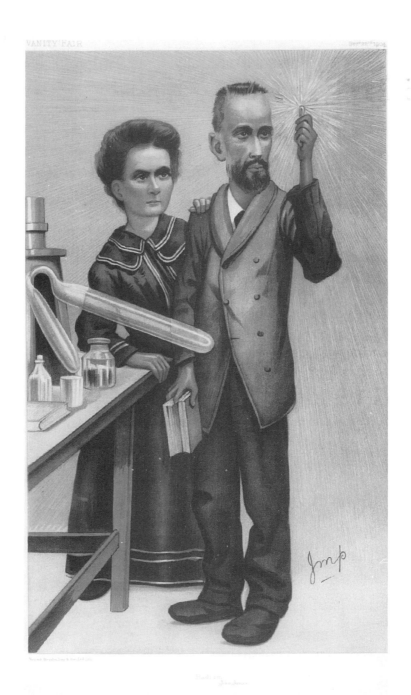

Pierre and Marie Curie (courtesy of Dr Frances MB Calman).

# Current Radiation Oncology

## Volume 2

*Edited by*

## Jeffrey S Tobias MD, FRCP, FRCR

*Clinical Director, Meyerstein Institute of Oncology,*
*Middlesex Hospital, London, UK*

*and*

## Patrick R M Thomas MB, FRCP, FRCR, FACR

*Professor and Chairman, Department of Radiation Oncology,*
*Temple University School of Medicine, Philadelphia, PA, USA*

A member of the Hodder Headline Group
LONDON • SYDNEY • AUCKLAND
Co-published in the USA by
Oxford University Press, Inc., New York

First published in Great Britain 1996 by
Arnold, a member of the Hodder Headline Group,
338 Euston Road, London NW1 3BH

Co-published in the United States of America by
Oxford University Press, Inc.,
198 Madison Avenue, New York, NY 10016
Oxford is a registered trademark of Oxford University Press

*British Library Cataloguing in Publication Data*
A catalogue record for this book is available from the British Library

*Library of Congress Cataloging-in-Publication Data*
A catalog record for this book is available from the Library of Congress

ISBN 0 340 61387 4 (hb)

Typeset in 10/11 pt Plantin by Anneset, Weston super Mare, Avon.
Printed and bound in Great Britain by St. Edmundsbury Press,
Bury St. Edmunds, Suffolk and Hartnolls Ltd, Bodmin, Cornwall.

This volume is dedicated to Pierre and Marie Curie

# Contents

# Contributors

**Mitsuyuki Abe** MD, Professor and Chairman, Department of Radiology, Faculty of Medicine, Kyoto University, Kyoto, Japan

**Søren M Bentzen** PhD, DSc, Senior Scientist, Danish Cancer Society, Department of Experimental Clinical Oncology, Aarhus, Denmark

**James D Bridges** MD, Head, Division of Radiation Oncology, National Naval Medical Center, Bethesda, Maryland, USA

**Juan A del Regato** MD, DSc, FACR, Emeritus Professor of Radiology, University of South Florida College of Medicine and Emeritus Distinguished Physician, Veterans Administration, Tampa, Florida, USA

**Nina Einhorn** MD, PhD, Professor of Oncology, Konung Gustaf V:S Jubileumsfond, Cancerforeningen I Stockholm, Stockholm, Sweden

**Richard Fisher** MB BS, BSc, PhD, Medical Statistician, Department of Radiation Oncology, The Prince of Wales Hospital, Randwick, New South Wales, Australia

**R J Michael Fry** MD, Consultant, Biology Division, Oak Ridge National Laboratory, Oak Ridge, Tennessee, USA

**Mark N Gaze** MD, MRCP, FRCR, Consultant Oncologist, The Meyerstein Institute of Oncology, The University College London Hospitals and The Hospital for Sick Children, Great Ormond Street, London, UK

**Eli Glatstein** MD, Chairman, Department of Radiation Oncology, Simmons Cancer Center, University of Texas Southwestern Medical Center, Dallas, Texas, USA

**Stuart L Goldberg** MD, Assistant Professor of Medicine and Assistant Director, Bone Marrow Transplant Program, Temple University School of Medicine, Philadelphia, Pennsylvania, USA

**Colin Hopper** FRCS(Ed), FDSRCS, Maxillofacial Surgeon, University College London Hospitals and the Eastman Dental Institute for Oral Health Care Sciences and Senior Lecturer, National Medical Laser Centre, University College, London, UK

**Iain Hutchison** MB, FRCS, FFDRCSI, Consultant Oral and Maxillofacial Surgeon, St Bartholomew's Hospital, London, UK

**James W Lynch Jr** MD, Assistant Professor, Division of Medical Oncology, Department of Medicine, University of Florida Health Science Center, Gainesville, Florida, USA

**Hedy Mameghan** MA, BM, BCh(Oxon), FRCR(Lond), FRACR (Sydney), Radiation Oncologist, The Prince of Wales Hospital, Randwick, New South Wales, Australia

**Nancy Price Mendenhall** MD, Professor and Chairman, Department of Radiation Oncology, University of Florida Health Science Center, Gainesville, Florida, USA

**Gerard Morton** MB, MRCPI, FFRRCSI, FRCPC, Radiation Oncologist, Department of Radiation Oncology, Toronto-Sunnybrook Regional Cancer Center and Lecturer in Radiation Oncology, University of Toronto, Ontario, Canada

**Yasumasa Nishimura** MD, Lecturer, Department of Radiology, Faculty of Medicine, Kyoto University, Kyoto, Japan

**R Timothy D Oliver** MD, FRCP, Professor of Medical Oncology, Medical College, The Royal Hospitals NHS Trust, Smithfield, London, UK

**Jens Overgaard** MD, DSc, FRCR, Professor and Chairman, Danish Cancer Society, Department of Radiation Oncology, Aarhus, Denmark

**Ajmel A Puthawala** MD, Clinical Professor, University of California and Associate Director, Long Beach Memorial Medical Center, Long Beach, California, USA

**Andrew G Robertson** PhD, FRCR, FRCP(Glas), Consultant in Clinical Oncology, Beatson Oncology Center, Glasgow, UK

**Chris Robertson** BSc, MSc, PhD, Senior Lecturer, Department of Statistics and Modelling, University of Strathclyde, Glasgow, UK

**Yuta Shibamoto** MD, DMSc, Associate Professor, Department of Oncology, Chest Disease Research Institute, University of Kyoto, Kyoto, Japan

**Craig L Silverman** MD, Associate Professor, Department of Radiation Oncology, Temple University Medical School, Philadelphia, Pennsylvania, USA

**A M Nisar Syed** MD, FRCS, Professor, King/Drew School of Medicine, Clinical Professor, University of California and Chairman, Department of Radiation Oncology, Long Beach Memorial Medical Center, Long Beach, California, USA

**Gillian M Thomas** MD, BSc, Professor of Radiation Oncology and Obstetrics and Gynaecology, and Head Division of Radiation Oncology, University of Toronto, Ontario, Canada

**Patrick R M Thomas** MB, FRCP, FRCR, FACR, Professor and Chairman, Department of Radiation Oncology, Temple University Medical School, Philadelphia, Pennsylvania, USA

**Jeffrey S Tobias** MD, FRCR, FRCP, Clinical Director, The Meyerstein Institute of Oncology, The Middlesex Hospital, London, UK

**Clare C Vernon** MA, FRCR, Consultant in Clinical Oncology, Hammersmith Hospital, Du Cane Road, London, UK

**Thomas E Wheldon** BSc, PhD, Radiation Biologist, Departments of Radiation Oncology and Clinical Physics, Alexander Stone Building, University of Glasgow School of Medicine, Glasgow, UK

**Catherine D Williams** MRCP, DipRCPath, Research Fellow in Multiple Myeloma, Department of Haematology, University College Hospital, London, UK

# Preface

Encouraged by the response to *Current Radiation Oncology Volume 1* (1994) we were anxious to complete Volume 2 for publication during 1995, the centenary year following the discovery of radium and artificial X-rays. What better introduction than the outstanding contribution from Dr Juan del Regato, doyen of senior radiation oncologists and highly esteemed world-wide for his major textbook and many original contributions? Dr del Regato's comprehensive outline of the first hundred years of radiation oncology is a *tour de force* which serves to remind us of the outstanding individuals who contributed to the specialty during its early years. As he aptly points out: 'In the penumbra of the past, the historian can more easily distinguish the bright gems from the ordinary pebbles'.

Which other modern specialties are more firmly rooted in experimental and applied science? Chapter 2 provides an outline of current thought in clinical normal tissue radiobiology, stressing the importance of normal tissue complications as a dose-limiting feature in modern radiotherapy. For the foreseeable future, radiobiological strategies will continue to inform and modify the views and techniques of radiation oncologists; in recent years, novel techniques such as hyperfractionated radiotherapy, integrated radiation-chemotherapy and tele-brachy-combinations are common illustrations of this theme.

Yet we have long been aware of the potential dangers of radiation either from medical exposure to X-rays, from military incidents, radiation accidents or low level background exposure. These areas are well reviewed by Dr Fry in Chapter 3. As radiation oncologists we also have to recognize the inevitable consequences, sometimes adverse, of the powerful treatment we offer. In Chapter 7, Iain Hutchison offers an orofacial surgeon's view of common complications of head and neck radiotherapy, with particular emphasis on critical long-term damage to the complex tissues of the head and neck, together with an outline of corrective therapy – a timely reminder of the teamwork between radiation oncologist and surgeon so essential for patient welfare.

Continuing our theme of covering important growth areas not reviewed in Volume 1, we were keen to invite authoritative overviews from acknowledged experts. The contributions of Drs Einhorn, Robertson and colleagues, Oliver and Gaze are models of lucidity and good sense, and should be of great value both to specialist and trainee alike.

Total body irradiation is now fully established as a treatment modality, in refractory non-Hodgkin lymphoma, acute and chronic leukaemia and other haematological conditions. In Chapter 14, Drs Silverman and Goldberg have provided an excellent overview of both the history and rationale for treatment as well as an outline of current radiation technique.

Finally, looking to the future, novel approaches are of course the lifeblood of any changing specialty. Three chapters in particular address important areas of novel research in intraoperative radiation therapy (Chapter 18), photodynamic therapy (Chapter 5) and hyperthermia (Chapter 19). All are written by highly experienced and expert practitioners.

We are grateful to all our contributors for providing up-to-date and lively discussion in areas we have selected as both topical and dynamic, particularly since many of these fields are scarcely covered in standard texts. Many words of celebration have been written during this centenary year since 1895 and we hope that, in some small way, this second volume of *Current Radiation Oncology* will help to illuminate the exciting growing points which could improve the outcome for future generations of cancer patients. As we pointed out in the Preface to Volume 1, radiation therapy has been regarded for too long as a somewhat uninteresting and over-technical specialty; recent years have certainly witnessed a change for the better.

We also gratefully acknowledge the help of our Editor at Arnold Ms Diane Leadbetter-Conway and extend our thanks to our ever-patient secretaries Ms Jayshree Kara, Ms Mauria Reich and Ms Catherine Barnes.

JS Tobias
PRM Thomas
1995

# 1 One hundred years of radiation oncology

*Juan A del Regato*

## 1895–1920

Three weeks after the public announcement of Roentgen's discovery, on 29 January 1896, Emil Herman Grubbé (1875–1960) initiated the irradiation (eighteen daily 1-hour exposures) of a patient with advanced recurrent cancer of the breast; the condition was relieved but she died shortly afterward from metastases.[1] In March, an accidental radiation epilation was observed and reported by Vanderbilt Professor of Physics John Daniel (1861–1950).[2] Seeking to utilize this radiobiological effect for therapeutic purposes, Leopold Freund (1868–1943), of Vienna, irradiated a 4-year-old girl with an extensive hairy naevus of the torso, in November 1896 (ten daily 2-hour exposures): the hair fell off but at the price of a severe radioepidermitis that took a long time to heal.[3] Freund proceeded to irradiate other skin conditions such as hypertrichosis, favus, sycosis, etc., for which he is often credited as the father of radiotherapy. However, Grubbé's priority is incontestable.

The early radiologists had to struggle with sources of power, generators, condensers, interrupters, filters, and tubes. The standard static, friction or influence generator was the Wimshurst machine (Fig. 1.1), originally operated by hand and later motorized. A modified model with twenty ebonite discs and increased velocity of rotation was favoured by some radiotherapists.[4] Another type had large glass discs, 183 cm in diameter, turning at 250 rpm.[5]

An induction coil like the one used by Roentgen was favoured by others. The Ruhmkorff coil was the standard model (Fig. 1.2), but there were numerous varieties of coil. Frequent breaking of the primary current enhanced the potential of the induced current; thus, automatic interrupters were used for this purpose. Interrupters were mechanical, chemical or elec-

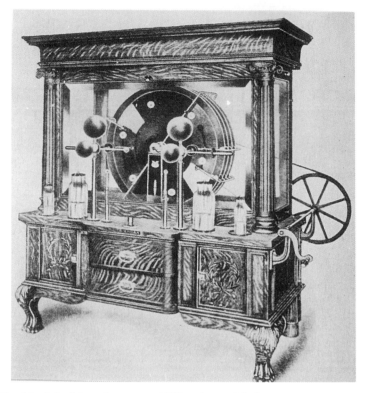

**Fig. 1.1**   Model of hand-operated Wimshurst friction generator.

trolytic; the use of condensers was eliminated by the electrolytic inter-rupters, but these had difficulties of their own. Where available, 'street' cur-rent was used, but also that provided by storage batteries and by a dynamo operated by a gasoline motor. Alternating currents had to be dealt with; at first, the reverse phase was eliminated and wasted, but later it was recti-fied. For this purpose, valve tubes (kenotrons) were widely used.[6] Theoretically, the induction coil could produce unlimited high voltages, but these were limited by insulation failures of the induced current or by the incapacity of the tubes to stand very high tensions. Spintermeters were used to avoid excessive charges on the tubes (Fig. 1.2). In time, the spark-gap became a means of measuring the peak voltage of the induced current and hence the lesser or greater ability of the X-rays to penetrate in depth.[7]

The Crookes' tube used by Roentgen had a simple pear shape (Fig. 1.3): with the anode out of its way, the cathode emitted a wide stream of cath-ode rays towards the glass wall where the X-rays were produced. The first innovations were:

1. the interposition of a target, the anticathode, usually made of platinum alloy or copper;
2. connection of the anode with the anticathode; and
3. giving the cathode a concave shape to focus its beam on the target (Fig. 1.4).

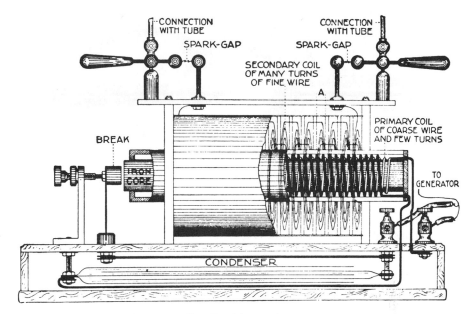

**Fig. 1.2**   Model of Ruhmkorff coil with spark-gap.

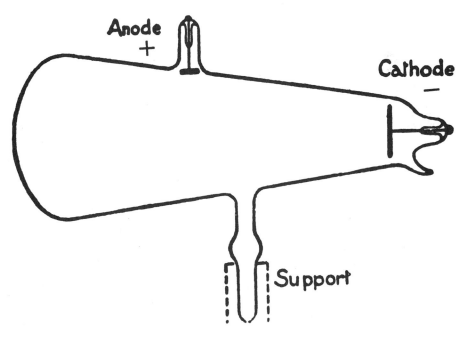

**Fig. 1.3**   Crookes' tube of the type used by Roentgen.

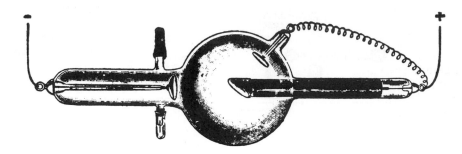

**Fig. 1.4** Tube with concave cathode and connection of the anode with the anticathode.

The manufacture of X-ray tubes became a veritable windfall to physicists, glass-blowers and electrical buffs: it gave wings to their imagination and provided an opportunity to participate in the new technology and to contribute to research. The result was a prodigious variety of ingenious tubes responding to various challenges.

Commercially available tubes were made with a moderate vacuum. With repeated use, the vacuum increased and the glass walls were metallized; as a consequence, the amount of X-rays produced was diminished and the tubes were said to have been hardened. 'Soft' tubes were preferred for radio-diagnostic use, so the hardened tubes were either discarded or returned to the manufacturer to reduce the vacuum. 'Hard' tubes yielded more penetrating radiations, so they were sometimes reserved for radiotherapy. A yellowish fluorescence of the tube was said to indicate softness while a greenish one indicated hardness. Tubes were also designed with an *osmoregulator*, an inbuilt palladium wire through the wall, that when heated on the outside released hydrogen inside the tube (Fig. 1.5). Also, the tubes could become excessively hot, and, to relieve this, some tubes were designed with circulating water around the target for cooling purposes. This was particularly useful in tubes used for roentgentherapy.[8]

Some tubes were produced for radiotherapy excusively; they were

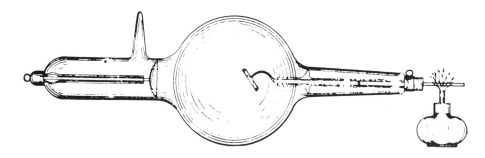

**Fig. 1.5** Tube provided with inbuilt osmoregulator.

characterized by a greater concern for the safety of the patient and operating personnel. Joseph Belot (1876–1953), of Paris, designed a tube, properly encased in ebonite with a localizing aperture reinforced with lead, for local irradiation (Fig. 1.6).[4] William Herbert Rollins (1852–1929), of Boston, a designer of numerous ingenious tubes, provided them with a special tube-holder coated with lead paint, and reinforced with lead plates having openings of various sizes (Fig. 1.7).[9] Henry Granger Piffard (1842–1910), of New York, designed a tube made entirely of lead glass with a small window of ordinary glass for the passage of X-rays and further collimation (Fig. 1.8). Eugene Wilson Caldwell (1879–1918), of New York, designed special tubes for intracavitary irradiation.[10]

The basic limitations of induction coils and gas tubes limited the production of X-rays to an estimated level of 60–70 kV and 1–2 mA. This was satisfactory for a variety of radiodiagnostic procedures that were rapidly investigated and put into practice; but the weak penetration of this range limited the radiotherapeutic possibilities. The pioneers of radiotherapy undertook to irradiate a number of skin diseases. The anti-inflammatory effects of radiations gave spectacular results in the treatment of such

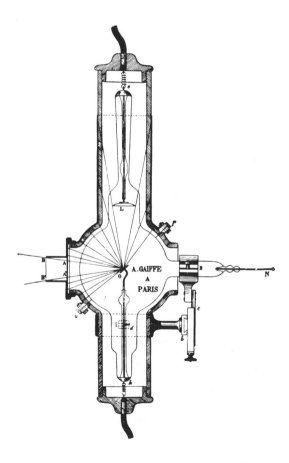

**Fig. 1.6**  Tube encased in ebonite designed by Belot for roentgentherapy.

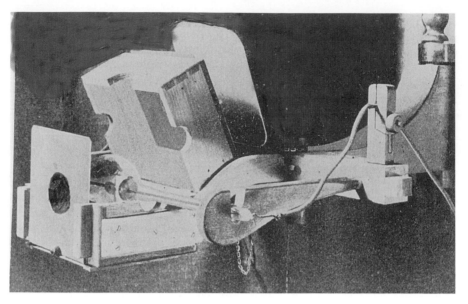

**Fig. 1.7**   Tube holder designed by Rollins with lead protection of walls.

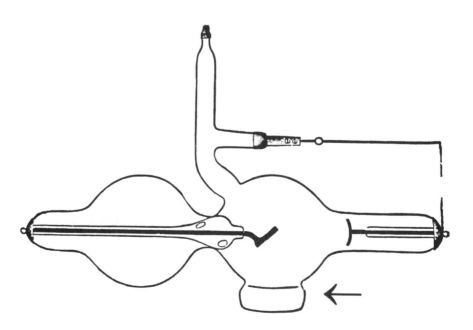

**Fig. 1.8**   Tube designed for roentgentherapy and made entirely of lead glass except for a portal of exit.

conditions as sycosis, eczema, etc., but radiotherapy was also applied to the treatment of chronic diseases such as psoriasis or lupus. The depilatory capability of X-rays became a long-sought-after solution to the age-old problem of tinea capitis, the contagious fungal infection of the scalp of children.

For a considerably long time, radiotherapy was carried out with the rays as they came out of the tubes, without the benefit of filtration. In an effort to provide means of comparison, the pioneers gave minute details of their generator, tube, distance from the tube and time of exposure. Often with equal technological details, the effects were quite different.

Not being able to measure the difference of quality and quantity of radiations delivered, the intensity of the effects on the skin were often ascribed to the type of generator, to the ozone produced by the electrical system, or to the ultraviolet rays that were assumed to accompany the X-rays. The author of one textbook recommended the routine preliminary testing of the beam's quality by the fluoroscopy of the radiologist's own hand (Fig. 1.9).[11]

Thor Stenbeck (1864–1914), of Stockholm, is credited with the first successful irradiation of a carcinoma of the skin in 1899. Contemporaneously, Francis Williams presented to the Boston City Hospital staff several cases of carcinoma of the skin and of the lower lip healed by fractionated irradiation.[9]

Heinrich Albers-Schönberg (1865–1921), of Hamburg, gave an accurate description of the successive manifestations of the irradiated skin: erythema, pigmentations, light oedema, excoriations and denudation of the dermis with eventual healing from the periphery.[12] Paul Oudin (1851–1923),

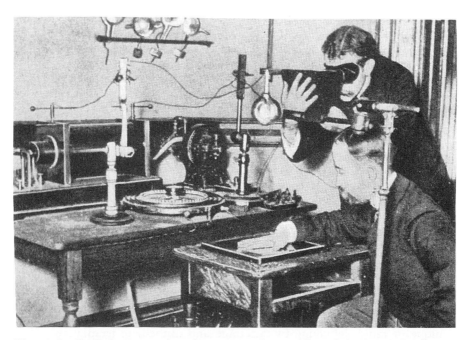

**Fig. 1.9** Radiologist testing the penetrating quality of the beam by fluoroscoping his own hand before operation.

Toussaint Barthelemy (1853–1906) and Jean Darier (1850–1938), of Paris, reported on an experimental study of the effects on the skin.[13] Various workers attempted to interpret the histological changes observed, but it was Walter Schölz (1871–1947), of Germany, who first undertook to correlate the clinical and histological studies of the effects of irradiation of the skin.[14]

Interest in radiophysiology gradually led to experimental studies in lower animals. Hermann Heineke (1878–1922), of Leipzig, discovered that other tissues of the body reacted and recovered more rapidly than the skin.[15] His study of the effects on the lymphoid tissues is a classic that has never been surpassed. In 1903, Albers-Schönberg reported that rabbits whose testes had been irradiated continued to have coitus but did not impregnate the females: in other words, they had been rendered sterile but not impotent.[16] Jean Bergonié (1857–1925) and Louis Tribondeau, of Bordeaux, verified the eventual azoospermia, although the mature spermatozoids in the seminal vesicles had not been affected. Claudius Regaud (1870–1940) and J Blanc, of Lyon, observed that the radiosensitivity of the various cells of the spermatogenic line was greater the more undifferentiated they were, with extreme radiosensitivity for the spermatogonia.[17] By 1906, Regaud and Blanc had already pointed out the importance of the observed difference for radiation oncology. Bergonié and Tribondeau expressed these facts in the form of what was long accepted as a law.

In the year that followed the discovery, over 1000 papers and fifty books were published on the subject of X-rays, and more followed. A few of these books are veritable historians' gems:

- In 1901, Francis Henry Williams (1852–1936), of Boston, published a book[9] that reveals his great resourcefulness, his exceptionally large static machine and illustrations of a great variety of tubes designed by William Herbert Rollins (1852–1939), as well as pictures of the earliest cures of carcinoma of the skin and lower lip treated by irradiation.
- In 1903, William Allen Pusey (1865–1940), a dermatologist of Chicago, and Eugene Wilson Caldwell (1870–1918), a physicist of New York, produced an excellent book[10] revealing great pragmatic insight and the first patient of leukaemia treated with X-rays.
- In 1904, Leopold Freund (1868–1943), of Vienna, published a book[18] that was promptly translated by GH Lancashire, of Manchester, and published in London and New York. The book gives an account of Freund's 4-year experience with radiotherapy of skin diseases, and, in addition, a thorough review of pertinent literature. The survey reveals a variety of views and conjectures in reference to the observed effects of irradiation. Freund puts to rest, by experimental laboratory work, the long-debated bactericidal properties of X-rays.
- In 1905, Joseph Belot (1876–1953), of Paris, published a book[4] on radiotherapy of skin diseases using a tube and localizer of his own design (Fig. 1.6). It contains photographs of patients treated with fractionated irradiation over periods of several weeks, with excellent aesthetic results. Nevertheless, Belot's name became subsequently attached to his technique of rapid debulking by curettage and immediate irradiation of the resulting wound base by a single exposure to unfiltered radiations.
- In 1907, Mihran Krikor Kassabian (1870–1910), of Philadelphia, a

dedicated pioneer who abridged his life-span by his excessive exposure to radiations, published his book.[19] In addition to a thorough presentation of the state of the art, Kassabian reported on an interesting survey that he had undertaken. He wrote to practitioners in England, Germany, France and the United States, requesting information as to their practice; the appendix of the book presents the replies: an amazing disparate collection of opinions in reference to indications for radiotherapy, details of technology and results.

Embraced primarily by dermatologists, radiotherapy was starting cautious incursions into the treatment of internal tumours. This made new demands on technology. Gradually empiricism gave in to rational methods. Louis Benoist (born 1856), a French physics teacher, invented a device that permitted the appraisal of the beam's penetrability for comparison with others (Fig. 1.10). Benoist's *radiochromometer* consisted of an aluminium disc, divided, as a clock, into sectors of twelve stratified thicknesses of 1–12 mm of aluminium and a central circle of 0.11 mm of silver. Exposed to the beam, its radiograph will show which sector and thickness of aluminium would match the tint of the silver circle (Fig. 1.10). Thus, the hardness of the

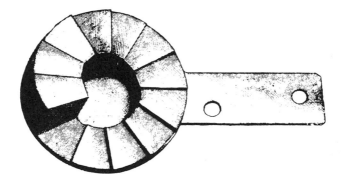

**Fig. 1.10** *Radiochromometer of Benoist.*

beam could be expressed on a scale of 1 to 12. An appraisal of quality, however, did not solve the remaining problem of the quantity of radiations delivered by a given exposure. Guido Holzknecht (1872–1931), of Vienna, presented his *chromoradiometer* at the Second International Congress of Medical Electrology, in Berne in 1902 (Fig. 1.11). Based on the photochemical effect and the consequent changes in colour of a mixture of sodium carbonate and potassium chloride, Holzknecht evaluated the dose that would produce a mild skin reaction and designated it as 3H.[20] The H unit became widely adopted as the only means of dosimetry for several decades. Since colour could also be affected by heat there was need of a control. In time, Holzknecht adopted the barium platinocyanide method proposed by the Parisian dermatologist Raymond Jacques Adrian Saboureaud (1864–1918). There were several other photochemical methods proposed,

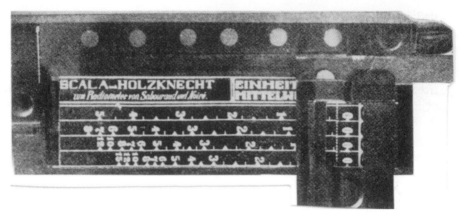

**Fig. 1.11** Chromoradiometer of Holzknecht using photochemical changes of colour for dosimetry.

including one by Robert Kienbock (1871–1953), of Vienna, who used strips of paper impregnated with silver bromide.

Pierre Curie (1859–1906) and Marie Sklodowska Curie (1867–1934) discovered radium in 1898.[21] It took 1 ton of pitchblende ore, 50 tons of water, 5 tons of chemicals and months of laborious effort to separate a few milligrams of radium, but they fitted easily in the vest pocket of Professor Antoine Henri Bequerel (1852–1909), to whom they were made a gift. Thus, on the skin of the professor's abdomen, the first radiobiological effects of radium were observed. Having verified the effects on his own forearm, Pierre Curie made available a few more milligrams to Alexander Danlos (1844–1922), a dermatologist who investigated its use in the treatment of skin diseases at the Saint Louis Hospital of Paris.[22]

Meanwhile, the reputation of radium as a potential agent against neoplasia had spread rapidly. Robert Abbé (1851–1923), a New York surgeon, obtained two tubes of radium which he used as a surgical adjuvant.[23] Margaret Abigail Cleaves (1848–1917), a New York electrotherapist, borrowed a sealed glass tube containing radium and introduced it in contact with an extensive carcinoma of the cervix.[24] Impressed by the response, she requested from Eugene Caldwell the manufacture of a special tube of X-rays to be introduced in the vagina (Fig. 1.12); to avoid burning of the vaginal wall by the heat of the tube, a water-containing jacket was added.[10] Francis Williams, the Boston pioneer who had worked with a weak source of radium chloride, went to Paris and purchased 200 mg of radium bromide; in 1904, he reported on the treatment of forty-two patients.[25] In 1904, Danlos handed over the borrowed radium to Louis Frederic Wickham (1861–1913), a dermatologist of the Saint Lazare Hospital of Paris, who, together with physicist Paul Desgrais (1874–1954), extended the research and produced new gadgetry including the first intrauterine and vaginal applicator for the treatment of cancer of the cervix (Fig. 1.13). They adopted the heavy metal filtration advocated by Henri Dominici (1857–1927). Wickham and Desgrais' 1909 book was translated and published in New York in 1910[26] and awoke renewed interest in radiumtherapy. Wickham also developed a Laboratoire Biologique du Radium at Gif,

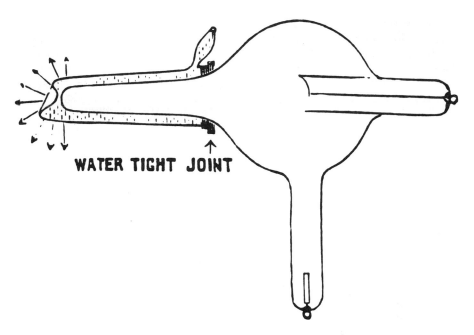

WATER TIGHT JOINT

**Fig.1.12** Tube designed by Caldwell for transvaginal irradiation of the cervix.

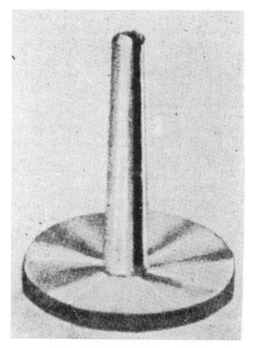

**Fig. 1.13** Early applicator for intrauterine and vaginal application of radium. The gadget was painted with a thick varnish containing radium and covered by an aluminium filter.

in the outskirts of Paris, where basic studies on the physical and biological properties of radium and radon were made by Dominici, Jacques Danne, H Rubens-Duval (1876–1924) and Henri Coutard (1876–1950).[27,28]

In 1909, Gösta Forssell (1876–1950), of Stockholm, reported on the treatment of thirty-two cancer patients using eight silver tubes containing 8 mg of radium sulphate.[29] Forssell, who coined the word 'brachytherapy', became a world leader of radiation oncology. In 1913, Neville Samuel Finzi (1881–1950), the resourceful English pioneer of radiation oncology, published a book on his radium therapeutics work from 1909. Finzi had made an early attempt at telecurietherapy with 600 mg of radium.[30]

In Lyon, Regaud had found that it was impossible to sterilize the testis of a laboratory animal by a single irradiation, no matter how large, whereas a smaller total dose divided into several applications over a period of days produced the desired results without affecting the tissues of the scrotum.[31] His student, Antoine Lacassagne (1884–1971) wrote his thesis on the biological effects of radiations on the ovary.[32]

In 1913, H Cheron and Rubens-Duval had already observed encouraging results in the treatment, with radium, of 152 patients with carcinoma of the cervix.[33] However, it soon became evident that only small lesions were healed. Walter Friedrich (1883–1968), of Freiburg im Breisgau,[34] and B Krönig, also of Germany, had already started to complement the treatment with external pelvic roentgentherapy.[35]

It should be evident from this chronicle that we owe a great debt to dermatologists who contributed importantly to the early development of roentgentherapy. Their interest in the treatment of malignant tumours led them to found special institutions such as the Skin and Cancer Hospitals of New York and of Saint Louis.

Research on the application of radium to patients with cancer, and the scarcity of the radioactive element, called for the creation of special institutions for research, where workers of various disciplines could cooperate in the development of pragmatic methods for its use. Most notable were the following:

- In 1910, with only 120 mg of radium, an institution properly named as a home, the Radiumhemmet of Stockholm, was founded with Gösta Forssell as director.
- In 1913, the Institut du Radium of the University of Paris was created, with a building for research in physics and chemistry under Madame Curie and another for radiophysiology and medicine under Regaud.
- In 1913, the final agreement was reached for the founding of the New York Memorial Hospital for the treatment of cancer and allied diseases, with an endowment of several grams of radium and James Ewing (1866–1943) as director.

These institutions, created to face the challenge of radiumtherapy, were to become the outstanding centres for the treatment of cancer in general. Regaud made seminal contributions to radiophysiology. Ewing became an authority in tumour pathology and Forssell was the leader on the social fight against cancer. They and their associates and students contributed in various ways to the nascent specialty of radiation oncology.

In 1912, Max von Laue (1879–1960), of Munich, discovered the diffraction of X-rays through crystals, proving the wave nature of the rays. This discovery permitted the measurement of wavelength and hence the quality of a given beam of rays.

Articles on the subject of radiotherapy were published in journals of general radiology in Europe and America. In 1912, the first journal devoted exclusively to radiotherapy was launched in Germany by Hans Meyer (1877–1944) of Kiel, Carl Joseph Gauss (1875–1967) of Freiburg, and Richard Werner (1875–1945) of Heidelberg: *Strahlentherapie* has recently added *und Onkologie* to its title.

Likewise, there were early societies of general radiology in Germany, England and the United States. But, in 1916, a group of interested physicians gathered in Philadelphia and founded the American Radium Society. Its membership grew, and, although the society refused jealously to change its name, it became a forum of multidisciplinary clinical oncology. The *American Journal of Roentgenology* added *and Radiumtherapy* to its title and became its official organ.

# 1920–45

Within days of his demobilization from the army, in March 1919, Regaud was back at work at the Radium Institute of Paris. He and his associate, Antoine Lacassagne (1884–1971), bicycled to the city's hospitals to try the possibilities of radiumtherapy. Within a relatively short time they developed the system of tandem plus colpostat applications for the treatment of carcinoma of the cervix (Fig. 1.14). With the help of the dedicated associates at their service in the Pasteur Hospital, they also perfected the technique of interstitial implantation (radiumpuncture) for carcinoma of the tongue.[31] Regaud and André Debièrne (1874–1935) developed a system of radium dosimetry in *millicuries destroyed*.[36]

William Duane (1872–1935), of Boston, developed a radium emanation extraction and purification plant; he compressed the radioactive gas into glass capillary tubes and proposed to cut them into small fragments to be imbedded into tumours; in view of the short half-life of radon, the glass *seeds* could be left to be sloughed. James Janeway (1873–1921), and other associates of James Ewing, in New York, used the procedure[37] in the treatment of cancer of the bladder, of the prostate and on metastatic lymph nodes. Gioacchino Failla (1891–1961), aware that the bare *seeds* were too caustic, developed the *gold seeds* which became very popular in the United States.[38]

Two important inventions gave great impetus to roentgentherapy in the postwar years. One of these was the cascade (or on-ladder) transformer of Friedrich Dessauer (1881–1963), of Frankfurt, that permitted higher voltages by by-passing the insulation difficulties of the ordinary transformer (Fig. 1.15). Equally important was the *hot cathode tube* of William Coolidge (1873–1975), of Schenectady, which eliminated the impertinence of gas tubes. These innovations were rapidly adopted by manufacturers on both sides of the Atlantic, and 200 kV units and their use was heralded as 'deep therapy' (tiefentherapie, radiothérapie profonde).[39] The gain in kilovoltage

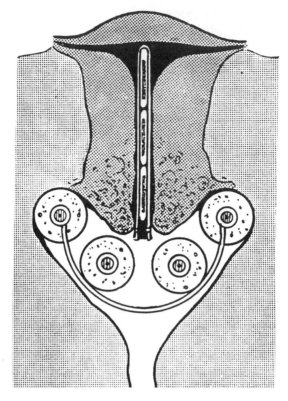

**Fig. 1.14**  Early arrangement of intrauterine sources in tandem and colpostats for intracavitary irradiation of cancer of the cervix.

was not accompanied by increased milliamperage (around 4 mA), and consequently the output remained low.

There were Austrian (Holtznecht's), German (Behnke's) and French
(Solomon's) units being used. At the First International Congress of
Radiology (present series), held in London in 1925, Antoine Béclère made
an impassioned plea for a defined and internationally accepted unit that
would permit standardization of techniques and comparison of results. An
impressive Commission of Units and Measures was charged with finding
the solution and was to render its report at the next congress.

The greater availability of equipment and the increased practice of radiotherapy created a need for sources of information. Iser Solomon
(1880–1939), of Paris, published a *Précis de Radiothérapie*.[39] Paul Lazarus,
of Switzerland, also wrote a *Handbuch der Gesamter Strahlenheilkunde*,[40]
including chapters by Hermann Holthusen (1886–1971) of Hamburg. Both
these books found large circulation in Europe and abroad. In the United
States, Isa Seth Hirsh (1880–1942), of New York, published *The Principles
and Practice of Roentgen Therapy*.[41] This latter book included a chapter contributed by Holtznecht, with a long list of indications and specific techniques for the treatment of innumerable diseases: from asthma, angina

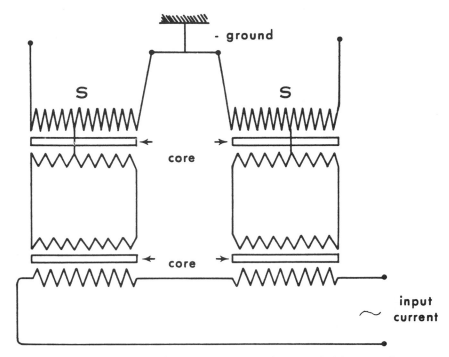

**Fig. 1.15**  Basic design of Dessauer's cascade or on-ladder transformer.

pectoris and arthritis to pulmonary tuberculosis and syringomyelia. This unwarranted empiricism was to bring disrepute from which it took a long time for radiotherapy to be free.

Quartered in the basement of the Pavillon Pasteur of the Radium Institute of Paris, Henri Coutard (1870–1950) had given himself to the study of roentgentherapy of cancer of the upper air passages. He made clinical observations of skin and mucous membrane reactions[42] and contributed an original radiographic study of the normal and cancerous larynx.[43] But it was his eventual report on roentgentherapy of cancer of the tonsil that awoke wide interest in his work.[44] Regaud had emphasized the importance of fractionation, but not beyond 10 days. Coutard had dared to extend the treatment of his patients to several weeks of daily exposure. His unprecedented results motivated great interest in what was called the Coutard method.[45] Hans Schinz (1891–1966) and Adolf Zuppinger (1904–92), of Zurich, made a personal inquiry and observed that Coutard treated his patients twice daily for sittings of over 1 hour (protraction) and that the total treatments lasted 6 or more weeks (fractionation); they dubbed Coutard's work the *protahiert fraktionierten methode*.[46]

Finally, in 1926, the Commission on Units and Measurements brought forth the **roentgen** at the Second International Congress of Radiology in Stockholm. It was truly an international unit, for it was based on ionization of air, as long-proposed by Paul Villard (1850–1934) of France, having similarities with the unit proposed by Hermann Behnken (1889–1945) of Germany, and was almost identical in its definition with the electrostatic unit long-used by William Duane (1872–1935) of the United States.

Commercially available ionization chambers were in wide use to calibrate the output and to measure doses delivered. Two models found practical acceptance: the German *Hammer* and the Austrian *Mekapion*; both could be used as integrometers to deliver a given dose for a sitting. The chamber was usually placed in the centre of the field of entry and registered the dose delivered plus the backscatter. In the US, John Victoreen (1902–  ) studied under Otto Glasser (1895–1964), long a student of ionization chambers. Victoreen produced a chamber bearing his name and used mostly for calibration.

There were reasonable means of measuring the dose administered at the portal of entry, but the dose delivered at any point in depth had to be calculated. Using photometric methods, Dessauer produced a series of *intensity charts* corresponding to fixed circumstances of kilovoltage, filter, focus–skin distance and size of field, which were widely adopted to estimate doses in depth (Fig. 1.16).[47] Others, working with water phantoms, also produced similar information that Glasser called *isodose charts*. In order to accumulate the desirable dose in depth, several portals of entry were used to converge on the tumour area. These calculations required precise anatomical measurements; the available charts often differed substantially. For a while, the accumulated dose at one point was registered as 'tumour dose', although the tumour could not be expected to be only at one point.

It had been empirically established that the complete destruction of a malignant tumour required the administration of a relatively large dose, equivalent to that required to produce radioepidermitis of the skin. But

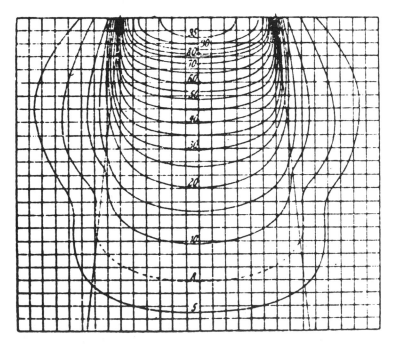

**Fig. 1.16** Sample of isodose chart.

there was no agreement or understanding as to the time in which that dose should be delivered. Ludwig Seitz (1872–1961), and Hermann Wintz (1887–1947) of Erlangen, advocated delivery of the total dose in the shortest possible time.[48] Clinically, the adoption of this view resulted in 'radiation sickness': nausea, vomiting, and malaise, particularly when large fields were used. Leopold Freund, of Vienna, advocated a division of the total dose into a great number of fractions, but without a rationale.[49] Biophysicists became interested in the effects on the skin as a model. Karl Stënstrom (1891–1973), then in Buffalo, found that identical reactions could be obtained by an *erythema dose* delivered in one sitting, or by 120% of it in four consecutive daily exposures, or 130% in 8 days.[50] Experimentalists became preoccupied with the rate of recovery. LB Kingery estimated that an initial irradiation lost half of its effectiveness in $3\frac{1}{2}$ days and proposed a *saturation method* based on this assumption.[51] Edith Quimby (1891–1982), of New York, found that recovery after each exposure was smaller than the precedent and that the assumption of a regular rate of recovery was unwarranted.[52] Magnus Strandqvist (1904–78), of Stockholm, undertook a study of over 200 patients who had been irradiated for carcinomas of the skin and lower lip. He plotted on double logarithmic graphs the total doses against the time in which they had been administered and found that the successfully treated cases followed a straight line, above which were all the cases of necrosis and below which were the cases of recurrence.[53]

The radiosensitivity of certain tumours became an important factor in their recognition, starting with Regaud's *lymphoépithéliomas* of the upper air passages, Ewing's *endotheliosarcomas* and Oberling's *reticulum-cell sarcoma* of bone, Berger's *ésthesioneuroépithéliomas*, and still others. Tumour pathologists were attracted by these facts and sought their explanation in morphology. Hugo Ahlbom (1900–52), a radiation oncologist of Stockholm, wrote an exemplary thesis on salivary gland tumours.[54] And Elis Berven, also a radiation oncologist of Stockholm, published a monograph on malignant tumours of the tonsil.[55.] Both of these epoch-making publications made it evident that knowledge of histopathology of tumours was an essential component of the intellectual strength of the radiation oncologist. A nexus had been established between the two endeavours.

The injurious effects of excessive irradiation of the skin had been recognized early in the development of radiotherapy.[56] The effects of the irradiation of lymphoid tissues and on the male and female gonads had been demonstrated also, and, as radiotherapy developed, interest arose about the effects on other tissues. Shields Warren (1898–1961), a pathologist of Boston, undertook, with several of his disciples, a series of separate studies of the effects of irradiation on various tissues.[57] Arthur Desjardins (1864–1944), a radiotherapist of the Mayo Clinic, made an exhaustive review of the literature on the effects of radiations on the eye and ear, published in three separate consecutive articles.[58] Knowledge of the radiophysiology of tissues and organs also became part of the intellectual requirement for the practitioner of radiation oncology.

Gustav Thoraeus (1895–1970), a physicist of Stockholm, developed the composite filter that bears his name. Theophil Christian (1873–1920), of Switzerland, introduced the concept of the *half-value layer* (HVL) as a means of expression of the quality of a beam of rays. Both the Thoraeus filter and the HVL appeared frequently in charts and reports of treatments.

In Germany, although radiology had remained subservient to other academic departments, roentgentherapy became popular, with Hans Holfelder (1871–1944) of Frankfurt as its leader. He advocated the multiportal approach for the irradiation of deeply seated tumours; the Holfelder 'cannon', of German manufacture, was very popular. In time, Hermann Holthusen (1886–1971), of Hamburg, a great advocate of the international **R-unit** led the development of a model department of radiotherapy that now bears his name.[59] In Sweden, James Heyman (1892–1945) extended the concept of the Stockholm method for the treatment of cancer of the cervix in three separate intracavitary applications of radium, 2 weeks apart. As chairman of a Committee of the League of Nations he promulgated the staging, and collated the results, of radiotherapy on cancer of the cervix.[60] He also developed the *packing* method of intrauterine irradiation for carcinoma of the endometrium. In England, the indefatigable Neville Finzi (1881–1968) organized the first comprehensive and well-equipped department of radiotherapy at the Saint Bartholomew's Hospital of London. He had a decisive influence in the subsequent development of radiation oncology in Great Britain.

Through the years, there had been isolated efforts to utilize radium in other than surface or intracavitary brachytherapy. Its high cost had limited these efforts to telecurietherapy units of 1–4 g of radium. The Radium Institute of Paris; the Radiumhemmet of Stockholm; the Westminster and the Royal Cancer Hospitals, as well as the Radium Beam Research, of London; and the Memorial Hospital of New York were the principals attacking these trials.[61] But the relatively small amounts of radium forced a short source-to-skin distance (SSD) to allow for reasonable times of exposure. For the protection of personnel, some of these units had pneumatic withdrawal of the sources to a safe distance; but no one claimed any advantageous results. Regaud believed that the shorter wavelength of the gamma rays offered a greater selectivity of effects between the tumour and the normal tissues, thus offering a greater margin of safety; he felt that telecurietherapy had to be carried out with the same careful fractionation and clinical control that had proven successful with roentgentherapy. He obtained a loan of 14 g of radium in 1934, and initiated a new trial. For these purposes, a floor of the new laboratory building of the Fondation Curie was equipped with six beds and a new 10-g unit; it required manual shifting for the beam at the beginning and end of the treatments (Fig. 1.17).[62] The project had to be discontinued when it was discovered that some of the sealed sources were leaking radon. Greater safety measures were introduced when the project was resumed, but no advantage was reported. The last trial of telecurietherapy took place at the Roosevelt Hospital of New York with 50 g of radium.[61]

In the nineteenth century, hospitals were created for the care of the incurables — where cancer patients went. These charitable institutions, such as the Christie Hospital for the Incurables of Manchester, had an understandably mournful reputation. It was the advent of X-rays and radium that motivated creation of new institutions to gather the scarce facilities and skills for the curative efforts in the treatment of cancer, but carefully avoiding the

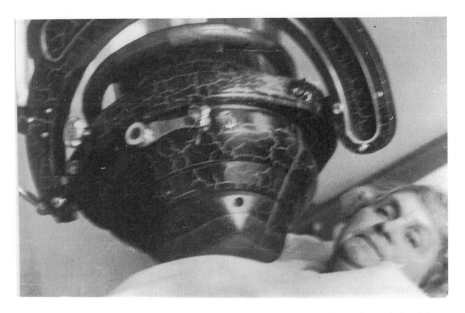

**Fig. 1.17** Patient under a 10 g telecurietherapy unit. Note the original lever for hand deviation of the beam.

use of the dreaded word. The Radium Institute, the Radiumhemmet, and the Memorial Hospital, mentioned above, became leading institutions for treatment and research in which radiation oncology made great strides. The Royal Cancer Hospital of London, founded in 1851 for the care of the hopeless, and its associated Cancer Research Institute, changed their names to the Royal Marsden and Chester Beatty Institute, respectively, honouring their founders. The Marie Curie Hospital of London, inaugurated in 1934, was named after a woman, staffed by women, for the exclusive treatment of cancer in women, thus avoiding a gender prejudice. And likewise, the Istituto dei Tumori of Milan and the Roswell Park Memorial Institute of Buffalo, attempted to keep from the public their true mission.

A contrary view was that of others who held that a frank use of the word 'cancer' would dissipate the public fear and counter the assumption that cancer was always incurable: the Instituto del Cancer of Havana (1929), and the Institut du Cancer of Villejuif (1934), in the outskirts of Paris, were examples of this alternative view. The Congress of the United States founded the National Cancer Institute (NCI) of Bethesda in 1937. The Ellis Fischel Cancer Hospital of Columbia, Missouri, also openly admitted its purposes.

At special institutions, regardless of their name, dedicated workers sought to improve the treatment of cancer patients and contributed to the strength and unbiased recognition of radiation oncology. In England, the radium officers originally appointed as custodians of the radioactive sources gradually became arbiters of their use and recognized radiotherapeutic experts. In the United States, the exclusive practice of radiotherapy found special obstacles. The radiological societies and the academic chairs of radiology considered radiotherapy only as a part of general radiology. Considerations of the exclusive practice of radiotherapy aroused fears of weakening the specialty and of harbingers of cessation. The use of radium was considered the province of oncologic surgeons.

Shortly after the First World War, British radiologists followed a brief course offered at Oxford and obtained a Diploma of Medical Radiology (DMR). This certification later qualified as a Diploma of Medical Radium Therapy (DMRT) was a recognized title of British radiation oncologists. The University of Paris offered a diploma of *Radiophysiologie et Radiothérapie* that required a previous 1-year course of electroradiology and four *stages* of 6-months duration at recognized departments of radiotherapy, and a final presentation of a thesis. The American Board of Radiology (ABR) was established in 1934. From its inception, the ABR offered certification in radiumtherapy and in therapeutic radiology but, since there were no centres of training, most of the early certifications went to surgeons who practised some radiumtherapy.[63]

In 1930, the cancer mortality in England had become alarming; private as well as government institutions took measures to improve facilities for the treatment of cancer patients. Allotment of radium to various institutions resulted in the search for trained radiotherapists. The Middlesex Hospital of London appointed a young Australian, Brian Windeyer (1904–1994), as radium officer. The Holt Radium Institute of Manchester put Ralston Paterson (1897–1981) in charge. Thanks to the efforts of David Smithers (1908–95), a department of radiotherapy was created and upgraded at the Royal Cancer Hospital.

In January 1934, working in the basement of the Pavillon Curie of the Radium Institute, Frederic Joliot (1905–57) and Irène Joliot-Curie (1902–56) discovered artifical radioactivity and opened the doors of 'nuclear medicine'. Their discovery gave new vistas to radiation oncology and resulted in transcendental consequences in the history of the world.

Although roentgentherapy had received its greatest radiobiological and clinical impulses in France, and seemed to have reached its apogee in Germany, there was no apparent hope of a progression to supervoltage in Europe before the Second World War. It was in the United States that the first million-volt units were produced. Some of these units were put in the hands of those interested in their physical properties, or of general radiologists who expected the higher voltages to compensate for their lack of clinical skills. There was frank antagonism to supervoltage, particularly from academic radiology. Professor Sherwood Moore (1894–1963), of Washington University, Saint Louis, stated his unswerving opposition to the use of supervoltage in the treatment of malignant tumours.[62] There were conservative defenders of the conventional. Leo Henry Garland (1903–66), a brilliant radiodiagnostician of Stanford University, then at San Francisco, declared 200 kV to be 'orthovoltage'; it is rather 'cacovoltage', quipped Franz Buschke, of the Swedish Hospital of Seattle. Nevertheless, in the early 1940s, Richard Dressser (1893–?) of the Huntington Memorial Hospital of Boston, Walter Murphy (1907–?) of the Roswell Park Institute of Buffalo and Milton Friedman (1903–83) of the Walter Reed Hospital of Washington, DC, were unanimous in their enthusiasm for the clinical advantages of supervoltage radiations.

Because of the lack of centres of instruction and training in therapeutic radiology in the United States, those interested followed special courses such as those offered by the Chicago Tumor Institute in the 1930s (Fig. 1.18). After the war the refresher courses of the Radiological Society of North America (RSNA) were increasingly attended; at first, they were concerned with dosimetry or were taught by surgeons, but gradually the society engaged radiation oncologists to cover all areas of clinical applications of radiotherapy. The scarcity of well-qualified radiotherapists obliged Leo Rigler (1896–1979), Professor of Radiology at the University of Minnesota, to entrust the service of radiotherapy to Karl Stënstrom (1891–1973), a biophysicist whose wife was a physician. Stënstrom acquitted himself of this challenge very well: he wrote a handbook on radiotherapy and was the earliest advocate of extended-field irradiation for Hodgkin's disease; he held the job for 25 years.

Having worked with Neville Finzi at Bart's and having an understanding of the challenges of clinical radiology, William Mayneord (1902–88) took a position as physicist at the Royal Cancer Hospital of London.[64] Frowned upon at first by his academic colleagues, Val Mayneord's talents and personality made medical physics respectable, and he became a role model to a generation of hospital physicists that contributed strength and authority

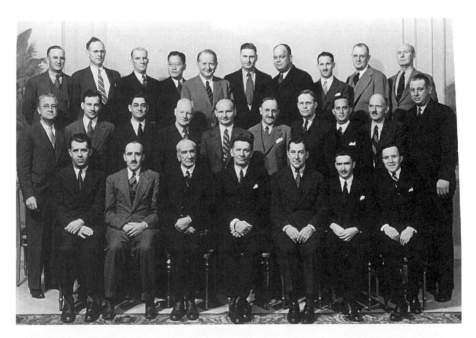

**Fig. 1.18** Attendants of one of the courses offered by the Chicago Tumor Institute in the summer of 1938. Seated in the front row was the faculty of instructors, from left to right: Ralph Caulk (radiologist), Ernest Woilan (physicist), Sir Lenthal Cheattle (surgeon), Henri Coutard (radiation oncologist), Max Cutler (pathologist), Juan del Regato (radiation oncologist), Louis Rosenthal (radiumtherapist). Missing on the front row were Franz Buschke and Sim Cantril, radiation oncologists.

to radiotherapy. He supported David (later Sir David) Smithers (1908–95) in the development of a department of radiotherapy and in the extension of radiotherapeutic research. In Manchester, Ralston Paterson (1897–1981) caused the physicist to become an integral element in the daily planning of treatments. With Herbert Parker (1910–84), he found a formula to express radium dosage in **r-units**; with Jack Meredith (1913–   ), he emphasized the importance of physics in everyday planning. Likewise, Gioacchino Failla (1891–1961) and Edith Quimby (1891–1982) contributed, in New York, to an understanding of the role of physics and organized the teaching of physics to young candidates of radiation oncology. X-rays and radium had brought the physicists out of their 'shops' and into the patients' wards to become partners in clinical endeavours.

Untoward effects of irradiation were observed promptly on the skin. Within the first decade following Roentgen's discovery, there were numerous cases of carcinoma of the skin on the hands and face of workers in radiology. Radium workers with unsuspected total exposure of their haemopoietic system developed aplastic anaemia with a terminal leukaemoid reaction often diagnosed as leukaemia. These martyrs of pioneer radiology are memorialized in a series of stelae which can be seen in the garden of the Sankt Georg Krankenhaus of Hamburg (Fig. 1.19).[65]

Untoward effects of irradiation of bones and other structures gradually were observed, particularly in young children successfully irradiated for malignant tumours. Side-effects on other tissues and organs, including kidneys, lungs, and spinal cord, were eventually recognized and related to dose and fractionation. Since 1925, the Commission on Protection of the International Congress of Radiology has formulated proper measures of pro-

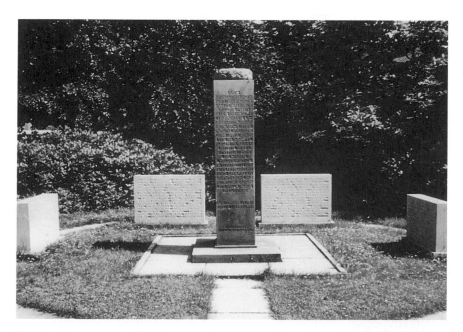

**Fig. 1.19**  Stelae with the carved names of martyrs of radiology from all nations, in the garden of the Sankt Georg Krankenhaus of Hamburg.

tection and limits of exposure for radiological workers.[66] Lauriston Taylor (1902–   ) and Gioacchino Failla were perennially reducing the estimated maximum permissible doses. During the Second World War, a number of scientists were engaged for the first time in research work with radiation in the Metallurgical Laboratory of Chicago. Robert Stone (1895–1955) was appointed to head a division of agents, mostly physicists, in charge of monitoring the various laboratories and to provide proper measures of protection. These agents were designated as *health physicists*.

The Archives of the Radium Institute of Paris appeared in the form of irregularly printed fascicles, published by the Presses Universitaires de France, from 1929 to 1938. Originally, they contained a thorough review of the world literature on radiobiology, but later also the contributions of the staff. These fascicles were gathered in three bound volumes entitled *Radiophysiologie et Radiothérapie*. This rare publication, long out of print, constitutes a rich historical source.

The Atomic Energy Research, intended for other purposes, brought a great demand for supervoltage units from which radiation oncology was to benefit. Generators of 1 million-plus volts became commercially available.

During the war, Lacassagne had made the observation that mice irradiated while in a state of asphyxia, and revived, were less affected by total body irradiation than those normally exposed.[67] This observation was to open important avenues of research on radiosensitivity in the years that followed. Lacassagne also invented the useful technique of autoradiography.

# 1945–70

In the postwar realignment of talents and facilities, the British Empire Cancer Campaign and the Medical Research Council (MRC) agreed to concentrate their clinical and laboratory research at the Hammersmith Hospital of London. Constance Wood (1897–1985) was appointed director and Louis Harold Gray (1905–65) was chosen as deputy director. Both were interested in the production of isotopes and on the building of a cyclotron and a linear accelerator. Connie Wood had definite clinical goals in mind whereas Hal Gray thought to utilize these sources for radiobiological research.

Many radiation physicists, following the example of Mayneord in England and Failla in the United States, were abandoning pure physical experimentation for the more promising field of radiobiology. Moreover, the development of mammalian cell culture resulted in great expansion of laboratory research using *in-vitro* techniques. This opened an opportunity to study the various phases of the cell cycle as it underwent chromosomal changes in preparation for mitosis. The DNA synthetic phase (S) has been studied with meticulous techniques involving radioactive tritium, thymidine and autoradiography, with a promise of better understanding of tumour growth, population kinetics and a hope of fruitful clinical application. These large vistas have resulted in an unprecedented bonanza for laboratory researchers.

Gray decided to pursue the investigation of the subject initiated by Lacassagne — the role of oxygen in radiosensitivity. He reported that tumours in mice that were made to breath oxygen showed increased radiosensitivity.[68] His work brought about considerable enthusiasm and trials for the use of hyperbaric oxygen in clinical radiotherapy.[69] It took years for the working party of the Medical Research Council to render its disappointing report.[70] But although hyperbaric radiotherapy was not the success that had been expected, it has left a legacy of innumerable avenues of research on the role of cellular hypoxia, on differences of radiation response and methods of surmounting them. As a consequence, there have been efforts to develop hypoxic cell radiosensitizers and an interminable series of other radiosensitizers. The laboratory worker often overlooks the fact that equal sensitization of normal and pathologic tissues is not helpful, and that what is needed is an enlargement of the margin of safety between the destruction of the tumour and the injury of surrounding structures. The volume of laboratory work in this area far exceeds any clinical demonstration of usefulness.

Isadore Lampe (1906–82), a self-taught radiation oncologist of Ann Arbor,[62] revealed the curability of medulloblastomas of the cerebellum by roentgentherapy.[71] Franz Buschke (1902–85), Simeon T Cantril (1908–59) and Herbert Parker (1910–84), of Seattle, published their book on supervoltage roentgentherapy,[72] demonstrating the unquestionable advantage of associating high voltages with clinical skills. Gradually, successful radiotherapy of a variety of tumours has become evident and also the development of new techniques which have added to the credit of radiation oncology.

The Atomic Energy Research brought forth cobalt-60, the artificially radioactivated metal, emitting rays of two very close wavelengths equivalent to 1.2 MeV. Cobalt sources of several curies became available for clinical use at 80 cm SSD. Cinical work with cobalt proved remarkably fruitful; it had only the disadvantage of a relatively short half-life.

The Fifth International Congress of Cancer was held in Paris in 1950, presided upon by Antoine Lacassagne, a prestigious radiation oncologist. A Cobalt-60 Unit was first exhibited there. A few days later, the Sixth International Congress of Radiology took place in London under the presidency of Ralston Paterson, another radiation oncologist.

In the United Kingdom, the physicians who had been appointed as guardians of radium, and consultants on its use, gradually became recognized as leading radiation oncologists. They undertook to visit each other and exchange views. The Radiotherapists Visiting Club was thus created; in time it became the first British society of therapeutic radiologists (Fig. 1.20).

In 1953, the Seventh International Congress of Radiology was held in Copenhagen under the honorary presidency of Niels Bohr (1885–1962). Jens Nielsen (1899–1964), a dedicated radiation oncologist, was vice-president in charge of the section on radiotherapy. Nielsen extended a personal invitation to all registered radiotherapists to join him for a luncheon at the Radium Centre of which he was director. At the end of the luncheon he rose to propose the creation of an International Club of Radiotherapists (ICR). With enthusiastic approval of all those present, a steering committee was elected and 2 days later we were invited to an evening meeting of the 'embryo' club at the Domus Medica. After discussion and changes, the

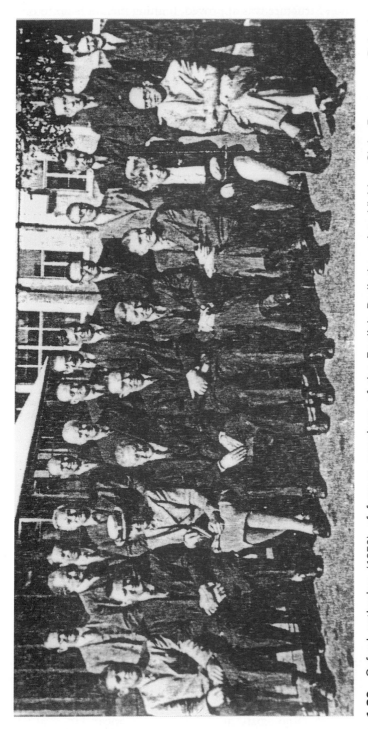

**Fig. 1.20** Oxford gathering (1950) of former members of the English Radiotherapists Visiting Club. Front row: Robert McWhirter (Edinburgh), Brian Windeyer* (London), Constance Wood* (London), Gioacchino Failla (guest), Ralston Paterson* (Manchester), Frank Ellis* (Oxford), John Nutthal* (London), Sylvia Widoger (Newcastle), Walter Levitt (London). Back row: AG Taylor (Southampton), Anthony Green (London), Robert Morrison (Birmingham), George Bloomfield (Sheffield), W Roy Ward (Northwood), AA Latouche (Leeds), George Binnie (Stoke-on-Trent), SP Raban (Bristol), Oliver Chance* (Dublin), FE Chester-Williams (Bradford), John Bromley (Birmingham), JA Fleming (London), AJ Durden-Smith (Northwood), Joseph Mitchell* (Cambridge). (The asterisk indicates membership in the International Club of Radiotherapists.)

proposed Organization Structure was approved, limiting membership to one hundred heads of departments of radiotherapy. Those in attendance nominated others in various countries to an initial total of seventy-seven. Ralston Paterson was elected as President, Nielsen as Secretary for Europe and Cantril as Secretary for the Americas (Fig. 1.21). American radiation oncologists were to benefit indirectly by this initiative.

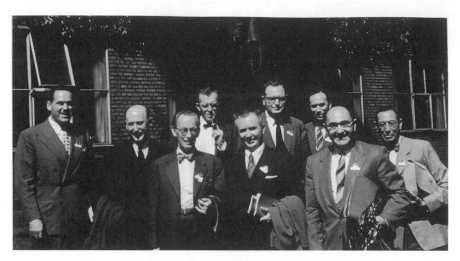

**Fig. 1.21**  Group of charter members of the International Club of Radiotherapists on the patio of the Radium Centre of Copenhagen (1953). Front row: Clifford Ash (Canada), François Baclesse (France), Elis Berven (Sweden), JA del Regato (USA), Bertram LowBeer (USA). Back row: James Nickson (USA), Simeon Cantril (USA), David Smithers (England), Bertil Ebenius (Sweden).

In the United States, even at the end of the Second World War there were only sixty physicians confining their practice to radiotherapy; they were mostly autodidactic or had received their training abroad. Even such experienced teachers as Isadore Lampe had not been permitted to train anyone in straight radiotherapy. In 1953, at a meeting of the American College of Radiology in Chicago, we made a plea for the creation of centres of training in therapeutic radiology.[73] The representative of radiology in the American Medical Association (AMA) Hospital Accreditation Committee vetoed any programme of training that did not include radiodiagnosis. In the 1940s such training was offered at the Ellis Fischel Cancer Hospital of Columbia, Missouri, but most of the candidates were general radiologists seeking only 6 months of exposure to complement their diagnostic training before certification. One such candidate, William T Moss, became the resident in straight radiotherapy and enhanced his experience in an additional year spent at the Radium Institute of Paris and the Holt Radium Institute of Manchester. In 1949, we organized the first comprehensive training programme for therapeutic radiologists at the Penrose Cancer Hospital of Colorado Springs, under a grant from the National Cancer Institute. In

1960, there were only twenty-five residents in training in therapeutic radiology in the United States; eight were in Colorado Springs.

For about 40 years, dosage of radiations was expressed in **roentgens** delivered at various points of the anatomy; this failed to recognize that what was important biologically was the dose absorbed, a point frequently pointed out by Holthusen. Herbert Parker originated the concept of **rep** (physical) and **rem** (biological) doses. In time, the **rad** (defined as 100 erg/g), was adopted; thereafter, doses were expressed in **R-units**.

In the United Kingdom, the Radiotherapists Visiting Club acquired the strength of a society and its members sought the companionship of their brethren in radiodiagnosis to found the Faculty of Radiology. In the United States, the national radiological societies accepted papers on radiotherapy but had repeatedly refused to form a section of therapeutic radiologists. Radiation oncologists joined the American Radium Society, where they met with a majority of surgical oncologists. The initiative was taken of inviting all American members of the International Club of Radiotherapists to a dinner during the annual meeting of the RSNA. The first one of these meetings took place in Chicago in December 1955 (Fig. 1.22). This innocent initiative aroused no alarm, but it was decided to invite other radiation oncologists as guests. As expected, these gatherings fostered the idea of an American Club of Radiotherapists with equal membership to all. We were prepared, and at the meeting of December 1958, a founder's agreement was proposed that was unanimously adopted by fifty-eight charter members of the American Club of Therapeutic Radiologists. Jealously groomed, the organization maintained an exclusive membership of radiation oncologists and by 1966 it had 252 members; these were mostly general radiologists

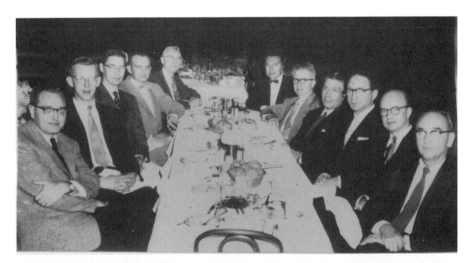

**Fig. 1.22** First dinner meeting of American members of the International Club of Radiotherapists and guests, Chicago, 1955. From left to right, clockwise: Simeon T Cantril (ICR), Charles J Ryan (guest), Bryan L Redd (guest), Robert Robbins (guest), Milford Schulz (ICR), Manuel Garcia (ICR), JA del Regato (ICR), E Dale Trout (guest), Milton Friedman (ICR), Don Mosser (guest), Gilbert Fletcher (ICR).

who had willingly rescinded their practice of radiodiagnosis and taken positions as radiotherapists. After the first decade, the membership voted to change the name and the club became the American Society of Therapeutic Radiologists (ASTR). It was incorporated under the laws of the state of Colorado, including a logo consisting of a crab surrounded by electronic orbits.

Linear accelerators became available in the 1950s for clinical work, first in England and later in the United States. As had been the case previously with any physical progress, the expectations of better results required skilful use and additional research. The expensive equipment was easier to get than the responsible talents required.

The rapid proliferation of departments or divisions of radiotherapy in the US promptly revealed the scarcity of specially trained technologists. Some academic institutions started to import English so-called *radiographers*, although radiography was precisely what they were not expected to do. One institution insisted on training graduated nurses as radiotherapeutic technologists. But a growing clinical practice created great demand for specially trained technologists to assist in radiation oncology.

To avoid the waste of valuable treatment time in the megavoltage units while discussing approaches to the treatment of patients, the idea of a special room devoted to treatment planning arose. Commercial manufacturers were prompt in offering *simulators*, which were gradually perfected to include position radiography. The planning and simulation of the treatment of each patient has become the opportunity for physicists, dosimetrists, technologists, imaging experts and radiation oncologists to cooperate on behalf of the patients.

The postwar discovery and development of cytotoxic drugs and the early success of vincristine in the control of acute leukaemia in children resulted in expectations of systemic treatment and cure of cancer patients. With the support of the wealth of special institutions, there was an increasing number of new cytotoxic drugs that had proven effective on lower animals and in clinical trials on cancer patients. As was to be expected, the claims were numerous and varied. Haematologists and other interninsts have become interested in oncology and created a new specialty—*Medical Oncology*.

In 1962, The British Empire Cancer Campaign decided to create a new centre for radiobiological research at the Mount Vernon Hospital in Northwood. Hal Gray, who had resigned his post at Hammersmith, was appointed director of the new centre. From very modest beginnings in a wooden hut, Gray expanded the project and gathered capable associates, developing an impressive research laboratory involving the use of neutrons and isotopes. He concentrated his work on cell biology, on the role of oxygen, on radiosensitizers, and on pulse-cytolysis. Gray was the guest speaker at the first meeting of the recently founded Radiation Research Society in Iowa City in 1959. He was also the first president of the International Congress of Radiation Research at Harrogate in 1962.

On the rapidly risen wave of enthusiasm for chemotherapy, the National Cancer Institute created a Clinical Studies Panel for consideration of cooperative trials of surgical adjuvants. The first US cooperative study involving radiotherapy was approved by this body: a comparison of postoperative radiotherapy or chemotherapy for cancer of the breast.[74] The Institute also created a Committee for Radiation Therapy Studies (CRTS) which initiated studies on chemotherapy and radiotherapy for cancer of the upper air passages and also on radiotherapy for inoperable cancer of the prostate. This committee later changed its name to the Radiotherapy Oncology Group (RTOG). In the UK, the Coordinating Committee for Cancer Research undertook equal cooperative studies on the value of chemotherapy.

# 1970–95

In the last quarter of the century following Roentgen's discovery there has been a remarkable expansion of radiation oncology services. As a medical specialty, radiation oncology has attained professional recognition and academic distinction. Laboratory as well as clinical researchers have engrossed the field and enriched its scientific contributions.

The increasing demands for radiotherapy services obliged David Smithers of the Royal Marsden Hospital of London to share his treatment obligations with two other competent radiation oncologists, Manuel Lederman (1911–84) and H Julian G Bloom (1923–88). At the Middlesex Hospital, within the Meyerstein Institute, a Nuclear Medicine Centre was developed under Brian Windeyer that became a model for other such centres in the United Kingdom. The Gray Laboratory and the Mount Vernon Centre for the treatment of cancer in the Marie Curie Wing at Northwood were also expanded. In Manchester, the Holt Radium Institute developed a network of satellite institutions. In Paris, the Fondation Curie added a several-storey Polyclinic and later the Hôpital Claudius Regaud at 26 rue d'Ulm. And the Institut du Cancer of Villejuif has developed and flourished under Maurice Tubiana into an admirable structure and staff for clinical and laboratory research—the Institut Gustave Roussy.

In the United States, community cancer centres were shunned as undesirable 'categorical' institutions when they were first advocated.[75] Once the exclusive domain of oncological surgeons, the treatment of cancer patients has increasingly required multidisciplinary consideration and approaches in centres where pathologists, surgeons, radiotherapists and medical oncologists collaborate on behalf of patients with a variety of malignant tumours. Thus, in recent years in the US, cancer centres have been improvised and some American cities claim more than one. Academic departments of radiology, once all inclusive, gradually allowed divisions of radiotherapy and, in time, chairs of radiation oncology. The first one of these was created in Portland, Oregon in 1968; presently, there are several dozens of such chairs in American medical schools.

In 1973, members of the International Club of Radiotherapists met in Madrid during the 17th International Congress of Radiology and elected Maurice Tubiana of France as their president. They also elected a committee to implement their decision to become an International Society of Radiotherapists. The committee failed to carry out their mission. Continental radiation oncologists were more interested in a European society and in separating radiotherapy from radiodiagnosis in the international congresses. In 1977, the members of the club met for the last time in Rio de Janeiro but no new officers were elected and the club was not to be heard of again. In 1989, in Paris, the international congress was finally split and the First International Congress of Radiation Oncology was held with François Eschwège of France as president. A second congress was held in Kyoto in 1993. The European Society of Radiation Therapy and Oncology (ESTRO) is now a working reality. Meanwhile, the American Society for Therapeutic Radiology and Oncology (ASTRO) has become the largest and most influential organization of radiation oncologists in the world, with over 3000 active members.

A great deal of the progress made by radiotherapy has been due simply to the greater implementation of knowledge and techniques that had long been available but are now in the hands of a greater number of well-trained practitioners. Time has helped to clarify views and to dispel doubts: a 20-year follow-up of inoperable patients with cancer of the prostate, adequately treated by radiotherapy, revealed that fewer died from metastatic cancer of the prostate than from intercurrent diseases proper to their advanced age.[76] But, in addition, radiation oncology has been progressively enriched by innumerable technological improvements now incorporated into everyday practice.

The new internationally adopted unit, the gray (Gy), is equivalent to 100 rad: 1 rad = 1 cGy. Computerized dosimetry is now a matter of course. Computerized axial tomography (CAT) has provided better assessment of thoracic and abdominal tumours. Magnetic resonance imaging (MRI) has proven most valuable in recognizing the limits of tumours of the central nervous system, the urinary bladder, and the prostate. *On-line imaging* verification of fields has been proposed.[77] As a result of advances in computerized imaging, permitting a greater precision of limits of the irradiated area, *three-dimensional* treatment planning and *conformal dosimetry* (3-D) has resulted.[78] Treatment of tumours utilizing charged particles remains a door open to investigation. The use of radium needles for interstitial implantation has been replaced by the use of gutters for afterloading with radionuclides; remote afterloading has also been proposed to diminish the exposure of personnel attending brachytherapy treatments.[79]

In an attempt to restrict the irradiation to the limits of a tumour, the procedure of surgical exposure and *intraoperative* irradiation has been investigated. But the elaborate procedure imposes a single massive irradiation, usually with electrons. Thus, the gain in precision loses the advantages of fractionation: the tolerance of tissues is much less for a single irradiation than for a fractionated series of exposures.

Treatment of tumours with protons and with heavy ions has been the subject of clinical appraisal in a limited number of institutions in England and in the United States. Trials have been carried out with the same fractionation models of megavoltage photons. Possibly a different fractionation for the use of these agents may be required and found.

Interest in radiosensitizers has resulted in a veritable avalanche of laboratory and clinical trials. Radiosensitizers abound but they usually affect normal as well as neoplastic tissues. What is desirable is a widening of the safety margin between the destruction of the tumour and the irreparable injury of the surrounding structures. Research in this area was initiated by hypoxic cell radiosensitizers: in particular, by *misonidazole* and *halogenated pyrimidine analogues*. The exact mechanism of action of these agents is not always understood and clinical trials have failed to show any benefit.[80]

Special techniques have been proposed for the destruction of very small tumours or malformations within noble structures such as the brain: *radiosurgery* or *stereotactic radiotherapy* requires precise utilization of multiple orbits of rotation therapy.[81] The destruction of tumour tissue by irradiation with specific wavelength light, *photodynamic therapy*, has been proposed for specific problems. Also proposed is the administration of biological modifiers such as *interferon* and *thymosin*. *Hyperthermia* alone is known to be able to destroy small superficial tumours; trials of hyperthermia in combination with radiotherapy have been limited by engineering difficulties. *Labelled tumour-associated antibodies* are hoped to target the specific tumour tissue but the uptake is often insufficient so it has not become a fruitful reality.[82]

The incessant development of new cytotoxic drugs and the large numbers of advocates of chemotherapy have motivated a marked change in the field of oncology. The drugs are definite poisons of growth, affecting not only the tumours but also vital physiological structures: in particular, those of the haemopoietic system. Unlike radiotherapists, who do not expect exciting overnight improvements, the medical oncologists receive periodical boosts of enthusiasm by the perennial advent of any new *drug du jour*. No drug or combination of drugs has been able to squelch one case of the major malignant tumours affecting man or woman. But since the drugs affect tumour growth, it is logical to expect that they may be useful surgical or radiotherapeutic adjuvants. Testing of this assumption requires seriously planned and carried-out clinical trials in a sufficient number of patients to justify biostatistical conclusions. Such requirements are not easily met at any single institution, and necessitate consideration of well-organized cooperative work by many institutions that agree to carry out a study in compliance with a common protocol. Such studies have been carried out by the Cancer Research Campaign in the United Kingdom and the National Cancer Institute in the United States. In 1993, the Radiation Therapy Oncology Group (RTOG), chaired by James D Cox, consisted of 203 institutions contributing 11 277 patients to thirty-four different cooperative studies frequently involving chemotherapy.[80]

In the penumbra of the past, the historian can more easily distinguish the bright gems from the ordinary pebbles. The distance helps him as it does the artist who steps back to better appreciate the nuances of a work of art, whereas at short range, his judgement becomes more difficult; uncertain of the eventual sanction of time, he is reduced to reporting.

# Envoi

The riddle of cancer is still with us. The mortality rate from cancer of the breast, the most common malignant tumour in American women, has not improved an iota since 1927, when Hugh Auchincloss proposed self-examination as a means of earlier diagnosis. The incidence and mortality of cancer of the stomach, once the most frequent cancer in American men, has persistently decreased for no recognizable reason. The increasing incidence rate of cancer of the prostate, particularly alarming in blacks, remains unexplained. These facts are the result of the inscrutable protean character of the disease rather than of any intelligent intervention, or lack of it, on our part.

# References

1. Hodges PC. *The Life and Times of Emil H. Grubbe.* Chicago: University of Chicago Press, 1964.
2. Daniel J. Depilatory action of X-rays. *Med Record* 1896; **49**, 595–6.
3. Freund L. Ein mit Roentgen-Strahlen behandelter Fall (von Nevus pigmentosus piliferus). *Wiener Med Wochenschrift* 1897; **47**, 856–7.
4. Belot J. *Radiotherapy in Skin Diseases.* New York, London: Rebman Co, 1905.
5. Williams FH. A large static machine. *Sci Am* 1899; **80**, 395–8.
6. Imboden HH. Progress in the development of Roentgen ray apparatus. *Am J Roentgenol* 1931; **25**, 517–23.
7. Béclère A. La mesure indirecte des pouvoirs de pénétration des rayons de Roentgen a l'aide du spintermètre. *Bull ASS franç d'Elwotroth* 1900; 7, 44–7.
8. Pfahler GE. A device for using a constant stream of water in a water-cooled tube. *Am J Roentgenol* 1913; **1**, 81–2.
9. Williams FH. *The Roentgen Rays in Medicine and Surgery.* New York: McMillan Co, 1901.
10. Pusey W, Caldwell E. *The Roentgen Rays in Therapeutics and Diagnosis.* Philadelphia: Saunders Co, 1903.
11. Beck C. *Practical Applications of Roentgen Rays.* Scranton: International Textbook Co, 1901.
12. Albers-Schönberg H. Beitrag zur therapeutischen Verwendung der Roentgenstrahlen in der Behandlung des Lupus. *Fortschritte a d Geb d Roentgen* 1897; **1**, 72–5.
13. Oudin P, Barthelemy T, Darier J. Accidents cutanés et visceraux consecutifs à l'emploie des rayons. *France Medicale* 1898; **48**, 113, 129, 162, 179.
14. Schölz W. Uber den Einfluss der Roentgenstrahlen auf die Haut in Gesunden und kranken Zustande. *Arch J Dermat und Syph* 1802; **59**, 27, 291, 422.
15. Heineke H. Ueber die Einwerkung der strahlen auf Tiere. *Munch Med Wochenschr* 1906; **50**, 2090–2.
16. Albers-Schönberg H. Ueber einer bisher unbekampte Wirkung der Roentgenstrahlen auf den Organismus der Tiere. *Munch Med Wochenschr* 1903; **60**, 1859–60.
17. Regaud C, Blanc J. Action des rayons X sur les diverses générations de la ligne spermatique; extreme sensibilité des spermatogonies à ces rayons. *Compt rend Soc Biol* 1906; **61**, 163–5.
18. Freund L. *Elements of General Radiotherapy for Practitioners.* London, New York: Riebman Ltd, 1904.
19. Kassabian MK. *Roentgen Rays and Electro-therapeutics.* Philadelphia, London: JB Lippincott, 1907.
20. Holtznecht G. Das Chromoradiometer. *Fortsch a d Geb d Roentgenstrah* 1902; **4**, 1–49.
21. Curie P, Curie M, Bemont G. Sur une nouvelle substance fortement radioactive contenue dans la petchblende. *Compt rend Acad Sci, Paris* 1898; **127**, 1215–17.
22. Danlos HA, Bloch P. Note sur le traitement du lupus erythemateux par les applications de radium. *Ann Dermat et Symph* 1901; **2**, 986–8.
23. Abbé R. Note on the physiologic and therapeutic action of radium. *Wash Med Ann* 1904; **2**, 363–77.

24. Cleaves MA. Radium; with preliminary note on radium rays in the treatment of cancer. *Med Record* 1903; **64**, 501–606.
25. Williams FH. Some of the physical properties and medical uses of radium salts; with report of 42 patients treated with pure radium bromide. *Med News* 1904; **164**, 241–6.
26. Wickham F, Desgrais P. *Radium Therapy*. New York: Funk and Wagnals Co, 1910.
27. Coutard H. Sur l'émanation du radium et son utilization en thérapeutique. *J Belge Radiol* 1912; **21**, 642–8.
28. Dominici H. Du traitement des tumeurs malignes par le rayonnement ultra-pénétrant du radium. *Bull Ass Franç, Étude Cancer* 1908; **1**, 124–56.
29. Forssel G. Quelques observations de radiumthérapie de tumeurs cancereuses. *Arch d'Éléctr Med Exper et Clin* 1910; **18**, 801–2.
30. Finzi NS. *Radium Therapeutics*. London: Oxford University Press, 1913.
31. Regaud C, Nogier T. Sterilization roentgenienne totale et definitive sans radio-dermite des testicules du belier adulte; conditions de la realization. *Compt rend Soc Biol* 1911; **70**, 202–3.
32. Lacassagne A. Étude histologique et physiologique des éffects produits sur l'ovaire par les rayons X. Thesis, Faculty of Medicine, Lyon, 1913.
33. Cheron H, Rubens-Duval H. Aperçu sur les resultats de la radiumthérapie des cancers de l'utérus et du vagin. *Bull Soc d'Obst et Gynec, Paris* 1913; **2**, 418–29.
34. Friedrich W. Ueber die Willenlange Roentgen und Gammastrahlen und ihre Bedingung fur die Strahlentherapie. *Deutsch Med Wochenschr* 1913; **32**.
35. Krönig B. Die Strahlentherapie in der Gynecologie. *Strahlentherapie* 1913; **3**, 429–36.
36. Debièrne A, Regaud C. Sur l'emploie de l'émanation condensée en tubes clos à la place des composés radifères et sur le dosage (en millicuries d'émanation detruite) de l'énérgie depensée pendant les applications radioactives locales. *Compt rend Acad Sci, Paris* 1915; **161**, 422–4.
37. Janeway JH. The use of buried emanation in the treatment of malignant tumors. *Am J Roentgenol* 1920; 7, 325–7.
38. Failla G. The development of filtered radon implants. *Am J Roentgenol* 1926; **15**, 507–25.
39. Solomon I. *Précis de Radiothérapie*. Paris: Masson et Cie, 1926.
40. Lazarus P. *Handbuch der Gesamter Strahlenheilkunde*. Hamburg: JF Bergmann, 1928.
41. Hirsch I. *The Principles and Practice of Roentgentherapy*. With dosage formulae and dosage tables by G Holtznecht. New York: Am X-ray Publ Co, 1925.
42. Coutard H. Sur les delais d'apparition et d'évolution des réactions de la peau et des muqueuses de la bouche et du pharynx provoquées par les rayons. *Compt rend Soc Biol, Paris* 1922; **88**, 1140–1.
43. Coutard H. Note preliminaire sur la radiographie du larynx normal et du larynx cancereux. *J Belge Radiol* 1924; **13**, 487–90.
44. Coutard H. Roentgenbehandlung des epithelialen Krebse der Tonsillengegund. *Strahlentherapie* 1929; **33**, 249–52.
45. Borak J. Uber die Coutardsche Methode des Roentgenbehandlung des Krebses. *Wien Med Wochenschr* 1941; **66**, 61–3.
46. Zuppinger A. Resultate der protahiertfraktionierten Roentgentherapie von malignant Tumoren. *Strahlentherapie* 1932; **43**, 701–18.
47. Glasser O. Isodose charts. *Am J Roentgenol* 1923; **10**, 405–7.
48. Seitz L, Wintz H. *Unsere Methode der Roentgenol-Tiefentherapie und Ihre Erfolge*. Berlin: Urban und Schwarzenberg, 1920.
49. Freund L. Du Gegenwartigen Methoden und Erfolge der Krebstrahlung mit verteilten Dosen. *Strahlentherapie* 1930; **17**, 795–7.

50. Stënstrom W. Study of skin reactions after divided Roentgen-ray dosage. *Am J Roentgenol* 1926; **15**, 513–19.
51. Kingery LB. Saturation in roentgentherapy; its estimation and maintenance. *Arch Dermat Syph* 1920; **1**, 423.
52. Quimby E, MacComb WS. Further studies on the rate of recovery of human skin from the effects of roentgen or gamma ray. *Radiology* 1937; **29**, 305–12.
53. Strandqvist M. Ueber die kumulative wirkung der Roentgenstrahlen bei Fraktionierung. *Acta Radiologica* 1944; Suppl 55.
54. Ahlbom H. Mucous and salivary gland tumors. *Acta Radiologica* 1935; **22**, 452.
55. Berven EGE. Malignant tumors of the tonsil; a special study with special reference to their treatment. *Acta Radiological* 1931; Suppl 11, 1–285.
56. Drury H. Dermatitis caused by Roentgen X-rays. *Br Med J* 1896; 1277–378.
57. Warren S, Gates O. Radiation pneumonitis; experimental and pathologic observations. *Arch Path* 1940; **30**, 440–60.
58. Desjardins AU. Action of Roentgen rays and radium on the eye and ear. Experimental data and clinical radiotherapy. *Am J Roentgenol* 1931; **28**, 643–79, 789–819, 923–42.
59. Holthusen H, Hamman A. Die Miterbeit des Krankenhauses bei der Krebsbekampfung. *Strahlentherapie* 1937; **60**, 70–81.
60. Heymann J. Annual report (League of Nations Health Organization) of the results of radiotherapy in cancer of the uterine cervix. *Acta Obstet Gynecol Scand* 1938; **18**, 1–94.
61. Wilson CW. Thirty years of telecurietherapy. *Br J Radiol* 1960; **33**, 69–81.
62. del Regato JA. *Radiation Oncologists, The Unfolding of a Medical Specialty.* Preston, VA: Radiology Centennial Inc, 1993.
63. del Regato JA. The American Board of Radiology. *Am J Roentgenol* 1975; **144**, 197–200.
64. Mayneord WV. Radiological physics: a retrospect. *Br J Radiol* 1973; **46**, 754–6.
65. Molineus W, Holthusen H, Mayer H. Ehrenbuch der Radiologen aller Nationen. Berlin: Blackwell Wissenchafts-Verlag, 1992.
66. Taylor LS. History of the International Commission on Radiologic Protection. *Health Physics* 1958; **1**, 97–104.
67. Lacassagne A. Chute de la radiosensibilité aux rayons X chez la souris nouveau-née en état d'asphyxie. *Compt rend Acad Sci* 1942; **215**, 231.
68. Gray LH, Conger AD, Ebert M, *et al.* The concentration of oxygen dissolved in tissues at the time of irradiation as a factor in radiotherapy. *Br J Radiol* 1953; **26**, 638–49.
69. Churchill-Davidson J, Sanger C, Thomlinson RH. High pressure oxygen and radiotherapy. *Lancet* 1955; **1**, 1091–5.
70. Windeyer BW. Hyperbaric oxygen and radiotherapy. *Br J Radiol* 1978; **51**, 875–94.
71. Lampe I, MacIntyre RS. Experiences in radiotherapy of medulloblastomas of the cerebellum. *Arch Neuro Psych* 1949; **62**, 322–9.
72. Buschke F, Cantril ST, Parker H. *Supervoltage.* Springfield: C. Thomas, 1950.
73. del Regato JA. Training Centers in Therapeutic Radiology. *Post Grad Med* 1953; **14**, 161–262.
74. del Regato JA. Radiotherapy as a post-operative surgical adjuvant in the management of cancer of the breast. *Radiology* 1979; **98**, 695–8.
75. del Regato JA. The Community Cancer Hospital. *Am J Roentgenol* 1970; **108**, 3–8.
76. del Regato JA. Twenty years follow-up of inoperable patients with carcinoma of the prostate (Stage C) treated by radiotherapy. Reports of a national cooperative study. *Int J Radiat Oncol Biol Phys* 1993; **262**, 197–201.
77. Wong JW, Yan D. On-line imaging radiotherapy; current status. In: JS Tobias,

PRM Thomas, eds, *Current Radiation Oncology*, Vol. 1. London: Edward Arnold, 1994; 24–35.

78. Lichter AS. Clinical experience with a three-dimensional treatment planning system. In: JS Tobias, PRM Thomas, eds, *Current Radiation Oncology*, Vol. 1. London: Edward Arnold, 1994; 36–50.

79. Almond P. Remote after-loading. In: AE Wright, AL Boyer, eds, *Advances in Radiation Therapy Treatment Planning*. New York: American Institute of Physics, 1989.

80. Cox JD. A brief history of cooperative clinical trials in radiation oncology (1994 RSNA Annual Oration in Radiation Oncology). *Radiology* 1995 (in press).

81. Ledermann JA. Radioimmunotherapy. In: JS Tobias, PRM Thomas, eds, *Current Radiation Oncology*, Vol. 1. London: Edward Arnold, 1994; 69–84.

82. Brada M, Graham JA. Stereotactic external beam radiotherapy in the treatment of glioma and other intracranial lesions. In: JS Tobias, PRM Thomas, eds, *Current Radiation Oncology*, Vol. 1. London: Edward Arnold, 1994; 86–100.

# Further reading

Clarkson JR, Mayneord WV. The 'quality' of high voltage radiations. *Br J Radiol* 1939; **12**, 168–80.

Cox JD (ed). *Moss' Radiation Oncology. Rationale, Technique, Results*, 7th edn. Saint Louis: Mosby, 1994.

del Regato JA. Historical changes in time–dose relationships. *Front Radiation Ther Oncol* 1968; **3**, 1–5.

Holfelder H. *Die Roentgen-Tiefentherapie*. Leipzig: Georg Thieme, 1938.

Lederman M. Cancer of the hypopharynx; results of radiotherapy. *Ann Otolaryngol, Paris* 1955; **72**, 506–27.

Lenz M, Coakley CG, Stout AP. Roentgentherapy of epitheliomas of the pharynx and larynx. *Am J Roentgenol* 1934; **32**, 500–7.

Oberling C. Les reticulosarcomes et les reticuloendothéliosarcomes de la moelle osseuse. *Bull Ass Franç p l'Étude du Cancer* 1928; **17**, 259–96.

Reverchon L, Coutard H. Lymphoépithéliome de l'hypopharynx traité par la roentgenthérapie sans réaction notable du pharynx ou du larynx. *Bull Med Soc Franc Otorhinol* 1922; 1–6.

# 2 Clinical normal-tissue radiobiology

*Søren M Bentzen and Jens Overgaard*

## Introduction

Radiotherapy is associated with a broad spectrum of side-effects and any choice of treatment schedule must represent a balance between the beneficial therapeutic effect and the deleterious effect of that schedule. Holthusen[1] was among the first radiotherapists to realize that there is no such thing as a well-defined tolerance dose in radiotherapy, a dose below which radiation complications are avoided. Rather, he noted, there is a broad dose range in which the probability of developing a specific radiation reaction rises from 0% to 100%. In his 1936 paper, Holthusen produced one of the most influential graphical presentations of this trade-off between tumour control and normal-tissue complications, a graph that has been reproduced over and over again in the literature, most often without proper acknowledgement of the source! Figure 2.1 shows a Holthusen-type graph of the dose–response curves for control of laryngeal tumours and persistent laryngeal oedema. If the positions and shapes of these dose–response curves were fixed for specific tumour histology and a given normal-tissue reaction, radiotherapy would be quite a dull medical specialty! Clinical research in radiotherapy would then be concerned with establishing these dose–response relationships, with the relatively simple task of optimizing the tumour control under some constraint on the acceptable risk of normal-tissue complications. In reality, a number of treatment and patient characteristics will change the position and/or the shape of these dose–response curves. It is thereby possible to improve the therapeutic ratio, i.e. to reduce the level of normal-tissue damage while keeping an unchanged or even increased tumour control. This optimization is the ultimate aim of clinical radiobiology, that is to say the radiation biology of human tumours, normal tissues, and organs, when

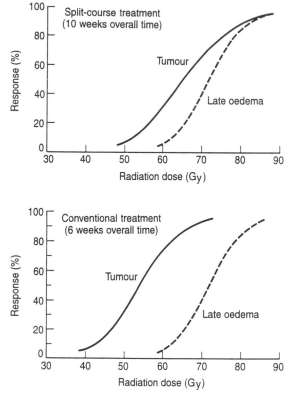

**Fig. 2.1** Dose–response curves estimated from the data by Overgaard *et al.*[116] for local control of laryngeal carcinoma and late laryngeal oedema after split-course (top) and conventional (bottom) radiotherapy. If the overall treatment time is protracted, a reasonable tumour control cannot be achieved without a high incidence of late oedema. The therapeutic ratio is improved when treatment time is shortened from 10 to 6 weeks.

exposed to the doses normally applied in radiotherapy.

As late as the early 1970s, it was generally believed that late reactions occurred mainly as a consequence of severe early reactions, that the therapeutic ratio between tumour control and normal-tissue tolerance did not depend on the number of fractions given, and that treatment protraction was the most efficient means of reducing normal-tissue sequelae. These assumptions formed the basis for the nominal standard dose (NSD) concept[2] and were reflected in its mathematical formulation. Clinical and experimental research over the past 15 years has shown that they are not generally valid for various tumour and normal-tissue endpoints, and that they are in fact wrong in most of the situations relevant for practical radiotherapy.[3] This has generated ideas for improving radiotherapy through altered dose-fractionation. At the same time, progress in biostatistics and biomathematical modelling has improved our ability to quantify radiobiological properties of human tumours and tissues. This again has improved the prospects for a rational design of controlled randomized trials.[4] A key parameter for achieving this is the steepness of the dose–response curve, which also has a bearing on the precision requirements for practical radiotherapy.

This chapter will briefly review some of the recent developments in clinical normal-tissue radiobiology. Recording and analysing data on normal-tissue sequelae will be discussed. The status of altered fractionation strategies will be summarized with special emphasis on the normal-tissue data needed for a rational trial of these strategies: repair half-times, the time factor for early- and late-responding normal tissues, and the steepness of the dose–response curve. The chapter will conclude with a discussion of the prospects for individualizing radiotherapy according to normal-tissue complication probability and the possibilities of ameliorating normal-tissue reactions by intervention in the pathogenic pathway.

# Recording of treatment-related morbidity

While the TNM (tumour, node, metastasis) system is widely accepted for staging human tumours, there is no general agreement on a uniform system for reporting normal-tissue complications. A recent survey by Dische et al.[5] of 166 papers reporting on the results of radiotherapy in the journals *Radiotherapy and Oncology* and *International Journal of Radiation Oncology, Biology, Physics* showed that 20% of these reports contained no information on morbidity and that another 23% contained only anecdotal accounts of treatment-related morbidity. Only 31% of the reports used a system for grading the severity of reactions. Few papers (12%) used a previously published system for reporting normal-tissue sequelae.[6] Another example is provided by Sismondi and colleagues,[7] who surveyed the classification employed in papers dealing with complications after treatment of carcinoma of the uterine cervix. The survey included ninety-six papers from twenty-four journals published in English, French or Italian between 1938 and 1986. Fifty-nine papers (61%) used no classification of the complications at all. Only thirty papers (31%) used a defined scale for grading the severity of complications, and among these papers only eight used a previously defined classification. It is also remarkable from a radiobiological point of view that only two reports distinguished between early and late complications (using < 6 months as the threshold).

Several comprehensive systems for reporting normal-tissue sequelae have been suggested[5,8–10] and more are under way.[11] These systems represent mainly a clinical perspective on normal-tissue reactions and none of them are ideal from a radiobiological point of view.[12] Clinically oriented systems most often mix up several different manifestations of injury in the same organ or tissue. As an example, the grading of late skin reactions in the RTOG/EORTC (Radiation Therapy Oncology Group/European Organization for the Research and Treatment of Cancer) system involves hair loss, telangiectasia, and atrophy/ulceration. Biologically, these manifestations of radiation injury occur in different tissues and they should be considered as three distinct endpoints for radiation effect. The grading of effects in a clinically oriented system is normally based on how severely the patient's life is affected by the reaction and/or the need for various types of medical treatment of the condition.[6]

Recently, the EORTC and the RTOG have formed two working groups with the purpose of updating their system for recording of late normal-tissue injury. The two groups have now agreed on a common system, the SOMA scale (subjective, objective, medical management, and analytical estimates).[11] The system reports measured values, whenever possible, so that a loss of information from grading is avoided, and it describes a set of recommended procedures for assessing normal-tissue injury. The SOMA scale will now undergo clinical evaluation before it may be recommended for general use.

It is indisputable that prospective recording of normal-tissue reactions is more reliable than retrospective recording, and, in general, the latter will tend to underestimate the incidence of sequelae. An example of this is the Villejuif studies on severe complications after brachytherapy in cervical carcinoma. A retrospective review[13] found a 4.7% incidence as compared to a prospective study[14] that found 8.8% incidence with exactly the same treatment. Scalliet et al.[15] have suggested that one possible difference between the two studies was that the prospective study recorded all events, whether or not they seemed attributable to the radiotherapy per se, whereas this was not the case in the retrospecive study.

Pedersen et al.[16,17] performed a retrospective study on complications after combined external beam and intracavitary radiotherapy in 442 patients with locally advanced carcinoma of the uterine cervix. The system used for recording of complications was based on retrospective evaluation of patient charts. Specific symptoms and objective signs were registered with emphasis on treatment-requiring morbidity.[16] Three important points are illustrated by this study.

1. Grading of complications involves a grouping of certain symptoms or signs into a single category. It is important, however, to record the specific expressions of damage which were actually observed. This will allow a subsequent analysis of these specific endpoints and/or a rescoring of the complication grade.
2. Recording of the maximum grade of reaction experienced by an individual represents a loss of information in the sense that the patient may have lived with a less-severe grade of reaction for a shorter or longer time.
3. Reporting accumulated frequencies rather than actuarial estimates may give an inaccurate impression of the toxicity of a specific treatment schedule (see below).

# Latent time

A specific expression of radiation injury to a tissue will occur after a characteristic time, the latent time. Biologically, the latent-time distribution depends mainly on the proliferative organization and the cellular turnover in the tissue.[18]

Latency has been studied in some detail for several late endpoints, in particular telangiectasia,[19-21] but also subcutaneous fibrosis[22] and impaired shoulder movement.[23] A rough characterization of the position of the latent-time distribution may be obtained from the median latent time or the 90th percentile of the latent-time distribution, $LT_{90}$, i.e. the time within which 90% of the expected ultimate incidence of complications has been seen. For subcutaneous fibrosis and impaired shoulder movement after postmastectomy radiotherapy, the $LT_{90}$ has been estimated at 3–4 years.[24] For telangiectasia, the latent period is generally longer than this but is strongly dependent on dose. An analysis of the Gothenburg series yielded an estimated median latent time increasing from 5 to 11 years as the dose was decreased from 70 Gy to 40 Gy with 2 Gy per fraction.[21]

## Follow-up and data analysis

Technically speaking, radiation reactions are response-time data. Estimating the level of late radiation reactions requires prolonged observation of the patient. The methodological problem in the analysis of such data springs from the fact that some individuals will have incomplete follow-up in the sense that they do not reach the endpoint before the time of the last observation. Prolonged observation in these subjects is not available/possible either because they have died from cancer or intercurrent disease, are lost to follow-up, or quite simply because they were still alive and well at the time of analysis. Such observations are said to be (time-) *censored* and for each patient the time for the last follow-up is called the *censoring time*. Patients who are still under observation at a given time after the end of treatment are said to be *at risk* at that time.

The statistical methods applied to failure-time problems must take censoring into account. Simply counting the number of patients who experience a normal-tissue complication or a tumour relapse will, in general, underestimate the true frequency of that event.[25,26] Here, 'true frequency' should be understood as the frequency that would have been observed if prolonged observation was possible in all patients. Another immediate consequence is that a quantity such as the median latent time for a radiation reaction will be downwardly biased (i.e. underestimated) if censoring is neglected.[27] The reason is that a reaction occurring after a short latent period will have a higher chance of being registered as such than a potential reaction with longer latent time. These points are illustrated in Fig. 2.2, which shows the cumulative incidence of moderate and severe bladder complications after combined intracavitary and external beam radiotherapy in patients with FIGO (Fédération Internationale Gynécologique et Obstetrique) Stage IIIb and IVa cervical cancer. The crude estimate, obtained as the ratio between the number of patients reaching the endpoint before a specific time and the total number of patients treated, is considerably lower than the actuarial estimate, and the difference increases with time. Intuitively, this is clear: assume that the risk of developing bladder complications is constant over time, say 10% per year. This will mean that the absolute number of events in the first year will be higher than the number of events in the fourth year, simply because there are more patients alive and under observation during the first year after the end of treatment than after 4 years of follow-up.

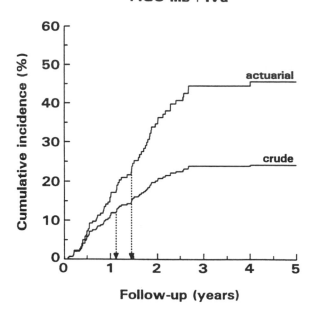

**Fig. 2.2** The cumulative incidence of moderate or severe bladder complications after radiotherapy for carcinoma of the uterine cervix. The crude incidence is the number of patients with complications as a function of the follow-up divided by all patients in the group. This should be compared with the actuarial curve which allows for the decrease in number of patients at risk with increasing time. The two arrows indicate the median latent times for the two methods of estimation. Data from the study by Pedersen *et al.*[17,130] where details of the radiotherapy regimens and the scoring of complications may be found.

Therefore, to obtain an estimate of the risk of complications after any specific radiotherapy schedule, special statistical methods, often called actuarial methods, must be used. These methods take into account the number of patients at risk at a given response time. Statistical methods are available for estimating the incidence of late normal-tissue reactions[28,29] or for multivariate regression analysis of such data.[30,31] The application of these methods in radiobiology has recently been discussed.[22,32-35]

It has been proposed that prevalence estimates rather than incidence estimates should be used when describing the toxicity of a radiotherapy schedule.[36] While the proportion of patients alive at a given time, with a certain grade of complications, is clearly relevant for the clinician, this may not be optimal in assessing biological injury because it reflects the management policy for complications as well as the incidence of these. We would, therefore, recommend that actuarial complication rates should be included in any report on normal-tissue injury.

# Early and late normal-tissue reactions

One of the most influential of radiobiological observations in the 1980s was the dissociation of the radiobiological properties of early- and late-responding tissues. Table 2.1 presents an overview of some of the biological and clinical characteristics of 'idealized' early and late radiation reactions. Biologically, this table should be taken with a grain of salt. Many exceptions exist; for example, the urothelium has the biological characteristics of an early-responding tissue but injury is expressed after a long latent period because of a very low cellular turnover in the tissue. Also, it is important to note that many organs and tissues develop more than one wave of overt damage; for example, two phases of damage may be recognized in the lung: radiation pneumonitis, occurring in humans some 3–8 months after irradiation, and lung fibrosis, developing after about 1 year. Nevertheless, the overall picture conveyed by the table is consistent with biological observations in both animals and humans. Most of our current thinking in clinical normal-tissue radiobiology is founded on these concepts and we will return to several of these in a little more detail in the following.

# Steepness of the dose–response curve

The steepness of the dose–response curve is of both basic and practical interest in radiation biology: basic, because it is a challenge to radiation biologists to explain the factors influencing not only the position but also the shape of the dose–response curve, and practical, because it turns out that this parameter is of immediate importance in considering the precision requirements in radiotherapy,[37] and in the design of clinical trials.[4]

## Quantifying the steepness of the dose–response curve

A quantitative measure of the steepness of the dose–response curve is the normalized dose–response gradient, $\gamma$, which has the simple interpretation of being the increase in percentage points of the response probability for a 1% increase in total dose.[37] Formally, $\gamma$ is defined as

$$\gamma_r = D_r \cdot p'(D_r) \tag{2.1}$$

where $p'$ denotes the derivative of $p(D)$ with respect to dose and the index, $r$, refers to the response probability at which $\gamma$ is evaluated. The standard practice has been to estimate $\gamma$ at the point of maximum steepness of the dose–response curve, which is the 37% or the 50% response level for a Poisson or a logistic dose–response relationship, respectively. It may be quite instructive to look at the explicit formula for $\gamma$ for one of the standard mathematical formulations of the dose–response relationship. As an example, the probability of response, $p(D,N)$, for a logistic dose–response relationship and a linear-quadratic dose–effect relation is defined by the equation

**Table 2.1** Idealized characteristics of early- and late-responding normal tissues

| Property | Early-responding normal tissue | Late-responding normal tissue |
|---|---|---|
| Latency | Few weeks to a few months; the latent time is independent of dose while the time for the injury to heal is dose dependent | 0.5 → 5+ years; the latent time is dose dependent |
| Examples of tissues | Mucosa, skin, intestinal epithelia, haemopoietic system | Liver, kidney, lung, CNS |
| Fractionation sensitivity[a] | Low | High |
| Time factor[b] | High | Very low |
| Tissue characteristics | Rapidly self-renewing, hierarchical organization: stem cells → functional cells | Slowly self-renewing, no well-defined hierarchical structure |
| Predominant defence against radiation injury | Regeneration | Repair of sublethal damage |
| Radiation pathogenesis | Stem cell depletion leading to functional breakdown | Loss of parenchymal cells, fibrosis, vascular damage |
| Clinical course | Transient, but consequential late reactions may occur | Irreversible, progressive, but functional compensation may occur |

[a] Change in isoeffect dose with changed dose per fractions.
[b] Dose recovered per day.
CNS: central nervous system.

$$p(D,N) = \frac{\exp\left(a_0 + a_1 \cdot D + a_2 \cdot \dfrac{D^2}{N}\right)}{1 + \exp\left(a_0 + a_1 \cdot D + a_2 \cdot \dfrac{D^2}{N}\right)} \tag{2.2}$$

where $D$ is the total dose, $N$ is the number of fractions, and $a_0$, $a_1$, and $a_2$ are model parameters to be estimated from a set of data. The coefficients $a_1$ and $a_2$ play a role similar to $\alpha$ and $\beta$ in the standard formulation of the linear-quadratic (LQ) model, and the ratio between these two parameters is equal to $\alpha/\beta$.

In clinical practice, two prototypical designs have been used in generating dose–response data. One is by addition of dose fractions of a constant size; the other is by escalation of the total dose with the number of fractions being fixed. For a dose–response curve resulting from varying the total dose while keeping the dose per fraction constant, the normalized dose–response gradient is denoted $\gamma_{d,50}$, and it may be shown[4] that

$$\gamma_{d,50} = -\frac{a_0}{4} \tag{2.3}$$

which is remarkable insofar as it does not depend on the dose per fraction or the $D_{50}$. This is a simplifying circumstance which makes it attractive to report this quantity as a characteristic of the dose–response curve for a specific endpoint. If, instead, the dose–response curve results from a change in dose with a fixed number of fractions, the corresponding dose–response gradient is denoted $\gamma_{N,50}$. The formula for this quantity is slightly more complex, but it can be shown that

$$\gamma_{N,50} = \gamma_{d,50} + \frac{a_2}{4} \cdot \frac{D_{50}^2}{N} \tag{2.4}$$

As $a_2 > 0$, the inequality $\gamma_{N,50} > \gamma_{d,50}$ holds up, independent of the value of $N$. It is also seen that the difference between the steepness of the dose–response curve in the two situations increases with decreasing $N$ or, in other words, with increasing dose per fraction (as this is equal to $D_{50}/N$). Also, which is intuitively clear, it depends on the magnitude of the coefficient of the dose-squared term in the logistic model.

The fact that $\gamma$ is greater for dose–response relationships obtained using a fixed number of fractions, rather than a fixed dose per fraction, may be seen as another reflection of what Withers[38] has named 'double trouble': when the total dose is increased but the number of fractions is kept constant this will cause an increase in both total dose and the dose per fraction.

## Clinical implications of the high $\gamma$

A few recent papers have been concerned with human data on $\gamma$.[4,39,40] Table 2.2 summarizes the experience from the Aarhus study on sequelae after postmastectomy radiotherapy. For $N = 22$, the $\gamma_{N,50}$ for subcutaneous fibrosis is estimated at 5.7 whereas reducing the number of fractions to one

**Table 2.2**   Steepness of the dose–response curve for various late endpoints after postmastectomy radiotherapy—the Aarhus experience

| Endpoint | Grade | $\gamma_{d,50}$ | $\gamma_{22,50}$ | $\gamma_{12,50}$ |
|---|---|---|---|---|
| Subcutaneous fibrosis[25] | ≥2 | 3.7 | 5.7 | 6.1 |
| Telangiectasia[25,70] | 3 | 2.2 | 3.2 | 3.4 |
|  | ≥2 | 1.0 | 1.4 | 1.5 |
| Frozen shoulder[23] | ≥2 | 4.8 | 6.6 | 7.2 |

is associated with an increase in $\gamma_{N,50}$ to 7.0. This illustrates the principal point that treating with large dose fractions will increase the precision requirements. On the other hand, this is a relatively modest change and it may be difficult to verify this prediction empirically. Indeed, Turesson[40] concluded from a study of dose–response curves for severe telangiectasia that the steepness was around 7, independent of fraction number, but this may very well be explained by the statistical problems in resolving a shift of the above magnitude. Another important observation is that, for a specific endpoint, the incidence of increasing grades of reaction follows increasingly steep dose–response curves.

The two parameters $\gamma_{d,50}$ and $\gamma_{N,50}$ are relevant for two different practical settings. The first situation is one in which the prescribed dose is escalated in an attempt to improve therapeutic efficacy. Historically, this has often been implemented as an increase in total dose while keeping the number of fractions constant. However, our current knowledge shows that the use of higher-than-standard dose fractions is associated with a loss of therapeutic ratio between late-responding normal tissues and at lease some of the tumour histologies such as squamous cell carcinoma. Therefore, a more attractive way to proceed is to add extra dose-fractions of the same size. In this case, the expected change in the incidence of a specific late endpoint may be approximated by multiplying the relative dose increment by $\gamma_{d,50}$. Similarly, to estimate the anticipated improvement in tumour control, the relevant parameter is $\gamma_{d,50}$ for the tumour. The second situation is for hot and cold spots in the irradiated volume, and for patients who are systematically over- or under-dosed. In these cases, the effect should be estimated from the $\gamma_{N,50}$. The effect of a hot spot may be overestimated if a substantial volume effect exists. This is because $\gamma_{N,50}$ will normally be estimated from clinical data where the field size is large compared to a typical hot-spot region in a therapeutic dose distribution, and shows a relatively limited variability.

The rather high values of $\gamma_{N,50}$ observed for late normal-tissue reactions put very strict limits on the required precision in radiotherapy. The often-quoted aim of being able to deliver the prescribed dose with a precision of ±5% seems to be insufficient for late reactions. A rough estimate is obtained by multiplying the γ-value from Table 2.2 by ±5, yielding a ±29 percentage point uncertainty in the incidence of subcutaneous fibrosis, e.g. from 21% to almost 79% incidence (a more precise calculation, allowing for the sigmoid shape of the dose–response curve, yields from 24% to 76%). The dose–response curve for telangiectasia was less steep in the Aarhus study (Table 2.2), but, as discussed above, in the Gothenburg study the maximum steepness of the dose–response curve for severe telangiectasia for a fixed number of fractions was around 7.

The maximum steepness of the dose–response curve will be influenced by organ structure, dosimetric heterogeneity, and patient-to-patient variability in the response to radiotherapy. As an example, radiation-induced lung damage is also characterized by a strong dose–reponse relationship, although somewhat weaker than for the above examples. A recent Dutch study[41] showed that the local measures of lung density, ventilation, and perfusion were strongly related to dose, with $\gamma_{N,50}$ for $N \approx 21$ being in the range 1.9–2.6. It should be noted that this is not necessarily equivalent to the steepness of a standard dose-incidence curve derived from reactions in individual patients. The latter has been assessed by computerized lung densitometry of routine chest X-rays[42] in a study of patients treated with postmastectomy radiotherapy in Aarhus. For $N \approx 22$, $\gamma_{N,50}$ for the endpoint marked early lung density changes was estimated at 2.3.

# Radiobiological strategies to improve radiotherapy

Several radiobiologically based strategies for improving the therapeutic ratio in radiotherapy are currently being investigated in clinical trials. Table 2.3 summarizes some of the main experimental therapies currently under investigation. For several of these, the biological rationale is not well established, in the sense that there are no convincing clinical data supporting the strategy. The ongoing trials in themselves will be of great value in providing more precise quantitative estimates of important biological properties of human tumours and normal tissues. In the following, some research areas in which more data are strongly needed will be briefly reviewed.

# Fractionation sensitivity of human normal tissues

Based on data from experimental animal studies, Thames *et al.*[43] proposed that the fractionation sensitivities of normal tissues could be quantified by the ratio, $\alpha/\beta$, of the parameters of the LQ model. In doing so, they observed that $\alpha/\beta$-values for early and late endpoints fell in two distinct ranges of 8–12 Gy and 1–5 Gy. This has subsequently been shown to hold up for human normal-tissue endpoints as well.[39,44,45] The status of available data on fractionation sensitivity may be summarized as follows. There are quite good estimates available for many late endpoints in humans. Here, the main problem is the confidence interval on $\alpha/\beta$, which for most published estimates is so wide that estimates of isoeffect dose can only be obtained in a rather narrow interval (±1 Gy) around the reference dose of 2 Gy per fraction.[4,39] There are fewer data available for early reactions, and the

**Table 2.3**  Radiobiological approaches to improve radiotherapy

| Strategy | Basic rationale | Current status |
|---|---|---|
| *Hyperfractionation:* reducing dose per fraction below 1.8 Gy | The increase in isoeffective dose for a reduced dose per fraction is larger for late-responding normal tissues than for (some) tumours (squamous cell carcinoma). This allows the tumour dose to be escalated without increased late reactions. Early reactions likely to increase | *Biological rationale:* well established for late reactions vs tumour control in the head and neck. Lack of good data for other tumours but the detrimental effect of large dose fractions is well established for many late-responding tissues *Randomized trials:* The EORTC trial[47] demonstrated an improved therapeutic ratio by hyperfractionation |
| *Accelerated fractionation:* rate of dose accumulation exceeding 10 Gy per week (biological equivalent dose in 2 Gy per fraction) | The dose recovered per day is greater in some tumours (e.g. squamous cell carcinoma of the head and neck and possibly the uterine cervix) than in late-responding normal tissues. Early reactions may become dose-limiting | *Biological rationale:* well-documented decrease of therapeutic ratio if treatment breaks are introduced in squamous cell carcinoma of the head and neck and uterine cervix.[61] Effect of shorter treatment is currently being tested *Randomized trials:* several large trials in progress |
| *Conformal therapy:* reducing the (high-dose) irradiated volume relative to some reference technique | Reducing the irradiated normal-tissue volume will reduce normal tissue complications and/or allow an escalation of the target dose | *Biological rationale:* mainly based on modelling. Clinical data on volume effect are scarce[81] *Randomized trials:* mostly Phase I/II studies |
| *Chemoradiotherapy:* combined chemotherapy and radiotherapy | The dominating rationale now is spatial cooperation, i.e. that chemotherapy might control micrometastases outside the radiotherapy target volume | *Biological rationale:* no strong support for this strategy although inducing rapid tumour shrinkage may be advantageous. Toxicity of combined therapy mainly studied experimentally[113] *Randomized trials:* several large trials completed, in general with no substantial benefit from combined therapy[114] |
| *Hypoxic modification:* sensitization of hypoxic cells by oxygen-mimetic or blood-flow-modifying drugs, gas breathing, changing oxygen pressure | Hypoxic cell sensitization is expected to increase the therapeutic ratio as hypoxic cells exist in human tumours but, in general, not in normal tissues | *Biological rationale:* well established although the role of reoxygenation remains controversial *Randomized trials:* more than twenty trials conducted in head and neck cancer alone. Most of these too small to resolve what appears from a meta-analysis to be the real magnitude of the gain from hypoxic modification |

incorporation of a time factor in the LQ model for early reactions has still not found a satisfactory solution.[46]

In the consideration of altered-dose-per-fraction schedules, the weak point is the tumour $\alpha/\beta$ where only crude estimates have been published so far. The resolution of these estimates is sufficient[4] to demonstrate, with statistical significance, that the EORTC hyperfractionation schedule delivering 80.5 Gy with 1.15 Gy per fraction, two fractions a day in an overall time of 7 weeks, should indeed be expected to improve the therapeutic ratio for local control of oropharyngeal carcinoma relative to late normal-tissue sequelae when compared to a conventional schedule delivering 70 Gy with 2.0 Gy per fraction, one fraction a day in the same overall time. Yet extrapolation of the dose being isoeffective with a reference schedule applying 2 Gy fractions is only feasible for doses per fraction in the range of 1.4–2.7 Gy if a ±5% limit on the 95% confidence interval is desired. The EORTC hyperfractionation trial has been closed and the final results have now been published;[47] from the outcome of this trial a rough estimate of the fractionation sensitivity of oropharyngeal carcinoma can be obtained. The 5-year local control rate was 19% higher (59% vs 40%) in the hyperfractionated arm of the trial. As this local-control range is close to the maximum steepness of the dose–response curve, a $\gamma$-value of around 2 would be expected from data in the literature.[4] Under this assumption, the biologically equivalent dose with 2 Gy per fraction in the hyperfractionation arm should be around 76.7 Gy, which again would mean that $\alpha/\beta$ is about 16 Gy.

## Repair half-time

Multiple fractions per day (MFD) schedules are normally designed under the assumption of complete repair between the two (or more) daily fractions. Yet human data on repair kinetics are sparse and most considerations of the interfraction interval, needed to reduce the unrepaired sublethal damage (SLD) to a clinically insignificant level, have relied on experimental animal data. Assuming monoexponential repair kinetics, the rate at which SLD repair proceeds may be characterized by its half-time, that is the time at which 50% of the SLD is repaired. There are data suggesting that repair does not follow simple monoexponential kinetics in the lung,[48] skin,[49] and kidney.[50] This means that more than one repair half-time is needed to describe the repair kinetics: typically two-component models have been fitted to the data and two distinct half-times in the ranges 0.1–0.2 hr and 2–5 hr have been estimated.

The available clinical data do not allow resolution of more than one repair component, and even data sets allowing analysis under the assumption of monoexponential repair kinetics are sparse. Turesson and Thames[51] estimated the repair half-time for telangiectasia at 3.4 hr with 95% confidence interval [2.8, 4.2] hr. There was some indication of two possible components of repair, but a biexponential model could not be fitted to the data. These authors also estimated repair half-times for erythema and moist desquamation at 1.3 hr and 1.1 hr, respectively, but with 95% confidence limits ranging from 0.5 hr to infinity.

For the oral mucosa there are two studies of interest, both providing a hint about the repair half-time in this tissue. One is the study from Warsaw[52] on sixty-five patients with supraglottic cancer who completed a course of concomitant boost radiotherapy between February 1988 and December 1989. The total dose ranged from 60 Gy to 76 Gy, with a median of 66 Gy. The daily dose during the first 4 weeks was 1.8 Gy and during the last 2 weeks it was 1.6 Gy twice daily, with 4- or (after September 1988) 6-hrs separation. Confluent membranous mucosal reaction was significantly more frequent in patients treated with a 4-hr interval (68%) than with a 6-hr interval (41%) between the daily fractions, the difference being 27% with 95% confidence interval [3.2, 50]%. This was an unexpectedly large effect of prolonging the interfraction interval by 2 hrs. However, this observation is supported by data from the RTOG 79-13 hyperfractionation study in advanced head and neck tumours.[53] A marked increase in the frequency of mucositis was seen when interfraction intervals of > 4.5 hr (28%) were compared with intervals of ≤ 4.5 hr (5%). The weighted averages of the interfraction interval were 5.5 hr and 3.9 hr, respectively. Also, the late reactions, both fibrosis and necrosis, were more frequent with the short interval between fractions.

The most intense debate on the importance of the interfraction interval in MFD has originated from the unexpected observation of four cases of radiation myelopathy in the continuous hyperfractionated accelerated radiation therapy (CHART) study at Mount Vernon Hospital[54,55] and a report on two additional cases from the Princess Margaret Hospital.[56] Application of the complete-repair LQ model with standard assumptions on the $\alpha/\beta$ ratio showed that the doses given in both studies should have produced a very low risk of spinal cord injury. This leaves two immediate possibilities, namely that the LQ model overestimates the sparing from low doses per fraction, or that the repair half-time is longer than previously assumed. Ang et al.[57] showed that in the rat spinal cord a significant repair still takes place between intervals of 8 hr and 24 hr. Model simulations[58] have shown that incomplete repair is a possible, though not very likely, explanation for the unexpected incidence of radiation myelopathy in the CHART trial. What puts a limit on the assumed half-time in this simulation study is the fact that, in the lung cancer patients treated with CHART, no patient developed radiation myelopathy. It is unknown at the time of writing which other biological mechanism might have played a role.

Taken together, the human data give a serious warning that interfraction intervals of 4 hr or less may be associated with an unexpected increase in early and late toxicity. It appears that intervals of 6 hr or more are preferable. Although the available data are rather sparse, and originate from studies where the interfraction interval was not assigned by randomization, the large difference between radiation reactions after 4-hr and 6-hr intervals suggests that sublethal damage repair may not be the sole explanation for the observed effects.

# The effect of overall treatment time on normal-tissue injury

Accelerated fractionation schedules employing shorter overall treatment times aim for improved tumour control with unchanged late effects. The crucial assumption here is that the dose recovered per day, $D_{rec}$, for late normal-tissue endpoints is less than for the tumour type being treated. If this is the case, a therapeutic advantage in terms of tumour control vs late morbidity should be obtainable by reducing overall treatment time. Quite a few estimates of $D_{rec}$ have been published for squamous cell carcinoma of the head and neck and they generally fall within the range 0.4–0.8 Gy/day.[59,60] In spite of a number of methodological problems in many of these studies,[61] this appears to be a fair estimate. For other tumour histologies and sites the data are sparse, but there is some evidence that the time factor is lower in most other cases.[60,61]

## Early endpoints

It is well established from both clinical and experimental studies that treatment protraction leads to reduced early reactions. This is due to compensatory proliferation of critical cell populations in the tissue. By analogy, accelerated fractionation with unchanged total dose and dose per fraction is expected to increase the incidence and severity of early reactions, as less time is available for regeneration during the treatment course. The classical data from Fletcher et al.[62] show that the dose equivalent of proliferation, $D_{rec}$, in the human oral mucosa is around 1.8 Gy/day towards the end of a 6-week radiotherapy course. Thus, the oral mucosa may become dose-limiting when treatment time is gradually reduced, as $D_{rec}$ is larger than the average value seen in squamous cell carcinoma of the head and neck.

Kaanders et al.[63] conducted a Phase I/II trial of concomitant boost radiotherapy in eighteen patients with $T_{1-3}N_xM_0$ squamous cell laryngeal carcinoma and compared the outcome with that of forty patients receiving conventional fractionation of 2 Gy per fraction, five fractions a week, total dose 64–70 Gy. The total dose and dose per fraction in the concomitant boost schedule were unchanged, whereas an average reduction in overall treatment time of 11 days was achieved by giving two fractions per day during the last part of the course. The application of a range of doses allowed estimation of dose–response relationships. The isoeffect dose for 50% incidence of confluent mucositis decreased from about 69 Gy to 66 Gy when the treatment time was reduced by 11 days. Thus, $D_{rec}$ for laryngeal mucosa is estimated at 0.3 Gy/day which is somewhat lower than for oral mucosa.

The fact that early-responding normal tissues, in particular the mucosa, are able to recover a quite substantial dose per day means that reactions in these tissues may become dose-limiting with accelerated fractionation schedules. One example of this is the CHART schedule,[64] where the very short and intense schedule used, $3 \times 1.5$ Gy/day for 12 consecutive days, requires a reduction of the total dose down to 54 Gy. This dose reduction means that the CHART schedule should be predicted to be very well tolerated with respect to late sequelae, but that some of the advantage from the short treatment time may be offset by the reduced total dose.[24] This has created interest in methods for overcoming or relieving mucositis (see below).

## Late endpoints

From a normal-tissue perspective, the crucial question is whether late normal-tissue injury will be unaffected by a shortening of overall treatment time. In recent years, most authors have assumed that changed overall treatment time will have no appreciable effect on the late-responding normal tissues because of the very low rate of cellular turnover. As an example, Hendry and Jen[65] estimated a 0.01–0.04 Gy/day equivalence of proliferation in the kidney, assuming a labelling index of 0.2%, an S-phase duration of 8 hrs, and a $D_0$ between 5 and 20 Gy. Although such estimates are somewhat speculative, it seems likely that target-cell proliferation cannot be the only, and perhaps not even the main, explanation of the dose sparing from protracted treatment time that has been reported by some authors. In all probability, repair of sublethal damage with a long half-time may also contribute. Recent reviews of experimental animal data have reached differing conclusions, some authors finding evidence for[65,66] and some finding no evidence for[67] a significant influence of overall treatment time on the incidence of late reactions.

The effect of overall treatment time is not well established from clinical data, but a few estimates have been obtained, as summarized in Table 2.4. Many of these studies have not allowed a direct estimation of the dose recovered per day, $D_{rec}$, but they all point in the same direction, namely that there is limited, if any, sparing of late endpoints from a protraction of overall treatment time. This is another area in which better data are urgently needed.

It is conceivable that recovery (or lack of it) during a treatment-free

**Table 2.4**  Time factor for late human endpoints

| Endpoint | Result | Reference |
|---|---|---|
| Telangiectasia | 'No recovery after a 3-week split' | Turesson and Thames[51] |
| Late laryngeal oedema | $D_{rec} = 0.10 \pm 0.22$ Gy/day | Overgaard et al.[116] |
| Fistula secondary to salvage surgery | $D_{rec} = 0.09 \pm ?^a$ Gy/day | Overgaard et al.[116] |
| Rectosigmoid complications | $D_{rec} < 0.15$ Gy/day | Bentzen et al.[117] |
| Parotid gland function | $D_{rec} \approx 0$ Gy | Leslie and Disch[68] |
| Bladder | 'Reduction of treatment time to 4 weeks gave no increase in bladder toxicity' | Moonen cited in Kaanders and Ang[76] |

[a]Not estimated.

interval might not be a valid representation of the effect of treatment acceleration/protraction with a constant temporal distribution of dose-fractions. In this context, the report by Leslie and Dische[68] on parotid gland function is of special interest as the data originate from a comparison between six patients treated with the strongly accelerated CHART schedule (54 Gy with 1.5 Gy per fraction delivered in 12 days) and two groups of patients receiving standard fractionation: one of them a group of twelve head and neck cancer patients receiving 60–66 Gy with 2 Gy per fraction in 6–7 weeks, the other a group of eight lymphoma patients receiving 35–40 Gy with 2 Gy per fraction in around 4 weeks. A significantly larger reduction in parotid function was seen in patients receiving conventional treatment for head and neck cancer as compared with the two other groups, whereas there was no demonstrable difference between the lymphoma patients and the patients treated with CHART. Assuming $\alpha/\beta = 3$ Gy for this endpoint, the biologically equivalent dose in 2 Gy fractions received by the CHART patients is around 48.6 Gy, which, when delivered in 12 days, resulted in a parotid gland function comparable to that seen after 40 Gy in 4 weeks. Due to the limited number of patients per group and a relatively large interindividual variation in the parotid function measure, the conclusion that the two schedules were isoeffective has a relatively low power.[4] If isoeffect is assumed, $\alpha/\beta$ for this endpoint would have to be < 1 Gy. Although this may not be realistic, it is clear that there is no room for any major influence of overall treatment time for this endpoint.

## Consequential late reactions

Consequential late reactions are a potential problem with strongly accelerated treatment schedules. This term refers to late reactions occurring as a consequence of severe early reactions.[69,70] Clinical examples are the occurrence of bone and soft tissue necrosis after severe mucosal denudation[71] or telangiectasia after moist desquamation.[70] Experimental studies show that severe early damage may also be a risk factor for subsequent development of reduced bladder capacity[72] and rectal stenosis.[73] Followill et al.[74] studied late colorectal obstruction in the mouse after various single doses or two equal doses. Both the early reactions and the late phase were documented by sequential histological studies. The main finding was that two patterns of late obstruction could be distinguished: a consequential form associated with persistent epithelial denudation and a generic late reaction characterized by development of fibrosis in the submucosa.

One clinical study[67] did find a significant time factor for late effects in the oral cavity and oropharynx. The $D_{rec}$ was estimated at 0.25 Gy with 95% confidence limits [0.19, 0.27] Gy. The authors speculated that the significant effect of time may have resulted from a consequential late effect as they found a rather strong correlation between early and late reactions in their patients. A previous study from the same centre on complications after radiotherapy for laryngeal carcinoma showed no significant influence of overall treatment time in the interval 4–7 weeks.[75]

All of the above suggest that an increased incidence of some of the late sequelae must be anticipated in schedules producing an intense early reaction. Strategies for amelioration of early effects[76] may be warranted, not only to improve early tolerance but also to reduce the risk of consequential late reactions.

# Conformal therapy

Conformal therapy is a loosely defined term referring to treatment techniques which aim for an improved matching of the dose distribution to the target volume, relative to what is obtained by some reference technique. The current interest in this field has been stimulated not so much by new biological concepts or data but rather by the great technological advances in diagnostic imaging and in treatment planning and delivery over the past two decades.[77] These advances have dramatically improved our technical ability to define the tumour volume and to deliver conformal therapy. Most conformal therapy strategies aim for an escalation of the dose to the target volume with a concomitant reduction in the irradiated volume of the dose-limiting normal tissues. This may not always be possible, as conformal therapy techniques often involve an increased number of treatment fields or 'dynamic therapy' with scanned elementary photon or electron beams and/or dynamic field shaping by computer-controlled multileaf collimators.[78] Thus, in practice, many conformal therapy techniques involve some trade-off between dose and volume, often visualized in a dose–volume histogram. The concept is that, if a normal-tissue volume receives a high dose, this should be compensated by the volume effect; similarly, in the case of a large irradiated volume, this should be balanced by a lowering of the dose to this tissue.

Biologically, there are several caveats to be considered in the simple rationale for conformal therapy. First of all, the expectation from an escalation of the target dose depends on the steepness of the dose–response curve.[4,79] As an example, a two-arm clinical trial of a 10% escalation of dose in patients with head and neck cancer should aim for inclusion of more than 200 patients.[4] For many other tumour histologies, relatively little is known about the steepness of the dose–response curve. It may seem indisputable that a dose escalation will reduce the in-field recurrence rate. Yet radiotherapy in Hodgkin's disease is an example in which substantial dose escalations have been tried without any demonstrable improvement in tumour control[80] and, although this disease would probably not be considered a candidate for conformal therapy, this observation illustrates that local control may not, in all cases, be dose-limited. Second, the dose–response relationship for late normal-tissue endpoints is generally steeper than for human tumours. This means that even small increments in the dose to critical normal tissues may strongly affect the complication rate. Finally, as discussed below, the volume effect for human normal tissues is still not well established.

## Treatment volume and normal-tissue complications

The discussion of the treatment volume effect for irradiation of normal tissue has been dominated by extensive modelling efforts and surprisingly few clinical data. Withers[38] pointed out the importance of realizing that there are several mechanisms contributing to the general clinical impression of a deleterious effect of large treatment volume. Table 2.5 summarizes some of these.

Most of the modelling studies have been concerned with probabilistic considerations of various organizations of a hypothetical tissue substructure called functional subunits (FSUs).[81,82] It has been proposed that in some organs, for example, the spinal cord, these FSUs are serially arranged, and that the failure of any one of these FSUs would lead to a radiation complication, say, a radiation myelitis. The idea underlying this model is well illustrated by frequent references to it as 'the sliced salami model'.[82] Experimental data from rat spinal cord have shown an increasing incidence of radiation myelitis with increasing length of spinal cord being irradiated,[83] an observation that was interpreted in terms of the serial FSU model. However, the investigators have questioned whether these results could be taken as support for the simple FSU concept.[84] Other tissues have a parallel organization of the FSUs: if one FSU is inactivated, this has no consequence for the functioning of the remaining units. Hybrid models of 'serial–parallel' tissue structures have also been proposed,[85] but again the resolution of the available data makes discrimination between alternative models very difficult. In most situations it is doubtful whether the FSU is a biologically realistic concept.

In clinical studies (see review by Withers *et al.*[81]), diverse results are found concerning the influence of treatment volume on the incidence of late radiation sequelae. Withers *et al.* came out with a negative result when looking for an effect of treatment volume on late sequelae after radiotherapy for head and neck cancer.[67] In contrast, a series of patients with laryngeal carcinoma[86] showed a marked increase in the frequency of late oedema with increasing field size after definitive radiotherapy. Although there were early attempts to use empirical models like the 'cube root rule' (see Cohen[87]) and also suggestions for mechanistic models,[81,88,89] there is a lack of quantitative radiobiological data relating to the effect of treatment volume. A recent study of late radiation injury to the small intestine[90] showed no significant volume effect for treatment volumes ranging from 45 cm³ to 390 cm³ . Larger volumes (on average 790 cm³) treated by anterior–posterior parallel opposing fields before 1983 had a markedly higher incidence of intestinal complications (37% vs 6%). It should be noted that all patients had undergone prior surgery. The authors also reviewed a number of studies from the literature and found a strong interaction between surgery for colorectal carcinoma and radiotherapy. It is difficult to rule out differences in surgical procedures and postoperative care of the patients treated before and after 1983. A study by the EORTC Radiotherapy Cooperative Group[91] found no significant correlation between irradiated volume of small bowel and the incidence of small bowel obstruction, whereas a volume effect was seen for chronic diarrhoea. This is the opposite of what would be expected from a simple serial FSU model, but illustrates well the difficulties in clinical testing of dose–volume models.

At the time of writing, the clinical data available do not allow a test of the underlying biological assumptions for current models of the treatment volume effect.

**Table 2.5** Proposed mechanisms behind a clinical volume effect

| Mechanism | Explanation | Clinical relevance |
|---|---|---|
| Increased cytotoxicity | Toxicity at the cellular level may increase if a large volume is irradiated | Tested experimentally but remains controversial[81,118] |
| Cell migration | Small injured volumes may effectively be rescued by migrating cells from the surroundings. Possibly also effect on revascularization and reinnervation | Experimentally verified for small lengths of spinal cord[84] and small areas of skin.[83] Not well documented in humans |
| Functional organization | Local loss of function may or may not impair organ function depending on the functional (parallel/serial) organization | Remains controversial to what extent these concepts are biologically relevant[81,119] |
| Physiological reserve capacity | Many organs (e.g. kidney, lung, liver) have a large physiological reserve capacity. Even if a partial volume shows complete loss of function this may not affect the patient | Well established, exploited in routine radiotherapy |
| Patient tolerance | A certain reaction, e.g. mucositis, may be less troublesome for the patient if confined to a small volume | Well established, exploited in routine radiotherapy |
| Diagnostic sensitivity | A large damaged area/volume may be more readily detected | Probably true for some diagnostic methods/types of reactions (radiological changes, palpation) |
| Dose heterogeneity | Hot spots in the absorbed dose in normal tissue may occur more frequently with large treatment volume | True in many situations, the clinical importance of this phenomenon is uncertain |

# Patient-to-patient variability in the response to radiotherapy

One of the recurring controversial themes in the history of radiotherapy is whether a substantial patient-to-patient variability in radiosensitivity exists. Throughout this century, it has been a common belief that dose–response relationships were relatively weak but that a very strong interindividual variation in radiosensitivity existed. As discussed above, the dose–response relationship, especially for late reactions, is very steep; so steep that small variations in absorbed dose at the relevant reference depth, which are likely to be undetected, may give rise to a markedly different clinical outcome. Thus, the dose–response relationship is so strong that it may seem impossible to predict which patients are likely to show a specific radiation reaction after radiotherapy. From a historical point of view, an interesting parallel of this argument is found in the review given by Wetterer in his textbook from 1908.[92] The notion of a pronounced patient-to-patient variability in radiosensitivity was strongly opposed by Holzknecht and Kienböck, among others, who claimed that the observations made by earlier investigators could simply be explained as dosimetric errors. Systematic studies using chemical dosimetry indicated that the sensitivity of individuals showed only modest, if any, variation but that the output from the X-ray tubes available at that time was indeed highly variable!

A refined analysis of this problem was presented by Holthusen,[1] who proposed a direct link between the shape of the dose–response curve and the patient-to-patient variability in radiosensitivity. He showed that the incidence of telangiectasia followed a well-defined sigmoid dose-response curve, but went one step further when he interpreted the shape of this curve as the cumulative distribution of the individual radiosensitivities of the patients. An alternative explanation of the shape of the dose–response curve originated from the work by Munro and Gilbert,[93] who interpreted this as a result of the random nature of radiation-induced cell kill. These two pictures are not mutually exclusive[94] and it is likely that the stochastic 'ideal' dose–response curve is strongly influenced by patient-to-patient variability in treatment and tumour/host characteristics. If this heterogeneity could be taken into account, our ability to optimize radiotherapy for the individual patient would drastically improve.

A number of factors have been suggested to alter the probability of expressing normal-tissue injury after a given treatment and these have recently been reviewed.[95] The conclusion of that review was that the effect of many of these factors is doubtful when tested critically in a well-designed study. For example, it has been proposed that comorbid conditions like collagen vascular diseases, diabetes mellitus, or hypertension might increase the risk of late complications after radiotherapy. However, for all of these the available data suggest that there is only minimal, if any, effect on the level of late sequelae. Factors that do have an impact on the incidence and severity of radiation reactions include infections/immunosuppression, age, and smoking habits. This, again, is an area where more data are needed, but the overall impression is that such factors are probably less important than has been generally believed.

## *In-vitro* radiosensitivity assays

In 1975, Taylor *et al.*[96] showed that normal skin fibroblasts from patients with the genetic syndrome ataxia–telangiectasia (AT) were hypersensitive to radiation *in vitro*. This has strongly stimulated research into *in-vitro* radiosensitivity assays, the hypothesis being that cancer patients without known genetic disorders might also show a genetic variation in their cellular (intrinsic) radiosensitivity and therefore in their response to radiotherapy. At the time of writing, several studies have been published and more are on the way.[95] There is considerable variation in the design of these studies, in the assays used, the assay conditions (e.g. high- or low-dose-rate irradiation, exponential or plateau-phase cells), and in the clinical endpoints. Most studies have been concerned with skin fibroblasts but lymphocytes and keratinocytes have also been investigated. One of the most important design differences is whether patients are selected to express atypically strong reactions (so-called 'over-reactors')[97] or whether they are unselected.[98–100] Over-reactors could be defined as cases with a more or less extreme response to radiotherapy but will typically constitute a very small fraction, less than 1%, of all cancer patients. Because of this very low prevalence, screening for over-reactors is not in itself a likely practical application of *in-vitro* assays. Therefore, the basic problem with this type of design is that it is difficult to evaluate the representativeness of the findings for prospective application of the assay on unselected patients.[95] Designs in which patients have been selected to show a broad range of responses[99] are subject to the same criticism as the over-reactor studies.

Three studies have looked for an association between *in-vitro* radiosensitivity and clinical radioresponsivenesss with respect to late reactions.[99–101] The Aarhus study[101] demonstrated, for the first time, a positive correlation between *in-vitro* radiosensitivity of skin fibroblasts and the clinical occurrence of fibrosis. The Houston study[100] used the RTOG grade of any late reaction in patients with head and neck cancer receiving definitive radiotherapy. A highly significant correlation was found between grade of reaction and *in-vitro* radiosensitivity. The study from Sutton found a suggestion of a significant correlation between *in-vitro* radiosensitivity of fibroblasts and telangiectasia.[99] No statistical test for significance was stated, and it is not clear if the selection of patients showing a broad range of reactions might have influenced the result. A relationship between the *in-vitro* radiosensitivity of fibroblasts and clinical occurrence of telangiectasia was looked for in the Aarhus study but no statistically significant correlation was found.

Four studies have looked at the possible correlation between early reactions and *in-vitro* radiosensitivity, and three of these, the Houston,[100] Amsterdam,[98] and Aarhus[101] studies, found no significant correlation. In contrast, the study by the Sutton group on six patients treated in Gothenburg showed a significant correlation between erythema and *in-vitro* radiosensitivity of fibroblasts.[99] A subsequent study by Brock and colleagues in Houston, including patients from the same institution, failed to find a significant correlation between *in-vitro* radiosensitivity of fibroblasts and early reactions (cited in West *et al.*[102]).

The picture emerging from these studies seems to be consistent with the result of clinical studies looking for a host factor in the expression of radiation injury in multiple treatment areas in the same individual. It has been demonstrated[70,103,104] that, for a specific normal-tissue endpoint, an atypically strong/weak response in one treatment area is correlated with a strong/weak response in another irradiated area in the same patient. However, when two different endpoints are analysed the within-patient correlation is no stronger than the between-patient correlation. Therefore, in unselected series of patients, clinical hypersensitivity appears to be tissue/endpoint specific and a predictive assay will therefore have to be aimed at a specific biological endpoint. Although this may subtract from the clinical value of *in-vitro* assays, there is little doubt that this research field will contribute much useful knowledge on the factors influencing treatment-related morbidity.

# Modification of the expression of normal-tissue injury

Manipulation of the dose–time-fractionation pattern has been the traditional method of trying to improve the therapeutic ratio in radiotherapy. An improved understanding of the radiation pathogenesis of human normal-tissue reactions has opened up the possibility of active intervention in the pathogenic pathway. Table 2.6 gives examples of some strategies that have been tried in the laboratory and/or the clinic. Although several of these seem promising in preclinical testing, it remains to be seen whether they will find a role in routine radiotherapy.

Most of these strategies have been applied to early-responding normal tissues and some were proposed many years ago. Until recently, the possibilities of modifying late radiation reactions were limited. However, this picture has already started to change. One example is radiation-induced fibrosis, which occurs in several human organs and tissues after irradiation

**Table 2.6** Examples of strategies for amelioration of the expression of normal-tissue damage after radiotherapy or chemotherapy (based on the review by Hendry[120])

| Strategy | Examples | Tissue/organ |
| --- | --- | --- |
| Proliferation modifiers: chemical stimulation | Local silver nitrate application | Mucosa[121,122] |
| Proliferation modifiers: cytokines | GM-CSF | Haemopoietic system,[123] mucosa[123] |
| | Interleukin-I | Intestine,[124] lung[125] |
| Antibiotics | | Intestine[126] |
| Prostaglandins | Arachidonic acid | Intestine[127] |
| Vascular modifiers | Angiotensin-converting enzyme inhibitors (captopril) | Lung,[128] kidney[129] |

GM-CSF: granulocyte–macrophage colony-stimulating factor.

and is one of the major causes of late radiotherapy-related morbidity. Histologically, fibrosis is characterized by an abnormal deposition of collagen in the irradiated tissue. Of the five major types of collagen, described by Altman,[105] the initial phase of collagen deposition is dominated by the relatively flexible Type III,[106] whereas, later on, deposition is also enhanced by the biomechanically more rigid Type I collagen.[105] The radiation-pathogenesis of fibrosis is poorly understood. The most prominent hypothesis in the late 1980s was the 'target-cell' hypothesis, namely that the grade of fibrosis should depend on the level of depletion of a specific target cell, *in casu* the fibroblast. This has provided the conceptual basis for studies of a clonogenic *in-vitro* sensitivity assay for prediction of radiation-induced fibrosis, and a correlation has been demonstrated between the *in-vitro* surviving fraction of fibroblasts in this assay and the clinical occurrence of subcutaneous fibrosis.[100] Although this observation is in accordance with the target-cell hypothesis, it seems counterintuitive that enhanced killing of the cell type thought to be responsible for the formation of radiation-induced fibrosis should lead to an increased severity of the clinical reaction.

All of the above have created interest in the induction and release of cytokines as mediators of radiation-induced fibrosis. At present, there are strong indications that the potent fibrogenic cytokine, transforming growth factor β (TGFβ), plays a key role in the process.[107, 108] An improved understanding of the pathogenesis of fibrosis opens up the possibility of preventing or ameliorating this radiation reaction. Indeed, preliminary studies have shown that TGFβ antagonists may inhibit or reduce the action of this growth factor in kidney,[109] skin,[110] and lung.[111]

# Conclusions

Our current practice of radiotherapy is largely empirically founded. However, many of the treatment techniques that are now accepted as standards have been optimized under serious technical constraints as well as an incomplete understanding of the underlying radiobiology. It seems likely that a rational approach to clinical radiobiology may lead to major advances in practical radiotherapy. The second line of development that will almost certainly revolutionize normal-tissue radiobiology is the increasing use of molecular biology techniques in the study of radiobiological problems. New insights into the biological mechanisms will produce new radiotherapy strategies that, in due course, must be subject to clinical trials.[112]

# References

1. Holthusen H. Erfahrungen über die Verträglichkeitsgrenze für Röntgenstrahlen und deren Nutzanwendung zur Verhütung von Schäden. *Strahlentherapie* 1936; 57, 254–69.
2. Ellis F. Dose, time and fractionation: a clinical hypothesis. *Clin Radiol* 1969; 20, 1–7.
3. Bentzen SM, Overgaard J. Time–dose relationships in radiotherapy. In: GG Steel, ed, *Basic Clinical Radiobiology*. London: Edward Arnold, 1993; 47–54.

4. Bentzen SM. Radiobiological considerations in the design of clinical trials. *Radiother Oncol* 1994; **32**, 1–11.

5. Dische S, Warburton MF, Jones D, *et al.* The recording of morbidity related to radiotherapy. *Radiother Oncol* 1989; **16**, 103–8.

6. Dische S. The uniform reporting of treatment-related morbidity. *Semin Radiat Oncol* 1994; **4**, 112–18.

7. Sismondi P, Sinistrero G, Zola P, *et al.* Complications of uterine cervix carcinoma treatments: the problem of a uniform classification. *Radiother Oncol* 1989; **14**, 9–17.

8. Perez CA, Brady LW. Overview. In: CA Perez *et al.*, eds, *Principles and Practice of Radiation Oncology*. Philadelphia: JB Lippincott Co, 1992; 1–63.

9. Miller AB, Hoogstraten B, Staquet M, *et al.* Reporting results of cancer treatment. *Cancer* 1981; **47**, 207–14.

10. Chassagne D, Sismondi P, Horiot JC, *et al.* A glossary for reporting complications of treatment in gynecological cancers. *Radiother Oncol* 1993; **26**, 195–202.

11. Pavy J-J, Denekamp J, Letschert J, *et al.* Late effects damage scoring: the SOMA scale. *Radiother Oncol* 1995 (in press).

12. Bentzen SM, Overgaard J. Clinical manifestations of normal-tissue damage. In: GG Steel, ed, *Basic Clinical Radiobiology*. London: Edward Arnold, 1993; 89–99.

13. Gerbaulet A, Kunkler I, Kerr G, *et al.* Combined radiotherapy and surgery: local control and complications in early carcinoma of the uterine cervix—the Villejuif experience 1975–1984. *Radiother Oncol* 1993; **23**, 66–73.

14. Lambin P, Gerbaulet A, Kramar A, *et al.* Phase III trial comparing two low dose rates in brachytherapy of cervix carcinoma: report at two years. *Int J Radiat Oncol Biol Phys* 1993; **25**, 405–12.

15. Scalliet P, Gerbaulet A, Dubray BM. HDR versus LDR gynecological brachytherapy revisited. *Radiother Oncol* 1993; **28**, 118–26.

16. Pedersen D, Bentzen SM, Overgaard J. Reporting radiotherapeutic complications in patients with uterine cervical cancer. The importance of latency and classification system. *Radiother Oncol* 1993; **28**, 134–41.

17. Pedersen D, Bentzen SM, Overgaard J. Early and late radiotherapeutic morbidity in 442 consecutive patients with locally advanced carcinoma of the uterine cervix. *Int J Radiat Oncol Biol Phys* 1994; **29**, 941–52.

18. Wheldon TE, Michalowski A, Kirk J. The effect of irradiation on function in self-renewing normal tissues with differing proliferative organisation. *Br J Radiol* 1982; **55**, 759–66.

19. Turesson I, Notter G. The predictive value of skin telangiectasia for late radiation effects in different normal tissues. *Int J Radiat Oncol Biol Phys* 1986; **12**, 603–9.

20. Turesson I. The progression rate of late radiation effect in normal tissues and its impact on dose–response relationships. *Radiother Oncol* 1989; **15**, 217–26.

21. Bentzen SM, Turesson I, Thames HD. Fractionation sensitivity and latency of telangiectasia after postmastectomy radiotherapy. A graded response analysis. *Radiother Oncol* 1990; **18**, 95–106.

22. Bentzen SM, Thames HD. Incidence and latency of radiation reactions. *Radiother Oncol* 1989; **14**, 261–2.

23. Bentzen SM, Overgaard M, Thames HD. Fractionation sensitivity of a functional endpoint: impaired shoulder movement after postmastectomy radiotherapy. *Int J Radiat Oncol Biol Phys* 1989; **17**, 531–7.

24. Bentzen SM. Quantitative clinical radiobiology. *Acta Oncol* 1993; **32**, 259–75.

25. Bentzen SM, Thames HD, Overgaard M. Latent-time estimation for late cutaneous and subcutaneous radiation reactions in the single-follow-up clinical study. *Radiother Oncol* 1989; **15**, 267–74.

26. Schultheiss TE, Thames HD, Peters LJ, *et al.* Effect of latency on calculated complication rates. *Int J Radiat Oncol Biol Phys* 1986; **12**, 1861–5.
27. Bentzen SM, Johansen LV, Overgaard J, *et al.* Clinical radiobiology of squamous cell carcinoma of the oropharynx. *Int J Radiat Oncol Biol Phys* 1991; **20**, 1197–206.
28. Berkson J, Gage RP. Survival curve for cancer patients following treatment. *J Am Stat Ass* 1952; **47**, 501–15.
29. Kaplan EL, Meier P. Non-parametric estimation from incomplete observations. *J Am Stat Soc C* 1958; **53**, 457–81.
30. Cox DR. Regression models and life-tables (with discussion). *J Roy Stat Soc B* 1972; **34**, 178–220.
31. Farewell VT. A model for a binary variable with timecensored observations. *Biometrika* 1977; **64**, 43–6.
32. Bentzen SM, Thames HD, Travis EL, *et al.* Direct estimation of latent time for radiation injury in late-responding normal tissues: gut, lung and spinal cord. *Int J Radiat Biol* 1989; **55**, 27–43.
33. Taylor JMG, Withers HR, Vegesna V, *et al.* Fitting the linear-quadratic model using time of occurrence as the endpoint for quantal response multifraction experiments. *Int J Radiat Biol* 1987; **52**, 459–68.
34. Taylor JMG, Kim DG. Statistical models for analyzing time-to-occurrence data in radiobiology and radiation oncology. *Int J Radiat Biol* 1993; **64**, 627–40.
35. Bentzen SM. Analysis and evaluation of clinical data: parameter estimation and model validation. In: D Baltas *et al.*, eds, *Modelling in Clinical Radiobiology*. Freiburg: Albert-Ludwigs Universität, 1995 (in press).
36. Haie-Meder C, Kramar A, Lambin P, *et al.* Analysis of complications in a prospective randomized trial comparing two brachytherapy low dose rates in cervical carcinoma. *Int J Radiat Oncol Biol Phys* 1994; **29**, 953–60.
37. Brahme A. Dosimetric precision requirements in radiation therapy. *Acta Radiol Oncol* 1984; **23**, 379–91.
38. Withers HR. Biologic basis of radiation therapy. In: CA Perez *et al.*, eds, *Principles and Practice of Radiation Oncology*. Philadelphia: JB Lippincott Co, 1992; 64–96.
39. Bentzen SM, Overgaard M. Early and late normal-tissue injury after post-mastectomy radiotherapy. In: W Hinkelbein *et al.*, eds, *Acute and Long-Term Side-Effects of Radiotherapy*. Berlin: Springer-Verlag, 1993; 59–78.
40. Turesson I. Dose–response relationships for late effects on skin and mucosa. In: W Hinkelbein *et al.*, eds, *Acute and Long-Term Side-Effects of Radiotherapy*. Berlin: Springer-Verlag, 1993; 49–57.
41. Boersma LJ, Damen EMF, de Boer RW, *et al.* Dose-effect relations for local functional and structural changes of the lung after irradiation for malignant lymphoma. *Radiother Oncol* 1994; **32**, 201–9.
42. Bentzen SM, Skoczylas JZ, Overgaard M, *et al.* Quantitative assessment of radiation-induced lung changes by computerized optical densitometry of routine chest x-rays. *Int J Radiat Oncol Biol Phys* 1995; **33** (in press).
43. Thames HD, Withers HR, Peters LJ, *et al.* Changes in early and late radiation responses with altered dose fractionation: implications for dose–survival relationships. *Int J Radiat Oncol Biol Phys* 1982; **8**, 219–26.
44. Thames HD, Bentzen SM, Turesson I, *et al.* Time–dose factors in radiotherapy. *Radiother Oncol* 1990; **19**, 219–35.
45. Bentzen SM, Overgaard M. Clinical radiobiology and normal-tissue morbidity after breast cancer treatment. In: KI Altman *et al.*, eds, *Advances in Radiation Biology*. San Diego: Academic Press, 1994; 25–51.
46. Tucker SL, Travis EL. Comments on a time-dependent version of the linear-quadratic model. *Radiother Oncol* 1990; **18**, 155–63.

47. Horiot JC, Le Fur R, N'Guyen T, *et al*. Hyperfractionation versus conventional fractionation in oropharyngeal carcinoma: final analysis of a randomized trial of the EORTC cooperative group of radiotherapy. *Radiother Oncol* 1992; **25**, 231–41.

48. Parkins CS, Whitsed CA, Fowler JF. Repair kinetics in mouse lung after multiple X-ray fractions per day. *Int J Radiat Biol* 1988; **54**, 429–43.

49. van den Aardweg GJ, Hopewell JW. The kinetics of repair for sublethal radiation-induced damage in the pig epidermis: an interpretation based on a fast and a slow component of repair. *Radiother Oncol* 1992; **23**, 94–104.

50. Millar WT, Jen YM, Hendry JH, *et al*. Two components of repair in irradiated kidney colony forming cells. *Int J Radiat Biol* 1994; **66**, 189–96.

51. Turesson I, Thames HD. Repair capacity and kinetics of human skin during fractionated radiotherapy: erythema, desquamation, and telangiectasia after 3 and 5 years' follow-up. *Radiother Oncol* 1989; **15**, 169–88.

52. Bujko K, Skoczylas JZ, Bentzen SM, *et al*. A feasibility study of concomitant boost radiotherapy for patients with cancer of the supraglottic larynx. *Acta Oncol* 1993; **32**, 637–40.

53. Marcial VA, Pajak TF, Chang C, *et al*. Hyperfractionated photon radiation therapy in the treatment of advanced squamous cell carcinoma of the oral cavity, pharynx, larynx, and sinuses using radiation therapy as the only planned modality: (preliminary report) by the Radiation Therapy Oncology Group (RTOG). *Int J Radiat Oncol Biol Phys* 1987; **13**, 41–7.

54. Dische S, Saunders MI. Continuous, hyperfractionated, accelerated radiotherapy (CHART): an interim report upon late morbidity. *Radiother Oncol* 1989; **16**, 65–72.

55. Dische S. Accelerated treatment and radiation myelitis. *Radiother Oncol* 1991; **20**, 1–2.

56. Wong CS, Van Dyk J, Simpson WJ. Myelopathy following hyperfractionated accelerated radiotherapy for anaplastic thyroid carcinoma. *Radiother Oncol* 1991; **20**, 3–9.

57. Ang KK, Jiang GL, Guttenberger R, *et al*. Impact of spinal cord repair kinetics on the practice of altered fractionation schedules. *Radiother Oncol* 1992; **25**, 287–94.

58. Guttenberger R, Thames HD, Ang KK. Is the experience with CHART compatible with experimental data? A new model of repair kinetics and computer simulations. *Radiother Oncol* 1992; **25**, 280–6.

59. Withers HR, Taylor JMG, Maciejewski B. The hazard of accelerated tumour clonogen repopulation during radiotherapy. *Acta Oncol* 1988; **27**, 131–46.

60. Withers HR. Treatment-induced accelerated human tumor growth. *Semin Radiat Oncol* 1993; **3**, 135–43.

61. Bentzen SM. Time–dose relationships for human tumors: estimation from non-randomized studies. In: HP Beck-Bornholt, ed, *Current Topics in Clinical Radiobiology of Tumours. Medical Radiology*. Berlin: Springer-Verlag, 1993; 11–26.

62. Fletcher GH, MacComb WS, Shalek RJ. *Radiation Therapy in the Management of Cancer of the Oral Cavity and the Oropharynx*. Springfield: Charles C Thomas, 1962.

63. Kaanders JH, van Daal WA, Hoogenraad WJ, *et al*. Accelerated fractionation radiotherapy for laryngeal cancer, acute, and late toxicity. *Int J Radiat Oncol Biol Phys* 1992; **24**, 497–503.

64. Saunders MI, Dische S. Radiotherapy employing three fractions in each day over a continuous period of 12 days. *Br J Radiol* 1986; **59**, 523–5.

65. Hendry JH, Jen Y-M. The time factor for late reactions in radiotherapy: repopulation or intracellular repair. In: W Hinkelbein *et al*., eds, *Acute and Long-Term Side-Effects of Radiotherapy*. Berlin: Springer-Verlag, 1993,

17–26.

66. Trott KR, Kummermehr J. The time factor and repopulation in tumors and normal tissues. *Semin Radiat Oncol* 1993; **3**, 115–25.
67. Maciejewski B, Withers HR, Taylor JMG, *et al.* Dose fractionation and regeneration in radiotherapy for cancer of the oral cavity and oropharynx. Part 2. Normal tissue responses: acute and late effects. *Int J Radiat Oncol Biol Phys* 1990; **18**, 101–11.
68. Leslie MD, Dische S. Parotid gland function following accelerated and conventionally fractionated radiotherapy. *Radiother Oncol* 1991; **22**, 133–9.
69. Peters LJ, Ang KK, Thames HD. Accelerated fractionation in the radiation treatment of head and neck cancer. A critical comparison of different strategies. *Acta Oncol* 1988; **27**, 185–94.
70. Bentzen SM, Overgaard M. Relationship between early and late normal-tissue injury after postmastectomy radiotherapy. *Radiother Oncol* 1991; **20**, 159–65.
71. Peracchia G, Salti C. Radiotherapy with thrice-a-day fractionation in a short overall time: clinical experiences. *Int J Radiat Oncol Biol Phys* 1981; **7**, 99–104.
72. Bentzen SM, Lundbeck F, Christensen LL, *et al.* Fractionation sensitivity and latency of late radiation injury to the mouse urinary bladder. *Radiother Oncol* 1992; **25**, 301–7.
73. Dubray BM, Thames HD. Chronic radiation damage in the rat rectum: an analysis of the influences of fractionation, time and volume. *Radiother Oncol* 1994; **33**, 41–7.
74. Followill DS, Kester D, Travis EL. Histological changes in mouse colon after single- and split-dose irradiation. *Radiat Res* 1993; **136**, 280–8.
75. Maciejewski B, Preuss-Bayer G, Trott KR. The influence of the number of fractions and of overall treatment time on local control and late complication rate in squamous cell carcinoma of the larynx. *Int J Radiat Oncol Biol Phys* 1983; **9**, 321–8.
76. Kaanders JH, Ang KK. Early reactions as dose-limiting factors in radiotherapy. *Semin Radiat Oncol* 1994; **4**, 55–67.
77. Tait DM, Nahum AE. Conformal therapy and its clinical application. In: JS Tobias, PRM Thomas, eds, *Current Radiation Oncology*, Vol 1. London: Edward Arnold, 1994; 51–68.
78. Brahme A. Design principles and clinical possibilities with a new generation of radiation therapy equipment. *Acta Oncol* 1987; **26**, 403–12.
79. Thames HD, Schultheiss TE, Hendry JH, *et al.* Can modest escalations of dose be detected as increased tumor control? *Int J Radiat Oncol Biol Phys* 1991; **22**, 241–6.
80. Brincker H, Bentzen SM. A re-analysis of available dose–response and time–dose data in Hodgkin's disease. *Radiother Oncol* 1994; **30**, 227–30.
81. Withers HR, Taylor JMG, Maciejewski B. Treatment volume and tissue tolerance. *Int J Radiat Oncol Biol Phys* 1988; **14**, 751–9.
82. Yaes RJ, Kalend A. Local stem cell depletion model for radiation myelitis. *Int J Radiat Oncol Biol Phys* 1988; **14**, 1247–59.
83. Hopewell JW, Morris AD, Dixon-Brown A. The influence of field size on the late tolerance of the rat spinal cord to single doses of X rays. *Br J Radiol* 1987; **60**, 1099–108.
84. Hopewell JW, van der Kogel AJ. Volume effect in spinal cord. Authors' reply. *Br J Radiol* 1988; **61**, 973–5.
85. Källman P, Aagren A, Brahme A. Tumour and normal tissue responses to fractionated non-uniform dose delivery. *Int J Radiat Biol* 1992; **62**, 249–62.
86. Hjelm-Hansen M, Jørgensen K, Andersen AP, *et al.* Laryngeal carcinoma. II. Analysis of treatment results using the Ellis model. *Acta Radiologica Oncol*

1979; **18**, 385–407.

87. Cohen L. The tissue volume factor in radiation oncology. *Int J Radiat Oncol Biol Phys* 1982; **8**, 1771–4.

88. Wolbarst AB, Chin LM, Svensson GK. Optimization of radiation therapy: integral-response of a model biological system. *Int J Radiat Oncol Biol Phys* 1982; **8**, 1761–9.

89. Schultheiss TE, Orton CG, Peck RA. Models in radiotherapy: volume effects. *Med Phys* 1983; **10**, 410–15.

90. Letschert JG, Lebesque JV, de-Boer RW, *et al*. Dose–volume correlation in radiation-related late small-bowel complications: a clinical study. *Radiother Oncol* 1990; **18**, 307–20.

91. Letschert JG, Lebesque JV, Aleman BM, *et al*. The volume effect in radiation-related late small bowel complications: results of a clinical study of the EORTC Radiotherapy Cooperative Group in patients treated for rectal carcinoma. *Radiother Oncol* 1994; **32**, 116–23.

92. Wetterer J. *Handbuch der Röntgentherapie*. Leipzig: Otto Nemnich Verlag, 1908; 322–4.

93. Munro TR, Gilbert CW. The relation between tumour lethal doses and the radiosensitivity of tumour cells. *Br J Radiol* 1961; **34**, 246–51.

94. Bentzen SM. Steepness of the clinical dose–control curve and variation in the *in vitro* radiosensitivity of head and neck squamous cell carcinoma. *Int J Radiat Biol* 1992; **61**, 417–23.

95. Bentzen SM, Overgaard J. Patient-to-patient variability in the expression of radiation-induced normal-tissue injury. *Semin Radiat Oncol* 1994; **4**, 68–80.

96. Taylor AMR, Harnden DG, Arlett CF, *et al*. Ataxia–telangiectasia: a human mutation with abnormal radiation sensitivity. *Nature* 1975; **258**, 427–9.

97. Loeffler JS, Harris JR, Dahlberg WK, *et al*. *In vitro* radiosensitivity of human diploid fibroblasts derived from women with unusually sensitive clinical responses to definitive radiation therapy for breast cancer. *Radiat Res* 1990; **121**, 227–31.

98. Begg AC, Russell NS, Knaken H, *et al*. Lack of correlation of human fibroblast radiosensitivity *in vitro* with early skin reactions in patients undergoing radiotherapy. *Int J Radiat Biol* 1993; **64**, 393–405.

99. Burnet NG, Nyman J, Turesson I, *et al*. Prediction of normal-tissue tolerance to radiotherapy from *in-vitro* cellular radiation sensitivity. *Lancet* 1992; **339**, 1570–1.

100. Geara FB, Peters LJ, Ang KK, Wike JL, *et al*. Prospective comparison of *in vitro* normal cell radiosensitivity and normal tissue reactions in radiotherapy patients. *Int J Radiat Oncol Biol Phys* 1993; **27**, 1173–9.

101. Johansen J, Bentzen SM, Overgaard J, *et al*. Evidence for a positive correlation between *in vitro* radiosensitivity of normal human skin fibroblasts and the occurrence of subcutaneous fibrosis after radiotherapy. *Int J Radiat Biol* 1994; **66**, 407–12.

102. West CML, Scott D, Peacock JH. Meeting report: Association for Radiation Research Workshop 21–23 March 1994. *Int J Radiat Biol* 1994; **66**, 231–4.

103. Bentzen SM, Overgaard M, Overgaard J. Clinical correlations between late normal-tissue endpoints after radiotherapy: implications for predictive assays of radiosensitivity. *Eur J Cancer* 1993; **29A**, 1373–6.

104. Tucker SL, Turesson I, Thames HD. Evidence for individual differences in the radiosensitivity of human skin. *Eur J Cancer* 1992; **28A**, 1783–91.

105. Altman KI. The effect of ionizing radiations on connective tissue. In: JT Lett *et al*., eds, *Advances in Radiation Biology*, Vol 10. New York: Academic Press Inc, 1983; 237–304.

106. Barcellos-Hoff MH. Radiation-induced transforming growth factor β and subsequent extracellular matrix reorganization in murine mammary gland. *Cancer*

*Res* 1993; **53**, 3880–6.

107. Sporn MB, Roberts AB, Wakefield LM, *et al.* Transforming growth factor-β: biological function and chemical structure. *Science* 1986; **233**, 532–4.
108. Canney PA, Dean S. Transforming growth factor beta: a promotor of late connective tissue injury following radiotherapy? *Br J Radiol* 1990; **63**, 620–3.
109. Border WA, Okuda S, Languino LR, *et al.* Suppression of experimental glomerulonephritis by antiserum against transforming growth factor β1. *Nature* 1990; **346**, 371–4.
110. Shah M, Foreman DM, Ferguson MW. Control of scarring in adult wounds by neutralising antibody to transforming growth factor β. *Lancet* 1992; **339**, 213–14.
111. Giri SN, Hyde DM, Hollinger MA. Effect of antibody to transforming growth factor β on bleomycin induced accumulation of lung collagen in mice. *Thorax* 1993; **48**, 959–66.
112. Coleman CN. Beneficial liaisons: radiobiology meets cellular and molecular biology. *Radiother Oncol* 1993; **28**, 1–15.
113. von der Maase H. Complications of combined radiotherapy and chemotherapy. *Semin Radiat Oncol* 1994; **4**, 81–94.
114. Tobias JS. Chemotherapy–radiotherapy combinations for advanced head and neck cancer. In: JS Tobias, PRM Thomas, eds, *Current Radiation Oncology*, Vol. 1. London: Edward Arnold, 1994; 231–49.
115. Overgaard J. Advances in clinical applications of radiobiology: Phase III studies of radiosensitizers and novel fractionation schedules. In: JT Johnson *et al.*, eds, *Head and Neck Cancer*, Vol III. Amsterdam: Elsevier, 1993; 863–9.
116. Overgaard J, Hjelm-Hansen M, Johansen LV, *et al.* Comparison of conventional and split-course radiotherapy as primary treatment in carcinoma of the larynx. *Acta Oncol* 1988; **27**, 147–52.
117. Bentzen SM, Pedersen D, Overgaard J. Clinical radiobiology of rectal complications after combined brachytherapy and external radiotherapy for cancer of the uterine cervix. ESTRO 11th Annual Meeting. *Radiother Oncol* 1992; **24** (Suppl), S21 (Abstract).
118. Chen F-D, Hendry JH. Effects of field size on the incidence of skin healing and the survival of epidermal colony-forming cells after irradiation. *Br J Cancer* 1986; **53** (Suppl VII), 73–4.
119. van der Kogel AJ. Dose–volume effects in the spinal cord. *Radiother Oncol* 1993; **29**, 105–9.
120. Hendry JH. Biological response modifiers and normal tissue injury after radiation. *Sem Radiat Oncol* 1994; **4**, 123–32.
121. Dörr W, Kummermehr J. Increased radiation tolerance of mouse tongue epithelium after local conditioning. *Int J Radiat Biol* 1992; **61**, 369–79.
122. Maciejewski B, Zajusz A, Pilecki B, *et al.* Acute mucositis in the stimulated oral mucosa of patients during radiotherapy for head and neck cancer. *Radiother Oncol* 1991; **22**, 7–11.
123. Vadhan-Raj S, Broxmeyer HE, Hittelman WN, *et al.* Abrogating chemotherapy-induced myelosuppression by recombinant granulocyte–macrophage colony-stimulating factor in patients with sarcoma: protection at the progenitor level. *J Clin Oncol* 1992; **10**, 1266–77.
124. Hancock SL, Chung RT, Cox RS, *et al.* Interleukin 1β initially sensitizes and subsequently protects murine intestinal stem cells exposed to photon radiation. *Cancer Res* 1991; **51**, 2280–5.
125. Dorie MJ, Bedarida G, Kallman RF. Protection by interleukin-1 against lung toxicity caused by cyclophosphamide and irradiation. *Radiat Res* 1991; **128**, 316–19.
126. Taketa ST. Water electrolyte and antibiotic therapy against acute (3 to 5 day) intestinal radiation death in the rat. *Radiat Res* 1962; **16**, 312–26.

127. Hanson WR. Radioprotection of murine intestine by WR-2721, 16,16-dimethylprostaglandin E2 and the combination of both agents. *Radiat Res* 1987; **111**, 361–373.
128. Ward WF, Molteni A, Ts'ao C-H, *et al.* Radiation pneumotoxicity in rats: modification by inhibitors of angiotensin converting enzyme. *Int J Radiat Oncol Biol Phys* 1992; **22**, 623–5.
129. Robbins MEC, Hopewell JW. Physiological factors affecting renal radiation tolerance: a guide to the treatment of late effects. *Br J Cancer* 1986; **53** (Suppl VII), 265–7.
130. Pedersen D, Bentzen SM, Overgaard J. Continuous or split-course combined external and intracavitary radiotherapy of locally advanced carcinoma of the uterine cervix. *Acta Oncol* 1994; **33**, 547–55.

# 3 Radiation carcinogenesis: current issues and future prospects

*R J M Fry*

## Introduction

Just 100 years ago Röntgen announced the discovery of X-rays,[1] and since that day the use of X-rays and radioactive material has increased in the practice of medicine, in research, and in industry. The application of X-rays to medicine was rapid after their discovery, more rapid than the rate of understanding of the effects that radiation had on tissues. Within a year, the effects on the skin, such as radiodermatitis, were being seen by the early workers. Considering the length of the latent periods for most radiation-induced carcinomas, the report of cancer of the skin associated with exposure to X-rays within a mere 7 years of their discovery reflects the very large doses that were incurred.[2]

Information about the carcinogenic effects of ionizing radiation accumulated slowly from observations on the effects of exposure on both humans and experimental animals. The discovery by Muller of the mutagenic effect of X-rays[3] concentrated the concern about exposure to radiation on the genetic effects of radiation. It was decades before it was appreciated that cancer was, in fact, the risk of concern after occupational exposures.

The question of the precise level of risk posed by exposure to ionizing radiation has been under continual examination by both international organizations such as the United Nations Scientific Committee on the Effects of Atomic Radiation (UNSCEAR) and the International Commission on Radiological Protection (ICRP), and national bodies such as the National Council on Radiation Protection and Measurements (NCRP), the National Radiological Protection Board (NRPB) and the Committees on the Biological Effects of Ionizing Radiations of the National Research Council (NRC), the so-called BEIR Committees.

No agent to which the population is exposed has had the attention of so many experts, from those working on the effects of radiation on DNA at a molecular level to those on international and national committees examining the quantification of risk posed by exposures in the home, in the workplace and from clinical procedures. Despite this remarkable effort the public's and, in particular, the news media's perspective about radiation risks is not a shining example of rational thought.

The interest in radiation effects not only is related to risk estimation based on epidemiological studies, but is in the elucidation of the mechanisms of the induction of cancer by radiation. A great deal is known about the deposition of energy by different types of radiation and about the precise damage induced in the DNA, how it is processed and how this is reflected in the behaviour of cells. This knowledge has made ionizing radiation a very useful tool for the investigation of the salient aspects of carcinogenesis.

# Exposure to radiation

Humans have evolved in a radiation environment with exposure to cosmic rays, terrestrial $\gamma$-rays, radionuclides and the progeny of radon. These natural sources account for about 80% of the total exposure experienced by the general population, man-made sources account for about 20% of the total, and the largest component of this source is from medical procedures. The total average equivalent dose from these sources is considered to be about 3600 µSv in the US[4-6] and about 2500 µSv in the UK.[7] Radon is the major source of background radiation. The exhortation to build on the rock and not upon the sand is good advice only if the rocks do not contain the radionuclides $^{238}$U and $^{226}$Ra. Radium-226 comes from the decay of $^{232}$U, and, in turn, it decays to radon, $^{222}$Rn, which emanates from the ground. Radon disperses and decays into short-lived isotopes that attach to particles of dust that are, in turn, deposited in the tracheobronchial tree, where the $\alpha$-particles that are emitted from the short-lived daughter products $^{218}$Po and $^{214}$Po reach cells that are at risk for carcinogenesis.[8] $\alpha$–Particles have some important characteristics; for example, the particle tracks are short but have a high linear energy transfer (LET) and a greater carcinogenic effect than X- or $\gamma$-rays, perhaps by a factor of about 20. The density of the ionization along the particle track increases the probability of locally multiply damaged sites in the DNA that are more difficult for the cell to process without some untoward effect.[9]

About one-third of the terrestrial and internal whole-body dose that comes from radionuclides is from $^{40}$K. Although $^{40}$K is in low abundance in the body in relation to its counterpart, stable potassium, it is ubiquitous in cells and fluids of the body.

Cosmic radiation consists of galactic cosmic rays and solar radiation. On Earth, we are shielded by the radiation belts and the atmosphere and are exposed mainly to secondary particles. The main components are muons, the electrons associated with their decay, and photons from $\gamma$-ray-emitting radionuclides. The dose from cosmic radiation varies considerably depending on solar cycle, latitude and particularly altitude. The average annual equivalent dose has been calculated to be about 260 µSv.[5] Since the dose rate of cosmic radiation is so dependent on altitude, this type of radiation exposure becomes of significance to air crews who spend much of their career on high-altitude transcontinental flights, and to astronauts involved in long sojourns in space and activities outside the space vehicle.

The question of whether the natural background contributes significantly to cancer rates in the general population is unanswered. Many estimates of the contribution of the naturally occurring radiation are based on assumptions that either have not been, or cannot be, verified. The question of what excess risk of cancer may be caused by exposure to background radiation over 50 years of the life-span, a total equivalent dose of about 0.15 Sv, is of importance in the attempt to put occupational and medical exposures in perspective.

## Occupational exposures

A large population associated with medicine is exposed occupationally to radiation: about 280 000 people in the US. The average annual equivalent dose is low (Table 3.1) but there are very large variations in the levels of exposure. For example, physicians involved in procedures requiring a considerable period of fluoroscopy have significantly higher exposures than the general staff.

**Table 3.1**   Annual worldwide occupational exposures to radiation of monitored workers 1985–9 (UNSCEAR, 1993)[10]

| Occupation | Annual average effective dose (mSv) |
|---|---|
| Medicine | 0.5 |
| Industry | 0.9 |
| Nuclear industry | 2.9 |

## Medical exposures

In the US, medical and dental procedures, such as diagnostic X-rays and those involving radionuclides, account for about 14% of the average total dose of radiation incurred by the US population.[6] The total annual number of diagnostic X-ray examinations in the US had reached 800 per 1000 persons in the years 1985–90, and this astonishing rate is below the average for highly developed countries.[10] The number of diagnostic radionuclide examinations in 1989 was estimated to be about seven million.[11] The doses incurred vary greatly, of course, but, unless repeated examinations are involved, the doses are small in comparison to those incurred from a lifetime of exposure to background radiation.

# Risk estimation

Estimation of potential risks resulting from exposure to radiation during diagnostic procedures is obviously important, however small the risks are perceived to be. Similarly, it is important to determine risk estimates of radiogenic cancer resulting from radiotherapy when the efficacy of different types of therapy is being considered. Risk estimates based on populations exposed to radiation in clinical procedures are all the more important now because the new estimates based on the atomic bomb survivors are about two- to four-fold greater than previously estimated. The recent estimates of UNSCEAR[12] and the National Academy of Sciences (NAS)/NRC (BEIR V)[13] are shown in Table 3.2 and compared to those of UNSCEAR in 1977.[14] Both ICRP[15] and NCRP[16] concluded that the best estimates for radiation protection purposes were a lifetime risk of cancer of $4 \times 10^{-2}$/Sv for the worker population and $5 \times 10^{-2}$/Sv for the general population, and a risk of about $1.0 \times 10^{-2}$/Sv for severe hereditary effects. On the basis of the background cancer rates in the United Kingdom, NRPB estimated the risks to be $5.9 \times 10^{-2}$/Sv for the general population and $5.0 \times 10^{-2}$/Sv for the worker population.[17] The question that the clinician may ask is, 'How well do these risk estimates reflect the clinical experience?'[7]

**Table 3.2** Estimates of risk of fatal cancer after a single dose[a]

| Source of estimate | Probability (%/Sv) |
|---|---|
| UNSCEAR (1977)[14] | 1.0[b]–2.5[c] |
| UNSCEAR (1988)[12] | 4.0[d]–11[e] |
| BEIR V (1990)[13] | 4.4[f] |

[a] Based on the general population.
[b] The estimate for low doses was based on the estimated lifetime risk for leukaemia multiplied by 5, on the assumption that the ratio of solid cancers to leukaemias induced by radiation would be about 5, and divided by 2.5 to allow for the difference of the risk at high and low doses. This reduction for low doses was justified on the evidence that the dose–response relationship for the induction of leukaemia was linear-quadratic.
[c] Estimate for high doses.
[d] Estimate based on additive model.
[e] Estimate on the more favoured multiplicative model.
[f] Estimate based on a multiplicative model modified for age at irradiation, sex and time after exposure. A reduction factor of 2 for low doses and dose rates has been applied to the BEIR V estimate in the case of solid tumours for which a linear dose response was assumed. Since a linear-quadratic model was used to fit the data for leukaemia, there was a reduction of about 2 in the estimated risk.

Estimates of the risk of cancer induction by radiation, for radiation protection purposes, are based almost entirely on the experience of the atomic bomb survivors. The results of the studies of patients who had radiotherapy were considered but were not used in those risk estimates. There are a number of reasons why estimates based on populations of patients are important and more appropriate for assessing risk involved in radiotherapy than the estimates based on the atomic bomb survivors.

1. The atomic bomb survivors were exposed to whole-body irradiation at a high dose rate, and the data from those exposed to high doses dominate the estimates. In contrast, in radiotherapy, with the exception of patients receiving irradiation prior to marrow transplants, the dose

received is localized to the tumour and the surrounding normal tissues. Other tissues receive much less exposure.

2. In the case of the bone marrow, a variable but small fraction of the active bone marrow is exposed, and therefore the number of cells at risk is considerably smaller than with whole-body irradiation incurred by the atomic bomb survivors.

3. Patients treated with radiation, with the exception of those with childhood cancer, are in the older age groups.

4. Those atomic bomb survivors who were young at the time of the bombing were at greater risk, and the estimation of their risk projected through their lifetime is a major contributor to the total risk estimate for the general population. Thus, the accuracy of this estimate is dependent on the appropriateness of the risk projection model.

5. The risk estimates based on the atomic bomb survivors have to be transferred from the Japanese population to those of the US and other countries. The correct way to make this transfer is unknown, but the results are influenced by the background rates in the two populations involved. It is of concern that the background rates of cancers differ markedly between countries. For example, in the US and UK, cancers of the oesophagus, stomach, small intestine, colon and rectum account for about 15–16% of the total cancer mortality, whereas in Japan these sites account for about 31% of the total. In the estimate by the ICRP[15] of excess cancer mortality resulting from exposure to radiation, the risk of cancer of the oesophagus, stomach and colon accounts for about 45% of the total risk, a surprisingly high figure. Another aspect of the problem of basing the risk estimates for patients on the data from atomic bomb survivors arises in the case of exposure to [131]I. The physical half-life of [131]I is 8 days and the radiation dose to the tissues is protracted and therefore at a lower dose rate than the exposures to radiation from the atomic bombs. The low dose rate is considered to be one of the factors involved in the finding that, if there is any excess of leukaemia in patients exposed to [131]I in diagnostic or therapeutic procedures, it is not more than 25% greater than the rate of leukaemia in unexposed persons.[18]

# Risk of radiogenic cancer

## Diagnostic procedures

Despite the uncertainties involved in estimating the risks of such low levels of radiation, attempts have been made, especially for the risk of leukaemia and lymphoma.[19–23] Evans *et al.*[20] reported that 1% of all cases of leukaemia might result from diagnostic radiography, but the confidence intervals are broad and the true estimate could be zero or greater than 1%. All these studies are plagued with the problems of low-probability events and relatively small numbers of cases. Hodgkin's disease and chronic lymphocytic leukaemia have not been associated with radiation exposure, and the evidence suggests that diagnostic X-ray procedures do not increase the risk of non-Hodgkin's lymphoma.[23]

Patients with pulmonary tuberculosis (TB) treated by pneumothorax were monitored with fluoroscopy examinations. The individual doses were small but the cumulative doses to the superficial tissues, such as the breast, were often large: about 3 Gy in the study in the US[24,25] and 10 Gy in Nova Scotia.[26,27] Over 100 000 such patients have been studied. A dose-dependent increase in breast cancer was noted that decreased from a relative risk per Gy of about 7.5 at about 10 years of age to little or no excess in women exposed at over 40–45 years of age.[27]

The dose response for breast cancer was also dependent on age at exposure in the atomic bomb survivors.[28] The estimated excess relative risk per Gy decreased from 5.3 for females exposed between 0 and 9 years of age to zero for those exposed between 40 and 49 years of age. The marked susceptibility of females in infancy[28,29] is particularly intriguing considering how few cells must be at risk in the breast of those so young.

It is somewhat surprising that the induction rate of breast cancer per unit dose is the same in the atomic bomb survivors and the TB patients, considering the marked differences in the baseline rates of breast cancer between the Japanese and US populations and the difference in characteristics of the exposures to radiation.[30] The natural incidence of breast cancer in the US is four to five times higher than in Japan. This suggests that whatever factors are responsible for the high breast cancer rates in the US do not appear to interact or be synergistic with radiation. The fact that the effect of the high-dose-rate single exposures in the case of the atomic bomb survivors and multiple small doses to the TB patient have the same carcinogenic effect on the breast per unit dose indicates that the fractionation of the doses from fluoroscopy did not reduce the effect.

In contrast, the estimates of risks of lung cancer are very different between the atomic bomb survivors[31] and the patients exposed to multiple fluoroscopic examinations.[27,32] In the study of the TB patients in Massachusetts, no lung cancers were noted despite average cumulative doses of about 0.8 Gy.[32] Similarly, in the Canadian study, no significant excess was found even with cumulative doses of about 2.0 Gy[27] (Table 3.3). It is of interest that the difference in the effect of fractionation on the induction of breast and lung cancers is consistent with the experimental findings.[33]

Weighed against about 25 000 cases of leukaemia and about 180 000 cases of breast cancer that occur in the general population, any potential risk of excess cancer after medical radiography is extremely small.

**Table 3.3** Lung cancer in persons exposed to external low-LET radiation

| Source | Excess relative risk | Reference |
| --- | --- | --- |
| Atomic bomb survivors | 0.63 | Shimizu *et al.* 1990[31] |
| TB patients (fluoroscopy) | −0.019 (males) | Howe 1992[27] |
|  | −0.12 (females) |  |

## Radiotherapy

The benefit of radiotherapy of a malignancy outweighs the risk of a radiation-induced secondary cancer; however, the estimate of that risk is important, especially when comparing the efficacy of different types of treatment.

The concerns about radiogenic cancer relate to the risk of cancer induction by low doses. It is, of course, for low doses that the estimates of risk are the least reliable, because it is difficult or impossible to estimate the risk directly. At doses of the order of 0.01 Gy, which is not uncommon in X-ray procedures, Land[34] has pointed out that to establish unequivocally an excess risk of breast cancer with exposure to 0.01 Gy would entail a sample size of 100 million women, obviously an impractical proposition. Thus, it has been necessary to derive the estimate of risk at low doses by extrapolation from data obtained at higher doses. The accuracy of such extrapolation depends on the validity of the model used for the dose–response relationship. In the case of leukaemia there is good reason to assume a linear-quadratic response, based on knowledge about the role of chromosome aberrations in the mechanism of induction. The current view is that, for solid cancers, a linear, no-threshold dose–response relationship is more probable. However, it is not known with any precision how such factors as multiple steps in the mechanism of carcinogenesis, repair and cell killing influence the shape of the dose–response curves. Many aspects of the carcinogenic process are ignored for the sake of simplicity and the lack of understanding of the component changes in the processes that result in a malignancy.

Leukaemia is the quintessential radiogenic cancer, accounting for 10–12% of the total risk after whole-body exposures to high doses. The relative importance of the risk of leukaemia after any type of cancer therapy compared to the risk of secondary solid cancers is increased by the shorter latent period found with leukaemias. Therefore, many of the studies of the potential risk of radiogenic cancers resulting from radiotherapy have concentrated on leukaemia.

The largest of the studies of patients exposed to radiotherapy was initiated in 1968 by Hutchison.[35] A cohort of about 150 000 patients treated for cervical cancer with either external radiation, brachytherapy or a combination of both has been followed for over 30 years.[36] There has been about a two-fold increase in the risk of all types of leukaemia except chronic lymphocytic leukaemia, a risk that is significantly less than the excess risk in the atomic bomb survivors and somewhat less than in the patients with ankylosing spondylitis[37] (Table 3.4). An increase in the incidence of leukaemia has been noted in patients treated for various cancers[38,39] and benign gynaecological disorders.[40,41] The risk of a radiation-induced

**Table 3.4**   Comparison of risk of radiation-induced leukaemia in different populations

| Population | Relative risk |
| --- | --- |
| Atomic bomb survivors (UNSCEAR[31]) | 9.4 |
| Ankylosing spondylitis patients[37] | 3.2 |
| Cervical cancer patients[36] | 2.5[a] |

[a]Maximum at 5 years after irradiation with about 2.5 Gy.

leukaemia associated with therapy varies with age at irradiation, the radiation field, the dose, the underlying disease and whether the radiation is combined with chemotherapy. In the case of Hodgkin's disease, the risk with radiotherapy alone is very small, but is significant when radiotherapy is combined with chemotherapy.[42]

# Radiation carcinogenesis

There is a broad range of susceptibility among tissues for the induction of cancer by radiation—from the radiosensitive progenitor cells in bone marrow to the stem cells of the crypts of Lieberkühn in the small intestine, which have a very low susceptibility. Susceptibility depends not only on the inherent genetic susceptibility but also on the age at exposure and, at least in some cancers, interactions with other agents. For example, skin exposed to ionizing radiation that is also normally exposed to sunlight is considerably more susceptible to the induction of non-melanoma skin cancer than skin not normally exposed to sunlight.[43]

Based on the mortality data for the atomic bomb survivors, significant excess risk occurs in leukaemias (except chronic lymphocytic leukaemia) and cancers of the stomach, colon, liver, lung, breast, ovary and bladder.[31] When cancer incidence is considered, the list of radiogenic cancers includes thyroid, salivary glands and non-melanoma cancer of the skin.[44] Studies of other organs in patients treated with radiotherapy or exposed to radionuclides have shown excess risk for brain, bone, and the epithelium of nasal sinuses and the mastoid.

The largest study of the risk of secondary cancer in radiotherapy patients is the international study[45,46] referred to previously in relation to leukaemia.[35,36] In this study, involving many hospitals and different types of radiation sources, dosimetry has not been easy, but tissues have been exposed to a broad range of doses extending up to several hundred grays. The organs close to the cervix received large doses; in the bladder, rectum and vagina, a significant excess risk was found. Organs such as the stomach, which received an average dose of about 2 Gy, showed a two-fold increase in risk. The results have been more surprising for the relatively[14] small increase or lack of increase in risk that has been found than for the increases noted. Only about 5% of all the secondary cancers that occurred in these patients could be attributed to the radiotherapy.

Over 14 000 patients with ankylosing spondylitis given a single course of X-rays during 1935 to 1954 have since been followed up. The lack of precise information about the organ doses has dogged this study from the beginning. Nevertheless, it has been possible to make estimates of the relative risk for a number of organs that received doses in excess of 1 Gy. For cancers other than leukaemia and cancer of the colon, it was concluded that the 28% mortality in excess of that of the general population could be attributed to the radiotherapy. The increased risk started about 5 years after exposure, reaching a maximum at about 10 years, and then appeared to decrease. Whether this apparent decrease is real and how the period of excess risk varies among various tissues are unknown.

The question of whether the risk of cancer remains in excess from the end of the latent period after exposure to the end of the life of the exposed person, or decreases at some stage, is central to the choice of the appropriate risk projection model. Previously, the data for solid cancers have been fitted using a single model. However, in the BEIR V report in 1990,[13] individual models were used in the analysis of the data for leukaemia, cancer of the respiratory system, cancer of the breast, cancers of the digestive system, other cancers, and all cancers other than leukaemia. These models took into account departures from a constant relative risk projection model.[13] If the excess risk of cancer in persons exposed at a young age lasts only 20–30 years, the current risk estimates[15,16] are overestimates. The excess risk of leukaemia does decline markedly with time after exposure but does not disappear. It is important that similar information be obtained for solid cancers.

The estimates of risk of radiogenic cancer, based on studies of secondary cancers after radiotherapy, appear to be lower than the estimates based on the atomic bomb survivors. A number of factors have to be taken into account in such a comparison. The age distribution of patients treated for cancer is skewed to the older age groups compared with those exposed to the atomic bombs. The combination of reduced susceptibility and the length of the latent period after exposure reduces the risk of those exposed at older ages. In radiotherapy, the exposed field is restricted, which reduces the number of cells at risk, and the doses are fractionated, which is thought to decrease the risk.

In a small number of cases there may be an increased susceptibility that has played a role in the origin of the cancer that is the reason for the therapy. In the BEIR V report, there is a good review of the various sources of information about the induction of cancer at specific sites by radiation, and in this chapter discussion will be restricted to a few organs of interest.

## Specific organs

The information about the molecular changes in cancer has outpaced the synthesis into models that cover all the aspects of the carcinogenic process and how radiation affects the various stages. However, much can be learned from the similarities and differences in the induction of cancer in different organs. In this section, some aspects of radiation carcinogenesis in the thyroid, breast and gut are discussed separately. Breast and thyroid are particularly susceptible tissues, especially in young persons. In the case of the thyroid, the question of the effect of dose rate is of importance in the assessment of any potential carcinogenic risk from radioiodine. Cancer of the gut is important because it is the major contributor to the estimated risk of cancer induction by radiation.[15]

### *Thyroid*

The most common type of thyroid cancer that occurs naturally and that is induced by ionizing radiation is classified as papillary, which is slow-growing and not aggressive. Perhaps this indolent nature explains why the association between exposure to ionizing radiation and thyroid cancer was not made until 1950.[47] Shore has reviewed the information available up to 1992,[48] and the recent report on the incidence of solid tumours in

the atomic bomb survivors[44] has provided further evidence about susceptibility.

In the atomic bomb survivors, the excess relative risk decreased from 9.5
for those exposed before the age of 9 years to virtually zero for those exposed
at $\geq$40 years of age.[44] In contrast to other studies, no evidence of dependency on sex was found, although the background rates were three times
greater in females than males.[44]

The sensitivity of the thyroid in the young for induction of thyroid cancer
is indicated by several studies (see Table 3.5), in particular, in the study by
Ron *et al.*[49] of over 10 000 children treated for ringworm of the scalp with
X-rays in which the average total thyroid dose was less than 0.1 Gy. Why
these children were apparently so susceptible to the induction of thyroid cancer is not known. A similar but much smaller study of children in New York
suggested a lower susceptibility.[50] When all of the relevant studies of children
whose thyroids were exposed during therapy for various conditions are considered, the conclusion is that exposure to low doses of radiation at a young
age is associated with a risk of cancer.[43] In adults the risk is greatly reduced,
and, as indicated above in the case of the atomic-bomb survivors, the risk is
not significant in those exposed at greater than 40 years of age.

**Table 3.5**    Estimated risks of thyroid cancer after acute external
irradiation (0–20 years of age)

| Source | Age at exposure (years) | Excess relative risk |
|---|---|---|
| Atomic-bomb survivors[44] | 0–9 | 9.5 at 1 Sv |
| Tinea capitis[49] | 0–15 | 27/Gy |
| Skin haemangioma[51] | 0–1 | 10.1/Gy |
| Childhood cancer[52] | 0–18 | 4.2/Gy |

There have been a number of studies of populations exposed to $^{131}$I.[53–57]
The impression is that the effect of irradiation at the lower rate with radioiodine is less than after acute high-dose exposures. In a study of 35 000
patients, followed on average for 20 years, Holm *et al.*[55,57] found no significant excess of thyroid cancer. Only 5% of the population was under 20
years of age at the time of exposure, and the small number of thyroid cancers did not allow a satisfactory comparison of the risk at high and low
dose rates in the susceptible younger age groups. When age at exposure is
taken into account and comparisons are made between appropriately
matched groups, it appears that the protracted irradiation from $^{131}$I is about
one-fifth to one-quarter as carcinogenic as acute external irradiation.[43] This
finding is important from two aspects. First, there are few data for humans
that can be used to examine the question of how much lowering the dose
rate of radiation lowers the risk. The evidence from experimental studies
indicates that the reduction varies for different types of cancer. Second, the
evidence that a reduction in the carcinogenic effectiveness by lowering the
dose rate is important, because it provides evidence that a reduction in carcinogenic effect may occur with low dose rates or protraction despite a
linear no-threshold dose–response curve after acute exposure.

## Breast

Cancers of the breast induced by radiation are histologically similar to breast cancers induced by other agents and those that occur naturally. The incidence of breast cancer, as noted above, varies markedly between races. The incidence in second-generation Japanese living in the United States is similar to the rate in the general US population, suggesting that the susceptibility is influenced by diet more than by genetic background. The risk of breast cancer in the 'high-risk' countries has been decreasing but has been increasing in the 'low-risk' countries, which also suggests that diet and lifestyle have an influence. That does not mean that genetic factors are unimportant; of considerable importance is the question of the existence and size of susceptible subpopulations.

The existence of a susceptible genetic subgroup is thought to be the explanation of the recent findings of Tokunaga *et al.*[58] They identified a number of women exposed before the age of 20 who developed breast cancer before the age of 35. The relative risk was several times greater than in women in whom the same diagnosis was made at later ages. The more common finding is that the radiation-induced cancers appear at ages similar to those of women who develop breast cancer in the unexposed population. Risk of breast cancer before the age of 35 is known to be associated with germline mutations of the *p53* tumour suppressor gene in the Li–Fraumeni syndrome.[59] However, the cases of early-onset breast cancer in the atomic bomb survivors do not have this syndrome. Perhaps the most likely candidate for the gene associated with the early onset in the atomic bomb survivors is the *BRCA-1* gene. It has been shown that a good many of the cases of breast cancers in the US that occur before the age of 35 are familial and are linked with a gene on chromosome 17q21.[60] It is not known whether a subpopulation that has a genetic predisposition for breast cancer is reflected in an increased susceptibility for induction by radiation, but the existence of subpopulations that are at increased risk for cancer induction is obviously of concern and their identification will be important.

The cells of patients with ataxia–telangiectasia are very radiosensitive[61] and the tissues of these patients show marked damage with standard therapeutic doses of radiation.[62] These patients are also cancer prone.[63] Although there is no unequivocal evidence that radiosensitivity for cell killing and susceptibility for induction of cancer by radiation are related, the association between the cancer proneness and the radiosensitivity of the patients who are homozygous for the ataxia–telangiectasia gene suggests the possibility of an increased susceptibility for the induction of breast cancer by radiation. The number of homozygotes is low, but about 1% of the US population are heterozygous for ataxia–telangiectasia. It has been reported that the risk of breast cancer is greater in heterozygotes[64] and that their cells are more radiosensitive than normal cells.[61] Swift *et al.*[65] have investigated the question of a relationship between exposure to radiation and breast cancer in persons heterozygous for the ataxia–telangiectasia gene, and they have suggested that exposure to radiation below 0.02 Gy and doses associated with diagnostic procedures such as mammography may increase the risk of breast cancers. This suggestion stimulated a quiver full of responses (see letters in *New England Journal of Medicine* 1992; **326**, 1357–60). The arguments against the contention of Swift *et al.*[65] that very low doses of radiation posed a risk for breast cancer in women heterozygous for ataxia–telang-iectasia ranged from methodological problems of the epidemiological study to the virtual lack of excess risk in women over 40 years of age, when mammography and other procedures would be most likely. It was pointed out that, based on the authors' own estimates, to incur the level of risk suggested by the authors, the dose to the heterozygotes exposed to medical radiation would have to be nearly 0.4 Gy, very many times greater than the cumulative dose from a few diagnostic procedures.

Although an unequivocal association between an increased susceptibility to radiation-induced breast cancer in females heterozygous for ataxia–telangiectasia has not been established, the solution to the question of whether heterozygotes for various genes associated with cancer are at an increased risk for radiation-induced cancer is of general importance.

## Gut

As yet there is no evidence that the risk of radiogenic cancer of the gut will be the same per unit dose independent of the background rate, as is the case for breast cancer. Since the risk of cancer of the gut is such a large component of the total risk estimate of cancer after exposure to radiation, and because the estimate may be biased because it is based on the experience of the atomic bomb survivors who have a high background rate, it is important to glean as much information as possible from studies of other populations.[66] In Table 3.6 the relative and absolute risks for cancer of the stomach are shown. It can be seen that relative risks based on the various populations differ very much less than the absolute risks, which for the Japanese population based on mortality are about six times greater than for those in the US and UK.

**Table 3.6**  Radiation-induced cancer of the stomach in humans

| Source | Mean dose (Gy) | Absolute excess risk (per $10^4$ PYGy) | Relative risk at 1 Gy |
|---|---|---|---|
| Atomic bomb survivors | | | |
| Incidence[44] | 0.73 | 4.68 | 1.30 |
| Mortality[31] | 0.23 | 2.02 | 1.22 |
| Radiotherapy | | | |
| Cervical cancer[46] | 2.00 | 0.37 | 1.54 |
| Ankylosing spondylitis[41] | 1.65 | 0.03 | 1.01 |
| Peptic ulcer[67] | 14.8 | 0.43 | 1.09 |

In the atomic bomb survivors, the estimates of risk of radiation-induced cancer of the oesophagus, colon and rectum are based on smaller numbers of observed cases; excess risk was noted for oesophagus and colon, but these organs were at considerably less risk than the stomach.[68] In the studies of both TB patients monitored with fluoroscopy and cervical cancer patients treated with radiotherapy, any excess risk that was found could be attributed to tobacco or alcohol but not to radiation. The doses in these two studies were relatively low and were either at low dose rate in the cervical cancer patients or in small multiple fractions in the TB patients. No excess in cancer of the rectum was found in the atomic bomb survivors, and excess risk of rectal cancers has been found only in the cervical cancer series where the rectal doses were enormous (30–60 Gy).[46] The most intriguing finding is the lack of radiogenic cancers of the small intestine, but, overall, malignant tumours of the small intestine are very rare.

The estimates of risk of induction of cancers of the gut in populations of the Western world would not satisfy the purists, but there seems little doubt that they suggest the estimates based on transfer of the risk from the atomic bomb survivors are too high.

Colorectal cancer has been a paradigm for modelling multistage carcinogenesis. The genetic analysis has provided the evidence of multiple mutations and some evidence of association of specific mutations with specific stages.[69] For example, it is suggested that the initial event leading to hyperproliferative epithelium in the colon results from mutations at the adenomatous polyposis coli (*APC*) and mutated in colon cancer (*MCC*) tumour suppressor genes; 15–20% of these benign colorectal tumours progress to malignancy. Loss of the deleted in colon cancer (*DCC*) and *p53* genes appears to be related to the progression. One of the difficulties in modelling carcinogenesis is the distinction of the roles of mutation and selection in tumour progression. Presumably, radiation is capable of inducing mutations at the several loci involved, but the probability that simultaneous mutation occurs with single exposures to radiation must be infinitesimally small. It is likely that radiation is involved in an increased risk of induction of initial events and that the subsequent changes are patterned on what happens in cancers that occur naturally. The discovery of mutation of *hMSH2*, the mismatch repair gene, in cases of hereditary non-polyposis colorectal cancer and cell lines has provided a possible explanation of the plethora of mutations. It has been established that the human mismatch repair gene *hMSH2* on chromosome 2 is involved in hereditary non-polyposis colon cancer (*HNPCC*).[70,71] A second gene that encodes a protein, human MutL homologue (*hMLH1*), has been assigned on the basis of linkage data to chromosome 3.[72] Deletions and insertions are characteristically found in microsatellite sequences that consist of dinucleotide repeats. This type of instability is found in cases of HNPCC and about 15% of the sporadic colorectal cancers. This instability is considered to be a mutator phenotype, and the loss of microsatellite stability may be an early event.

The questions relevant to radiation carcinogenesis of the colon are, 'Which genes are the targets involved?' and 'Does radiation affect stages other than initial events?' The discovery of a dominant mutation named *Min* (because it results in multiple intestinal neoplasia), which causes a phenotype reminiscent of inherited colon polyposis syndromes[73] in the human, has provided a long-awaited animal model for probing the genetics of cancer of the gut. It was shown that the murine homologue of the *APC* gene was linked to the *Min* locus and the mutation in this gene was analogous to that found in familial adenomatous polyposis in humans and in sporadic colorectal cancers.[74] It should now be possible to establish how such genetic predisposition influences radiation induction of intestinal tumours and, most importantly, how radiation influences progression from adenomas to carcinoma.

The epidemiological data suggest that, whatever factors are involved in the high background rates of cancer of the stomach in the Japanese population, they interact with radiation, resulting in the high incidence in the atomic bomb survivors. It is important to determine whether the factors involved in the comparatively high rates of colon cancer in the US also interact with radiation. To date, the evidence that cancer of the gut poses a marked risk after exposures that are likely to occur clinically is not compelling.

## Mechanisms of radiation carcinogenesis

The role of chromosomal aberrations in the development of malignancy has long been invoked in the descriptions of the development of both naturally occurring and radiation-induced cancers, especially leukaemias. While the evidence does not suggest that radiation is a powerful carcinogen, its ability to cause mutation in somatic cells and to influence gene expression underline its potential to induce cancers, a fact that is well documented, at least for doses greater than 0.2–0.5 Gy.

As indicated in the discussion about colon cancer, it is conventional these days to consider that carcinogenesis is a multistage process. Most of the studies of the mechanism of the induction of cancer by radiation have concentrated on the changes that are associated with the initial events, or so-called initiation. The major effect of the mutations identified in the development of cancers, such as loss of tumour suppressor genes and the activation of oncogenes, is on the control of cell proliferation. Obviously, a change in control of cell proliferation is central to carcinogenesis, but it is only one aspect of the process. Initiation is a prerequisite for the development of a cancer, but it is the factors that influence whether those initial events get expressed and lead to malignancy that determine the probability of a cancer and the excess risk due to radiation. Experimental evidence suggests that initiation is relatively common and few initiated cells proceed to the development of a clinically detected malignant tumour.

It is presumed that stem cells are the cells at risk, but, in tissues that consist of what appear to be differentiated cells, it is not clear whether only a very small subpopulation that have the properties of stem cells are the only susceptible cells or if dedifferentiation can be induced. Which of these possibilities is, in fact, the case makes a large difference to the estimate of risk based on a per-cell basis. Radiation-induced chromosome aberrations have been shown to be an initial event in the induction of myeloid leukaemia in mice.[75,76] The apparently specific chromosome aberration is the same in the leukaemias that are induced by radiation or that occur naturally. This suggests an underlying condition that predisposes the sequences to the deletion and rearrangement in chromosome 2 that occurs as an early event in leukaemogenesis.[76] Telomere-like repeat sequences, which may have a high rate of recombination, may constitute a fragile site[77] and be the target for the effect of radiation. It is likely that other changes are also involved in the development of leukaemia but such changes as angiogenesis that are essential to solid cancers are not required.

The question of whether radiation induces specific mutations that can be distinguished from those induced by other agents is not only intriguing from the point of view of mechanisms, but also important for determining whether exposures to low doses do cause cancers. The investigations of this question have concentrated on mutations of the p53 gene, which are very common in solid cancers. Vähäkangas *et al.* examined the spectrum of mutations in the p53 gene of cells from lung cancers in uranium miners and found clusters of mutations between codons 141–161 and 195–208 that they interpreted as hot spots for mutation caused by alpha particles from exposure to radon, and that the spectrum was different from that caused by tobacco.[78] More recently, Taylor *et al.* have reported mutations in codon 249 that they consider may be a marker for lung cancer induced by radon daughters.[79]

These divergent results raise both hope and concerns: hope that specific mutations may be identified and concern that an unequivocal association of a specific cancer to a specific causal agent may be elusive. In the case of human hepatocellular carcinomas, thought to be associated with hepatitis B virus and aflatoxin $B_1$, the spectrum of mutations in the p53 gene was distinct from that associated with radon.[80]

Different carcinogenic agents may affect different target cells. For example, squamous cell carcinomas of the lung have long been associated with cigarette smoking.[81] Land *et al.*[82] found that adenocarcinomas are more frequent in atomic bomb survivors than in uranium miners, in whom small cell carcinomas predominate. Another example of a cancer whose very nature suggests the identity of the causative agent is carcinoma of the mastoid. All such rare tumours appear to have been due to irradiation by α-particles from radium deposited in the bone below the epithelium of the air space. Such tumours were found in radium dial painters.[83]

In solid cancers there are clear-cut rate-limiting stages, namely altered control of cell proliferation, angiogenesis and capability of invasion of neighbouring tissues and metastasis. Based on cancer death rates in relation to age, Armitage and Doll, as long ago as 1954, suggested that carcinogenesis was a 'multistage' process and that there were about six stages.[84] It was pointed out in the discussion of the multistage model for colon cancer that about six mutations had been identified but that all of them appeared to be associated with genes involved in cell proliferation. Whether or not these mutations are steps in a stage, the later changes that involve vascularization of the tumour and invasion and metastasis are likely to be stages predicted by the Armitage–Doll model.

# Summary

The risks of radiation-induced cancer are known to a considerable degree of accuracy for single high-dose-rate exposures. The risks resulting from multiple small doses are less well known and may be overestimated. However, more precise estimates must await either developments such as the unequivocal identification of the cause of a specific tumour based on specific mutations, or a fuller understanding of the mechanisms. For certain types of tumours, such as those of the gut, epidemiological data for radiogenic cancers in populations in the western world are needed.

There is good evidence that there are inherited factors that influence predisposition to the induction of cancer by radiation. It is thought that the number of persons in any susceptible population is small, but obviously the ability to identify them would be a great advantage to both the clinician and the epidemiologist.

It is the young who are at the greatest risk and require the most concern in relation to exposures. The reasons for the age dependency of susceptibility for induction of certain cancers by radiation are not understood, and any model of carcinogenesis worth its salt must be able to explain age and sex dependency. The discoveries of the molecular changes in DNA associated with cancer and with exposure to radiation are occurring at a rate that suggests many of the aspects of the mechanism of radiation carcinogenesis will soon be known, but understanding the complete process of radiation carcinogenesis will require more than molecular biology.

# Note

The culmination of the search for the AT gene came with the announcement[85] in *Science* that a gene *ATM* that is mutated in ataxia–telangiectasia had been identified on chromosome 11q22–23. The evidence suggests that it is the sole gene responsible for the disorder. This discovery will spawn many studies. Two areas are of particular interest. The first is the role of the *ATM* gene in breast cancer, especially in women of families with a high incidence of breast cancer but not linked to *BRCA1*, *BRCA2* or *P53* genes. Second, it should be possible to test the contention of Swift *et al.* that patients with even one defective *ATM* gene are more susceptible to the induction of breast cancer by radiation.[65]

# Acknowledgements

It is a pleasure to acknowledge the help of Mrs S Allen.

The research was sponsored by the Office of Health and Environmental Research and the Office of Epidemiology and Health Surveillance, US Department of Energy, under contract DE-AC05-84OR21400 with Martin Marietta Energy Systems, Inc.

# References

1. Röntgen WC. Ueber eine neue Art von Strahlen. Proceedings of the Würzburg Physio-Medical Society 1895. For an account of the discovery of X-rays see Grigg ERN. *The Trail of the Invisible Light*. Springfield, IL: Charles C Thomas, 1965.
2. Frieben A. Demonstration eines Cancroids des rechten Handrückens, das sich nach langdauernder Einwirkung von Röntgenstrahlen entwickelt hat. *Fortschr Röentgenstr* 1902; **6**, 106–11.
3. Muller HJ. Artificial transmutation of the gene. *Science* 1927; **66**, 84–7.
4. NCRP (National Council on Radiation Protection and Measurements). Ionizing

radiation exposure of the population of the United States. NCRP Report No 93. Bethesda: NCRP, 1987.

5. NCRP (National Council on Radiation Protection and Measurements). Exposure of the population in the United States and Canada from natural background radiation. NCRP Report No 94. Bethesda: NCRP, 1987.

6. NCRP (National Council on Radiation Protection and Measurements). Exposure of the U.S. population from diagnostic medical radiation. NCRP Report No 100. Bethesda: NCRP, 1989.

7. Hughes JS. The radiation exposure of the UK population, 1988 review. Chilton NRPB—R227. HMSO: London, 1988.

8. NAS/NRC (National Academy of Sciences/National Research Council) Committee on the Biological Effects of Ionizing Radiations. *Health Risks of Radon and Other Internally Deposited Alpha Emitters,* BEIR IV. Washington: National Academy Press, 1988.

9. Ward JF. Some biochemical consequences of the spatial distribution of ionizing radiation produced free radicals. *Radiat Res* 1981; **86**, 186–95.

10. UNSCEAR (United Nations Scientific Committee on the Effects of Atomic Radiation). *Sources and Effects of Ionizing Radiation*. Report to the General Assembly, with Scientific Annexes, New York: United Nations, 1993.

11. NCRP (National Council on Radiation Protection and Measurements). Misadministration of radioactive material in medicine—scientific background. NCRP Commentary, No 7. Bethesda: NCRP, 1991.

12. UNSCEAR (United Nations Scientific Committee on the Effects of Atomic Radiation). Annex F: Radiation carcinogenesis in man. In: *Sources, Effects and Risks of Ionizing Radiation*. Report to the General Assembly, with Annexes, Publication E.88.IX.7. New York: United Nations, 1988.

13. NAS/NRC (National Academy of Sciences/National Research Council). Committee on the Biological Effects of Ionizing Radiations. *Health Effects of Exposure to Low Levels of Ionizing Radiation*, BEIR V. Washington: National Academy Press, 1990.

14. UNSCEAR (United Nations Scientific Committee on the Effects of Atomic Radiation). *Sources and Effects of Ionizing Radiation*. Report to the General Assembly, with Annexes, Publication E.77.IX.1. New York: United Nations, 1977.

15. ICRP (International Commission on Radiological Protection). *1990 Recommendations of the International Commission on Radiological Protection*. ICRP Publication 60, Annals of the ICRP 21. Elmsford, New York: Pergamon Press, 1991.

16. NCRP (National Council on Radiation Protection and Measurements). Limitation of Exposure to Ionizing Radiation. NCRP Report No 116. Bethesda: NCRP, 1993.

17. Muirhead CR, Cox R, Stather JW, *et al.* Estimates of late radiation risks to the UK population. *Documents of the NRPB*, Vol 4, No 4. Chilton: NRPB, 1993.

18. Hall P, Boice JD Jr, Berg G, *et al.* Leukemia incidence after iodine exposure. *Lancet* 1992; **340**, 1–4.

19. Boice JD Jr, Land CE. Adult leukemia following diagnostic x-rays? *Am J Public Health* 1979; **69**, 137–45.

20. Evans JS, Wennberg JF, McNeil BJ. The influence of diagnostic radiography on the incidence of breast cancer and leukemia. *N Engl J Med* 1986; **315**, 810.

21. Preston-Martin S, Thomas DC, Yu MC, *et al.* Diagnostic radiography as a risk factor for chronic myeloid and monocytic leukaemia (CML). *Br J Cancer* 1989; **59**, 639–44.

22. Boice JD Jr, Morin MM, Glass AG, *et al.* Diagnostic x-ray procedures and risk of leukemia, lymphoma and multiple myeloma. *JAMA* 1991; **265**, 1290–4.

23. Boice JD Jr. Radiation and non-Hodgkin's lymphoma. *Cancer Res* 1992; **52**

(Suppl); 5489s–91s.
24. Boice JD Jr, Monson RR. Breast cancer in women after repeated fluoroscopic examinations of the chest. *J Natl Cancer Inst* 1977; **59**, 823–33.
25. Boice JD Jr, Preston D, David FG, *et al*. Frequent x-ray fluoroscopy and breast cancer incidence among tuberculosis patients in Massachusetts. *Radiat Res* 1991; **125**, 214–22.
26. Miller AB, Howe GR, Sherman GJ, *et al*. Mortality from breast cancer after irradiation during fluoroscopic examinations in patients being treated for tuberculosis. *N Engl J Med* 1989; **321**, 1285–9.
27. Howe GR. Effects of dose, dose-rate and fraction on radiation-induced breast and lung cancers: the Canadian fluoroscopy study. In: *Proceedings of the International Conference on Radiation Effects and Protection*. Tokyo: Japan Atomic Energy Research Institute, 1992; 108–13.
28. Tokunaga M, Land CE, Yamamoto T, *et al*. Incidence of female breast cancer among atomic bomb survivors. Hiroshima and Nagasaki, 1950–1980. *Radiat Res* 1987; **112**, 243–72.
29. Hildreth NG, Shore RE, Dvoretsky PM. The risk of breast cancer after irradiation of the thymus in infancy. *N Engl J Med* 1989; **321**, 1281–4.
30. Land CE, Boice JD Jr, Shore RE, *et al*. Breast cancer risk from low-dose exposures to ionizing radiation. Results of parallel analysis of three exposed populations of women. *J Natl Cancer Inst* 1980; **65**, 353–76.
31. Shimizu Y, Kato H, Schull WJ. Studies of the mortality of A-bomb survivors. 9. Mortality, 1950–1985, Part 2. Cancer mortality based on the recently revised doses (DS86). *Radiat Res* 1990; **121**, 120–41.
32. Davis FG, Boice JD Jr, Kelsey JL, *et al*. Cancer mortality in a radiation-exposed cohort of Massachusetts tuberculosis patients. *Cancer Res* 1989; **49**, 6130–6.
33. Ullrich RL, Jernigan MC, Satterfield LC, *et al*. Radiation carcinogenesis: time–dose relationships. *Radiat Res* 1987; **111**, 179–84.
34. Land CE. Estimating cancer risks from low doses of ionizing radiation. *Science* 1980; **209**, 1197–203.
35. Hutchison G. Leukemia in patients with cancer of the cervix uteri treated with radiation. A report covering the first 5 years of an international study. *J Natl Cancer Inst* 1968; **40**, 951–82.
36. Boice JD Jr, Blettner M, Kleinerman RA, *et al*. Radiation dose and leukemia risk in patients treated for cancer of the cervix. *J Natl Cancer Inst* 1987; **79**, 1295–311.
37. Darby SC, Doll R, Gill SK, *et al*. Long term mortality after a single treatment course with X-rays in patients treated for ankylosing spondylitis. *Br J Cancer* 1987; **55**, 179–90.
38. Boivin JF, Hutchison GB, Evans FB, *et al*. Leukemia after radiotherapy for first primary cancers of various anatomic sites. *Am J Epidemiol* 1986; **123**, 993–1003.
39. Tucker MA, Meadows A, Boice JD Jr, *et al*. Cancer risk following treatment of childhood cancer. In: JD Boice Jr, JF Fraumeni Jr, eds, *Radiation Carcinogenesis: Epidemiology and Biological Significance*. New York: Raven Press, 1984; 211–24.
40. Inskip PD, Kleinerman RA, Stovall M, *et al*. Leukemia, lymphoma, and multiple myeloma after pelvic radiotherapy for benign disease. *Radiat Res* 1993; **135**, 108–24.
41. Darby SC, Reeves G, Key T, *et al*. Mortality in a cohort of women given X-ray therapy for metropathia haemorrhagica. *Int J Cancer* 1994; **56**, 793–801.
42. Curtis RE, Boice JD Jr, Stovall M, *et al*. Risk of leukemia after chemotherapy and radiation treatment for breast cancer. *N Engl J Med* 1992; **326**, 1745–51.
43. Shore RE. Overview of radiation-induced skin cancers in humans. *Int J Radiat Biol* 1990; **57**, 809–27.
44. Thompson DE, Mabuchi K, Ron E, *et al*. Cancer incidence in atomic bomb survivors, Part II: Solid tumors, 1958–1987. *Radiat Res* 1994; **137**, S17–67.

45. Boice JD Jr, Day NE, Andersen A, *et al.* Second cancers following radiation treatment for cervical cancer. An international collaboration among cancer registries. *J Natl Cancer Inst* 1985; **74**, 955–75.
46. Boice JD Jr, Engholm G, Kleinerman RA, *et al.* Radiation dose and second cancer risk in patients treated for cancer of the cervix. *Radiat Res* 1988; **116**, 3–55.
47. Duffy BJ, Fitzgerald P. Thyroid cancer in childhood and adolescence. Report of 28 cases. *J Clin Endocrinol Metab* 1950; **10**, 1296–308.
48. Shore RE. Issues and epidemiological evidence regarding radiation-induced thyroid cancer. *Radiat Res* 1992; **131**, 98–111.
49. Ron E, Modan B, Preston D, *et al.* Thyroid neoplasia following low-dose radiation in childhood. *Radiat Res* 1989; **120**, 516–31.
50. Shore RE, Hempelmann L, Woodward E. Carcinogenic effects of radiation on the human thyroid gland. In: A Upton, R Albert, F Burns, R Shore, eds, *Radiation Carcinogenesis*. New York: Elsevier, 1986; 293–309.
51. Furst CJ, Lundell M, Holm L. Tumors after radiotherapy for skin hemangioma in childhood. *Acta Oncol* 1990; **29**, 557–62.
52. Tucker MA, Jones P, Boice JD Jr, *et al.* Therapeutic radiation at a young age is linked to secondary thyroid cancer. *Cancer Res* 1991; **51**, 2885–8.
53. Hoffman DA. Late effects of I-131 therapy in the United States. In: JD Boice Jr, JF Fraumeni Jr, eds, *Radiation Carcinogenesis: Epidemiology and Biological Significance*. New York: Raven Press, 1984; 273–80.
54. Edmonds CJ, Smith T. The long-term hazards of the treatment of thyroid cancer with radioiodine. *Br J Radiol* 1986; **59**, 45–51.
55. Holm L-E, Wiklund KE, Lundell G, *et al.* Cancer risk in populations examined with diagnostic doses of $^{131}$I. *J Natl Cancer Inst* 1989; **81**, 303–6.
56. Robbins J, Adams W. Radiation effects in the Marshall Islands. In: S Nagataki, ed, *Radiation and the Thyroid*. Amsterdam: Excerpta Medica, 1989; 11–24.
57. Holm L-E, Hall P, Wiklund K, *et al.* Cancer risk after iodine-131 therapy for hyperthyroidism. *J Natl Cancer Inst* 1991; **83**, 1072–7.
58. Tokunaga M, Land CE, Nishimori I, *et al.* Incidence of female breast cancer among atomic bomb survivors. 1950–1985. *Radiat Res* 1994; **138**, 209–23.
59. Li FP, Garber JE, Friend SH, *et al.* Recommendations on predictive testing for germ line p53 mutations among cancer-prone individuals. *J Natl Cancer Inst* 1992; **84**, 1156–60.
60. Hall JM, Lee MK, Newman B, *et al.* Linkage of early-onset familial breast cancer to chromosome 17q21. *Science* 1990; **250**, 1684–9.
61. Taylor AMR, Harnden DG, Arlett CF, *et al.* Ataxia–telangiectasia: a human mutation with abnormal radiation sensitivity. *Nature* 1975; **258**, 427–9.
62. Cunliffe PN, Mann JR, Cameron AH, *et al.* Radiosensitivity in ataxia–telangiectasia. *Br J Radiol* 1975; **48**, 374–6.
63. Morell D, Cromartie E, Swift M. Mortality and cancer incidence in 263 patients with ataxia–telangiectasia. *J Natl Cancer Inst* 1986; **77**, 89–92.
64. Swift M, Reitnauer PJ, Morrell D, *et al.* Breast and other cancers in families with ataxia–telangiectasia. *N Engl J Med* 1987; **316**, 1289–94.
65. Swift M, Morrell D, Massey RB, *et al.* Incidence of cancer in 161 families affected by ataxia–telangiectasia. *N Engl J Med* 1991; **325**, 1831–6.
66. Boice JD Jr, Fry RJM. Radiation carcinogenesis in the gut. In: CS Potten, JH Hendry, eds, *Radiation and Gut*. Amsterdam: Elsevier Science BV, 1995; 291–305.
67. Griem ML, Kleinerman RA, Boice JD Jr, *et al.* Cancer following radiotherapy for peptic ulcer. *J Natl Cancer Inst* 1994; **86**, 842–9.
68. Nabatsuka H, Shimizu Y, Yamamoto T, *et al.* Colorectal cancer incidence among atomic bomb survivors. *J Radiat Res* 1992; **33**, 342–61.
69. Fearon SR, Vogelstein BE. A genetic model for colorectal tumorigenesis. *Cell*

1990; **61**, 759–67.

70. Fishel R, Lescoe MK, Rao MRS, *et al*. The human mutator gene homolog *MSH2* and its association with hereditary nonpolyposis colon cancer. *Cell* 1993; **75**, 1027–38.

71. Leach FS, Nicolaides NC, Papadopoulos N, *et al*. Mutations of a *mut*S homolog in hereditary nonpolyposis colorectal cancer. *Cell* 1993; **75**, 1215–25.

72. Bronner CE, Baker SM, Morrison PT, *et al*. Mutation in the DNA mismatch repair gene homologue *hMLH1* is associated with hereditary non-polyposis colon cancer. *Nature* 1994; **368**, 258–61.

73. Moser AR, Pitot HC, Dove WF. A dominant mutation that predisposes to multiple intestinal neoplasia in the mouse. *Science* 1990, **247**, 322–4.

74. Su L-K, Kinzler KW, Vogelstein B, *et al*. Multiple intestinal neoplasia caused by a mutation in the murine homolog in the APC gene. *Science* 1992; **256**, 668–70.

75. Hayata I, Seki M, Yoshida K, *et al*. Chromosomal aberrations observed in 52 mouse myeloid leukemias. *Cancer Res* 1983; **43**, 367–73.

76. Breckon G, Papworth D, Cox R. Murine radiation myeloid leukaemogenesis: a possible role for radiation sensitive sites on chromosome 2. *Genes Chromosom Cancer* 1991; **3**, 367–75.

77. Bouffler SB, Silver A, Papworth D, *et al*. Murine radiation myeloid leukaemogenesis: the relationship between interstitial telomere-like sequences and chromosome 2 fragile sites. *Genes Chromosom Cancer* 1993; **6**, 98–106.

78. Vähäkangas KH, Samet JM, Metcalf RA, *et al*. Mutations of *p53* and *ras* genes in radon-associated lung cancer from uranium miners. *Lancet* 1992; **339**, 576–80.

79. Taylor JA, Watson MA, Devereux TR, *et al*. *p53* mutation hotspot in radon-associated lung cancer. *Lancet* 1994; **343**, 86–7.

80. Hsu IC, Metcalf RA, Sun T, *et al*. Mutational hotspot in the *p53* gene in human hepatocellular carcinomas. *Nature* 1991; **350**, 427–8.

81. Lubin JM, Blot WJ. Assessment of lung cancer risk factors by histologic category. *J Natl Cancer Inst* 1984; **73**, 383–9.

82. Land CE, Shimosato Y, Saccomanno G, *et al*. Radiation-associated lung cancer: a comparison of the histology of lung cancers in uranium miners and survivors of the atomic bombings of Hiroshima and Nagasaki. *Radiat Res* 1993; **134**, 234–43.

83. Rowland RE, Lucas HF Jr. Radium dial workers. In: JD Boice Jr, JF Fraumeni Jr, eds. *Radiation Carcinogenesis: Epidemiology and Biological Significance*. New York: Raven Press, 1984; 231–40.

84. Armitage P, Doll R. The age distribution of cancer and a multi-stage theory of carcinogenesis. *Br J Cancer* 1954; **8**, 1–12.

85. Savitsky K, Bar-shifa A, Gilad S, *et al*. *Science* 1995; **268**, 1749–53.

# 4   Current brachytherapy techniques

*A M Nisar Syed and Ajmel A Puthawala*

## Introduction

Brachytherapy, or endocurietherapy, is a term used for the treatment of cancer by radioactive sources, either by keeping close to (brachy) or directly within (endo) the tumour. Although Dr LA Danlos treated skin lesions using radium surface applicators as early as 1901,[1] it was in 1931 that Dr G Forssel first called this 'brachytherapy'[2] and in 1977 we popularized this technique as 'endocurietherapy'.[3] From 1901 until 1963, radioactive sources including radium, radon and gold seeds, caesium-137 and cobalt-60 had been used in needles and capsules in the treatment of different cancers including cancer of the cervix, endometrium, head and neck, etc. The radioactive sources were utilized for interstitial, intracavitary or surface applicators with some unavoidable exposure to personnel, i.e. using preloaded techniques. Afterloading implants were performed as early as 1903 by Dr H Strebel by implanting a guide tube into the tumour and then afterloading it with a radium source.[4] Several surgeons and radiation oncologists used different radioactive sources ($^{60}$Co,$^{137}$Cs, $^{226}$Ra seeds, etc.) using afterloading techniques.[5-12] In 1953, Dr Ulrich Henschke popularized afterloading techniques by implanting plastic catheters or applicators into tumours in the operating room, and localization films were performed with inactive dummy sources. Appropriate radioactive iridium-192 or caesium - 137 sources were then loaded into these catheters or applicators in the patient's room.[13] This minimized the exposure to personnel in the operating and recovery rooms, during localization films and during transportation of the patient to the room. However, it did not eliminate the radiation exposure to the persons entering the patient's room.

Remote afterloading techniques are being utilized more frequently to reduce, and almost eliminate, the exposure to personnel.[14-20] The high, medium or low activity radioactive sources are loaded into the guides using remote control, which transports the source from the shielded container to the patient. The remote afterloading technique is almost a standard in most institutions in Europe for the treatment of carcinoma of the cervix. Remote afterloading techniques for interstitial implants are now being used more frequently in the treatment of cancer of the bronchus, breast, prostate and cervix.[2]

# Techniques

There are basically two types of implant technique in clinical use: permanent and temporary. Temporary implants are used in superficial and easily accessible tumours. Permanent implants are utilized in deep-seated tumours. There are five main types of temporary implant technique: plastic tube and button, gold button, template, intracavitary, and intraluminal.

# Temporary implant techniques

### Plastic tube and button

The plastic tube and button technique involves the insertion of plastic tubes in and around the tumour.[3] Most of the implants are of the planar type. The spacing of the tubes is critical with 1 cm separation in a single plane, 1.5–2 cm in two planes and 2 cm in more-than-two-plane implants. It is important to encompass the tumour with at least 1-cm margins around it if this is technically feasible. This technique is often used in the treatment of cancer of the breast, head and neck, sarcomas of the extremities, etc.[21-26] The tumour is marked on the skin with a skin marker. The entrance and exit points for the needles are marked with appropriate spacing. Hollow stainless steel guides are then inserted through the tumour and the thin ends of the plastic tubes are inserted through the guides. The guide needles are then removed. The plastic tubes are then pulled until the wider end of the tube lies in the tumour. The tubes are secured in position by threading plastic buttons through the narrow end of the plastic tubes. The tubes are cut 2–3 cm from the skin and the excess portions of the tube are discarded.

There are four types of plastic tube and button technique: simple plastic tube and button, gold button, loop and arch.

#### *Simple plastic tube and button*

This is the most commonly used temporary implant technique for cancer of the breast, neck, sarcomas of the extremities, etc. The technique of implantation is as described above except the plastic tubes are sealed at one end with a plastic button affixed, and the other end is narrow (Fig. 4.1).

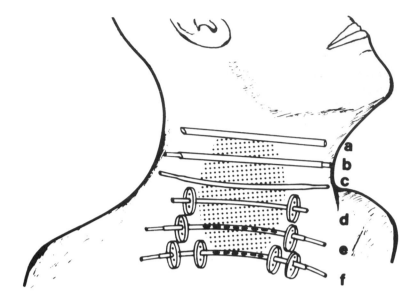

**Fig. 4.1**   Plastic tube and button technique.

### Gold button

This technique involves gold buttons in addition to the plastic buttons intra-orally to protect the overlying tissues (Fig. 4.2a,b). This method is used for cancers of the oral cavity, nasopharynx, oropharynx and hypopharynx.

### Loop

The loop technique is used in interstitial implantation of the alveolus, anterior floor of the mouth and retromolar trigone (Fig. 4.3). The technique involves insertion of a pair of 17-gauge hollow needles, with one needle on either side of the mandible, and threading plastic catheters with 'narrow both ends' through the intraoral ends of the needles. The needles are removed and both ends of the plastic tubes are pulled until the wider part of the tube lies on the alveolus. The plastic catheters are secured in position by threading plastic buttons through the narrow ends of the plastic tubes. The buttons are placed close to the skin and both ends of the tube are cut 2 cm from the skin.

### Arch

The arch technique is used in the interstitial implantation of the soft and hard palate and tonsillar pillars. The technique involves insertion of pairs of 17-gauge hollow needles on either side of the neck and cheek through the anterior–posterior tonsillar pillars, soft and hard palate (Fig. 4.4). The needles are brought out of the mucosa in the midline intraorally. Plastic tubes with 'narrow both ends' are threaded through the intraoral ends of

a

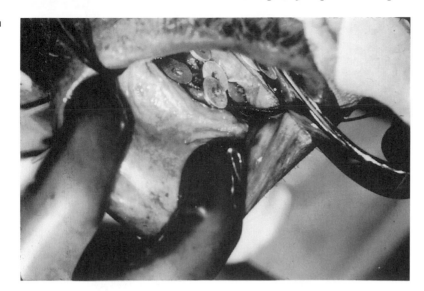

b

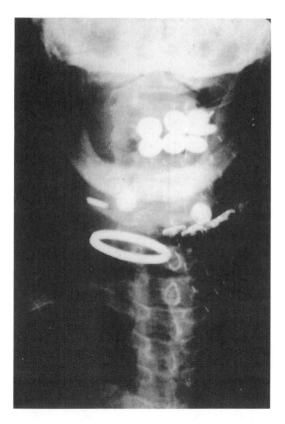

**Fig. 4.2** (a) Gold button technique in floor of mouth. (b) X-ray localization film with dummy sources.

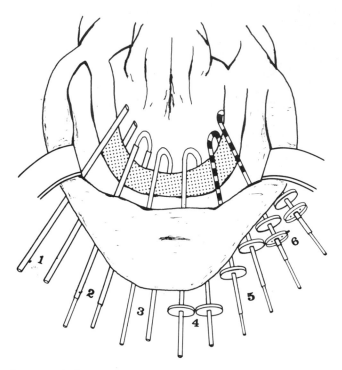

**Fig. 4.3**  Loop technique.

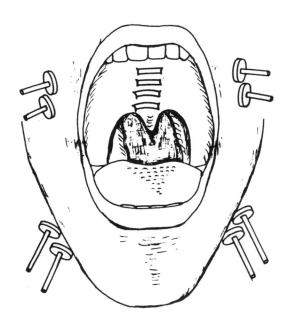

**Fig. 4.4**  Arch technique.

the needles. The needles are then removed and the plastic tubes are pulled from both ends until the wider ends of the tubes appear on the skin. The tubes are secured in the usual manner. The implants are removed in the operating room under general anaesthetic after delivering the appropriate dose.

## Template

Template techniques are used in relatively deep-seated tumours where the deep portion of the tumour is not accessible, i.e. cancer of the cervix, vagina, rectum and prostate.[27-37] This technique involves insertion of 17-gauge hollow stainless steel guides through a plastic template held against the skin close to the tumour (Fig. 4.5). The depth of the insertion of the

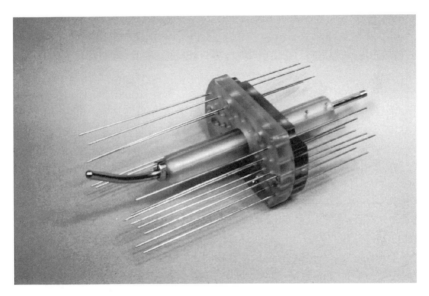

**Fig. 4.5**  Syed–Neblett gynaecological template.

guides is 1 cm beyond the tumour. The guide needles are tapered and closed at the tip. The template and needles are soaked in alcohol for easy insertion as alcohol acts as a lubricant. The guide needles are fixed in position when the alcohol evaporates from the template. The template is then secured in position by silk sutures through the skin and anterior two corners of the template. The space between the skin and template is filled with gauze soaked in antibiotic cream. In cancer of the cervix, vagina and prostate, barium-soaked gauze is inserted in the rectum and the Foley balloon is filled with Hypaque for X-ray localization films (Fig. 4.6a,b). The loading and unloading of the radioactive sources is either performed manually or with remote afterloaders. The implant is removed by cutting the sutures and pulling away the template with all the needles. Minimal bleeding from the skin is stopped by gentle pressure with gauze for 2–3 minutes.

a

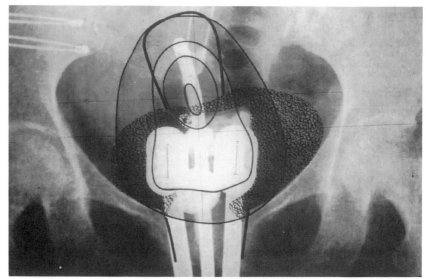

b

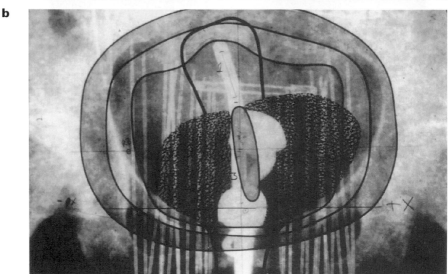

**Fig. 4.6** (a,b) Localization film with dosimetry plot using Fletcher applicator in carcinoma of the cervix, Stage IIIb.

The Foley catheter is then removed and the patient can be ambulating within an hour of the implant removal.

### Intracavitary

The intracavitary implant technique is routinely used in the treatment of carcinoma of the cervix, vagina and endometrium.[38-40] Intracavitary implants are used as a part of primary irradiation in combination with external beam radiotherapy in carcinoma of the cervix and vagina. The most commonly used applicators are Fletcher and Henschke. The radioactive sources can be loaded manually or by remote afterloader. Conventional low-dose-rate, medium- and high-dose-rate applications (LDR, MDR and HDR) have proven to be equally effective.

Intracavitary brachytherapy in the treatment of carcinoma of the cervix consists of insertion of an intrauterine tandem into the endometrial canal and two colpostats (ovoids) in the vagina, against the cervix. The vagina is then packed with gauze soaked in antibiotic cream. One can choose any of the tandems with different curvatures and colpostats from three different sizes, i.e. small, medium and large, and occasionally mini-ovoids if the vagina is particularly narrow.

After obtaining localization radiographs, radioactive sources are then loaded into the tandem and colpostats, either manually or by remote afterloader. Three sources of $^{137}$Cs, 15, 10, 10 mg Ra eq are usually loaded into the tandem and 20 mg Ra eq source into each of the two colpostats. Two applications, 2 weeks apart, following 45–50 Gy external irradiation deliver 40–45 Gy to Point A.

The International Commission on Radiation Units (ICRU) now recommends a 60-Gy dose to the target volume and reporting of specific rectal and bladder doses.[41] The number of applications using high-dose-rate brachytherapy varies from five to nine.

Preoperative irradiation with Heyman's technique in endometrial cancer is now rarely utilized. However, postoperative vaginal vault irradiation utilizing intracavitary ovoids, Delclos applicator or transvaginal mould is well established, with or without external irradiation.

### Intraluminal

Intraluminal implants are mainly utilized in the treatment of carcinoma of the oesophagus, bronchus and bile ducts[42–49] as a boost in primary tumours, or as a sole treatment in recurrent tumours. Most of these implants are palliative. Each site requires either a special applicator or a catheter. The applicator or plastic catheters are inserted into the oesophagus, bronchus or bile ducts and the radioactive sources are then inserted into these applicators. The dose delivered is estimated at 0.5–1 cm from the surface of the applicator, which is usually in close contact with the tumour. Each application can deliver 15–25 Gy with low-dose-rate brachytherapy or 7.5–10 Gy with high-dose-rate brachytherapy.

# Permanent implants

The permanent implant technique is usually used in deep-seated, surgically unresectable tumours or after debulking surgery, i.e. cancer of the pancreas, lung, brain, recurrent pelvic cancers, etc.[50–55] Most of the permanent implants are palliative, except in patients with localized cancers who are medically unfit to undergo surgical resection, i.e. cancer of the lung and prostate. The most commonly used radioactive sources are iodine-125 and palladium-103 with 60 and 17 days half-life and 28 KeV and 20 KeV energy, respectively. There are two types of permanent implant technique: applicator (Mick or Scot applicators) and seed-suture (radioactive sources in Vicryl material).

### Seed-suture technique

Radioactive sources ($^{125}$I or $^{103}$Pd) are placed 1 cm apart in absorbable Vicryl suture material with a needle attached at the non-radioactive end (Fig.4.7). The Vicryl suture with radioactive sources is loaded in a stainless steel ring as a shield. This can be sterilized before implanting. This technique can be utilized in minimal residual tumour in cancer of the lung, bladder, and pelvic recurrences.

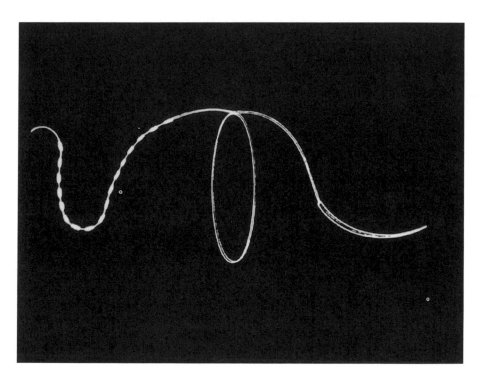

**Fig. 4.7**   Iodine-125 seeds in Vicryl suture.

### Applicator technique

Single and multiple seed inserters using the Scot applicator are rarely used. The most commonly used applicator for permanent implants is the Mick applicator. This applicator allows radioactive seeds to be implanted at desired depths by a ratchet mechanism (Fig. 4.8). The radioactive [125]I seeds are loaded into a magazine, which is inserted into the 'slot' on the Mick applicator. The applicator is attached to individual needles, and seeds are implanted into the tumour by pushing the stylet. The stylet pushes the seed from the magazine into the needle and then beyond the tip of the needle into the tumour. The ruler on the applicator helps to implant the seeds at desired depths. The needle is withdrawn 0.5–1 cm and another seed is implanted. Usually two to five seeds are implanted through each needle depending upon the size of the tumour.

This technique is used in the implantation of cancer of the lung, prostate and brain. Usually 0.4–0.5 mCi activity seeds are used. However, the total activity received is calculated using the average dimension method.[56] The total millicurie activity of [125]I seeds required is five times the average dimension in centimetres. The Memorial Nomograph for [125]I is used to determine the number of seeds and spacing required.[57]

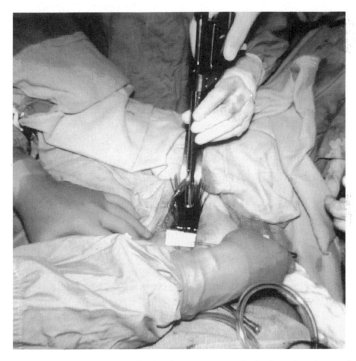

**Fig. 4.8** Mick applicator with iodine-125 seeds being implanted into the prostate.

## Localization films and dosimetry

Inactive dummy sources are loaded into the afterloading catheters or guide needles. Anteroposterior (AP) and lateral orthogonal X-ray localization films are obtained for computerized isodose distribution plotting and volume analysis. The tumour is outlined on the films, the isodose plots are overlaid on the AP and lateral films, and the isodose line encompassing the tumour is chosen to deliver the minimum tumour dose. The isodose line centrally encompassing a significant volume is identified as the maximum tumour dose. The minimum and maximum tumour doses determine the tumour control and complications, respectively. The doses to different vital structures around the implant, i.e. mandible, spinal cord, rectum and bladder, are evaluated.

In selected implants, a computed tomography (CT) scan of the implant can be obtained to determine the dose distribution more precisely. Several computer dosimetry systems are commercially available for dose calculations, isodose distribution plotting, dose volume histograms, etc.[58]

## Loading and unloading

Radioactive sources can be loaded manually using long tissue forceps with appropriate use of a loading shield. The sources are secured by crimping stainless steel buttons on the plastic tubes. However, remote afterloading is essential for high-dose-rate (HDR) and medium-dose-rate (MDR) applications. It is desirable but not mandatory to use remote afterloaders for low-dose-rate (LDR) applications.

The radioactive sources are removed after irradiation is completed and the implant is removed under sterile precautions.[3]

## Radioactive sources

The most commonly used radioactive sources for temporary interstitial and intracavitary implants are iridium-192 and caesium-137 (Table 4.1).[59] Radioactive iodine-125 (low intensity) and palladium-103 sources are best suited for permanent implants. Americium-241 may prove to be equally useful for permanent implants. High intensity iridium-192 (5–10 Ci) is the most commonly used source for HDR and pulse irradiation.

## Clinical evaluation

The irradiation dose required for microscopic disease is 50 Gy and 70–100 Gy for increasing size of tumour (T1 to T4).[60] External radiation alone can deliver 68–72 Gy with acceptable morbidity, which has less than 50% chance of local control for T3 and T4 lesions.

Conformal therapy and multiple daily fractions may further improve local control. However, combination of external and interstitial irradiation can deliver tumour doses as high as 90–100 Gy, depending upon the target volume. We have reported 92% locoregional control in patients with T3 and T4 (Stage III) breast cancer.[61] Overall tumour control of 84% was observed in patients with squamous cell carcinoma of the tonsillar fossa.[25] Sixty-two out of eighty patients (78%) had locally advanced tumours (Stage IV); 49% had clinically palpable lymphadenopathy. (Fig. 4.9, Table 4.2). Treatment-related complications, i.e. soft tissue and osteoradionecrosis, occurred in 6% of patients.

We have reported 89% local control in T1 and T2 lesions and 73% local

**Table 4.1** Physical parameters of radium substitutes

| Radionuclide | Half-life | Dose-rate constant ($mGy \cdot m^2 \, hr^{-1} \cdot GB^{-1}$) | Photon energy (MeV) | Beta energy, maximum (MeV) | HVT in lead (mm) | HVT in water (cm) | Filtration (mm) | Production process | Physical form | Maximum activity concentration used in practice ($GBq/mm^3$) |
|---|---|---|---|---|---|---|---|---|---|---|
| $^{137}$Cs | 30 years | 0.0768 | 0.662 | 0.51 (95%) 1.17 (5%) | 5.5 | 8.2 | 0.5 Pt Ir or 0.5 SS | Nuclear fission | Insoluble ceramic or glass | 1.2 |
| $^{60}$Co | 5.26 years | 0.307 | 1.17, 1.33 | 0.33 | 10.5 | 10.8 | 0.3 Pt, Ir | $^{59}$Co (n,r) $^{60}$Co | Metal | 44 |
| $^{192}$Ir | 74 days | 0.109 | 0.296–0.612 (Av. 0.37) | 0.24–0.67 | 2.2 (1st) 2.8 (2nd) | 6.3 (1st) | 0.1 Pt, Ir | $^{191}$Ir (n,r) $^{192}$Ir | Metal | 330 |
| $^{198}$Au | 2.7 days | 0.0548 | 0.412 | 0.96 | 3.0 | 7.0 | 0.15 Pt, Ir | $^{197}$Au (n,r) $^{198}$Au | Metal | 7.4 |
| $^{125}$I | 60 days | 0.0339 | 0.027–0.035 (Av. 0.028) | EC | 0.025 | 2.0 | 0.05 Ti | $^{124}$Xe + n (reactor) | Iodide ion | 3.7 |
| $^{182}$Ta | 115 days | 0.162 | 0.66–1.29 (Av. 0.67) | 0.18–0.514 | 10 | 8.3 | 0.1 Pt, Ir | $^{181}$Ta (n,r) $^{182}$Ta | Metal | 0.185 |
| $^{252}$Cf | 2.65 years | 2.0 µGy/µg | 0.8 | 2.35 (neutron energy) | 16.3 cm | 4.3 cm (polyethylene) | 0.15 Pt, Ir | $^{239}$Pu (13n,f) $^{252}$Cf | Metal | 0.0197 GBq/g |
| $^{103}$Pd | 17 days | 0.025 | 0.0209 | EC | 0.01 | 1.0 | 0.05 Ti | $^{102}$Pd (n,r) $^{103}$Pd | Metal | ~75 GBq/seed |
| $^{169}$Yb | 32 days | 0.0427 | 0.05–0.308 (Av. 0.0931) | 0.004–0.30 | 0.2 (1st) | 4.0 | 0.05 Ti | $^{168}$Yb (n,r) $^{169}$Yb | Metal | 350 |
| $^{241}$Am | 432 years | 0.0003 | 0.06 | — | 0.125 | 4.0 | 1.0 Ti | — | AmO² + Al powder | 0.34 |
| $^{145}$Sm | 340 days | 0.0275 | 0.038–0.061 | — | 0.06 | 4.0 | 0.05 Ti | $^{144}$Sm (n,r) | Metal | 72.8 |
| $^{75}$Se | 118.5 days | 0.046 | 0.066–0.4 (Av. 0.218) | — | 1.2 | 6.0 | 0.25 Y | $^{74}$Se (n,r) $^{75}$Se | Powder | 5476 |

HVT: half-value thickness; SS: stainless steel; EC: electron capture.
Reprinted with permission, from Iyer and Shanta, *Endocuriether/Hypertherm Oncol* 1994; **10**, 163.[59]

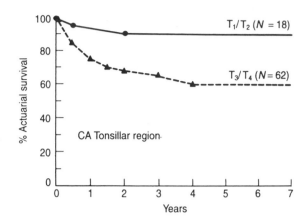

**Fig. 4.9**  Actuarial survival for patients with primary carcinoma of the tonsillar region and soft palate. (Reprinted, with permission, from Puthawala AA, Syed AM, Gates TC. Iridium–192 implants in the treatment of tonsillar region malignancies. *Arch Otolaryngol* 1985; **3**, 814.)

**Table 4.2**  Primary carcinoma of the base of the tonsillar region; tumour control according to TNM distribution.[a]

|       | N0          | N1         | N2           | N3         | Total              |
|-------|-------------|------------|--------------|------------|--------------------|
| T1    | 3/3         | —          | —            | —          | 3/3                |
| T2    | 12/12       | 1/1        | 1/2          | —          | 14/15              |
| T3    | 16/19       | 5/6        | 8/13         | 3/5        | 32/43              |
| T4    | 5/7         | —          | 3/4          | 3/8        | 11/19              |
| Total | 36/41 (88%) | 6/7 (86%)  | 12/19 (63%)  | 6/13 (46%) | 60/80 (75%)[b]     |

[a]Minimum follow-up period of 24 months to maximum of 84 months (median, 40 months).
[b]Seven patients failed in neck only. Therefore, primary was controlled in 67/80 (84%) of patients.
Reprinted, with permission, from Puthawala and Syed, *Int J Radiat Oncol Biol Phys* 1985; **11**, 1596.[25]

control in T3 and T4 lesions of the base of the tongue with overall loco regional control of 77% in seventy patients; osteoradionecrosis occurred in only two patients (Table 4.3).[23]  Locoregional control of 75% was achieved in sixty patients, with 58% 5-year disease-free survival in patients with either locally advanced carcinoma of the cervix or unsuitable for intra-cavitary applications due to anatomical distortion (Fig. 4.10).[28]  Similar results have been published by Aristizabal *et al.*[62] and Martinez *et al.*[63]

An overall 5-year actuarial survival rate of 85% with acceptable complications was observed in 200 patients with adenocarcinoma of the prostate, using a combination of interstitial and external irradiation with staging pelvic lymphadenectomy (Fig. 4.11).[35]

The role of interstitial irradiation in the treatment of soft tissue sarco-

**Table 4.3**   Carcinoma of the base of the tongue; tumour control according to TNM distribution.[a]

|      | N0          | N1          | N2          | N3        | Total          |
|------|-------------|-------------|-------------|-----------|----------------|
| T1   | —           | —           | 2/2         | —         | 2/2            |
| T2   | 7/7         | 3/3         | 4/5         | 0/1       | 14/16 (87.5%)  |
| T3   | 6/8         | 9/12        | 12/15       | 3/5       | 30/40 (75%)    |
| T4   | 3/4         | 1/1         | 3/5         | 1/2       | 8/12 (67%)     |
| Total| 16/19 (84%) | 13/16 (81%) | 21/27 (78%) | 4/8 (50%) | 54/70 (77%)[b] |

[a]Minimum follow-up period of 2 years to maximum of 10 years (median, 5 years).
[b]Seven patients failed at the primary site as well as in the neck; five patients failed at the primary site only and four in the neck only.
Reprinted, with permission, from Puthawala *et al. Int J Radiat Oncol Biol Phys* 1988; **14**, 845.[23]

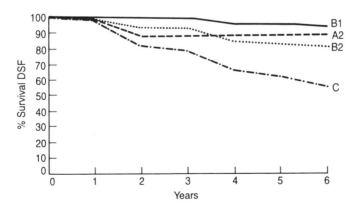

**Fig. 4.10**   Survival curves according to stages of carcinoma of the cervix. (Reprinted, with permission, from Syed *et al., Endocuriether/Hypertherm Oncol* 1986; **2**, 7.)

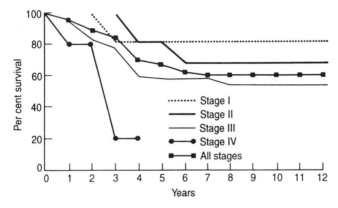

**Fig. 4.11**   Actuarial survival according to stage in adenocarcinoma of the prostate. (Reprinted, with permission, from Syed *et al., Cancer* 1992; **69**, 2522.)

mas in the extremities, with limb preservation, has been documented by Shiu *et al.*[64]

We believe that the majority of permanent interstitial implants are palliative, except for carcinoma of the prostate.   Whitmore, Hilaris and Nori have published long-term follow-up data in the treatment of carcinoma of the prostate with permanent iodine-125 techniques.[65] However, Blasko and others have achieved better results by using transrectal ultrasound-guided transperineal implant techniques using permanent iodine-125 and palladium-103 seeds.[66]

The permanent iodine-125 implant technique has yielded excellent palliation in carcinoma of the pancreas (Fig. 4.12).[49] We achieved 13 months median survival in unresectable carcinoma of the pancreas by combining permanent iodine-125 implantation of the pancreas and parapancreatic metastatic lymph nodes.[50] Interstitial irradiation has a significant role in the treatment of recurrent cancers following initial irradiation, with or without surgery and chemotherapy. We have reported 60% local control both in recurrent head and neck and pelvic cancers.[67,68] Cherlow *et al.*[69] and Fontanesi[70] have published papers on the important role of interstitial irradiation in paediatric cancers.

## Dose rate

Most clinical experience and data for local control and complications is based on the LDR technique (0.4–0.8 Gy/hr). However, HDR intracavitary application in the treatment of carcinoma of the cervix is now well established.[71,72] Integration of external beam pelvic and intracavitary irradiation has not been standardized.  The number of HDR intracavitary applications has ranged from three to nine.[71,72] Initially complications were higher in HDR applications than LDR applications but recent improvements in technique, dosimetry dose optimization and proper number (four to five) applications has reduced the complication rate without compromising the local control.[73]

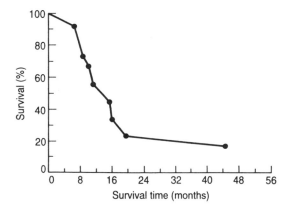

**Fig.   4.12** Actuarial survival in unresectable pancreatic carcinoma. (Reprinted, with permission, from Syed *et al.*, *Cancer* 1984; **52**, 811.)

HDR application in interstitial irradiation is still considered experimental and should be used only in palliative cases, i.e. recurrent carcinoma of the bronchus, oesophagus, etc., until sufficient data become available to warrant its use in curative cancers. The dose-rate effect on tissues both early and late in endocurietherapy has been thoroughly discussed by Hall and Brenner,[74] Fowler[75] and Fu and Phillips.[76]

# References

1. Danlos LA. Sur l'action physiologique et therapeutique du radium. *Bull Sci Pharmacol* 1904; **9**, 65–74.
2. Forssel G. La lutte sociale contre le cancer. *J Radiol* 1931; **15**, 621–34.
3. Syed AMN, Feder BH. Techniques of afterloading interstitial implants. *Radiol Clin* 1977; **46**, 458–75.
4. Strebel H. Vorschlaege zur radiumtherapie. *Deutsche Medizinal Zeitung* 1903; **24**, 11–45.
5. Abbe R. Radium in surgery. *J Am Med Assoc* 1906; **47**, 183–5.
6. Hames F. A new method in the use of radon seeds. *Am J Surg* 1937; **38**, 235–8.
7. Mead KW, Stevens KA. Methods of increasing accuracy in radon and radium implants. *Med J Australia* 1955; **2**, 232–5.
8. Mowatt KS, Stevens KA. Afterloading, a contribution to the protection problem. *J Fac Radiol* 1956; **8**, 28–31.
9. Morton JL, Callendine GW, Myers WG. Radioactive $^{60}$Co in plastic tubing for interstitial radiation therapy. *Radiology* 1951; **56**, 560–3.
10. Pierquin B, Chassagne D. La preparation non radioactive en curietherapie interstitielle et de contact. *J Radiol Electrol Med Nucl* 1962; **43**, 65–9.
11. Fletcher GH, Shalek RJ, Wall JA. A physical approach to the design of applicators in radium therapy of cancer of the uterine cervix. *Am J Roentgenol* 1952; **68**, 935–49.
12. Henschke UK. Afterloading applicator for radiation therapy of carcinoma of uterus. *Radiology* 1960; **74**, 834.
13. Henschke UK, Hilaris BS, Mahan GD. Afterloading in interstitial and intracavitary radiation therapy. *Am J Roentgenol Radium Ther Nucl Med* 1963; **90**, 386–95.
14. Decoulon G. Cervitron II, an apparatus for intracavitary radiotherapy. In: *Afterloading in Radiotherapy*, DHEW Publication No 72–8024. Washington DC: Supp. of Doc, Department of Health, Education and Welfare, 1971; 485–7.
15. Henschke UK, Hilaris BS, Mahan GD. Remote afterloading for intracavitary applicators. *Radiology* 1964; **83**, 344–5.
16. Joslin CAF, Smith CW. The use of high activity $^{60}$Co sources for intracavitary and surface mould therapy. *Proc Roy Soc Med* 1970; **63**, 1029–34.
17. Walstum R. Remotely controlled afterloading apparatus. *Acta Radiol Ther* 1965; Suppl 236, part II, 84.
18. Mundinger F, Sauerwein K. Gamma med ein gerut zur bestrahlung von hingeschwulsten mit radioisotopen. *Acta Radiol* 1966; **5**, 48–52.
19. Wakabayashi M, Osawa T, Mitsuhashi H, *et al.* High dose rate intracavitary radiotherapy using the Ralston introduction, part I: treatment of carcinoma of the uterine cervix. *Nippon Acta Radiol* 1971; **31**, 340–78.
20. van Hooft E. The selectron. In: DR Shearer, ed, *Recent Advances in Brachytherapy Physics*, AAPM Monograph No 7. New York, NY: American Institute of Physics, 1981; 167–77.
21. Seegenschmiedt MH, Grabenbauer GG, Lotter M. Clinical experience with a new remote afterloading system for low dose rate brachytherapy.

*Endocuriether/Hypertherm Oncol* 1994; **10**, 237–44.

22. Syed AMN, Feder BH, George FW III, *et al*. Iridium-192 afterloaded implant in the treatment of head and neck cancers. *Br J Radiology* 1978; **51**, 814–20.

23. Puthawala AA, Syed AMN, Eads DL, *et al*. Limited external beam and interstitial iridium-192 irradiation in the treatment of carcinoma of the base of the tongue: a ten–year experience. *Int J Radiat Oncol Biol Phys* 1988; **14**, 839–48.

24. Puthawala AA, Syed AMN, Neblett D, *et al*. The role of afterloading iridium-192 implant in the management of carcinoma of the tongue. *Int J Radiat Oncol Biol Phys* 1981; 7, 407–13.

25. Puthawala AA, Syed AM, Eads D, *et al*. Limited external irradiation and interstitial [192]iridium implant in the treatment of squamous cell carcinoma of the tonsillar region. *Int J Radiat Oncol Biol Phys* 1985; **11**, 1595–602.

26. Syed AMN, Puthawala AA, Orr LE, *et al*. Primary irradiation in the management of early and locally advanced carcinoma of the breast. *Br J Radiol* 1984; **57**, 317–21.

27. Syed AMN, Neblett DL. Interstitial–intracavitary applicator in the management of gynecologic malignancy. *Proceedings of the Pacific Endocurietherapy Society Winter Meeting*, Mazatlan, Mexico, 5–7 December 1979; 10.

28. Syed AMN, Puthawala AA, Neblett D, *et al*. Transperineal interstitial–intracavitary 'Syed–Neblett' applicator in the treatment of carcinoma of the uterine cervix. *Endocuriether/Hypertherm Oncol* 1986; **2**, 1–13.

29. Fleming PA, Syed AMN, Neblett DL, *et al*. Description of an afterloading [192]Ir interstitial–intracavitary technique in the treatment of carcinoma of the vagina. *Obstet Gynecol* 1980; **55**, 525–30.

30. Disaia PJ, Syed AMN, Puthawala AA. Malignant neoplasia of the upper vagina. *Endocuriether/Hypertherm Oncol* 1990; **6**, 251–6.

31. Syed AMN, Puthawala AA, Tansey LA. Management of prostate carcinoma: combination of pelvic lymphadenectomy, temporary [192]Ir implantation and external radiation. *Radiology* 1983; **149**, 829–33.

32. Syed AMN, Puthawala AA, Tansey LA, *et al*., Temporary interstitial irradiation in the management of carcinoma of the prostate: current status of a new approach. *Inter Med Spec* 1984; **5**, 146–61.

33. Tansey LA, Shanberg AM, Syed AMN, *et al*. Treatment of prostatic cancer by pelvic lymphadenectomy, temporary [192]Ir implant and external radiation. *Urology* 1983; **21**, 594–8.

34. Puthawala AA, Syed AMN, Tansey LA. Temporary iridium-192 implant in the management of carcinoma of the prostate: an analysis of treatment results and complications in the first one-hundred patients. *Endocuriether/Hypertherm Oncol* 1985; **1**, 25–34.

35. Syed AMN, Puthawala AA, Austin PA, *et al*. Temporary iridium-192 implant in the management of carcinoma of the prostate. *Cancer* 1992; **69**, 2515–24.

36. Syed AMN, Puthawala AA, Neblett DL, *et al*. Primary treatment of carcinoma of the lower rectum and anal canal by a combination of external irradiation and interstitial implant.*Radiology* 1978; **128**, 199–203.

37. Feder BH, Syed AMN, Neblett DL. Treatment of extensive carcinoma of the cervix with 'transperineal parametrial butterfly'. *Int J Radiat Oncol Biol Phys* 1978; **4**, 735–42.

38. Delclos L, Fletcher GH. Gynecologic cancers. In: SH Levitt, FM Khan, RA Potish, eds, *Levitt and Tapley's Technological Basis of Radiation Therapy: Practical Clinical Applications*, 2nd edn. Philadelphia, PA: Lea and Febiger, 1992; 263–88.

39. Perez CA, Camel HM, Galakatos AE, *et al*. Definitive irradiation in carcinoma of the vagina: long-term evaluation of results. *Int J Radiat Oncol Biol Phys* 1988; **15**, 1283–90.

40. Heyman J, Reuterwal O, Benner S. Radium-Hemmet experience with radiotherapy in cancer of corpus of uterus: classification, method of treatment and

results. *Acta Radiol* 1941; **22**, 11–98.

41. ICRU. *Dose and Volume Specification for Reporting Intracavitary Therapy In Gynecology: ICRU Report No. 38.* Bethesda, MD: International Commission on Radiological Units and Measurements, 1985; 1–15.

42. Syed AMN. Combination of external and intraluminal irradiation in the treatment of carcinoma of the esophagus. *Proceedings of the Fourth Annual Mid-Winter Meeting, American Endocurietherapy Society*, Maui, Hawaii, December 1981; 10.

43. Syed AMN, Puthawala AA, Severance SR, *et al.* Intraluminal irradiation in the treatment of esophageal cancer. *Endocuriether/Hypertherm Oncol* 1987; **3**, 105–13.

44. Moorthy CR, Nibhanupudy J, Ashayeri E. Intraluminal radiation for esophageal cancer: a Howard University technique. *J Natl Med Assoc* 1982; **74**, 261–6.

45. Gelb AF, Puthawala AA, Syed AMN, *et al.* Endobronchial brachytherapy for resistant lung cancer. *Endocuriether/Hypertherm Oncol* 1989; **5**, 161–7.

46. Seagren SL, Harrell JH, Horn R. High dose rate of intraluminal irradiation in recurrent endobronchial carcinoma. *Chest* 1985; **88**, 810–14.

47. Herskovic AM, Engler MJ, Noell KT. Radical radiotherapy for bile duct carcinoma. *Endocuriether/Hypertherm Oncol* 1985; 1, 119–124.

48. Abe M, Kitagawa T. Treatment of esophageal cancer with high dose rate intracavitary irradiation. *Tohoku J Exp Med* 1981; **134**, 159–67.

49. Speiser BL, Spratting L. Remote afterloading brachytherapy for the local control of endobronchial carcinoma. *Int J Radiat Oncol Biol Phys* 1993; **25**, 579–87.

50. Syed AMN, Puthawala AA, Neblett DL. Interstitial iodine-125 implant in the management of unresectable pancreatic carcinoma. *Cancer* 1984; **52**, 808–13.

51. Hilaris BS, Nori D, Martini N. Intraoperative therapy for non-resectable disease. In: NC Delarue, H Eschapasse, eds, *International Trends in General Thoracic Surgery*, Vol 1. Philadelphia, PA: WB Saunders Co, 1985; 207–16.

52. Hilaris BS, Nori D, Martini N. Results of radiation therapy in stage I and II unresectable non-small-cell lung cancer. *Endocuriether/Hypertherm Oncol* 1986; **2**, 15–21.

53. Puthawala AA, Syed AMN, Fleming PA, *et al.* Re–irradiation with interstitial implant for recurrent pelvic malignancies. *Cancer* 1982; **50**, 2810–14.

54. Gutin PH, Phillips TL, Hosobuchi Y, *et al.* Permanent and removable implants for the brachytherapy of brain tumors. *Int J Radiat Oncol Biol Phys* 1981; **7**, 1371–81.

55. Mundinger F. The treatment of brain tumors with interstitially applied radioactive isotopes. In: Y Wang, P Pasoletti, eds, *Radionuclide Applications in Neurology and Neurosurgery*. Springfield, IL: Charles C Thomas, 1970; 199–265.

56. Henschke UK, Cevc P. Dimension averaging: a simple method of dosimetry of interstitial implants. *Radiobiol Radiother* 1968; **9**, 287–98.

57. Anderson LL. Spacing nomograph for interstitial implants of iodine-125 seeds. *Med Phys* 1976; **3**, 48–51.

58. Neblett DL, Syed AMN, Puthawala AA, *et al.* An interstitial implant technique evaluated by contiguous volume analysis. *Endocuriether/Hypertherm Oncol* 1985; **1**, 213–22.

59. Iyer PS, Shanta A. Update of radionuclides used in endocurietherapy. *Endocuriether/Hypertherm Oncol* 1994; **10**, 161–5.

60. Fletcher GH. Keynote address: the scientific basis and present and future practice of clinical radiotherapy. *Int J Radiat Oncol Biol Phys* 1983; **9**, 1073–82.

61. Puthawala AA, Syed AMN, Sheikh KM, *et al.* Combined external and interstitial irradiation in the treatment of stage III breast cancer. *Radiology* 1984; **53**, 813–16.

62. Aristizabal SA, Surwit EA, Valencia A, *et al.* Treatment of locally advanced carcinoma of the cervix with transperineal interstitial irradiation. *Int J Radiat Oncol Biol Phys* 1983; **9**, 1013–17.

63. Martinez A, Edmundson GK, Cox RS, *et al.* Combination of external beam irradiation and multiple site perineal applicator (MUPIT) for treatment of locally advanced or recurrent prostatic, anorectal and gynecologic malignancies. *Int J Radiat Oncol Biol Phys* 1985; **2**, 391–8.

64. Shiu MH, Nori D, Hajdi S, *et al.* Control of locally advanced extremity soft tissue sarcomas by function-saving resection and brachytherapy. *Cancer* 1984; **53**, 1385–92.

65. Whitmore WF. Interstitial implantation of the prostate: 10 year results. In: BJ Hilaris, D Nori, eds, *Brachytherapy Oncology Update*. New York, NY: Memorial Sloan–Kettering Cancer Center, 1986; 69–77.

66. Blasko JC, Razde H, Schumacher BS. Transcutaneous I–125 implantation for prostatic carcinoma using transrectal ultrasound and template guidance. *Endocuriether/Hypertherm Oncol* 1987; **3**, 131–9.

67. Puthawala AA, Syed AMN, Rafie S, *et al.* Interstitial hyperthermia and interstitial irradiation (thermoendocurietherapy) in the treatment of recurrent and/or persistent head and neck cancers. *Endocuriether/Hypertherm Oncol* 1990; **6**, 203–10.

68. Puthawala AA, Syed AMN, Fleming PA, *et al.* Reirradiation with interstitial implant for recurrent pelvic malignancies. *Cancer* 1982; **50**, 2810–14.

69. Cherlow JM, Syed AMN, Puthawala AA, *et al.* Endocurietherapy in pediatric oncology. *Am J Ped Hematol Oncol* 1990; **12**, 155–9.

70. Fontanesi J. Update of St. Jude's children's research hospital experience. *Endocuriether/Hypertherm Oncol* 1993; **9**, 60.

71. Perez CA. Uterine cervix. In: CA Perez, LW Brady, eds, *Principles and Practice of Radiation Oncology*. Philadelphia, PA: JB Lippincott Co, 1992; 1166–78.

72. Haie–Meder C, Kramer A, Lambin P, *et al.* Analysis of complications in a prospective randomized trial comparing two brachytherapy low dose rates in cervical carcinoma. *Int J Radiat Oncol Biol Phys* 1994; **29**, 953–60.

73. Dale RG. The use of small fraction numbers in high dose rate gynaecological afterloading: some radiobiological considerations. *Br J Radiol* 1990; **63**, 290–4.

74. Hall EJ, Brenner D. The dose-rate effect in interstitial brachytherapy: a controversy resolved. *Br J Radiol* 1992; **65**, 242–7.

75. Fowler JF. The radiobiology of brachytherapy. In: A Martinez, CG Orton, RF Mould, eds, *Brachytherapy HDR and LDR*. Columbia, MD: Nucletron Corp, 1990; 121–37.

76. Fu KK, Phillips TL. High dose rate versus low dose rate intracavitary brachytherapy for carcinoma of the cervix. *Int J Radiat Oncol Biol Phys* 1990; **19**, 791–6.

# 5 Oncological applications of photodynamic therapy

*Colin Hopper*

## Introduction

Photodynamic therapy (PDT) is a complex treatment modality that relies on the interaction of a photosensitizer, an appropriate wavelength of light, and oxygen. The photosensitizing agent is applied (either topically or systemically) and light is introduced in close proximity. Although neither has any direct tissue effect, the two in combination with oxygen result in a nonthermal reaction which results in tissue necrosis. There is increased retention of photosensitizer in tumour tissue (as opposed to normal tissue), raising the possibility of achieving selective tumour-tissue necrosis with preservation of adjacent normal structures. Despite a small degree of selective retention, it is difficult at present to turn this into selective necrosis. However, ratios at least ten times background can be achieved, particularly with tumours in the central nervous system,[1] so it is hoped that selectivity of antitumour effect may yet be possible.

Unlike radiotherapy, which is limited by tissue tolerance, no cumulative toxicity has been found with PDT. It seems, therefore, that PDT can be repeated regularly, if necessary over many years, without the danger of long-term tissue damage such as endarteritis obliterans associated with conventional radiotherapy.

## Historical perspective

There has been documentation of photochemotherapy as early as 1400 BC in India. The Hindus practised a technique for the repigmentation of vitiliginous skin with psoralins and sunlight. Attempts were made to utilize photodynamic therapy as a treatment for skin tumours and skin carcinomas in the early part of the twentieth century.[2] However, it is only with the advent of laser technology that adequate light doses have been available for delivery to tissues in sufficient quantity to precipitate an adequate level of cell killing.

## Mechanism of damage

In order for a photochemical reaction to be triggered, it is necessary for there to be an adequate accumulation of the photosensitizer intracellularly within the target organ.[3] This agent can be activated by light of a wavelength matched to its absorption peak. On activation, the photosensitizer will undergo a series of intermolecular energy transfers resulting in the formation of singlet oxygen, which is highly reactive. This produces short-lived cytotoxic effects resulting in cell death, and oxygen is a fundamental prerequisite for this reaction.[4] When light falls upon the sensitizer in its ground state, one of three competing processes (points 1–3 below) can then occur (Scheme 5.1).

1.  The activated photosensitizer molecules can react with tissue oxygen to produce a singlet oxygen which causes the cellular toxicity.
2.  The activated molecules can fluoresce and then return directly to the ground state.
3.  The activated molecules can go through a different process of photodegradation in which they are destroyed by the same activating light.[4]
4.  PDT has been shown to cause cytotoxicity to a variety of cell types and PDT resistance does not seem to be a major consideration, although some cell lines have acquired PDT resistance following chronic repeated exposure. Porphyrins have been shown initially to bind within the plasma membrane and subsequently to migrate to intracellular organelles. There appears to be specific mitochondrial damage with inhibition of

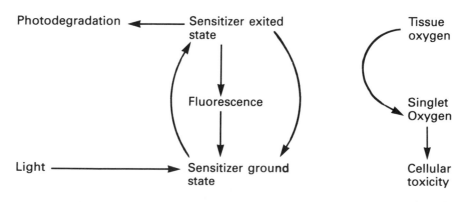

**Scheme 5.1**

oxidative phosphorylation, and interference with DNA synthesis has also been shown. There is also evidence from arterial work that there might possibly be a degree of precipitation of apoptosis.[5]

# Prerequisites for PDT

## 1 Oxygen

Oxygen is essential, not surprisingly, as the cytotoxicity of PDT is mediated through a photo-oxidative reaction, and oxygen is required to be present at levels in excess of 2% in order to trigger this effect. Oxygen tissue tension has been observed to fall during treatment and it may in the future be possible to monitor the PDT effect by serial measurements of tissue oxygen tension.

## 2 Photosensitizers

All of the currently available photosensitizers have drawbacks. Ideally, a sensitizer should

1. demonstrate a powerful photochemical cytotoxic effect;
2. be selectively distributed within tumour tissue so that selective tumour necrosis can be affected; and
3. should either be activated by light of such a wavelength that phototoxicity is not triggered by exposure to daylight or sunlight, or, alternatively, should be a compound that is short-lived.

Below are described the currently available photosensitizers which are in clinical use or soon to be employed.

### *Porphyrins*

The earliest and most widely available photosensitizers are the porphyrins. These tend to be ill-defined mixtures of porphyrins but it is the dihaematoporphyrin ether/ester mixture (available in the commercial form Photofrin) that seems to be in most common use. The absorption peak often used to carry out clinical PDT using porphyrins is in the red part of the spectrum at about 630 nm. This drug, when administered to humans, is well tolerated, the only significant side-effect being photosensitivity for about 4 weeks. It is essential that patients are advised to stay well away from sunlight for a period of 4–6 weeks. This advice has to be followed very seriously, especially where sunlight exposure is significant; this constitutes the only major toxic effect of this drug thus far.

There is a great deal of debate as to the exact mechanism of cell killing with this drug. It is thought to act by a combination of vascular effects, causing tumours to undergo necrosis secondary to a failure in their blood supply, plus some evidence of direct tissue destruction. With this group of porphyrins there is relatively little in the way of tumour selectivity, with the exception of intracranial tumours.

## Aminolaevulinic acid (ALA)

A number of other photosensitizers have been under investigation. One of the most exciting of these is aminolaevulinic acid. This is a precursor of protoporphyrin IX (PPIX) in the haem biosynthetic pathway (Scheme 5.2). Conversion of PPIX into haem is relatively slow; therefore, overloading the cellular metabolism with exogenous ALA results in a build-up of intracellular PPIX.[6]

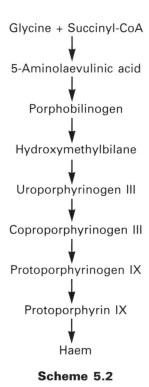

Glycine + Succinyl-CoA

↓

5-Aminolaevulinic acid

↓

Porphobilinogen

↓

Hydroxymethylbilane

↓

Uroporphyrinogen III

↓

Coproporphyrinogen III

↓

Protoporphyrinogen IX

↓

Protoporphyrin IX

↓

Haem

**Scheme 5.2**

This photosensitizer has been studied in a number of different tumours but seems most concentrated in tumours originating from the epidermis (basal and squamous cell carcinomas). It can be used as a sensitizer for skin tumours by topical application, or for internal surface tumours by systemic administration. There can be significant changes in liver enzymes but these are reversible in a few days. Patients receiving this drug remain photosensitive for only 24 hrs; hence, it has a significant advantage over the first-generation photosensitizers, e.g. Photofrin. After systemic administration, tissue level reaches a peak at about 5 hrs. When applied topically, optimum levels for therapy are reached after 3–6 hrs. In rats, neurotoxicity has been suggested with exceptionally high doses, but to date no such reports appear in humans.

### Meta-tetrahydroxyphenylchlorin (mTHPC)

This is a 'second-generation' photosensitizer which is much more active than the porphyrin derivatives. Initial evidence suggests that it can exert a PDT effect consistently in excess of that with porphyrin, and it is possible that depths of a centimetre can be recorded using light doses of 20–30 J/cm$^2$. The drug is administered intravenously at a dose of approximately 0.15 mg/kg by slow infusion, and the photochemical reaction is activated by light of 652 nm wavelength at about 4 days after administration. Treatment times are typically short, of the order of 2–3 min/cm$^2$ of tumour treated. A period of approximately 6 weeks probably needs to be left between repeated treatment courses. One might expect that with favourable drug concentrations in tumour tissue, compared with normal tissue, some degree of selectivity could be anticipated. There have been a number of claims that this is, in fact, the case but there is no histological evidence that supports this view.

As with the porphyrins, a great deal of care must be taken to avoid excessive light exposure, since full thickness burns have been recorded after using this drug, when inadequate protection has been taken during the sensitivity period. It is a very powerful sensitizer and care must even be taken when using the helium neon laser present in a pulse oximeter, as this can also cause burning if left on for any period of time.

### Phthalocyanines

These drugs would appear to have advantages over porphyrins. They are clean substances which are relatively easy to synthesize and to purify. They have strong absorption peaks in the 600–750 nm portion of the spectrum and theoretically should be capable of high yields of singlet oxygen. Because there is low absorption at visible wavelengths shorter than 600 nm, cutaneous photosensitivity is likely to be reduced. Animal experiments with aluminium chlorosulphonated phthalocyanine (AlSPc) have shown a degree of tumour selectivity similar to that of the porphyrins—results that are promising enough to warrant clinical trials, which are shortly to commence.

### Combination therapy

There is some evidence that by using multiple photosensitizers and light wavelengths a synergistic PDT effect can be gained, reducing the drug dose used and possibly also reducing side-effects.

# Light

A number of light sources can be used to precipitate the PDT effect. For management of basal cell carcinomas, for example, a high-energy projector lamp system has been used to great effect.

Since the development of medical lasers by Maiman in the early 1960s, there has been an enormous increase in the types of laser available. They come in a variety of shapes and sizes with the ability to deliver different levels of energy, density and wavelength. The advantages of laser light are that it is monochromatic and confluent. Commonly used systems for delivering 630 nm of light are pumped dye lasers and metal vapour lasers. The light delivery system is conducted via fibres to the delivery point where a microlens system can be used to distribute light evenly in a forward direction, or alternatively a bulbous tip can be used to diffuse light over a larger area. The depth of penetration of light is a function of wavelength—the longer the wavelength, the greater the depth of penetration. Hollow organs present something more of a problem in ensuring that light dosimetry is even, but it is possible to use a medium such as intralipid to reflect the light internally in a solution to get a predictable surface light dosimetry within an uneven organ. At present, lasers tend to be large and unwieldy but it is anticipated that with the development of the diode laser both the cost and weight will decrease.

# Animal experimentation

A variety of experiments have been carried out on animals to ascertain the safety of the treatment and the direct effects and distribution of drugs in various systems in the animal model.

## Trials of photosensitivity

There have been few studies to assess the degree of photosensitivity of sun-exposed sites. One study compares mouse skin photosensitivity with dihaematoporphyrin ether and aluminium sulphonated phthalocyanine; this seems to lend weight to the theoretical concept that photosensitivity is less with phthalocyanines than with dihaematoporphyrin ether. This appears to be the case both in terms of reaction to a given amount of light, and also for the duration of the photosensitivity.[7]

# PDT effects on normal tissues

There are few satisfactory studies on nervous tissue using any of the photo-sensitizers; however, on a theoretical basis, the nervous system is the most attractive site for the use of PDT as the relative concentration of sensitizer in tumour to that in normal tissue is so favourable. As far as mucosa is concerned, PDT effects result in an immediate necrosis of mucosal tissue, but healing appears to progress normally, with complete mucosal regeneration.[8] Cartilage seems to be relatively immune to PDT effects, probably because of its low vascularity. Bone does not seem to be significantly damaged, though the vascular elements within it obviously are. One study in the rabbit jaw was strongly suggestive that PDT effects on bone were negligible.[8] Salivary glands seem to be slightly resistant to PDT injury. It is possible that the initial reaction is to undergo necrotizing sialometaplasia but it seems likely that the tissues then return to normal.

With regard to vascular structure, studies examining PDT in normal rats are strongly suggestive that arteries treated with PDT (using disulphonated aluminium phthalocynanine and aminolaevulinic acid) undergo extensive cell death but with preservation of mechanical integrity. The long-term patency of the vessel seems to be unimpaired and PDT is probably safe in tumour therapy affecting blood vessels.[9] Finally, muscle seems to be the most vulnerable tissue when subjected to PDT. However, experiments with mouse limbs show that good function is restored to striated muscle even after extensive necrosis. Treatment of the bladder shows healing but with considerable impairment of function.[10,11]

# Human studies

## 1 Head and neck cancer

There is a wealth of anecdotal evidence within the literature to support the use of PDT in this clinical setting. Zhao and colleagues reported long-term results in seventy-two cases of cancers in the head and neck region, with good results.[12] However, the drug and light doses used in this study were not particularly well controlled and some of the responses might have been due to tissue heating as much as to a pure PDT effect. There is paucity of objective scientific data and little is known about the basic effects of PDT in the human. Attempts have been made to address this problem where areas of oral squamous cell carcinoma were treated with PDT and excised. One study, in particular, showed a marked variation in the depth of PDT effect, from 3 to 12 mm.[13] The histological evaluation of the tissue excised in this study did show that healing of the oral mucosa took place with minimal scarring, and it was suggested that this was because of the collagen and elastin that was preserved in the connective tissue (Fig. 5.1). From a variety of studies in the mouth, it would appear that the primary role of PDT (using Photofrin) would be in thin or superficial disease limited to the mucosa. There does not appear to be any limit to the area of the oral cavity that can be treated using this technique so it would seem ideally suited to condemned mucosal disease.[14] It should be noted, however, that patients with field cancerization will continue to develop new lesions so that considerations of disease-free intervals may be grossly misleading due to the development of metachronous as well as synchronous tumours. The repeatability of treatment makes it ideal for these patients, who would otherwise suffer the insult of progressive mutilation due to the ablative surgery, or permanently dry mouths from extensive and radical dose irradiation to the oral mucosa.

### *Treatment of early squamous cell carcinomas of the pharynx, oesophagus and tracheobronchial tree*

In a study on a group of ENT (ear, nose and throat) patients suffering synchronous second primaries, Monnier *et al.*[15] looked at a group of forty-

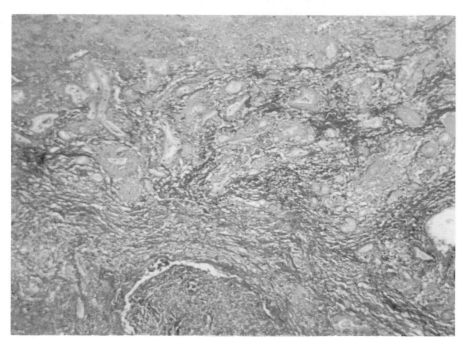

**Fig. 5.1** Squamous cell carcinoma of the mouth following photodynamic therapy, clearly showing preservation of collagen and elastin in the absence of tumour tissue.

one early squamous cell carcinomas of the pharynx, oesophagus and tracheobronchial tree. In this study, Photofrin I and II (dihaematoporphyrin ether/ester mixtures) were used with controlled light doses. Tumour ablation was successful in all cases but a series of complications was observed, resulting from lack of selectivity of the treatment. These included three cicatricial stenoses, two fistulae and one severe sunburn.

### Treatment of laryngeal tumours

PDT may well have a role both in the treatment of radiotherapy failures and also as primary treatment in tumours of the larynx. There are two studies which show encouraging results; one[16] in a group of eight patients who remained disease-free up to 13 months after treatment, and the second,[17] a larger series of forty-one, showing complete response (at 5 years) in thirty patients. The treatment was well tolerated without significant dysphonia and may well offer a slight advantage over conventional radiotherapy.

## 2 Urological tumours

The dihaematoporphyrin ether/ester (Photofrin) is now licensed for prophylactic use in recurrent bladder tumours in Canada. The potential for this type of treatment was demonstrated by Kelly and Snell[18] in 1976 and high complete response rates in patients with carcinoma *in situ* and invasive disease have been demonstrated, albeit in fairly small series as reported by Benson.[19,20] However, in addition to the usual complications of phototoxicity, the reduction in bladder capacity can be quite dramatic, often in excess of 50%.[21]

## 3 Gastrointestinal tract

Loh *et al.*[22] have demonstrated successful treatment of villous adenomas of the colon and rectum using Photofrin- or haematoporphyrin-derivative photodynamic therapy. This treatment was carried out in combination with debulking using an Nd-YAG (neodymium–yttrium aluminium garnet) laser. The treatment was carried out without any complications except for a little phototoxicity, and appears to be an effective way of treating flat lesions which are not suitable for treatment by thermal methods due to the risk of perforation. PDT, however, does not rely on a thermal effect and the mechanical strength of the colon is preserved, even in the presence of full-thickness necrosis. In this study, complete eradication of the adenoma was seen in six out of eight patients.

### *Treatment of pancreatic tumours*

In experimental studies,[23] aminolaevulinic acid PDT was used to treat pancreatic cancer in Syrian golden hamsters, resulting in a prolonged survival time. This could be an interesting new approach to treating small pancreatic tumours. Preliminary clinical trials are planned for the treatment of bile duct tumours.

## 4 Thoracic cavity

There are currently several studies which involve PDT treatment in a variety of tumours of the lung and pleura. These include a multicentre trial of photodynamic therapy for early-stage lung cancer[24] which claimed an 85.9% complete remission rate in fifty-seven patients with superficial early-stage tumours treated with Photofrin. PDT has also been used as adjunctive intra-operative photodynamic therapy in mesothelioma of the lung. In a group of patients treated at the Royal Melbourne Hospital, median survival was improved from 250 to 713 days in PDT patients versus controls.[25] However, some authors suggest that the complication rate from this is unacceptable; in one series, postoperative complications were noted in more than 50% of patients.[26]

## 5 Neurosurgery

One of the most exciting areas for the use of photodynamic therapy is in adjunctive treatment of brain tumours. Unfortunately, there is no respectable prospective study in this situation but on a theoretical basis[1] the concentrations of photosensitizers in tumours compared with normal tissue reach high ratios of 28:1. This means that it should be ideal for treatment of brain tumours, and early clinical results in uncontrolled studies suggest that this may, in fact, be the case. In a group of 115 patients with cerebral glioma, median survival time in patients with brain tumours was three times that of historical controls.[27] This is obviously an area in which more work needs to be done.

## 6 Kaposi's sarcoma

With the advent of acquired immune deficiency syndrome (AIDS) this has become a significant problem. Radiotherapy or chemotherapy may cause an even greater degree of immunosuppression in these patients and the vascular nature of the tumour and ease of access to the multiple cutaneous sites have made this condition ideally suited to PDT treatment. Although there is little data from large series, there are a number of reports to suggest that this early promise might be confirmed,[28] with complete responses in four and partial responses in three patients, and further large-scale studies planned.

## 7 Breast cancer

There are reports of the control of recurrent cutaneous carcinoma of the breast with PDT. Clearly, the long-term prognosis remains gloomy but at least locally fungating tumours might be better controlled. Larger-scale studies are awaited.

# Future developments

## Aminolaevulinic acid

ALA has been systemically administered to a group of patients and its dose–time distribution profile has now been evaluated using fluorescence microscopy.[29] This has clearly demonstrated that, when administered systemically, there is a clear peak of fluorescence at about 5 hrs postingestion, confined to epithelium (Fig. 5.2). Subsequent studies using a group of patients with intramucosal squamous cell carcinoma and severe dysplasias have shown that treatment has been effective in 'normalizing' this tissue. There have, however, been problems in achieving an adequate depth of effect for this treatment, though these may partly be overcome by fractionating the light dose or by supplementing the oxygen supply during treatment.

ALA can now be applied topically for sensitization of cutaneous basal cell carcinomas for PDT. Using this technique, Kennedy and Pottier have demonstrated successful tumour destruction in 79% of over 300 cases.[30] The greatest potential for treatment of basal cell carcinomas by ALA–PDT may lie in the management of patients with multiple lesions.

## PDT as a means of photodetection

Dihaematoporphyrin ethers have been shown to fluoresce under a Woods

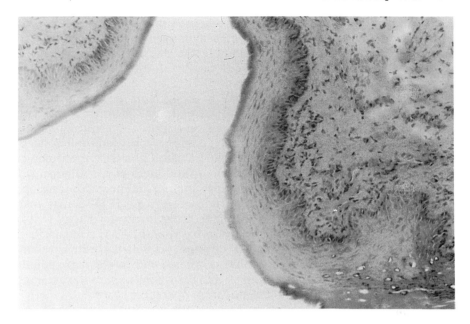

a

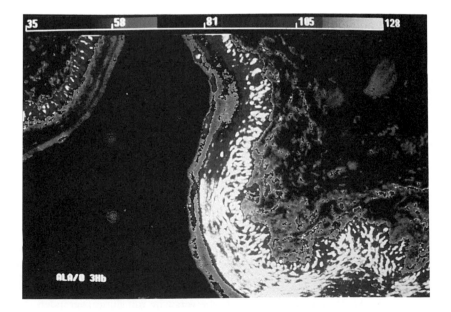

b

**Fig. 5.2** (a) Histopathological section and (b) charged coupled device image of ALA fluorescence to show concentration in the epithelial layer.

lamp, a technique which has recently been used to map out tumours. With more recent advances, ALA and *in-vivo* fluorescence measurements show considerable promise for tumour mapping. As yet, there is no evidence of correlation between fluorescence and degree of dysplasia, but this will clearly be an area for future investigation.

In summary, photodynamic therapy is an evolving treatment modality where new changes occur on an almost weekly basis. There are now a large number of new photosensitizers coming on-stream for clinical usage. It would appear that some of these, at least, could radically alter our concepts about treatment of several neoplastic conditions. The best current clinical indications are for controlling small tumours and areas of premalignancy in accessible organs such as the aerodigestive tract. PDT may also develop a role as an adjunct to surgery. New sensitizers such as *m*THPC may make it possible to destroy larger tumours up to 1 cm in depth. It may well be that with some sensitizers it could be possible to re-treat on a regular basis and slowly slice away the tumour. It also seems possible that extensive local disease in head and neck cancers could be treated with surgery and adjunctive PDT. A practical problem here is that we would require a wavelength of activation that could be filtered out from operating lights.

Some of the new photosensitizers are very powerful agents and it is anticipated that with increased light penetration through the surface it should be possible to effect cell killing to a much greater depth. A great deal of work needs to be done on real-time monitoring, to establish the depth and extent of tumours before treatment. If changes could be observed that indicated tumour killing, then the effectiveness of PDT could be much more effectively monitored. At present, one problem that seems to be hindering the proper evaluation of PDT is overenthusiasm and rapid service application, a poor substitute for scientific assessment of treatment effects. It is therefore essential that this treatment should still be confined, as far as possible, to the small number of centres carrying out clinical research in these challenging diseases.

# Acknowledgement

Grateful thanks to my coworkers, Mr WE Grant, Miss K Fan, Dr P Speight and Professor SG Bown in the preparation of this chapter.

# References

1. Wharen RE, Anderson RE, Laws ER. Quantitation of hematoporphyrin derivative in human gliomas: experimental central nervous system tumours and normal tissues. *Neurosurgery* 1983; **12**, 446.
2. Tappenier H, Jesionek A. Therapeutische versuche mit fluoreszierenden stoffe. *Muench Med Wochenschr* 1903; **1**, 2042.
3. Auler H, Banzer G. Untersuchungen uber die Rolle der Porphyrine Bein Geschwulstkranken Menschen und Tieren. *Krebsforsch* 1942; **53**, 65–8.
4. Weishaupt KR, Gomer CJ, Dougherty TJ. Identification of singlet oxygen as the cytotoxic agent in photoactivation of a murine tumour. *Cancer Res* 1976;

**36**, 2326–9.

5. Pass HI. Photodynamic therapy in oncology mechanisms and clinical use. *J Natl Cancer Inst* 1993; **85**, 443–56.

6. Kennedy JC, Pottier RH, Pross DC. Photodynamic therapy with endogenous protoporphyrin IX: basic principles and present clinical experience. *J Photochem Photobiol B: Biol* 1990; **6**, 143–8.

7. Tralau CJ, Young NPJ, Walker DI, *et al.* Mouse skin photosensitivity with dihaematoporphyrin ether (DHE) and aluminium sulphonated phthalocyanine (AlSPc): a comparative study. *Photochem Photobiol* 1989; **49**, 305–12.

8. Meyer M, Speight P, Brown SG. A study of the effects of photodynamic therapy on the normal tissues of the rabbit jaw. *Br J Cancer* 1991; **64**, 1093–7.

9. Grant WE, Hopper C, MacRobert AJ, *et al.* Photodynamic therapy of normal rat areries: microscopic fluorescence distribution and response to PDT using disulphonated aluminium phthalocyanine and aminolaevulinic acid induced protoporphyrin IX sensitisation. *Br J Cancer* 1994; **70**, 72–8.

10. Chevretton EB, Berenbaum MC, Bonnett R. The effect of photodynamic therapy on normal skeletal muscle in an animal model. *Lasers Med Sci* 1992; **7**, 103–10.

11. Pope AJ, Bown SG. The morphological and functional changes in the rat bladder following photodynamic therapy with phthalocyanine photosensitisation. *J Urol* 1991; **145**, 1064–70.

12. Zhao FY, Zhang KH, Jiang F, *et al.* Photodynamic therapy for treatment of cancers in oral and maxillofacial regions: a long-term follow up study in 72 complete remission cases. *Lasers Med Sci* 1991; **6**, 201–4.

13. Grant WE, Hopper C, Speight P, *et al.* Photodynamic therapy of the oral cavity: response of normal tissues and squamous carcinomas. In: T Spinelli, M Dall Fante, R Marchesini, eds, *Photodynamic Therapy and Biomedical Lasers*, ICS 1101. Amsterdam: Elsevier Science Publishers (Excerpta Medica), 1992; 638–41.

14. Grant WE, Hopper C, Speight PM, *et al.* Photodynamic therapy of malignant and premalignant lesions in patients with 'field cancerisation' of the oral cavity. *J Laryngol Oncol* 1993; **107**, 1140–5.

15. Monnier Ph, Savary M, Fontolliet Ch, *et al.* Photodetection and photodynamic therapy of 'early' squamous cell carcinomas of the pharynx, oesophagus and tracheo-bronchial tree. *Lasers Med Sci* 1990; **5**, 149–68.

16. Biel MA. Photodynamic therapy and the treatment of neoplastic and non-neoplastic disease of the larynx. In: T Spinelli, M Dall Fante, R Marchesini, eds, *Photodynamic Therapy and Biomedical Lasers*, ICS 1101. Amsterdam: Elsevier Science Publishers (Excerpta Medica), 1992; 647–52.

17. de Corbiere S, Ouayoun M, Sequert C, *et al.* Use of photodynamic therapy in the treatment of vocal cord carcinoma. In: T Spinelli, M Dall Fante, R Marchesini, eds, *Photodynamic Therapy and Biomedical Lasers*, ICS 1011. Amsterdam: Elsevier Science Publishers (Excerpta Medica), 1992; 656–61.

18. Kelly JF, Snell ME. Haematoporphyrin derivative: a possible aid in the diagnosis and therapy of carcinoma of the bladder. *J Urol* 1976; **115**, 150–1.

19. Benson RC. Integral photoradiation therapy of multifocal bladder tumours. *Eur Urol* 1986; **12** (Suppl 1), 47–53.

20. Benson RC. Treatment of bladder cancer with haematoporphyrin derivatives and laser light. *Urology* 1988; **31** (Suppl), 13–17.

21. Jocham D, Beer M, Baumgartner R, *et al.* Long-term experience with integral photodynamic therapy of Tis bladder carcinoma. In: G Bock, S Harnett, eds, *Photosensitising Compounds: Their Chemistry, Biology and Clinical Use*, Ciba Foundation Symposium 146. Chichester: Wiley, 1989; 198–208.

22. Loh CS, Bliss P, Bown S, *et al.* Photodynamic therapy for villous adenomas of the colon and rectum. *Endoscopy* 1994; **26**, 243–6.

23. Regula J, Ravi B, Bedwell J, *et al.* Photodynamic therapy using 5-amino laevulinic acid for experimental pancreatic cancer—prolonged animal survival. *Br J Cancer* 1994; **70**, 248–54.
24. Kato H, Okunaka T, Furuse K, *et al.* Multicentric clinical trial of photodynamic therapy for early stage lung cancer. *5th International Photodynamic Association Biennial Meeting, Abstracts* 1994; 179.
25. Knight SR, Clarke CP, Daniel FJ, *et al.* Photodynamic therapy for malignant pleural mesothelioma. *5th International Photodynamic Association Biennial Meeting, Abstracts* 1994; 66.
26. Takita H, Mang TS, Loewen GM, *et al.* Surgery and intracavitary photodynamic therapy for malignant pleural mesothelioma. *5th International Photodynamic Association Biennial Meeting, Abstracts* 1994; 65.
27. Kaye A, Hill J. Photodynamic therapy for brain tumours. *5th International Photodynamic Association Biennial Meeting, Abstracts* 1994; 59.
28. Schweitzer VG, Visscher D. Photodynamic therapy for treatment of AIDS-related oral Kaposi's sarcoma. *Otolaryngol Head Neck Surg* 1990; **102**, 639–49.
29. Grant WE, Hopper C, MacRobert AJ, *et al.* Photodynamic therapy of oral cancer: photosensitisation with systemic aminolaevulinic acid. *Lancet* 1993; **342**, 147–8.
30. Kennedy JC, Pottier RH. Endogenous proto-porphyrin-IX, a clinically useful photosensitiser for photodynamic therapy. *J Photochem Photobiol B: Biol* 1992; **14**, 275–93.

# 6 Applying sound radiobiology principles to the management of carcinoma of the larynx

*A G Robertson, Thomas E Wheldon and C Robertson*

## Introduction

Communication is a very important aspect of life. The loss of the power of speech is a shattering blow to most people. For this reason, the larynx has been regarded as a testing area for radiotherapists.[1] Even though the introduction of speech valves[2] has helped improve the quality of life in patients who have had a laryngectomy,[3] they still do not restore life to normal. As early as 1928, Finzi and Harmer[4] and other clinicians showed that radiation treatment was extremely important in the management of early glottic tumours. As radiotherapy techniques have improved, the place of surgery has shifted and now should be reserved for salvage of recurrences following radiotherapy,[5] or in the management of the node positive neck, though induction chemotherapy may reduce the need for elective neck dissections in node positive patients.[6] Conservation surgery[7] and laser surgery[8] are still used in the management of small glottic tumours despite the excellent results that can be obtained by radiotherapy.

Carcinoma of the larynx is a disease which develops more in males than females (ratio in Scotland 4:1;[9] England and Wales 9:1[10]), the incidence varying quite sharply from centre to centre. Although it can arise in all age groups it tends to be more common at around 60 years of age. The commonest cause of squamous carcinoma of the larynx is heavy smoking associated with high alcohol consumption.[11] Recently, other agents such as asbestos [12,13] and marijuana[14] have been identified as aetiological factors. The vast majority of tumours are squamous carcinomas. Other histologies — including lymphomas and sarcomas — have been identified, though very infrequently. A biopsy is always mandatory to establish diagnosis.

The larynx is divided into three subareas: the glottis, the supraglottis and the subglottis. Each has its own lymphatic system and pattern of spread (Fig. 6.1).[5] The glottis has a very poor lymphatic system and these tumours tend to remain localized, especially early ones. The supraglottic and subglottic regions have better-developed lymphatic systems and tumours here metastasize to lymphatics more readily. Tumour spread beyond the head and neck region is relatively infrequent, as with most tumours arising in the head and neck region, and local control is a vital factor in achieving tumour cure.[15]

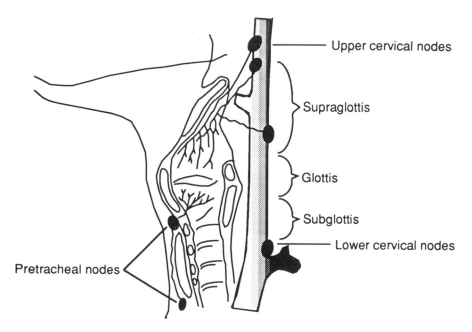

**Fig. 6.1**    Lymphatic spread in the larynx.

# Prognostic factors

The role of ploidy status as a prognostic factor in head and neck carcinomas is controversial,[16] some doubt having recently been cast on its value.[17]. Nonetheless, Westerbeek *et al.*[18] investigated its significance in T1 glottic lesions and reported a significantly higher risk ($P = 0.018$) of local recurrence in aneuploid tumours compared with diploid ones. Other tumour markers have been investigated as possible prognostic markers in head and neck carcinomas, including laryngeal tumours, and not found to be of value.[19] Sex and patient performance may be predictors of response. Female patients with tumours arising in the larynx[20] have been found to have a better prognosis than males. Any patient with a reduced Karnofsky score is likely to show a reduced response to radiotherapy.[21]

# Staging

Tumours are staged by the criteria of either the Union Internationale Contre le Cancer (UICC)[22] or the American Joint Committee on Cancer (AJCC).[23] These systems are now very similar for stratification of both lesions at the primary site and neck nodes. Staging depends on both clinical evaluation of involvement of structures in the larynx and mobility of the cords along with radiological assessment of spread of the tumour. Clinical examination involves first examining the neck for palpable nodes, then assessing the larynx with a mirror. Where a good image cannot be obtained the patient should be assessed with a nasendoscope. Fibreoptic equipment has become an essential tool for those treating laryngeal carcinoma. Radiological assessment involves tomography, computed tomography (CT)[24] and magnetic resonance imaging (MRI).[25] Early glottic lesions, T1 and T2 tumours, can be adequately assessed by conventional tomography, a technique which will confirm the size of more advanced lesions but does not adequately demonstrate invasion of cartilage or extralaryngeal extension. CT scanning is also limited and may fail to show tumour infiltration of cartilage or extralaryngeal tissues. MRI scanning with and without gadolinium contrast is now an important means of assessing laryngeal tumours. Laryngeal tumours, especially supraglottic lesions, extend submucosally; MRI identifies such spread. T2 lesions may be overestimated because of granulomatous tissue; however, T3 and T4 lesions tend to be more accurately staged. Care must be taken in assessing the neck as the incidence of false negative and false positive results is still high enough to make the results of the investigation valueless when it comes to making a treatment decision. There are software packages available to estimate the volume of the tumour present. These may be of value in staging the tumour and may influence management policy. CT scanning assists in detecting laryngeal tumours invading the pre-epiglottic and paraglottic spaces, laryngeal cartilages and soft tissues. In the past, conventional tomography was used to assess the subglottic region, the ventricles and the pyriform fossa with reasonable success. Ali *et al.*[26] felt that conventional tomography overestimated ventricular and false cord involvement and underestimated invasion of laryngeal structures. Although CT scanning is more expensive, it gives important information which improves tumour staging and treatment planning. Finally, a biopsy under anaesthetic is required to confirm the diagnosis.

Despite a number of reports in the literature describing the prognostic value of impaired mobility of the cords in Stage T2 for local tumour control there have been no moves to subdivide the group T2 formally into subgroups T2a and T2b.[27-29] Harwood and coworkers[27] from Princess Margaret Hospital (PMH), Toronto, Wang[28] from Boston and Slevin *et al.*[29] from Christie Hospital, Manchester all report significant differences in local tumour control rates between those with T2 disease who have impaired cord mobility (50–64%) and those with normal cord movement (79–80%) treated by radiotherapy alone. These results suggest that there are two subgroups of Stage T2 disease, possibly with a significantly different prognosis following radical treatment.

## Carcinoma *in-situ*

The role of radiotherapy in the management of these tumours is still controversial. The natural history of these lesions appears to be progressive, though the percentage that eventually become invasive is unknown. Progression of disease may be associated with incomplete excision. If surgery is adopted as the means of treatment, the patient has to be followed-up regularly with frequent biopsies or strippings of the cord, ultimately affecting the quality of voice. The best approach would appear to be to strip the cord initially and irradiate after the first recurrence,[30] giving a radical dose of radiotherapy. Although there have been reports that recurrence rates after primary radiation are high,[31] many have found that the local control rates are in the region of 70–95%.[31,32,33]

## Radiotherapy

All patients with Tis and small glottic lesions — $T_1N_0M_0$, $T_2N_0M_0$ — should be treated with small parallel-pair wedged fields (Fig. 6.2). These lesions rarely metastasize to the lymph nodes (0–5%).[14] An oblique wedged pair is used to treat $T_1N_0M_0$ lesions in some centres. The field size varies from 4.5 × 4.5 cm to 7 × 7 cm. Where the anterior commisure is involved it is best to build up the middle centimetre with 1 cm of wax to ensure that the dose distribution is optimum in that region.

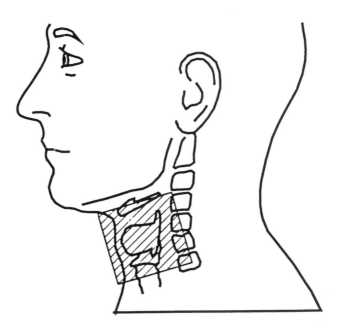

**Fig. 6.2** Field arrangement for treatment of $T_1N_0M_0$ laryngeal tumours.

Early series suggested that field size affected outcome.[34] Harwood's group in Toronto in the 1970s noted that recurrence rates were higher in patients treated using 5 × 5 cm fields than those treated with 6 × 6 cm fields. The tumours received 55 Gy in twenty-four to twenty-six fractions over 5 weeks, but patients were only immobilized using a compression technique. More recently Teshima and coworkers[35] reported a randomized trial where patients were treated with either a 5 ×5 cm or a 6 × 6 cm field. They received 60 Gy in 6 weeks with X-rays. All were immobilized using beam-directed shells (BDS) (Fig. 6.3). The local control rates were the same for each group (93% vs 96%) although the acute mucosal reactions were more severe in the group treated with the larger field. $T_1N_0M_0$ lesions can be treated safely with 5 × 5 cm fields if the patient is immobilized using a BDS, without the worry of recurrence due to a geographic miss.[36] Even the motion of swallowing should only reduce the dose to the larynx by 0.5%.[37] Robertson and coworkers have also presented results which suggest that immobilization of the patient with a BDS during treatment increases the local control rate, especially where the patient is being treated with a small field.[38] They found that where patients with $T_1N_0M_0$ disease had been immobilized using a BDS, an increase in effective dose over the range 55–65 Gy resulted in an increase in local tumour control. This observation was

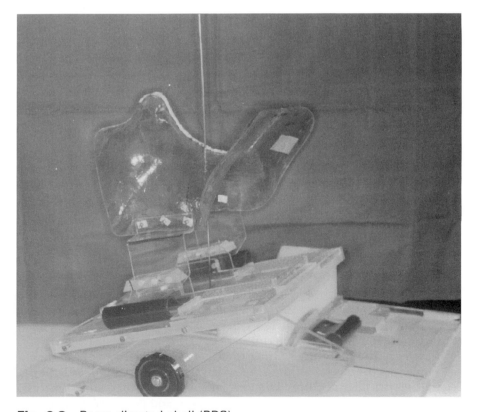

**Fig. 6.3** Beam-directed shell (BDS).

contrary to the results presented by Harwood and Tierie,[39] who showed no change in control rate as biological dose was increased. Harwood and Tierie assumed that the optimum dose for treatment of $T_1N_0M_0$ lesions had been reached; however, their patients had not been immobilized with a BDS. When Robertson et al.[38] analysed their results for all patients with $T_1N_0M_0$ lesions, i.e. those treated with a BDS and those treated without, their results were similar to those of Harwood and Tierie. They assumed that where patients were not treated with a BDS there was a high risk of a geographical miss, confounding the results and leading to the erroneous observation that for T1 lesions there was no association between dose and local control. It would appear, therefore, that all patients with laryngeal cancer receiving radiotherapy should be treated wearing a BDS. Patients with more advanced T3/T4 disease, those with nodal involvement or those with supraglottic tumours should be treated with larger fields incorporating Levels II and III cervical nodes.

# Radiobiological models

Over the past 30 years, a number of mathematical models have been evolved in an attempt to compare different radiation treatment schedules, starting with Ellis's nominal standard deviation (NSD) formula.[40] Later, Kirk et al. developed the cumulative radiation effect (CRE) formula,[41] and more recently the linear-quadratic (LQ) formula[42] has been found to be of value in quantifying the effect of treatment schedules in achieving local tumour control and in producing both acute and chronic morbidity. An LQ analysis assumes a linear-quadratic dependence of log cell survival ($S$) on dose (for each fractional dose) and exponential proliferation of surviving cells. The final surviving fraction of cells after $N$ treatments, each of dose $d$ extending over total time $T$, is then given by

$$\ln(S) = -N(\alpha d + \beta d^2) + \gamma T \tag{6.1}$$

where $\alpha$ and $\beta$ are the parameters of the linear-quadratic survival curve and $\gamma$ is the specific growth rate of the repopulating tumour cells. This can also be written as

$$\ln(S) = -D(\alpha + \beta d) + \gamma T \tag{6.2}$$

where $D = Nd$ is the total given dose. Therefore, the biological expectation is that treatment outcome (which is closely related to $\ln(S)$) should be governed by an equation with a term in $D$, a term in $Dd$ and a term in $T$. Conceptually, the problem of fitting the clinical data consists of estimating the numerical parameters of these three terms, and in asking how well the relevant model then performs as a predictor of clinical outcome. One can then consider the estimation of the parameters $\alpha$ and $\beta$, and $N$, from radiotherapeutic data.

# Radiobiological analysis of radiotherapeutic data

In practice, it is convenient to rearrange the algebra for the ease of statistical analysis. Maciejewski *et al.*[43] and Robertson *et al.*[38] introduced the 'biologically effective dose', $D_{eff}$, for a given treatment schedule as that dose which, if given as 2-Gy fractions and in the same overall time as the actual schedule, would have the same biological effect as the actual schedule. By equating the $\ln(S)$ values for an actual schedule, and an equivalent schedule composed of 2-Gy fractions, one obtains

$$D_{eff} = D(\alpha/\beta + d)/(\alpha/\beta + 2) \qquad (6.3)$$

$$\therefore \quad D = D_{eff}(\alpha + 2\beta)/(\alpha + d) \qquad (6.4)$$

Substituting $D$ in $\ln(S)$ gives

$$\ln(S) = -\gamma_1 D_{eff} + \gamma_2 T \qquad (6.5)$$

where $\gamma_1 = \alpha + 2\beta$ and $\gamma_2 = \gamma$. Therefore,

$$S = \exp\left(-\gamma_1 D_{eff} + \gamma_2 T\right) \qquad (6.6)$$

Local control is said to occur if the patient is disease free for at least 5 years. This is taken to imply that there are no cells remaining after treatment. Now, on the statistical theory of cell survival, $S$ gives the *average* surviving fraction following treatment, the actual surviving fraction in any one treatment being distributed in accordance with a Poisson distribution. If there were $M_0$ clonogenic cells initially, then at the end of treatment there will be $SM_0$ clonogenic cells remaining on average. The number of cells remaining is assumed to follow a standard Poisson distribution with a mean of $SM_0$. This gives the probability of local control, denoted $P_c$, as the probability that there are no surviving cells, which is given by

$$P_c = \exp(-SM_0) \qquad (6.7)$$

The surviving fraction is assumed to be based on a linear-quadratic dose model with exponential repopulation. Substituting for $S$ in the equation for $P_c$ above, and after rearranging, the final equation is reduced to

$$\ln[-\ln(P_c)] = \gamma_0 - \gamma_1 D_{eff} + \gamma_2 T \qquad (6.8)$$

The parameter $\gamma_2$ measures the rate of accelerated repopulation of clonogens and is expected to have a positive sign as longer treatment times give the tumour the opportunity to regenerate during treatment. In fact, $\ln(2)/\gamma_2$ is a valid estimate of the doubling time of the tumour. The parameter $\gamma_1$ measures the effect of $D_{eff}$ on the probability of local control. It should be positive as an increase in the effective dose is associated with an increased local control rate. Parameter $\gamma_0$ is associated with the estimated probability of local control for a patient receiving a standard dose schedule.

One of the disadvantages of this analysis is that the $\alpha/\beta$ ratio has to be known. This is assumed to be 10–15 Gy for acute-reacting tissues and 3 Gy for late-reacting tissues.

# Time–dose relationships in clinical experience

Over the past 10 years, data have accumulated which show that time–dose relationships are very important in achieving local tumour control in head and neck tumours in general, including all stages of laryngeal tumours. In 1979, using an analysis based on the NSD model, Harwood and Tierie[39] reported that the dose–cure curve for glottic lesions was flat over the range 1650–2050 ret, with the risk of complications increasing over 2050 ret. Robertson *et al.*,[38] on the basis of LQ analysis, suggested that for $T_1N_0M_0$ lesions an effective dose of 62 Gy given as 2-Gy fractions is necessary to achieve optimal local control.

Schwaibold *et al.*[44] reported local failure in seven out of twenty-eight patients with $T_1N_0M_0$ lesions treated to 66 Gy with 1.8-Gy fractions compared to none out of twenty-eight receiving similar doses at 2-Gy fractions. Although it was assumed that the fraction size of 1.8 Gy might be too low, four of the seven patients treated with this fraction size had breaks in their treatment and this is more likely to be the cause of any reduction in local tumour control. Mendenhall *et al.*,[45] however, assumed that fraction size was the important factor and increased their fraction size to 2–2.25 Gy per day. Maciejewski *et al.*,[46] reviewing the results of treating 310 patients with $T_{3/4}N_0M_0$ lesions using 200 kV X-rays, found that larger dose fractions (>2.3 Gy) increased the incidence of late morbidity. Naturally, here the field sizes were larger than one would use to treat $T_1N_0M_0$ or $T_2N_0M_0$ lesions. Slevin *et al.*,[29] in a review of results from Manchester, concluded that the large dose fraction used routinely at the Christie Hospital did not appear to affect overall late morbidity. It was felt that the 4.1% serious morbidity rate reported was due, in part, to the high tumour biological dose delivered. This was seen in the associated high local control rate reported. This conclusion is in keeping with the findings of the later British Institute of Radiology (BIR) study.[47] The latter study actually reported that the patients treated over the shorter period of time, and who therefore received the larger dose fraction, had the lower incidence of late radiation damage. There was no statistical difference between the two groups when the incidence of acute reactions was considered.

# Relevance of overall treatment time

It is becoming obvious that one of the important factors involved in achieving local tumour control is overall treatment time. Until recently, the practice of prolonging radiotherapy treatments by a few days to deal with acute reactions, machine failures, machine servicing, or public holidays had not been thought serious. The introduction of a gap in the middle of treatment was actually advocated as therapeutic practice at one time.[48] A review of non-randomized data, where some patients had been given a 2-week break in the middle of treatment and others had not, showed that the gap greatly reduced the level of local tumour control achieved.[49] Overgaard *et al.*[49] reviewed 308 patients with carcinoma of the larynx treated over 6–8 weeks. Those receiving 60 Gy in 6 weeks achieved 78% control; those treated with 72 Gy over 8 weeks achieved the same local control but with increased late morbidity, which was unacceptable. Fowler and Lindstrom[50] calculated that the loss of local control that would have arisen if a dose compensation had not been added is in the region of 45%. Barton *et al.*[51] reviewed 1012 patients with carcinoma of the larynx treated radically at Princess Margaret Hospital in Toronto. By mathematical modelling, using linear-quadratic analysis, they estimated that a gap in treatment of 1 day could result in the level of local control being reduced by 4.8%. The 4-year local control rate for the whole data set treated with no interruption was 63.3%, and where there was a gap of 1 day the local control rate was reduced to 61.9%. Fowler and Lindstrom[50] had previously estimated that for a gap of a week the local control rate is reduced by 14% (range 3–25%). Application of the method of Fowler to the more recent results reported by Robertson *et al.*[38] for $T_1N_0M_0$ (Fig. 6.4) and $T_2N_0M_0$ laryngeal tumours gave a predicted reduction in local control, for 1 week prolongation, of between 7% and 16% depending on stage.[52] It should be noted that the importance of unplanned gaps *per se* lies in causing a prolongation of total treatment time. There is no evidence that planned gaps (e.g. radiation-free days at weekends) have any adverse effect on outcome. In most of the theoretical models considered here, it does not matter whether radiation-free days occur or not: the important factor is overall time. (It is of course possible that radiation-free days in themselves do have some independent influence on outcome but

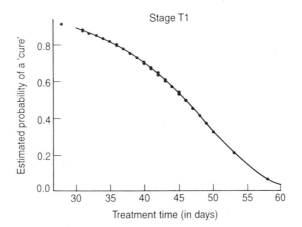

**Fig. 6.4** Relationship between probability of achieving local tumour control and overall treatment time in days for patients with $T_1N_0M_0$ tumours of the larynx.

there is no theoretical justification for this hypothesis and no published evidence which would allow the influence of radiation-free days to be separated from that of overall time.)

The BIR study comparing three fractions of radiotherapy a week with five fractions a week showed a significant improvement in local control in those treated five times a week.[53] It was also noted that those receiving treatment five times a week had a slightly higher incidence of late reactions. Perhaps the dose reduction of 11–13% for those being treated three times a week was just a little too large and allowed more tumour repopulation in the time period between fractions than was optimal.

It is generally assumed that the reduction in local control is due to repopulation that occurs during the gap period. *In-vivo* studies using bromodeoxyuridine (BUDR) estimate that the potential doubling time for squamous cell carcinomas of the larynx is in the region of 4.2 days.[54] Calculations using the linear-quadratic equation estimate that the potential doubling time ($T_{pot}$) is about 6 days for $T_1N_0M_0$ lesions.[38]

Using the linear-quadratic equation, one can determine what dose is required to compensate for the cell repopulation that occurs during an unscheduled gap in treatment. Barton *et al.*[51] calculated that 0.7 Gy per day should be added to each remaining daily treatment. Slevin *et al.*[55] estimated that the dose increment required to maintain a constant local control was between 0.5 and 0.6 Gy per day. It should be noted that there is an apparent decrease in local control with increasing total dose.[56] This is shown in Fig. 6.5 which shows a reanalysis of our previous data[38] presented in the same fashion as Lindstrom and Fowler's.[56]

Fowler and Lindstrom[50] raised the important question: 'With protracted treatment reducing local control rates, should treatment schedules be shortened to 4 or 3 weeks as recommended by the BIR trial[47] and followed as routine therapy in the Christie Hospital, Manchester?'[29]

The treatment of T3 and T4 lesions is still controversial. The relative roles of surgery and radiotherapy are not well delineated. The treatment options available are irradiation alone (with salvage laryngectomy for recurrence), total laryngectomy, or extended hemilaryngectomy. There is a 15–20% risk of nodal involvement with an approximately 15% incidence of subclinical disease[14] in these cases. When radiotherapy is used, these lesions are treated with larger fields incorporating Node levels II and III (Fig. 6.6). An alternative is to use an anterior–posterior field arrangement with a 4:1 weighting delivering 45 Gy to the lesion and then to replan and bring the dose to 66 Gy using a standard lateral parallel pair to the neck.[57] Using radiotherapy as first-line treatment allows patients a chance to retain their natural voice. Laryngectomy has other effects on the ultimate quality of life including loss of the sense of taste. Where radiotherapy is first-line treatment, close follow-up is mandatory to detect early recurrence or persistent disease; these patients should proceed to laryngectomy immediately if recurrent tumour is detected.

The reported tumour control results achieved with conventional radiotherapy are relatively poor, ranging from 30% to 55%.[58–60] 'Conventional radiotherapy' (2 Gy/fraction, given five times a week) treatment regimens were adopted because they give a tolerance dose for late effects with an acceptable level of acute morbidity. Such a regimen, however, is not always

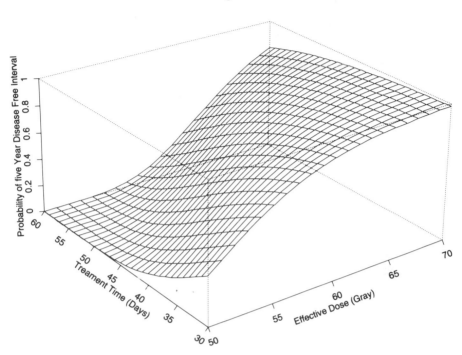

**Fig. 6.5** Relationship between probability of achieving local tumour control, effective dose in grays and overall treatment time in days for patients with $T_1N_0M_0$ lesions of the glottis.

the most ideal for treating certain tumours. In an effort to improve local tumour control rates in advanced lesions, variations in fractionation schedules have been introduced, including an accelerated fractionation, hyperfractionation, and a combination of both.

## Accelerated fractionation

Accelerated fractionation is where the overall time that the total dose is delivered in is shorter than a 'conventional' schedule. This is achieved by giving the dose in two or three fractions daily. Fraction size is usually conventional, and total dose may be the same or slightly reduced.

## Hyperfractionation

This is where the fraction sizes are smaller than 'conventional' doses (2 Gy in most centres). The fractions are given two or three times a day. Usually the total dose is increased and is given over the same period of time.

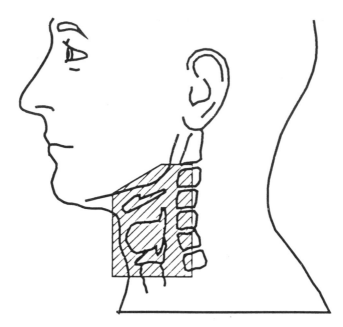

**Fig. 6.6**　Field arrangement for patients with supraglottic carcinoma.

### Accelerated hyperfractionation

Schedules such as continuous hyperfractionated accelerated radiotherapy (CHART)[61] are a combination of these variations in fraction where the fraction size and total dose are reduced to give the schedule over a shorter period of time and omit the normal breaks in treatment on Saturdays and Sundays.

## Radiobiological factors in tumour control

The four 'Rs' of radiation biology — repopulation, reoxygenation, repair and redistribution — all contribute to the outcome of a dose–time-fraction schedule.

### Repopulation

Repopulation of stem cells during a 'conventional' radical schedule of radiotherapy contributes to the differential sparing of early-responding tissues relative to both slow responding normal tissue and (possibly) most tumours. There is a delay between initial exposure to radiation and the commencement of cell regeneration in both tumours and acute-responding normal tissues. This is related to the proliferation kinetics of the cells, the size of the fraction dose and the duration of fractionation. Where dose is protracted over a number of weeks, the delay in tumour regeneration is longer than for acute-responding normal mucosa. Clonogenic cells arising in the larynx proliferate rapidly — the potential cell-doubling time is in the region of 4–6 days.[38,54] There should therefore be a gain in local control by administering treatment over a shorter period of time. By accelerating treatment, the opportunity for tumour cells to proliferate is reduced. The rapid proliferation rate of laryngeal tumours, and head and neck tumours in general, is the reason why split-course treatment is so ineffective unless the gap can be compensated for, by increasing the dose.[49]

## Reoxygenation

Reoxygenation allows hypoxic cells in the tumour mass to be sensitized. It has been suggested that shorter treatment times may not allow time for reoxygenation. It has also been hypothesized that the oxygen enhancement ratio may be reduced in hyperfractionated schedules when dose per fraction is reduced. This may be therapeutically beneficial. The possibility of reduced time for reoxygenation should also be a cautionary consideration in accelerated regimens when overall treatment time is reduced.

## Redistribution

The sensitivity of cells to radiation varies throughout the cell cycle. After each dose of radiation, cells in resistant phases (e.g. late S phase) survive preferentially, resulting in some degree of synchronization of surviving cells; but, given time, these will again redistribute themselves over all the phases. This phenomenon of redistribution can increase the sensitivity of both tumour and normal cells. Target cells for late sequelae are slow growing and will therefore not undergo changes in distribution in the cell cycle to any great extent. A multifractionated regimen should therefore spare late effects more than acute effects. Tumours are less homogeneous in biological features than are normal tissues. Response to radiation therefore varies. Sensitization due to synchronization of cell division in tumour cells is the same as in normal tissues. Tumour masses have large numbers of cells in G0 phase, and, as proliferating cells die, a number of the cells in G0 phase become active again, starting to proliferate and hence becoming sensitized. Multifraction schedules increase this phenomenon and therefore increase sensitivity.

## Repair

Clinical and laboratory studies suggest that the repair capacities of acute- and late- responding normal and tumour tissues vary widely. Lengthening treatment times have allowed radiotherapists to give large doses in fraction sizes of 1.8–2 Gy without causing excessive acute normal-tissue reactions. Tolerance doses depend upon acute- and late-responding tissues, the actual organs and areas being treated and the volume of tissue encompassed by the radiation fields. Late-responding tissues are more able to repair sublethal damage than acute tissues. Experimental evidence suggests that as the dose per fraction is reduced then the total dose required to produce a late effect is increased. The repair capacities of tumour cells are not greatly different from those of normal tissues. There is no evidence that they are capable of more repair than normal cells. With altered fractionation schedules, where therapy is given twice a day or more, it is important that Elkind repair[62] is completely achieved, or about 90–95%, between fractions.[63] If this degree of repair occurs then there should be little change or a small acceptable increase in the severity of the acute effects. A minimum time interval of 6 hrs between schedules is required. The response of the slowly cycling target cells for late effects should be unchanged.

# Clinical experience with unconventional schedules

The introduction of these new treatment schedules required modification of traditional fraction sizes. Withers[64] calculated that, compared with 'conventional' therapy, the dose for hyperfractionated therapy should be increased by 15–25% per day, i.e. from 2 Gy to 1.2 Gy twice a day. The overall total dose is increased from 66 Gy in thirty-three fractions to 79.2 Gy in sixty-six fractions. This schedule has been adopted by a number of centres in Europe and America. At the University of Florida, a study using the above hyperfractionated schedule[65] reported that the local tumour control rate for $T_3N_0M_0$ tumours of the larynx was 70%. Although the time between daily fractions was between 4 and 6 hrs, the acute reactions were more brisk, with 20% of patients requiring nasogastric feeding and some patients requiring 2–3 months before complete healing of the mucosa occurred.

Accelerated fractionation involves delivering a radical dose of radiation in a shorter period of time than that in which a 'conventional' dose would be given. This is not a new concept in radiation therapy since it was widely practised in the early years of this century.[66] To deliver a radical dose and avoid unacceptable morbidity, the dose fraction size is reduced and treatment given two or three times a day. Withers[64] stated that the fraction size should be the same as in 'conventional' treatments when fractionation was accelerated. Peracchia and Salti[67] adopted this approach, treating forty-seven patients with head and neck tumours and giving 2 Gy three times a day, 5 days a week over 9–11 days. The time interval between fractions was 4 hrs. General and local early tolerance were satisfactory; however, 68% developed necrosis, with 55% developing high-grade necrosis. Within 2 years, 25–30% died because of necrosis alone or in combination with recurrence. Peracchia and Salti concluded that repair from a fraction dose of 2 Gy was not completed in 4 hrs.

Other groups adopted alternative accelerated fractionation schedules. Horiot et al.[68] and Wang et al.[69] treated patients with advanced head and neck tumours with a twice-a-day regimen. They gave 1.6 Gy (using megavoltage equipment) twice a day for 12 days, with a time period between fractions of a minimum of 4 hrs. All fields were treated at each session. Once the patients had received 38.4 Gy they were given a 2-week rest period to allow acute reactions to subside. After the 2-week break, treatment was recommenced, usually using a reduced field giving 1.6 Gy twice a day to a total dose of 67.2–72 Gy. For $T_{3/4}N_0M_0$ lesions of the head and neck region, Wang's group[69] reported an increase in local control rate from 40% with 'conventional' therapy to 59% with accelerated therapy. The increases noted in those with nodal involvement were much more significant — in $T_{3/4}N_{1/3}M_0$ cases, from 16% to 60%.[68]

Johnstone *et al.*[70] adopted the technique of treating patients with a concomitant boost, using a conventional fraction (1.8 Gy/fraction) to the treatment field, combined with a boost of 1.8 Gy given 4–6 hrs after the first treatment to a reduced field during part of the treatment course. Patients were randomized to a conventional or an accelerated arm. Those in the conventional arm received 66–72 Gy by conventional therapy using doses of 1.8–2 Gy/fraction each day over 7–8 weeks. The whole neck received 50 Gy, the dose to the cord was limited to 40–45 Gy, and the tumours were boosted through reduced fields to a total dose of 66–72 Gy. Those treated with the concomitant boost schedule–accelerated arm received 1.8 Gy/fraction to 50.4 Gy. During the boost phase, a second fraction was delivered 4–6 hrs after the first, given over a period of three consecutive weeks on a Monday, Wednesday and Friday, through reduced portals to a volume covering all detectable disease. The fraction size for the boost was 1.6 Gy. In this way, a dose of 68.4–73.8 Gy was given in 42–45 days, 10 days less than a 'conventional treatment' schedule would have taken. Patients with advanced squamous carcinomas arising at many sites in the head and neck region were included in this study. Locoregional tumour control was 62% for the group receiving the boost schedule and 33% for those treated 'conventionally' ($P = 0.003$). All thirteen patients with tumours arising in the larynx (glottis and supraglottis) were controlled by the concomitant boost schedule whereas only five out of nine were controlled by 'conventional' scheduling.

Saunders *et al.*[61] introduced the CHART schedule, in which patients receive 1.6 Gy three times a day, with a minimum of 6 hrs between treatments. Treatment is given continuously for 12 days with no break. After twenty-five treatments the field size should be reduced if necessary. Results from an earlier pilot study showed that there was a significant difference between those treated three times a day, and the control arm in which patients received 66 Gy in thirty-three fractions, 5 days a week. The large National CHART Head and Neck study continues to recruit and the results will not be available for some time. This includes patients with $T_2N_0M_0$ glottic carcinomas, as well as those with more advanced disease.

The CHART schedule is very labour intensive. It is very demanding of a busy radiotherapy unit to treat patients three times a day, even if the numbers are small. Furthermore, to treat on Saturdays and Sundays is also difficult for paramedical and other staff, and greatly increases the cost of running a department.[71]

The concomitant boost technique allows an aggressive treatment schedule to be delivered to the tumour and limits the volume of normal tissue receiving twice daily therapy. Prolonged treatment interruptions are therefore avoided, as are planned gaps.[68]

# Supraglottic lesions

The prognosis for those with supraglottic lesions is considerably worse than for those with glottic cancer. Adjusted survival rates for supraglottic carcinomas is in the region of 46% compared with 83% for glottic lesions.[72] The poorer overall survival rates may be due to a number of factors. The presenting symptoms for those with supraglottic tumours are different from those with glottic lesions. Hoarseness, which often leads to early detection of glottic lesions, is not as common in patients with supraglottic carcinomas, especially where the tumour arises in the epilarynx. Tumours arising in the epilarynx as opposed to the lower supraglottic region frequently present with dysphagia, referred throat pain or otalgia. Such tumours are often very advanced at time of diagnosis.[73]

The supraglottic region also has a rich lymphatic system[74] and the incidence of nodal involvement reported ranges from 32% to 73%. Even where local control is achieved, a number of patients will die of metastases, second primaries or diseases related to their excessive smoking and drinking habits.[75,76] Tumours of the supraglottic region may be more aggressive than those arising in the glottic area and may be more comparable with tumours arising in the posterior third of the tongue. The staging of supraglottic lesions is not as precise as that for glottic lesions. The criterion for T3 lesions is 'deep invasion' but there is no definition of the methods to be used to identify this invasion. Staging will therefore vary from centre to centre depending upon their imaging and other facilities. This will obviously influence the results reported and make it difficult to compare treatment outcomes.

Of patients with T1 supraglottic lesions, 17% have been reported as having nodal involvement, though only 0–5% of patients with T1 lesions arising in the glottis have nodal involvement. Of patients with T2–T4 lesions of the supraglottis 47% have nodal involvement at the time of presentation.[74] Because of the relatively high incidence of node involvement in the neck and the inability of imaging techniques to accurately identify nodal disease, the neck should be treated prophylactically in N0 cases. The field size is therefore larger than that used for glottic lesions (Fig. 6.6), a difference which has been found to increase local control rates.[73] A recent review of patients treated at a Dutch centre showed that the field size certainly affected the incidence of locoregional tumour control.[77] There is clearly a volume effect and the effective safe total dose[38] that can be given is less than that given to a glottic lesion, in order to avoid excessive acute reactions. A recent report from Japan reviewing the results in 100 cases of early ($T_1N_0M_0$ and $T_2N_0M_0$) supraglottic carcinoma treated on telecobalt gave 5-year local control rates of 77% for T1 lesions and 62% for T2 lesions.[78] Hoekstra et al.[77] reported a 5-year relapse-free survival rate of 53% for T2 lesions, though in this group of 212 patients only 165 received radical radiotherapy and 109 of these were treated using a split course schedule. As already stated, prolongation of treatment leads to tumour repopulation which affects local tumour control rates.[46,51] Fowler and Lindstrom[50] estimated that a gap of a week results in loss of local control by about 12–15%. Van den Bogaert et al.[73] reported a difference in survival for T1 and T2 lesions in the epilarynx and lower supraglottic region (53% vs 68%; $P = 0.15$), though this was not statistically significant. Mendenhall et al.[79] reported no significant difference in control rate as a function of site within the supraglottis. Inoue *et al.*,[78] on the other hand, reported a significantly higher local control rate in epilaryngeal lesions compared with those arising in the lower supraglottis.

Advanced lesions, especially those arising in the supraglottis, do not respond favourably to radiotherapy as the sole form of treatment. One group reported a relapse free survival rate for T3/T4 lesions in the range of 39%.[80] Million[14] has identified a selected group of T3 squamous carcinomas of the supraglottic region: 'A lesion that is relatively exophytic with the vocal cords mobile'. These are staged T3 on the basis of pre-epiglottic space invasion or limited extension to the medial wall of the pyriform sinus or the post-cricoid area, and are thought to be more responsive to radiotherapy than other T3 lesions. He also states that T4 lesions with limited cartilage or soft tissue extension, or base of tongue invasion, can respond favourably to radiation therapy. Cartilage invasion is common in epiglottic tumours and should not be considered a contraindication to radiotherapy. Experience in managing these tumours is very varied, possibly due to difficulties in staging. The larger volume of tissue that has to be treated makes it more difficult to deliver an adequate radiation dose without interrupting the treatment schedule and these factors may well contribute to the poor results reported.

Million states that bulky endophytic T3 lesions with cord fixation should be treated primarily by surgery — total or partial laryngectomy, as appropriate[7] — radiotherapy being given postoperatively, if required. Hoekstra *et al.*,[77] on the other hand, in view of the poor results obtained in treating advanced lesions with conventional radiotherapy alone (T3/T4, 39% relapse-free survival rate), have suggested that results may be improved by giving treatment with no unscheduled interruptions and also by using a multiple fraction-per-day schedule. Wang and coworkers have advocated hyperfractionation schedules as a means to increase local control.[81] They have used a treatment protocol of: 1.6 Gy/fraction, two fractions per day, with a minimum of 4 hrs between fractions, 5 days per week for 12 treatment days, to a dose of 38.4 Gy. Patients are rested for 2 weeks, then treatment of 1.6 Gy twice daily is resumed, using a shrinking field technique, to a total dose of 64 Gy over 6 weeks and occasionally 67.2 Gy. This was compared with a 'conventional' schedule of 1.8 Gy per day, 5 days per week, given continuously, to a total dose of 65 Gy in 7 weeks. If there was residual disease in the neck at the end of treatment, a radical neck dissection was carried out. Although there is a gap in the twice daily schedule after 2–3 weeks, the treatment is still accelerated. The 3-year actuarial local control rates for T1 and T2 lesions were 88 vs 63.5% for twice and once a day, respectively. The results for T3 and T4 lesions were 66 vs 33%, respectively. The differences were statistically significant in both groups.

Surgery can sometimes be voice-sparing. Supraglottic laryngectomy[7] can be used successfully for selected lesions involving the epiglottis, the aryepiglottic fold and the false cord. If the true cords or both arytenoids are involved, then a total laryngectomy is required with loss of voice. Following supraglottic laryngectomy, all patients have difficulty swallowing and a tendency to aspirate. The vast majority, however, learn to swallow again very quickly. Voice quality is generally normal. Total laryngectomy, on its own, has a high rate of success for the management of T3 laryngeal lesions. Postoperative radiotherapy should only be included where margins are close or positive, or where there is invasion of soft tissues of neck, cartilage, or subglottis. Radiotherapy is also indicated where there is nodal involvement, especially if there is extracapsular spread.

## Adjuvant therapy

Over the last two to three decades there have been a number of attempts to enhance the effects of radiotherapy. Henk *et al*.[82] were among the first to use hyperbaric oxygen in the treatment of head and neck tumours. They showed a significantly increased local control rate in those treated in oxygen compared with those treated in air. Logistics make it almost impossible to use this technique routinely in any busy radiotherapy department. More recently, there has been interest in the value of agents such as misonidazole which have been identified as radiation sensitizers. Misonidazole has been used in several trials[83] but the results have so far shown no therapeutic advantage. There are early unpublished reports that a compound closely related to misonidazole may be of value as a radiosensitizer.

Chemotherapy is introduced into the treatment of cancer for two reasons: to improve local control and to reduce the incidence of distant metastases, both of which affect overall survival. Early results reported encouraging response rates to chemotherapy, though in cases where chemotherapy was given synchronously with radiotherapy the side effects were often severe,[84] resulting in prolongation of the radiation schedule. Other reports are less encouraging and Stell and Rawson's [85] overview leaves many sceptical as to the value of such therapy in the management of head and neck tumours. They detected only a 0.5% overall improvement in cancer mortality. Since the recognition that chemotherapy was of value in treating certain cancers, more than fifty chemotherapeutic agents have been identified. Until recently methotrexate — the agent first identified as being active against leukaemia — was considered the most active against head and neck cancer. One report from India suggested that bleomycin might also be of value.[86] Yosef and colleagues[9] also recorded activity for this agent when given in association with radiotherapy in the management of T3 laryngeal cancer, though these findings have not always been noted in other studies. More recently, cisplatin-based combinations have been reported as producing the best overall response rates, though interpretation of results is still controversial.[87]

Gupta *et al.*,[88] from Manchester, gave methotrexate concurrently with radiotherapy, administering 100 mg/m$^2$ on Days 0 and 14 of a 22-day course of radiotherapy. The randomized comparison arm consisted of radiotherapy alone. Patients with tumours arising in the oropharynx derived a survival advantage over the control arm. Patients with tumours arising in the larynx did not show any increase in local control or survival. On the basis of these and the South-East Co-operative Oncology Group's (SECOG)[89] results, a British trial has now been set up.[90]

In the USA, the Veterans Association established a trial comparing induction chemotherapy plus radiation versus surgery plus radiation in patients with advanced laryngeal cancer.[91] The induction chemotherapy was 100 mg/m$^2$ cisplatinum as a bolus, followed by 1 g/m$^2$ fluorouracil per day for 5 days. Chemotherapy was repeated on Days 2 and 43. Patients then received radiotherapy: 66–76 Gy to the primary site and 50 Gy to the neck if N0, or 66 Gy if the nodes were < 2 cm and 70 Gy if they were >2 cm. Fraction size was 1.8–2.0 Gy. The other group of patients had the lesion excised and received 50–57.4 Gy. Where there was thought to be residual disease, a boost of 15–23.8 Gy was delivered. There were 166 patients with Stage III or IV laryngeal cancer in each arm. Survival rates were identical. Disease-free interval was better for those treated by surgery and radiotherapy; however, 66% retained a functioning larynx in the chemotherapy arm. There was no improvement in preservation of the larynx between this group and historical groups treated by radiotherapy alone. It was concluded that the role of chemotherapy was still unresolved.

Prior to this, the National Cancer Institute (NCI) set up a trial to compare chemotherapy as induction therapy plus surgery and postoperative radiotherapy vs surgery plus radiotherapy plus maintenance chemotherapy vs surgery plus radiotherapy.[92] Again, there was no difference in survival, though there was a reduction in distant metastases in the group receiving maintenance chemotherapy (consisting of 100 mg/m$^2$ cisplatin as a bolus and 15 mg/m$^2$ bleomycin on Days 3, 7 and 14). Chemotherapy is still of uncertain value in head and neck tumours except in cases of palliation, and all patients receiving chemotherapy with curative intent should be entered into a clinical trial.

# References

1. Lederman M. Carcinoma of the larynx. *Br J Radiol* 1971; **44**, 569–78.
2. Singer MI, Blom ED. Medical techniques for voice restoration after total laryngectomy. *CA* 1990; **40**, 166–73.
3. Miller S. The role of the speech language pathologist in voice restoration after total laryngectomy. *CA* 1990; **40**, 174–82.
4. Finzi NS, Harmer D. Radium treatment of intrinsic carcinoma of the larynx. *BMJ* 1928; **2**, 886–9.
5. Candela FC, Shah J, Jaques DP, *et al.* Patterns of cervical node metastases from squamous carcinoma of the larynx. *Arch Otolaryngol Head Neck Surg* 1990; **116**, 432–5.
6. Armstrong J, Pfister D, Strong E, *et al.* The management of the clinically positive neck as part of a larynx preservation approach. *Int J Radiat Oncol Biol Phys* 1993; **26**, 759–65.
7. Robertson JB, Fee WE Jr. Conservation surgery for laryngeal carcinoma. *Ann Acad Med Singap* 1991; **20**, 656–64.
8. Silver CE, Moisa II. The role of surgery in the treatment of laryngeal cancer. *CA* 1990; **40**, 134–49.
9. Robertson AG, Boyle P, Yosef HM, *et al.* Cancer of larynx in west of Scotland. *Am J Clin Oncol* 1982; **5**, 527–33.
10. Parkin DM, Muir CS, Whelan SL, *et al.*, eds. *Cancer Incidence in Five Continents*, Vol VI. Lyon: IARC Scientific Publications, No. 120, 1992.
11. Wynder EL, Covey LA, Mabuchi K, *et al.* Environmental factors in cancer of the larynx (a second look). *Cancer* 1976; **38**, 1591–601.
12. Doll R, Peto J. *Effects on Health of Exposure to Asbestos.* London: Her Majesty's Stationery Office, 1985.

13. Stell PM, McGill T. Exposure to asbestos and laryngeal cancer. *J Laryngol Otol* 1975; **89**, 513–17.
14. Million RR. The larynx . . . so to speak: everything I want to know about laryngeal cancer I learned in the last 32 years. *Int J Radiat Oncol Biol Phys* 1993; **23**, 691–704.
15. Suit HD. Potential for improving survival rates for the cancer patient by increasing the efficacy of treatment of the primary lesion. *Cancer* 1982; **50**, 1227–34.
16. Stell PM. Ploidy in head and neck cancer: a review and meta-analysis. *Clin Otolaryngol* 1991; **16**, 510–16.
17. Cooke LD, Cooke TG, Forster G, *et al.* Flow cytometric analysis of DNA content in squamous carcinoma of the tongue: the relationship to host and tumour factors and survival. *Clin Otolaryngol* 1994; **19**, 131–4.
18. Westerbeek HA, Mooi WJ, Hilgers FJM, *et al.* Ploidy status and the response of T1 glottic carcinoma to radiotherapy. *Clin Otolaryngol Allied Sci* 1993; **18**, 98–101.
19. Walther EK, Dahlmann N, Gorgulla HT. Tumour markers in the diagnosis and follow up of head and neck cancer: role of CEA, CA 19-9, SCC, TK, and DTTASE. *Head and Neck* 1993; **15**, 230–5.
20. Harwood AR, Deboer G, Kazim F. Prognostic factors in T3 glottic cancer. *Cancer* 1981; **47**, 367–72.
21. Griffin TW, Pajak TF, Gilliespie BW, *et al.* Predicting the response of head and neck cancers to radiation therapy with a multivariate modelling system: an analysis of the RTOG head and neck registry. *Int J Radiat Oncol Biol Phys* 1984; **10**, 481–7.
22. UICC (Union Internationale Contre le Cancer). Larynx. In: P Hermanek, LH Sobin, eds, *TNM Classification of Malignant Tumours*, 4th edn. Berlin: Springer-Verlag, 1987; 23–6.
23. AJCC (American Joint Committee on Cancer). *Manual for Staging of Cancer* 3rd edn. Philadelphia: JB Lippincott Co, 1988.
24. Gerristen GJ, Valk J, van Velzen DJ *et al.* Computed tomography: a mandatory investigational procedure for the T-staging of advanced laryngeal cancer. *Clin Otolaryngol* 1986; **11**, 307–16.
25. Vogl TJ. Hypopharynx, larynx, thyroid and parathyroid. In: DD Stark, WG Bradley Jr, eds, *Magnetic Resonance Imaging*, Mosley Year Book, 2nd edn. St Louis, MO: Mosley, 1992; 1197–1220.
26. Ali YA, Saleh EM, Mancuso AA. Does conventional tomography still have a place in glottic cancer? *Clin Radiol* 1992; **45**, 114–19.
27. Harwood AR, Beale FA, Cummings BJ, *et al.* T2 glottic cancer: an analysis of dose–time–volume factors. *Int J Radiat Oncol Biol Phys* 1981; 7, 1501–5.
28. Wang CC. Factors influencing the success of radiation therapy for T2 and T3 glottic carcinoma. *Am J Clin Oncol* 1986; **9**, 517–20.
29. Slevin NJ, Vasanthan S, Dougal M. Relative clinical influence of tumour dose versus dose per fraction on the occurrence of late normal tissue morbidity following larynx radiotherapy. *Int J Radiat Oncol Biol Phys* 1993; **25**, 22–8.
30. Fein D, Mendenhall WH, Parsons JT, *et al.* Carcinoma in situ of the glottic larynx. *Int J Radiat Oncol Biol Phys* 1993; **27**, 379–84.
31. Miller AH, Fisher HR. Clues to the life history of carcinoma in situ of the larynx. *Laryngoscope* 1971; **81**, 1475–80.
32. MacLeod PM, Daniel F. The role of radiotherapy in in situ carcinoma of the larynx. *Int J Radiat Oncol Biol Phys* 1990; **18**, 113–17.
33. Doyle PJ, Flores A, Douglas GS. Carcinoma in situ of the larynx. *Laryngoscope* 1976; **86**, 310–16 .
34. Harwood AR, Hawkins NV, Rider WD, *et al.* Radiotherapy of early glottic cancer. *Int J Radiat Oncol Biol Phys* 1979; **5**, 473–6.
35. Teshima T, Chatani M, Inoue T. Radiation therapy for early glottic cancer

$(T_1N_0M_0)$: II. Prospective randomized study concerning radiation field. *Int J Radiat Oncol Biol Phys* 1990; **18**, 119–23.

36. Fletcher GH, Lindberg RD, Hamberger A, *et al*. Reasons for irradiation failure in squamous cell carcinoma of the larynx. *Laryngoscope* 1976; **86**, 987–1003.

37. Hamlet S, Ezzell G, Aref A. Larynx motion associated with swallowing during radiation therapy. *Int J Radiat Oncol Biol Phys* 1993; **28**, 467–70.

38. Robertson AG, Robertson C, Boyle P, *et al*. The effect of differing radiotherapeutic schedules on the response of glottic carcinoma of the larynx. *Eur J Cancer* 1993; **4**, 501–10.

39. Harwood AR, Tierie A. Radiotherapy of early glottic cancer — II. *Int J Radiat Oncol Biol Phys* 1979; **5**, 477–82.

40. Ellis F. Dose, time and fractionation: a clinical hypothesis. *Clin Radiol* 1969; **22**, 1–7.

41. Kirk J, Gray WM, Watson ER. Cumulative radiation effect, part 1: fractionated treatment regimes. *Clin Radiol* 1971; **22**, 145–55.

42. Fowler JF. The linear-quadratic formula and progress in fractionated radiotherapy. *Br J Radiol* 1989; **62**, 679–94.

43. Maciejewski B, Withers HR, Taylor JMG, *et al*. Dose fractionation and regeneration in radiotherapy for cancer of the oral cavity and oropharynx. Part 1. Tumour dose response and regeneration. *Int J Radiat Oncol Biol Phys* 1989; **16**, 831–43.

44. Schwaibold F, Scariato A, Nunno M, *et al*. The effect of fraction size on control of early glottic cancer. *Int J Radiat Oncol Biol Phys* 1988; **14**, 451–4 .

45. Mendenhall WM, Parsons JT, Million RR, *et al*. T1–T2 squamous cell carcinoma of the glottic larynx treated with radiation therapy: relationship of dose–fraction factors to local control and complications. *Int J Radiat Oncol Biol Phys* 1988; **15**, 1267–73.

46. Maciejewski B, Preuss-Bayer G, Trott K-R. The influence of the number of fractions and of overall treatment time on local control and late complication rate in squamous cell carcinoma of the larynx. *Int J Radiat Oncol Biol Phys* 1983; **9**, 321–8.

47. Wiernik G, *et al*. Final report on the second British Institute of Radiology fraction study: short versus long overall treatment times for radiotherapy of carcinoma of the laryngo-pharynx. *Br J Radiol* 1991; **64**, 232–41.

48. Sambrooke D. Clinical trial of a modified (split course) technique of X-ray therapy in malignant tumours. *Clin Radiol* 1968; **36**, 369–72.

49. Overgaard M, Hjelm-Hansen M, Vendelbo JL, *et al*. Comparison of conventional and split-course radiotherapy as a primary treatment in carcinoma of the larynx. *Acta Oncol* 1988; **27**, 147–61.

50. Fowler J, Lindstrom MJ. Loss of local control with prolongation in radiotherapy. *Int J Radiat Oncol Biol Phys* 1992; **23**,457–67.

51. Barton MB, Keane TJ, Galla T, *et al*. The effect of treatment time and treatment interruption on tumour control following radical radiotherapy of laryngeal cancer. *Radiother Oncol* 1992; **24**, 137–43.

52. Fowler JF, Chappell R. Effect of overall time and dose on the response of glottic carcinoma of the larynx to radiotherapy. *Eur J Cancer* 1994; **30**, 719–21.

53. Wiernik G, *et al*. Final report of the general clinical results of the British Institute of Radiology fraction study of 3F/wk versus 5F/wk in radiotherapy of carcinoma of the laryngo-pharynx. *Br J Radiol* 1990; **63**, 169–80.

54. Begg AC, Hofland I, Moonen L, *et al*. The predictive value of cell kinetic measurements in a European trial of accelerated fractionation in advanced head and neck tumours: an interim report. *Int J Radiat Oncol Biol Phys* 1990; **19**, 1449–53.

55. Slevin NJ, Hendry JH, Roberts SA, *et al*. The effect of increasing the treatment time beyond three weeks on the control of T2 and T3 laryngeal cancer using

radiotherapy. *Radiother Oncol* 1992; **24**, 215–20.

56. Lindstrom MJ, Fowler JF. Re-analysis of the time factor in local control by radiotherapy of T3/T4 squamous cell carcinoma of the larynx. *Int J Radiat Oncol Biol Phys* 1991; **21**, 813–17.

57. Doppke K, Novack D, Wang CC. Physical considerations in the treatment of advanced carcinomas of the larynx and pyriform sinuses using 10 MV X-rays. *Int J Radiat Oncol Biol Phys* 1980; **6**, 1251–5.

58. Hunter RD, Palmer MK. An analysis of the fate of patients treated radically for glottic carcinoma of the larynx. *Clin Radiol* 1980; **31**, 449–52.

59. Simpson D, Robertson AG, Lamont D. A comparison of radiotherapy and surgery as primary treatment in the management of $T_3N_0M_0$ glottic tumours. *J Laryngol Otol* 1993; **107**, 912–15.

60. Mendenhall WM, Parsons JT, Stringer SP, *et al.* Stage T3 squamous cell carcinoma of the glottic larynx: a comparison of laryngectomy and irradiation. *Int J Radiat Oncol Biol Phys* 1992; **23**, 725–32.

61. Saunders MI, Dische S, Hong A, *et al.* Continuous hyperfractionated accelerated radiotherapy in locally advanced carcinoma of the head and neck region. *Int J Radiat Oncol Biol Phys* 1989; **17**, 1287–93.

62. Elkind MM, Sutton H. X-ray damage and recovery in mammalian cells in culture. *Nature* 1959; **184**, 1293–5.

63. Denekamp J, Harris SR. Studies of the processes occurring between two sessions in experimental mouse tumours. *Int J Radiat Biol* 1976; **1**, 421–30.

64. Withers R. Biological basis for altered fractionation schemes. *Cancer* 1985; **55**, 2086–95.

65. Parsons JT, Mendenhall WM, Cassisi NJ, *et al.* Hyperfractionation for head and neck cancer. *Int J Radiat Oncol Biol Phys* 1988; **14**, 649–58.

66. Barkley HT. Accelerated treatment. *Cancer* 1985; **55**, 2112–17.

67. Peracchia G, Salti C. Radiotherapy with thrice-a-day fractionation in a short overall time: clinical experiences. *Int J Radiat Oncol Biol Phys* 1981; 7, 99–104.

68. Horiot JC, Le Fur R, N'Guyen T, *et al.* Hyperfractionated compared with conventional radiotherapy in oropharyngeal cancer: an EORTC randomised trial. *Eur J Cancer* 1990; 26, 779–80.

69. Wang CC, Blitzer PH, Suit HD. Twice-a-day radiation therapy for cancer of the head and neck. *Cancer* 1985; 55, 2100–4.

70. Johnston CR, Schimidt-Ullrich RK, Wazer DE. Concomitant boost technique using accelerated superfractionated radiation therapy for advanced squamous cell carcinoma of the head and neck. *Cancer* 1992; 69, 2749–54.

71. Southampton University Hospitals — NHS trust. A review of linear accelerator capacity — cancer care. Botley, Southampton: Salter Baker and Assoc, 1994.

72. Silvestri F, Bussani R, Stanta G, *et al.* Supra glottic versus glottic laryngeal cancer: epidemiological and pathological aspects. *Otorhinolaryngology* 1992; **54**, 43–8.

73. Van den Bogaert W, Ostyn F, van der Schueren E. The different clinical presentation, behaviour and prognosis of carcinomas originating in the epilarynx and the lower supraglottis. *Radiother Oncol* 1983; **1**, 117–31.

74. Neiderer J, Hawkins NV, Rider WD, *et al.* Failure analysis of radical radiation therapy of supraglottic laryngeal carcinoma. *Int J Radiat Oncol Biol Phys* 1976; **2**, 621–9.

75. Schmidt W, Popham RE. The role of drinking and smoking in mortality from cancer and other causes in male alcoholics. *Cancer* 1981; **47**, 1031–41.

76. Robin PE, Olofsson J. Tumours of the larynx. In: Scott-Brown, ed, *Textbook of Otolaryngology*, 5th edn. London: Butterworths, 1987, 186–234.

77. Hoekstra CJM, Levendag PC, van Putten LJ. Squamous cell carcinoma of the supraglottic larynx without clinically detectable lymph node metastases: problem of local relapse and influence of overall treatment time. *Int J Radiat Oncol*

*Biol Phys* 1990; **18**, 13–21.
78. Inoue T, Matayoshi Y, Inoue T, *et al.* Prognostic factors in telecobalt therapy for early supraglottic carcinoma. *Cancer* 1993; **72**, 57–61.
79. Mendenhall WM, Parsons JT, Stringer SP, *et al.* Carcinoma of the supraglottic larynx; a basis for comparing the results of radiotherapy and surgery. *Head Neck* 1990; **12**, 204–9.
80. Leyendag PC, Hoekstra CJM, Eykenboom WMH, *et al.* Supraglottic larynx cancer T1–T4N0 treated by radical radiation therapy: the problem of neck relapse. *Acta Oncol* 1988; **27**, 253–60.
81. Wang CC, Suit HD, Blitzer PH. Twice-a-day radiation therapy for supraglottic carcinoma. *Int J Radiat Oncol Biol Phys* 1986; **12**, 3–7.
82. Henk JM, Kunkler PB, Shah NK, *et al.* Hyperbaric oxygen in radiotherapy of head and neck carcinoma. *Clin Radiol* 1970; **21**, 223–31.
83. EORTC (European Organization for the Research and Treatment of Cancer) Cooperative Group of Radiotherapy: early results of the EORTC randomised clinical trial on multiple fractions per day (MFD) and misonidazole in advanced head and neck cancer. *Int J Radiat Oncol Biol Phys* 1986; **12**, 587–91.
84. Clifford P, O'Connor AD, Durden-Smith J, *et al.* Synchronous multiple drug chemotherapy and radiotherapy for advanced (Stage III and IV) squamous carcinoma of the head and neck. *Antibiot Chemother* 1978; **24**, 60–72.
85. Stell PM, Rawson NSB. Adjuvant chemotherapy in head and neck cancer. *Br J Cancer* 1990; **61**, 779–87.
86. Rangakumar G, Shanta V. Larynx cancer: a therapeutic policy at the Madras Cancer Institute. *J Surg Oncol* 1978; **10**, 183–9.
87. Eisenberger M, Krasnow S, Ellenberg S, *et al.* A comparison of carboplatinum plus methotrexate versus methotrexate alone in patients with recurrent and metastatic head and neck cancer. *J Clin Oncol* 1989; **7**, 1341–5.
88. Gupta NK, Pointon RCS, Wilkinson PM. A randomised clinical trial to contrast radiotherapy with radiotherapy and methotrexate given synchronously in head and neck cancer. *Clin Radiol* 1987; **38**, 575–81.
89. SECOG Participants. A randomised trial of combined multidrug chemotherapy and radiotherapy in advanced squamous cell carcinoma of the head and neck. *Eur J Surg Oncol* 1986; **12**, 289–95.
90. Tobias JS. Has chemotherapy proved itself in head and neck cancer? *Br J Cancer* 1990; **61**, 649–51.
91. The Department of Veterans Affairs Laryngeal Cancer Study Group. Induction chemotherapy plus radiation compared with surgery plus radiation in patients with advanced laryngeal cancer. *N Engl J Med* 1991; **324**, 1685–90.
92. Final report of the Head and Neck Contracts Program. Adjuvant chemotherapy for advanced head and neck squamous carcinoma. *Cancer* 1987; **60**, 301–11.

# 7 Complications of radiotherapy in the head and neck: an orofacial surgeon's view

*Iain Hutchison*

## Introduction

Most patients with cancers in the head and neck are treated with radiotherapy at some point in their illness. The constant challenge for radiotherapists is how best to eradicate the tumour whilst minimizing damage to normal tissues. In order to prevent and treat this damage it is important to understand both the fundamentals of radiobiology and the methods of administering radiotherapy that are currently employed.

The biological effects of radiation-induced cellular disruption may be manifested in three main ways:

1. in acutely responding cells, cell division may fail either at the first mitosis or after several subsequent mitoses (reproductive death);
2. non-proliferating cells may suffer interphase death and apoptosis; or,
3. cells may remain viable but be unable to perform their normal functions.[1-3]

In the head and neck, early complications at sites of radiotherapy are mainly caused by damage to the acutely responding radiosensitive stem cells of the oral mucosa and skin, although the intermediate-responding salivary acinar cells exhibit damage by the middle of the course of treatment.[4,5] Chronic complications are caused by two mechanisms. First, intermediate-responding cells and tissues such as fibroblasts, periosteum, bone cells and salivary cells suffer damage. Second, presumably due to endothelial cell damage, the intima of small arterioles thickens, reducing the lumen of the vessel.[6] The tissues served by these vessels are therefore inadequately perfused and become hypoxic.

## Radiation techniques and regimens

There are many variations to the standard radiotherapy regime for head and neck squamous cell carcinoma (SCC). The clinician dealing with radiotherapy complications should appreciate these subtle differences which result in ostensibly equivalent regimens producing different levels of morbidity.

Radiotherapists may prefer larger or smaller field sizes, use different numbers of portals for delivering the radiotherapy, provide prophylactic irradiation for node-negative necks, arrange planned breaks in the treatment for rest or surgery, and increase or reduce the total dose by a few grays. The simulation and scanning facilities vary enormously between hospitals. With the most sophisticated equipment, it is possible to reduce the volume of normal tissue treated so that a higher tumour dose can be delivered more accurately.

Some units use markedly different regimens. For example, the Christie Hospital in Manchester, UK, serves a large area in the north-west of England with a population of four million. Partly for logistic reasons, they have pursued a shortened course of treatment, delivering 55 Gy in sixteen fractions over 3 weeks.[7] Recent work analysing cell doubling time with labelled bromodeoxyuridine[8] has prompted studies on continuous hyperfractionated accelerated radiotherapy (CHART), in which 1.5 Gy fractions are given three times a day for 12 days continuously, to a total dose of 54 Gy.[9]

Hypoxic tumour cells are relatively resistant to X-irradiation and radiotherapists and radiobiologists have sought techniques which overcome this factor. Two centres in the UK have employed fast-neutron particulate radiation, which has a better oxygen enhancement ratio (OER) than X-irradiation.[10] Hypoxic cell sensitizers, such as the nitroimidazoles, have also been used in conjunction with conventional X-irradiation.

In addition to the external beam (teletherapy) methods, brachytherapy, using interstitially placed sources, may be used either as an alternative or as a supplement to deliver low-dose-rate radiotherapy within the tumour. Various sources have been used, including radium, caesium, gold and iridium.

Gold, with its short half-life, may be left in the tissues permanently, whilst iridium is left in the tumour for the time of treatment only. Afterloading techniques allow more accurate planning of treatment. Interstitial therapy is particularly useful for tumours in the mobile anterior two-thirds of the tongue, but when tumours are situated close to bone it should be avoided.

In the attempt to unify data, clinicians have developed factors representing the time course of radiotherapy, dose per fraction and total dose as total dose fractionation (TDF),[11] or biologically effective dose (BED).[12] The situation may be complicated further as many centres use adjuvant chemotherapy.[13-15]

All the modifications in radiotherapy mentioned above have been planned. However, there are also sources of human error to be considered. Cobalt-60 decays, and mistakes have been made with the recalibration of this source, resulting in under- and over-dosage of tumours and adjacent tissues.[16]

Radiotherapy is an innovative branch of medicine. However, the major chronic complications of radiotherapy often occur several years after treatment. Caution should therefore be observed in claiming low morbidity for new regimens until this time has elapsed.

## Tumours of the head and neck

Radiotherapy has been used to treat virtually all tumours in the head and neck, and also a group of benign conditions such as postparotidectomy gustatory sweating (Frey's syndrome) and keloid scarring. In situations where surgery is considered technically impractical, radiotherapy may also be recommended for the treatment of tumours such as recurrent skull-base ameloblastoma, which some would regard as radioresistant.

The commonest tumour in the head and neck, squamous cell carcinoma, is radiosensitive. The larynx, floor of the mouth and mobile tongue are the most commonly affected sites in cigarette smokers. However, patients with tobacco- or betel-chewing habits develop tumours where the 'quid' is held in the mouth, commonly the inside of the cheek.

Salivary gland tumours constitute the next commonest group affecting the head and neck, ranging from the benign pleomorphic adenoma to the intermediate-grade mucoepidermoid carcinoma on to the more malignant adenoid cystic and adenocarcinomas. Tumours at the benign end of the range are relatively radioresistant but the adenocarcinomas may be relatively radiosensitive. Lymphomas occurring in the head and neck region are usually radiosensitive. The whole range of sarcomas may occur in the head and neck; these exhibit variable radiosensitivity. Rarer malignancies such as odontogenic tumours and mucosal melanoma are frequently radioresistant.

## Normal-tissue effects

The key to recognition, understanding and treatment of radiation damage in the head and neck is the effect of radiotherapy on normal tissues. All tissues that lie within the radiotherapy field or beam will be affected. Tissues outside the field may also be affected indirectly. For example, teeth outside the field will have a higher incidence of caries (decay) because of the effects of xerostomia on plaque accumulation and oral microflora.[5,17] The damage sustained will vary in relation to total dose, fractionation, field size and placement, radiation source and the radiosensitivity of the specific tissue.

Acute-responding tissues of the stem type, such as oral mucosa and skin, are affected first, suffering reproductive death. When superficial epithelial cells die there are no immediate replacements so, typically, ulceration occurs. Radiotherapy also stimulates an initial inflammatory response with erythema and oedema, which ultimately interferes with blood flow and healing in this early phase.[18]

Intermediate-responding tissues such as salivary acinar cells are affected later, as the total dose of radiotherapy rises. Osteoblasts, osteocytes, fibroblasts, odontoblasts and cementoblasts (hard-tissue-forming cells of the teeth) all fall into this group. They tend to suffer both interphase and reproductive death, which can occur long after the completion of radiotherapy. Vascular endothelial cells are also affected, resulting in intimal thickening (endarteritis obliterans). This contributes significantly to late radiation damage, and the vascular effects are permanent and progressive.

Hard, calcium-containing tissues such as bone and teeth absorb relatively high amounts of radiation in the orthovoltage range because the photoelectric effect predominates. In the megavoltage range, this effect is reduced (the so-called 'bone-sparing' effect of megavoltage radiotherapy). However, bone scatters the radiation beam unpredictably in the large soft-tissue marrow spaces, which may result in excessive doses at these sites.[19]

Closed static populations such as muscle cells suffer late interphase death with fibrosis and shortening of muscle fibres. Nerve cells, if they lie within the radiation beam, will suffer a similar fate. This is particularly relevant when tumours lie close to the brain, spinal cord and eye, and meticulous planning is essential to protect these tissues.

Certain patients seem exquisitely sensitive to radiotherapy. An extreme example of this is the ataxia–telangiectasia syndrome.[20] It may be that other genetic susceptibilities to radiation will be discovered. *In-vitro* studies on the radiosensitivity of patients' fibroblasts offer some hope of detection of susceptible individuals.[21]

# Early radiotherapy complications and their management

These occur during the course of treatment and usually resolve 2–3 weeks after completion of therapy.

## Oral mucositis

Although this complication lasts for only a few weeks, the pain and dysphagia may be so severe that the patient needs admission to hospital for nutritional support. The course of radiotherapy may have to be stopped.

Prior to starting radiotherapy, there are several risk factors for oral mucositis which should be identified and remedied so that this complication is reduced in severity. Patients must be advised to stop smoking and drinking alcohol throughout their course of radiotherapy as continuation of these habits will exacerbate mucositis. Patients may present in a poor nutritional state because of self-neglect or pain from the tumour. A full haematological screen including iron, ferritin and folic acid levels can identify treatable deficiencies but all patients should receive dietary advice and nutritional supplements at the time of diagnosis and treatment planning.

Once radiotherapy has started, soreness may limit tooth cleaning. An oral hygienist should therefore be consulted for the cleaning of all teeth and education in effective self-cleaning prior to radiotherapy. At this appointment, custom-made fluoride carriers should be constructed so that the patient can apply topical fluoride gel (1% neutral sodium fluoride) to the teeth on alternate days. If the patient wears dentures, they should be advised to leave these out of their mouths, except when eating, for the whole radiotherapy course.[22]

Changes in the oral microflora occur during radiotherapy,[5] and gram-negative bacilli and their endotoxins have been implicated in severe mucositis.[23] As a prophylactic measure, Jansma *et al.*[22] recommend a regimen using a combination lozenge of polymyxin, tobramycin, and amphotericin B, four times daily, prior to and during radiotherapy. Joyston-Bechal[24] advises twice-daily mouthwashes with a 0.1–0.2% chlorhexidine solution. Patients should certainly use frequent oral rinses with salt–bicarbonate solutions during radiotherapy to remove viscous secretions.[25] Saliva substitutes and coating agents such as sucralfate suspension[26] will reduce discomfort, and topical anaesthetic agents such as viscous lignocaine or benzydamine rinses[27] are used to reduce pain.

### Radiation dermatitis

This rarely causes such severe problems in the head and neck that radiotherapy must be discontinued.

Barrier and steroid creams, and analgesic and sedative lotions have all been used with mixed success. When moist desquamation develops, topical antiseptic agents, such as aqueous betadine, are applied. Some success in symptom control and wound healing has been reported with hydrocolloid dressings.[28] Occasionally, systemic infection may develop after moist desquamation and contamination with pathogens. Skin cultures determine appropriate antibiotic treatment.

# Late radiotherapy complications and their management

These problems affect the patient for the rest of their life and may be progressive. Their development should be anticipated and preventive strategies introduced before starting radiotherapy.

### Xerostomia (dry mouth)

This complication is fundamentally important not only because of the discomfort associated with dry oral mucosa, but also because of its secondary effects on the oral flora, and dental decay.

Initial symptoms of viscous, sticky saliva may develop after a dose as low as 10 Gy has been administered,[17] and correlate with damage to salivary gland tissue, particularly the serous acinar cells.[4] Both the symptoms and salivary gland structural damage increase with progressively increasing doses of radiotherapy.[29–31] In young patients, salivary secretion may recover to a certain degree, over several years,[32] but in most patients the xerostomia is a permanent effect.[33,34]

The end result is a profound reduction in both resting and stimulated salivary flow, increased salivary viscosity, and a reduction in the pH of saliva into the acidic range.[17] The consequences of this include loss of the normal mechanical cleansing effect of saliva on teeth and a dramatic change in the oral flora, with overgrowth of cariogenic organisms such as *Lactobacillius* spp. *Streptococcus mutans* and *Candida* spp.[5] Plaque deposits containing high concentrations of cariogenic micro-organisms adhere to the cervical margins (necks) of teeth, causing tooth decay at these classic sites. The plaque also irritates the gingiva and periodontium (gums) causing chronic inflammation and destruction of the supporting bone of the teeth.

Xerostomia, in conjunction with direct radiation damage to the taste buds, alters and dulls taste perception. Patients are often unable to tolerate sharp, acidic or spicy foods and fail to perceive all but the highest concentration of sucrose solutions. They may only be able to manage semisolid foods, either because of oral mucosal discomfort, or because of surgical alteration to their teeth, jaws and tongue. In turn, this will restrict them to a bland, liquid diet, denying them one of life's pleasures — interesting food.

It is vital that all patients should see an oral hygienist prior to, during, and at regular intervals after radiotherapy. Their teeth should be scaled and polished by the hygienist regularly, and with the help of disclosing tablets they should be educated in correct, efficient cleaning techniques.[35,36] Specially constructed flexible trays should be made for patients to apply 1% neutral fluoride gels to their teeth for 5 mins on alternate days.[22,34,37] If there is residual functioning salivary tissue, flow may be increased by tactile stimuli such as sugar-free chewing gum, or systemic stimulation using cholinergic agents such as carbacholine[38] or pilocarpine.[39]

Alternatively, neutral pH saliva substitutes containing carboxymethyl cellulose (CMC) or mucin,[40] and applied with atomizers, as required, may reduce the unpleasant symptoms of dryness. Novel modifications include mucin lozenges and reservoirs within dentures. Solutions of 0.1–0.2% chlorhexidine[24] and 5% chlorhexidine gel[41] have been recommended to reduce the volume of oral pathogens, and antifungal lozenges are used intermittently as fungal overgrowth occurs.[5] Recently, butter or vegetable oils have been suggested as coatings for the oral mucosa.[42] The plethora of 'folk' remedies such as salt and soda solutions, camomile and old brown ale attest to the overall failure of conventional therapy.

Strategies aimed at minimizing the initial salivary gland damage have been studied in animals. The preradiotherapy administration of glutathione, a scavenger of free radicals, has reportedly minimized both acute and chronic radiation injury in rat parotid glands.[43]

## Teeth

There is no doubt that the rate of tooth decay and periodontal disease increases dramatically after radiotherapy to the oral cavity, but there has been disagreement over both the pathogenesis of radiation caries and the management of teeth in the radiation field.

It was thought that radiotherapy damaged the hard and soft tissues of the teeth directly, causing increased susceptibility to tooth decay.[44,45] Poyton[46] postulated that radiotherapy might denature the organic component of teeth which would predispose to dissolution of the calcified elements. Gowgiel's study on the macaque rhesus monkey,[47] and Nathanson and Backstrom's[48] research on rabbits demonstrated radiotherapy-induced pulpal fibrosis, but a causal link between this effect and dissolution of the calcified superficial enamel and dentine would be hard to develop.

In fact, Shannon *et al.*'s[49] study on cobalt-60-irradiated enamel and

Hutton *et al.*'s[50] research on irradiated dental pulps in monkeys showed no direct effect of radiotherapy on tooth substance. Furthermore, Frank *et al.*[17] showed that there was no increased incidence of caries if radiation was restricted to the teeth, and the salivary glands were excluded from the fields. Conversely, incidence of caries increased dramatically when the parotid glands were irradiated. The direct effect theory also fails to explain the increased incidence of caries affecting teeth outside the radiation fields. Most authorities now agree that the increased rate of dental decay is caused indirectly by the alterations in salivary flow and composition mentioned in the section 'Xerostomia' above.[37,51]

Radiotherapy directly affects the supporting structures of the teeth, the gingiva, periodontal ligament and bone.[52] The fibres of the periodontal ligament, anchoring the tooth to its adjacent alveolar bone, become hyalinized and irregular, losing their distinctive spatial organization. There is a marked reduction both in cellularity, including osteoblasts and cementoblasts, and also in the numbers and internal diameters of blood vessels.[53] These effects conspire with the increased plaque, and toxins from the microorganisms contained therein, to produce chronic periodontal disease with steady destruction of the bone that supports the teeth.[54] Unless careful attention is given by the patient to the elimination of plaque with correct toothbrushing technique, this chronic disease will cause tooth loss and 'spontaneous' osteoradionecrosis.

If a decision is made to preserve teeth, after careful preradiotherapy planning, four measures must be instituted immediately to reduce late radiation decay and periodontal disease:

1. The patient should be put on a low-sugar diet.
2. Customized fluoride carriers should be made and the patient should apply 1% neutral fluoride gel to their teeth using these carriers for 5 mins on alternate days.
3. The patient should rinse their mouth twice daily with 0.1% chlorhexidine solution to reduce levels of cariogenic oral flora.
4. The patient should see a hygienist for oral care and education, weekly during radiotherapy and monthly thereafter for the first year, relaxing to 3-monthly if the patient's oral hygiene is satisfactory.

Ideally, all these measures should be continued throughout the patient's life.

The next controversy centres on the necessity for tooth extractions. The traditional theory that all teeth in the radiation field should be extracted[55] has long since been discarded as both unnecessary and unacceptable to patients.[56–58] It is impossible to prescribe an absolute regimen for all. The patient's age, existing state of oral hygiene, incidence of caries, and expectations should all be taken into account in planning dental treatment at the preradiotherapy appointment.

All carious teeth should be restored with good-quality amalgam restorations — no overhangs or ledges which trap plaque should be tolerated. It is unwise to perform sophisticated crown or bridgework as radiotherapy increases the risk of restorative failure and osteoradionecrosis (ORN).[59] In exceptional circumstances, effective root canal therapy may be acceptable.[60] Tooth removal is often indicated, but extractions either before,[61] during, or following[62] radiotherapy have all been implicated as major aetiological factors in the pathogenesis of ORN. As a result, there has been considerable debate over the correct timing of extractions in relation to radiotherapy.

Occasional reports have suggested higher incidences of ORN when extractions are performed before radiotherapy, but most experts report that ORN is increased when extractions are carried out at any time after radiotherapy commences, when compared with preradiotherapy extractions.[63-65] Therefore, all teeth which are severely diseased should be extracted at the preradiotherapy planning appointment. Furthermore, it is important to anticipate which teeth might develop problems in the ensuing years; these should also be removed at this pretreatment stage (Fig. 7.1).

Experimental work has demonstrated that it takes 3 weeks for osteoid to form in the sockets, and epithelial repair to be complete after extractions.[66-68] Some authorities therefore advise that 3 weeks should elapse from the time of extractions to the start of radiotherapy.[2] This may be unacceptable to radiotherapists and patients. There have been clinical reports of sockets not healing and ORN developing after a gap of 2 weeks between extractions and radiotherapy. However, in most cases, unless very high doses of radiation are planned, or the patient proves particularly radiosensitive, 2 weeks represents a safe extraction–radiotherapy interval with an acceptably low risk of ORN.[69] This period does not cause undue delay in starting radiotherapy, as planning and mould room work are likely to occupy much of this time. The prescribed guidelines are therefore that a minimum of 2 weeks should elapse between extraction and radiotherapy in all cases, and, wherever possible, this should be extended to 3 weeks.

Most authorities advocate a technique of alveolectomy at extractions.[57,62,69,70] This technique eliminates much of the dead space of the socket; eliminates sharp bony spicules at the edges of sockets which may lacerate oral mucosa; removes alveolar bone which will resorb eventually; and permits edge-to-edge apposition of the oral mucosa which can heal rapidly by first intention. The mucoperiosteum overlying the alveolar bone to be removed must be elevated, but absolutely no more periosteal elevation should be done as this will prejudice the blood supply of the underlying bone. No relieving incisions are necessary or advisable. The historical alternative of simple 'atraumatic' tooth extraction demands organization of the haematoma in the socket and epithelial healing by second intention over a distance of 1 cm above this organizing haematoma. It is clear that this second technique expends more energy, takes a longer time and is likely to result in a higher complication rate than alveolectomy and primary closure.

Despite all precautions, some patients will present with decaying or periodontally involved teeth following radiotherapy. It is possible to perform conventional root canal therapy at this stage without incurring an increased risk of infection in the bone at the apex of the root.[60] The tooth may be decoronated and the root preserved, obviating the need for extraction with its attendant risk of ORN, and improving access to the gingival crevice for effective cleaning. Overdentures can be made to rest on these decoronated roots.[71]

If teeth are affected by chronic periodontal (gum) disease after radiotherapy, then creeping epithelialization may accompany granulation tissue formation in the socket of the tooth. The tooth often exfoliates spontaneously, or with finger pressure by the patient, leaving a full cover of

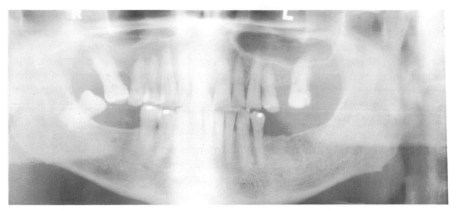

a

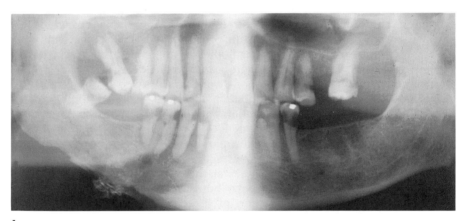

b

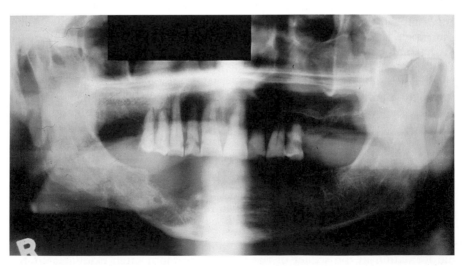

c

epithelium over the shallow socket. However, periodontal disease may also be a source of aggressive bone destruction and ORN.[54]

When teeth must be extracted after radiotherapy, the same process of alveolectomy and primary mucosal closure should be attempted. This is difficult to achieve with single teeth and in the molar regions of the mandible. In these circumstances, it is often necessary to extract several teeth in order to achieve closure. All surgeons agree that such extractions should be performed by the most senior staff experienced in the problems of ORN,[59] and that the operation should be covered by a period of antibiotic therapy, usually lasting 1–4 weeks.[37] Coffin[59] recommended long courses (1 year) of the bone-seeking antibiotic tetracycline. However, when sockets do not heal this probably reflects failure of oral mucosal healing secondary to radiation-induced hypovascularity and tissue hypoxia, rather than bone infection.

Marx *et al.*[72] demonstrated that prophylactic hyperbaric oxygen therapy improved extraction wound healing when compared with antibiotics. However, they had very high levels of ORN following extraction in both groups — 5.4% for the hyperbaric group and 29.9% for the antibiotic group. It is interesting to note that they did not perform an alveolectomy and primary closure was not attempted.

Maxymiw *et al.*[73] advocated the use of non-lignocaine, low adrenaline concentration local anaesthetic for extractions, with antibiotic cover provided preoperatively and for 1 postoperative week. They reported no cases of ORN. However, lignocaine and adrenaline have a local tissue effect for a very short period only and neither substance is likely to prejudice permanent wound healing in the head and neck.

To summarize, all teeth that require extraction should be removed with alveolectomy and primary closure at least 2 weeks before radiotherapy is commenced. After radiotherapy, teeth should be conserved, where possible, using endodontics and periodontal disease control. If tooth extraction is necessary, this should be covered with antibiotics for 2–4 weeks, alveolectomy should be performed and primary closure achieved. If hyperbaric oxygen is available, its use should be considered before, and for a short period following, tooth removal.

Dentures may cause mucosal irritation and ulceration leading to ORN.[74] After tooth extraction, at least 9 months should elapse for bone remodelling before new dentures are fitted.[69] During radiotherapy, the patient should only wear dentures for meals.[22] Soft-lining materials may be counterproductive because they drag on the oral mucosa[69] and are colonized by, and act as a reservoir for, oral flora.

**Fig. 7.1**  This sequence of radiographs was taken at yearly intervals on a patient who underwent external beam radiotherapy to a total dose of 60 Gy over 6 weeks for a floor-of-mouth carcinoma. (a) This orthopantomogram (OPG) was taken prior to radiotherapy. It was considered that no teeth required extraction. (b) The patient was not scrupulous in his oral hygiene and by 1 year postradiotherapy he had developed marked radiation caries and spontaneous osteoradionecrosis of the right mandibular body. (c) Two years following radiotherapy his teeth were removed. By this stage he had developed an orocutaneous fistula and marked separation at a pathological fracture site.

## Trismus (limitation of mandibular opening)

Radiotherapy fields used in the management of tumours of the pharynx, maxilla and posterior oral cavity (e.g. base of the tongue) invariably pass through the muscles of mastication, notably the masseter, medial pterygoid and temporalis. Although muscle cells are resistant to reproductive death, they suffer interphase death at higher radiation doses. This damaged tissue is repaired with dense, disorganized collagen. The result is progressive fibrosis and limitation of mandibular opening.

If patients develop severe restriction of jaw movement they will be unable to maintain good oral hygiene, thereby compounding the risk of radiation caries and subsequent ORN. Their diet will also be impoverished.

The best management of this problem is prevention. At the preradiotherapy appointment, the patient should be educated in mouth-opening exercises. Simple wooden spatulae may be used as wedges between the canine and premolar teeth, if these are present. Alternatively, spring-loaded devices are available.[75] These operate with an opening force which the patient has to resist with their mouth-closing muscles. The advantage of this method is that it can be used in edentulous patients. The exercises should be performed twice daily throughout the patient's life.

If the patient does develop shortening of the working length of the muscles, then exercises will not increase this opening. There is no effective medical treatment for this condition, although electrotherapy and hyperbaric oxygen have been tried.[76] The only option at this stage is surgical. I recommend bilateral mandibular coronoidectomies (to detach temporalis from the mandible) and division of fibrous bands on the deep surface of the masseter to increase mandibular opening. This increase must be maintained using painful intensive opening exercises for 5 mins every hour for the first 2 weeks postoperatively, reducing to 2-hourly for the next 4 weeks. The frequency of exercises may be reduced gradually over the next 5 months until the patient needs to exercise only twice a day to maintain their mouth opening.

## Soft tissue necrosis

This refers to late ulceration of soft tissue where no underlying bone is exposed. Sites affected include the tongue and cheek mucosa. The adjacent area is often indurated because of radiation fibrosis of the underlying connective tissues, sometimes causing diagnostic confusion since the ulcer may be mistaken for recurrent squamous cell carcinoma. It is wise not to proceed immediately with biopsy, but to wait 1–2 weeks to see whether the lesion is progressive. If there is continued doubt, then a small biopsy should be taken from the margins of the ulcer. The fibrosis may occasionally cause reduced mobility — for example, if the cheek is affected, the patient may not be able to open the mouth widely.

Historically, carotid artery rupture was a life-threatening example of soft tissue necrosis. It would usually be heralded by small bleeds prior to massive haemorrhage and exsanguination. With modifications in neck incisions (such as the MacFee approach) and cover with vascularized muscle flaps, this terrifying complication is now exceedingly rare.

The pathogenesis is mainly tissue hypoxia secondary to endarteritis obliterans and reduced vascularity. Ulcers may develop spontaneously if cell replacement cannot keep pace with cell loss. Alternatively, minor trauma from roughened teeth or dentures may precipitate an increased demand for energy to repair the tissue, which cannot be met, and a chronic wound develops. The ulcer may epithelialize eventually, but the correct tissue contour is rarely restored and tissue pits remain. Topical anaesthetic solutions, such as viscous lignocaine, can be used to control pain, and topical antiseptics, such as 0.1% chlorhexidine, should be used to reduce bacterial colonization.

Hyperbaric oxygen has been used successfully to heal pelvic soft tissue radionecrosis,[77] although its use in the head and neck has been mainly limited to osteoradionecrosis.[78] A pilot study using pentoxifylline, an agent which improves blood flow through capillaries, has shown promising results in healing soft tissue necrosis in the oral cavity.[79]

Other chemical and physical methods of promoting neovascularization have been studied in animals, with mixed results. Eppley *et al.*[80] conducted research on basic fibroblast growth factor in irradiated rabbit mandibles. They demonstrated increased blood vessel density in the soft tissues around graft sites. Rezvani *et al.*[81] studied the effect of multiwavelength light on radiation-induced dermal necrosis in the pig. This technique had little success.

## Osteoradionecrosis (ORN)

ORN is the most devastating complication of radiotherapy in the head and neck. It affects the mandible most frequently, but all bones within the radiation beam can be affected including the maxilla, temporal bone82 and zygoma. It can cause intractable pain, necessitating opiates for its control, and the patient may develop pathological fractures and orocutaneous fistulae. Deaths have been reported due to ORN.2,83 This section will describe ORN of the mandible unless otherwise stated. The principles of management of ORN at all sites are much the same.

### *Definition*

The earliest reports simply described the symptoms, signs and pathology of ORN. Titterington provided one of the first definitions in 1971: 'Osteomyelitis of irradiated bone'.84

In 1979, Beumer et al.69 redefined mandibular ORN as follows: 'When bone in the radiation field was exposed for at least 2 months in the absence of local neoplastic disease'; however, in 1983, they modified their own definition to: 'bone exposure of at least 3 months duration at an extraction site following removal of teeth within the radiation field'.64 Morrish et al., in 1981,85 included mucosal ulceration in their definition, and supported a minimum duration of 3-months jaw bone exposure.

Marx, in his seminal paper on the pathophysiology of ORN, defined ORN as 'an area greater than 1 cm. of exposed bone in a field of irradiation that had failed to show any evidence of healing for at least 6 months'.86 However, Marx and Johnson modified the definition later: 'An exposure of non-viable irradiated bone which fails to heal without intervention'.2 Both Beumer and Marx commented that the definition required clarification. In 1990, Friedman recognized that the substitution of signs and symptoms for a tight definition, and the lack of a universally accepted definition, created problems with incidence recording.87 The absence of an unequivocal diagnostic test (see also section 'Investigation', below) means that the definition must be based solely on symptoms and signs. Agreement and understanding of the pathogenesis (see section 'Pathogenesis', below) helps in formulating a definition.

The few authors who have defined ORN have provided several consistent criteria in their definitions: previous irradiation to the site; absence of recurrent neoplasia at the site; and mucosal breakdown or failure to heal, resulting in bone exposure.

The major difference in definition has been over the minimum time course of bone exposure before ORN can be said to exist. It occurs after trauma such as tooth extraction, other surgical procedures, irritation from dentures, or even spontaneously when there has been no history of trauma. The normal healing time of extraction sockets, or other surgical wounds, in non-irradiated tissue varies with age and general health, but is normally completed after 1 month. There should therefore be no bone exposure after this period. It is unreasonable to defer a diagnosis of, and therefore treatment for, ORN until 6 months have elapsed. Conversely, if the minimum period of bone exposure is too short, ORN will be overdiagnosed in patients where spontaneous healing might still occur. Small mucosal dehiscences can still be associated with bone destruction. In my own view, the definition of ORN should therefore be 'exposed bone in the mouth or on the face for more than two months in a previously irradiated field in the absence of recurrent tumour.'[88]

This definition only applies to the maxilla or mandible. The temporal bone may be exposed either onto the face and head or into the ear. Other bones that lie within thick soft tissue integuments, such as the pelvis or femur, may develop symptomatic ORN without being exposed.

Patients may develop a pathological fracture of the mandible after irradiation, with no overlying bone exposure. The patient will experience pain when the two bone ends move against each other. This condition, when no mucosal dehiscence occurs, represents an exceedingly rare exception to the definition. As the bone ends resorb, the patient's pain diminishes.

## Classification of severity

There is a spectrum of disease severity in ORN. Some cases heal spontaneously, whilst others exhibit progressive destruction. Once again, the lack of an adequate investigative tool has prevented objective assessment of the volume and degree of tissue damage. All attempts at classification have therefore relied on the history and clinical progression of the disease, or its response to treatment. These necessitate prolonged periods of observation or the empirical use of treatment protocols.

Daly *et al.* staged bone necrosis in 1972 but omitted to mention how they classified these stages.[74] Marx, in 1983, used a staging classification for treatment.[89] Morton subdivided ORN into *minor, moderate* and *major.*

*Minor* 'consisted of ulceration with exposed bone . . . which healed spontaneously over a period of months'. *Moderate* 'healed spontaneously or with conservative treatment within 6 months to a year'. *Major* involved 'large areas of exposed bone . . . often rapidly progressive lasting in excess of one year and often requiring radical treatment'.[7]

Epstein *et al.*, in 1987, classified ORN into Stages I–III, where I represents healed ORN, II is chronic persistent ORN, and in III the disease process is active with progressive destruction. They subdivided these stages according to whether a pathological fracture was (a) absent or (b) present.[90]

### Incidence

Reported incidences have varied from 1% to 44%.[59,91] Although certain tumour sites in the mouth are associated with relatively high incidence rates, and different radiotherapy and oral prevention regimens contribute to alterations in incidence rates between centres, other factors may affect these figures.

No clinician relishes complications, and courage is required to report these on one's own patients. The absence of a widely accepted definition allows confusion in the recognition of ORN which may contribute to underreporting at some centres.

Patients may be lost to follow-up, particularly since ORN may develop many years after radiotherapy. In these cases, there is often a failure to report the complication. This potential confusion is best illustrated by a series of papers from the MD Anderson Hospital, Houston, TX, which examined overlapping groups of patients from 1964 to 1975 and yet recorded incidence rates of ORN varying from 14% to 34%.[56,58,61] Larson et al. commented that 'this discrepancy appears to be related to our longer follow-up period and a smaller number of anatomic sites'.[56]

The most reliable reports on incidence are therefore likely to be prospective studies rather than retrospective case findings. Horiot *et al.* examined the effects of their preventive protocol in minimizing complications in [528] patients, and recorded an incidence of ORN of 2%.[37] Morrish *et al.* conducted a prospective study on 100 patients and noted a 22% incidence of ORN.[85] However, the minimum follow-up on these patients was only 6 months, which is inadequate to pick up all cases of ORN. Kluth *et al.* followed up patients for 18 months and reported a 10% rate of ORN.[92]

With careful preradiotherapy assessment and treatment and intensive post-therapy oral hygiene, it should be possible to reduce the incidence rate of ORN to between 5% and 10%.

### Pathogenesis

The titles given to ORN in the past illustrate the evolution of theories on its pathogenesis and treatment. Radiation osteomyelitis,[93] septic osteoradionecrosis,[94] radio-osteomyelitis,[95] and osteomyelitis secondary to radiation,[84] all imply an infective process of bone.

Early workers studied the histology of end-stage ORN. They noted the bone changes of reduced cellularity, loss of osteocytes and osteoblasts, and replacement of marrow with fibrous tissue, concluding that these were the primary pathogenic factors.[47,52,96] It was thought that trauma to the ovelying soft tissues then allowed the ingress of oral micro-organisms which grew apace in this hypocellular environment, producing a virulent osteomyelitis. This theory of radiation, trauma and infection[93] formed the basis of the original medical and surgical treatments. Long courses of antibiotic therapy were used, particularly with bone-seeking antibiotics such as tetracycline, with mixed results. When this medical treatment failed, the surgical philosophy was to eradicate all the infected and potentially infected bone by mandibulectomy.[97] However, studies on the progression of radiation damage prior to ORN have resulted in a dramatically altered theory of the pathogenesis of ORN.[6] MacLennan regarded avascularity and necrosis as primary events in ORN and mentioned endarteritis as a pathognomonic sign of radionecrosis.[55] Hart and Mainous, in 1971,[98] stated that ischaemia from progressive endarteritis obliterans was the primary cause for radiation necrosis. Marx, in 1983,[86] challenged the concept of an infective osteomyelitis in irradiated bone. Although micro-organisms could be demonstrated in superficial exposed bone, he was unable to culture any micro-organisms from deep mandibular bone specimens in patients with ORN. However, his work was opposed in the same year by Happonen et al., who used immunocytochemistry to show Actinomyces israelii in all five of their specimens of ORN.[99] In my own studies on deep bone from ORN patients, irradiated non-ORN patients, and ORN patients with orocutaneous fistulae, no Actinomyces spp. were found. The only difference in cultures from non-ORN and ORN bone specimens was a slight increase in Candida spp. in ORN bone specimens (Fig. 7.2). Staphylococcus aureus was isolated in more of the cases with fistulae. It was concluded that ORN was not an infective osteomyelitis.[100,101]

Marx proposed that the primary event in the development of ORN was

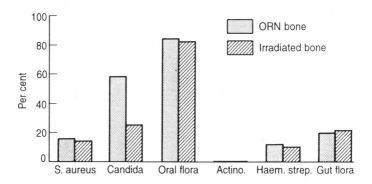

**Fig. 7.2**   This bar chart depicts the culture results from deep mandibular ORN specimens and from deep, irradiated but non-ORN mandible removed at surgery. All bone specimens will have been contaminated by oral flora at surgery. No Actinomyces spp. were cultured from any specimen. There was no difference in cultures of pathogens such as Staphylococcus aureus, haemolytic streptococci and gut flora between the two groups of specimens. Candida spp. were grown from more ORN specimens. We concluded from these results that ORN was not an osteomyelitis of deep bone.

endarteritis obliterans causing reduced vascularity and tissue hypoxia. The combination of hypoxia, and radiation-induced reproductive and interphase cell death conspired to produce a hypocellular environment. He postulated that tissues were either unable to maintain normal cell turnover when a spontaneous wound resulted, or that the tissues were unable to meet the increased energy demands posed by trauma.[86] Any wound would therefore exhibit slow or absent healing. He believed that micro-organisms only acted as superficial contaminants.

Although this theory has gained wide acceptance, and medical treatment is now aimed at improving vascularity, there is still a belief that ORN is primarily a disease of radiation-damaged bone. This is reflected in current surgical management. Continuity-violating resections of the mandible (hemimandibulectomy) are still the standard treatment.[89,102] The logic for this is unclear if the bone is not infected, but merely superficially contaminated.

I have proposed an alternative hypothesis, drawing on the reduced vascularity theory, but suggesting that ORN is mainly due to radiation damage of the soft tissue integument resulting in soft tissue breakdown and bone exposure.[101,103] All tissues that lie within the radiation field will become hypovascular and hypocellular. The mandible and maxilla have only a very thin covering of mucoperiosteum intraorally, which is easily breached. When these soft tissues break down, the cariogenic micro-organisms found in the irradiated mouth can then destroy superficially exposed bone by acid production in a manner analogous to tooth decay. I believe that the symptoms of ORN — pain, bad odour and bone destruction — are all due to the bone exposure created by soft tissue damage. In fact, most authorities have noted that breakdown of the soft tissues overlying bone is a prerequisite for the development of ORN.

From the point of view of treatment, this theory requires only restoration of soft tissue cover; there is no need for wholesale resection of bone. Superficial necrotic bone is debrided and the remaining mandibular rim is covered with vascularized soft tissue flaps which have a well-defined axial blood supply. This method has been applied successfully even in ORN patients with pathological fractures and orocutaneous fistulae (Figs 7.3 and 7.4).[103]

## Aetiology

The factors responsible for the development of ORN fall into three main categories: tumour-related; radiotherapy-related; and trauma-related.

There is debate over whether tumour size is directly proportional to the risk of developing ORN. Bedwinek et al.[61] and Rankow and Weissman[70] found that larger tumours were associated with a higher incidence of ORN, whilst Murray et al.[58] and Epstein et al.[62] found no correlation at all. All clinicians agree that if the tumour is adjacent to bone, such as on the alveolus or in the mouth floor, there is an increased incidence of ORN.

There is universal agreement that high total doses, short regimens using high doses per fraction, large field sizes, and the delivery of radiotherapy through a single homolateral field are all associated with an increased risk of ORN. Morrish et al.[85] found no cases of ORN when the total radiation dose to bone was less than [65] Gy. Murray et al.,[58] studying tumour doses,

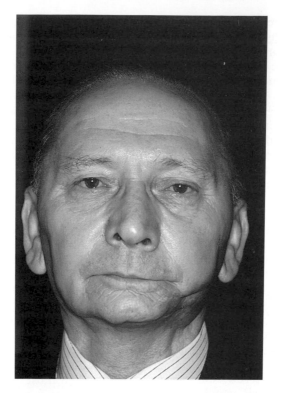

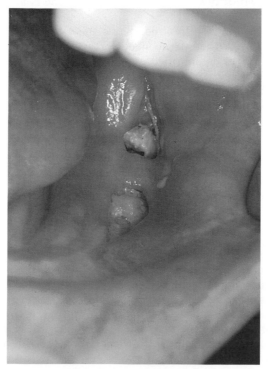

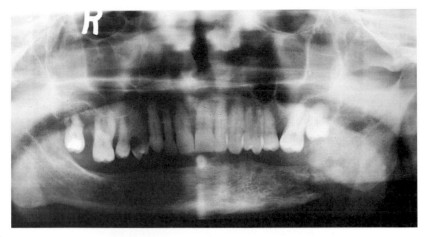

c

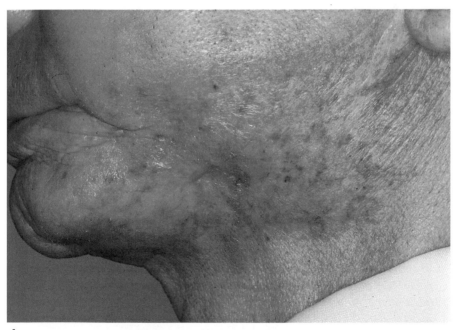

d

**Fig. 7.3**  This patient developed ORN at the left mandibular angle 10 years after fast neutron therapy for a mucoepidermoid tumour of the tongue. He suffered pain and developed a pathological fracture with an orocutaneous fistula through his papyrus-like skin. (a) Full face; (b) intraoral view of exposed bone; (c) OPG showing pathological fracture; (d) view of left face and neck with fistula. Medical treatment was unsuccessful. He underwent debridement of necrotic bone (not mandibulectomy). Intraoral cover was achieved with a temporalis muscle flap and the facial skin was replaced with a superficial temporal island flap which was tunnelled subcutaneously.

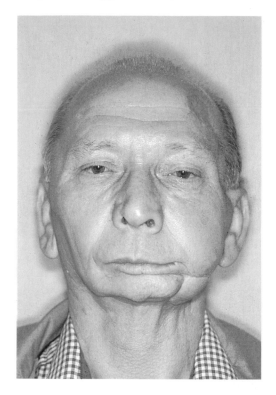

a

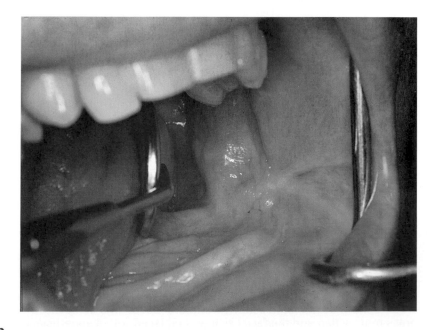

b

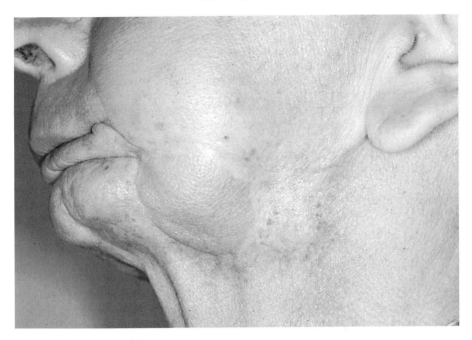

c

**Fig. 7.4** Photograph of patient taken 5 years after surgery. He has remained free of pain and has been able to eat a relatively normal diet over this period. He has no exposed bone or fistulation but his fracture has not united. (a) Full face; (b) intraoral; (c) close-up view of left side of the neck.

saw no cases of ORN with doses less than 40 Gy, and an incidence of 6% with doses between 40 and 50 Gy, increasing to 14% from 50 to 60 Gy. Low energy radiation has caused increased incidence rates of ORN. Although interstitial therapy is safer than external beam when tumours are situated well away from bone, it is associated with an exceedingly high incidence of ORN when used in tumours immediately adjacent to bone.

The use of fast neutrons is now known to cause very high rates of particularly severe ORN and soft tissue necrosis, which is almost impossible to manage medically.[10,104] Hypoxic cell sensitizers such as hyperbaric oxygen and the nitroimidazoles have been associated with an increased risk of ORN. Inaccurate planning and calibration of sources, and inadequate shielding of normal tissues all predispose to an increased risk of normal-tissue damage.[105,106]

Poor oral hygiene and periodontal (gum) disease have been noted as significant risk factors in dentate patients.[92] This may account for some cases of spontaneous ORN. Trauma from dentures accounts for a small percentage of ORN cases in most series. Marunick and Leveque noted trauma from unusual masticatory habits as a cause in three cases of ORN.[107]

The combination of radical neck dissection, either pre- or postradiotherapy, has been regarded as a surgical factor precipitating mandibular ORN.[51] This is because the facial artery, which is usually ligated in the radical neck dissection, supplies a significant proportion of the mandibular blood supply in the older age group, through periosteal vessels.[108,109] Mandibulotomy, when the mandible is divided at the beginning and fixed with metal plates at the end of the operation, is a well-recognized means of gaining access to oral tumours.[110] The siting of the mandibulotomy in the middle of the radiation field in either the pre- or postradiotherapy patient is a recipe for disaster (Fig. 7.5). In posterior tumours, a midline mandibulotomy is safe; with anterior tumours, mandibulotomy should be avoided.

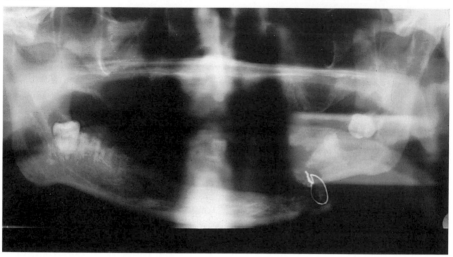

**Fig. 7.5** This man underwent surgery to remove recurrent tumour from the left floor of his mouth several months after radical radiotherapy. A manibulotomy was used in the middle of the radiation field directly over the recurrent tumour. This mandibulotomy failed to heal and resulted in an oro-cutaneous fistula and facial deformity.

The major surgical cause of ORN is dental extraction, carried out either less than 1 week before starting radiotherapy, or after the conclusion of radiotherapy (see section 'Teeth', above). Radiation contributes to this problem in two ways: first, xerostomia predisposes to a greatly increased rate of tooth decay; and second, when teeth are removed, the endarteritis obliterans reduces the tissue's ability to heal.

Kluth *et al.* have noted a significantly increased risk of ORN in those patients who continue to smoke tobacco and imbibe large amounts of alcohol after radiotherapy.[92]

### Investigation

The ideal investigation would determine the degree and extent of radiation damage of bone and soft tissue quantitatively. This would allow objective comparison of the damage caused by different radiotherapy regimens, exact determination of the risk of development of ORN, monitoring of the progress of ORN or its treatment, and comparison between different ORN treatment regimens. It might also determine those patients who would ultimately need surgical treatment for their ORN so that prolonged, ineffective medical treatment could be avoided in these patients.88

Unfortunately, plain radiography always underestimates the extent of radiation-damaged bone. Ardran noted that 30% of bone mineral must be lost before any radiographic change can be seen.111 Furthermore, several authorities have recognized that the extent of radiation-damaged bone is far greater than the visible ORN. Parulekar and Paonessa described this irradiation damage as osteoradioatrophy; aseptic osteoradionecrosis denoted more advanced pathology, and if the bone became exposed (ORN), allowing the introduction of micro-organisms, they used the term septic osteoradionecrosis.94 Marx and Johnson commented that ORN represented the end-product of radiation tissue injury.2 The irradiated but non-ORN bone is at risk of developing ORN itself. It would be useful to quantify this risk.

Two main methods of investigation are currently used: imaging and biological studies. The cheapest and most readily available image is the orthopantomogram (OPG) which can be supplemented by a variety of intraoral and extraoral radiographs.

Computed tomography (CT) scanning offers little more information than conventional radiography in ORN of the mandible and maxilla, but is of help with deep-seated ORN such as that affecting the temporomandibular joint and temporal bone. Magnetic resonance imaging (MRI) is helpful with soft tissue problems and deep-seated ORN, but once again provides little more information on mandibular bone damage than the OPG.

Claims have been made that positron emission tomography (PET) can differentiate between ORN and recurrent tumour.[112] This may be possible in some cases, but my personal experience has been that the results are often equivocal.

The radionuclide technetium methylene diphosphonate ($^{99m}$Tc-MDP) is thought to localize at sites of actively mineralizing bone with a good blood flow.[88] Cox has shown that uptake of $^{99m}$Tc-MDP falls to subnormal levels as little as 7 months after radiotherapy has finished.[113] However, ORN is marked by an increased rate of uptake and total uptake of $^{99m}$Tc-MDP relative to adjacent bone (Fig. 7.6).[88] This would normally imply that ORN bone has a good blood supply and is actively forming new bone, neither of which hold true. It is clear that some, as yet unexplained, mechanism accounts for this anomaly. The radionuclide bone scan is non-specific.

Marx used transcutaneous oxygen measurements to document improved tissue perfusion after hyperbaric oxygen therapy.[89] However, this cannot provide information on the whole tissue volume affected.

Near infrared spectroscopy (NIRS) has shown that sites of ORN are marked by decreased levels of deoxygenated haemoglobin (Fig. 7.7).[114] In the future, NIRS could be used to record sites of ORN but the technique is not readily available. It might also be possible, using the Fick principle and with increased refinement, to measure blood flow *in vivo* non-invasively.

Currently, the only investigation that provides consistent, well-recognized changes in mandibular ORN is plain radiography.

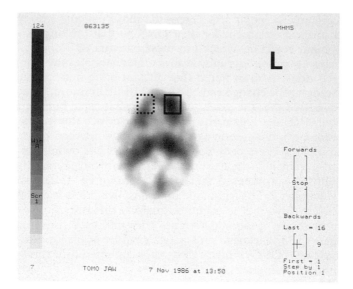

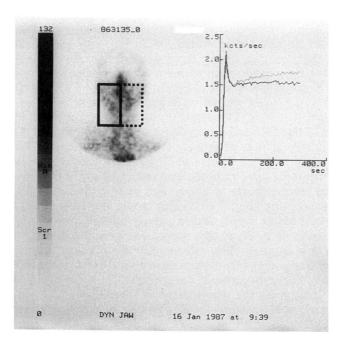

**Fig. 7.6**   The uptake of [99m]Tc-MDP can be quantified allowing more objective comparison between ORN and non-ORN sites. (a) Absolute uptake can be counted in two comparable sites in the mandible using cuts 1 pixel thick. This shows increased uptake, even at the centre of ORN, on the patient's left side. (b) Incremental measurement of uptake can be acquired at 5-s intervals for 5 mins. From these data, the rate of uptake of radionuclide can be measured and recorded graphically. ORN sites are marked by an increased rate of uptake compared with normal.

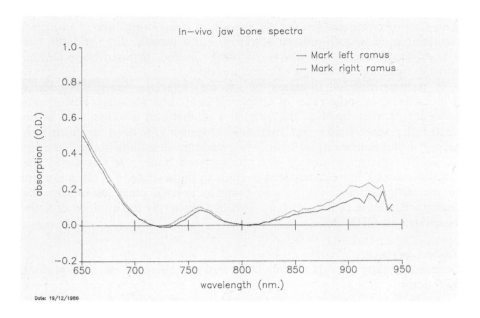

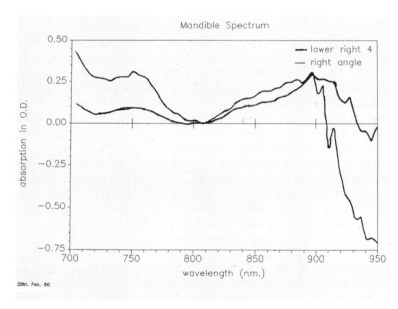

**Fig. 7.7** Absorption spectra produced by transmitting light in the near infrared band (700–1200 nm) through the facial tissues show peaks at 760 nm (deoxygenated haemoglobin) and 900 nm (oxgenated haemoglobin). (a) In this normal subject, spectra taken from opposite sides of the mandible show coincident peaks at 760 nm. (b) In this patient, the 760 nm peak (deoxygenated haemoglobin) is reduced at the site of osteoradionecrosis (ORN) compared with a non-ORN site. ORN seems to be marked by reduced amounts of deoxygenated haemoglobin compared with normal tissues.

### Treatment

The aims of treatment are the elimination of pain, improvement in mouth function (good speech and an ability to eat a normal diet) and the prevention of deformity (all fistulae should be closed, exposed bone covered and the mandible should be of normal shape).

It has been difficult to assess the success of various treatments because it is known that some cases of ORN will heal spontaneously. Historically, medical treatment involved the avoidance of chemical irritants, such as hot drinks and spicy foods, and mechanical trauma, for example from dentures.[70] Long courses of antibiotics were administered and topical antiseptic sedative dressings applied over the exposed bone.[70] It was noted that ORN bone took inordinately long periods to sequestrate.[115] This is not due to the indigestibility of irradiated bone as normal chick osteoclasts can resorb ORN bone *in vitro*.[116] It is probably caused by the absence of active osteoclasts in ORN bone.

### Medical treatment

Current therapy can be subdivided into pharmaceutical and physical methods.

Antibiotics still have a role as a prophylactic measure at the time of dental extractions and surgery, and for treatment of frank infection which is manifested by pronounced erythema of the soft tissue, discharge of pus and orocutaneous fistulae. Antibiotics rarely, if ever, cure ORN.

Promising results have been reported from preliminary studies on drugs which improve blood flow, or stimulate new vessel formation and bone growth. Basic fibroblast growth factor, when given prior to bone grafting, was shown to improve vascularity in the irradiated soft tissue bed, in the bone graft placed in this bed, and to reduce the risk of bone graft failure in rabbits.[80] Pentoxifylline has been used to heal the wounds of soft tissue radionecrosis of the oral mucosa.[79] Dambrain and Barrelier have reported success with calcitonin treatment in ORN.[117]

The physical methods have been chosen on the basis of their ability to stimulate angiogenesis, promote collagen formation and maturation, and to improve wound healing. Hyperbaric oxygen therapy (HBO) has been subject to the closest scrutiny and all reports have been favourable. Hart and Mainous treated forty-six patients with mandibular ORN using adjunctive tetracycline and α-tocopherol. The patients received oxygen at 2 atmospheres pressure, 2 hours daily, for sixty treatments. Of these patients, 80% were symptom-free at the end of this treatment; 11% required a further twenty treatments. However, 9% of their patients had a mandibulectomy and 41% of patients required some form of surgery for symptom control.[98]

Mansfield *et al.* treated twelve patients with oxygen at 2.4 atmospheres pressure, 90 mins daily, for an average of seventy-five treatments. Eight patients required sequestrectomy and one needed a bone graft.[118] Marx used a protocol with three stages of treatment. In Stage I, the patient received thirty HBO treatments, at 2.4 atmospheres, for 90 mins daily. If healing did not occur, an alveolectomy was performed with mucosal closure and the patient received a further thirty HBO treatments in Stage II. All failures of Stage II and those patients who presented with pathological fracture or orocutaneous fistulae received thirty treatments, mandibular resection and later bone graft reconstruction (Stage III). Of 58 patients, 15% were cured in Stage I, 14% in Stage II and 70% in Stage III (percentages are as quoted in the original article). In other words, the majority of patients underwent mandibular resection for cure.[89]

McKenzie *et al.* noted a 50% resolution of ORN with HBO treatment, but over half of these patients had undergone a mandibulectomy in conjunction with HBO to achieve this resolution.[119]

It is clear that HBO does not cure all cases of ORN. Furthermore, it is expensive, labour-intensive, hazardous and not readily available.[120] The use of HBO is contraindicated in some conditions, such as chronic obstructive airways disease. Therefore, the search has continued for a therapy which is cheaper and more practicable.

Harris has reported successful treatment of ORN with ultrasound therapy.[121] However, in a randomized study on sixteen ORN patients, comparing antibiotics alone with antibiotics and ultrasound, I found no objective improvement in healing with ultrasound. Barak *et al.* reported on a single case of ORN treated with electromagnetic stimulation.[122]

There has been no published prospective study on ORN therapy. This is partly because there is no objective measure of the severity of disease and no non-invasive quantitative assessment of tissue blood flow and viability by which the success of treatment could be measured. In the absence of a completely successful medical treatment for ORN, all new therapeutic techniques merit investigation. However, until universally accepted criteria for successful treatment can be stated, it will be difficult to evaluate these new therapies.

*Surgical treatment*

The sequence of surgical treatment is usually as follows. Loose bony sequestra are removed with minimal force.[45] This is augmented in some cases by advancement of the local soft tissues to achieve primary closure. The wound thus created frequently breaks down exposing further bone.[123]

The next stage in treatment is debridement of the superficial bone until bleeding cancellous bone is encountered. The cortical plates never bleed in ORN patients. Granulations form over these pockets of viable marrow and occasionally the surface of these granulations slowly epithelializes to achieve mucosal closure. Hahn and Corgill developed this further by drilling multiple holes through necrotic cortical plates until bleeding occurred. They reported this technique in two patients, one of whom required a distant soft tissue flap to achieve closure.[124]

If ORN persists, the full thickness of mandible is then resected back to healthy bone (mandibulectomy).[70] In these cases, collapse of the face can create severe functional disability and deformity if no reconstruction is performed, although the irradiated fibrotic soft tissues do help in reducing this tendency to collapse.[123]

Marx and Ames have listed criteria for successful bone grafting of the ensuing defect: restoration of bony continuity, alveolar height, facial form and osseous bulk which is maintained over time; and the elimination of soft tissue deficiencies so that dentures can be worn.[125] Obwegeser and Sailer used an intraoral approach to perform immediate reconstruction with autogenous decorticated bone grafts from the iliac crest and rib.[95] They ultimately achieved success in seven out of ten patients, although five of these seven patients had graft-threatening complications. Marx carried out delayed reconstruction supported by preoperative hyperbaric oxygen therapy. An extraoral approach was used to graft particulate bone and marrow in stainless-steel or allogeneic bone cribs. He reported complete success in all forty-one of his cases.[89]

Over the past two decades, the axial blood supply of muscles, bones and skin has been recognized, studied and applied surgically. There is now a vast armamentarium of cutaneous, myocutaneous, myo-osseous and osteocutaneous flaps which can be transposed over long distances as pedicled flaps. Alternatively, their vascular pedicle can be divided and the artery and vein can be anastomosed to recipient vessels in the neck (microsurgical revascularization or free flaps). These flaps are chosen from sites that have not been irradiated. They have a guaranteed blood supply which will improve the perfusion of the irradiated tissue bed into which they are placed.[126,127] They can therefore be used for immediate or delayed reconstruction without any adjunctive HBO therapy.

Baker reported the successful use of the pectoralis major myocutaneous pedicle flap with and without later bone graft reconstruction after hemimandibulectomy for ORN.[127] Pearlman *et al.* used pedicled pectoralis major and fifth rib, or trapezius and spine of scapula to reconstruct sites of ORN after hemimandibulectomy,[128] whilst Maruyama *et al.* reported on latissimus dorsi and rib.[129]

The literature is replete with microsurgical revascularization techniques for the treatment of ORN after hemimandibulectomy. Iliac crest flaps on the deep circumflex iliac vessels, radial forearm flaps on the radial vessels, scapular flaps on the circumflex scapular vessels and fibula flaps on the peroneal vessels all have their advocates.[130] However, all these reconstructive techniques have presupposed that it is essential to resect the mandible to cure ORN. If ORN represents superficially contaminated bone with soft tissue radionecrosis as the major contributor to bone exposure and symptoms (see section 'Pathogenesis', above), then the aim of treatment can be limited to vascularized soft tissue cover of the bone. The temporalis muscle flap, supplied by the deep temporal vessels, can be used for the posterior oral cavity, whilst the nasolabial flap, supplied by the terminal branch of the facial artery, provides satisfactory cover in the anterior oral cavity. They must not be used if their blood supply has been compromised by previous surgery, and their pedicles should never be divided. If these flaps are not available for use or are impractical, then distant myocutaneous flaps, or occasionally free microvascular cutaneous flaps may be used to cover the bone.

The advantage of retaining the patient's own mandible is maintenance of the correct facial form. The irradiated underlying mandible can behave variably; it may continue to resorb or it may form new bone. The disadvantage compared with bone grafting is inadequate osseous bulk and alveolar height to support denture wearing. Also, it is possible to use metal implants (osseointegration) in vascularized bone flaps to increase denture retention. This is not advisable in the patient's own mandible because of the risks of precipitating ORN once again, and it may not be possible because of lack of bone.

## Cartilage necrosis

Laryngeal necrosis occurs less frequently than ORN. Hyperbaric oxygen therapy has been used with some success, but the patient may ultimately require laryngectomy in severe cases. For a detailed discussion, the reader is referred to Berger *et al.*,[131] Oppenheimer *et al.*,[132] and Feldmeier *et al.*[133]

## Central nervous system necrosis

Radiation necrosis of the eye, brain and spinal cord may occur following radiotherapy for extracranial head and neck neoplasia.[134,135] Fortunately, these complications are rare as the nerve cell necrosis is irreversible. They are prevented by careful planning and shielding of the central nervous system.

# Prevention

ORN probably occurs in about 10% of irradiated patients with head and neck cancer. Its investigation is rudimentary, medical treatment used alone without surgery has limited success, and surgical treatment is technically difficult and expensive. The best management of all radiotherapy complications in the head and neck is prevention.

Prosthetic techniques which shield normal tissue with lead, or pull it out of the radiation beam, should be employed wherever possible.[105,106] Multiple fields should be used in preference to single fields, and, if practical, the major salivary glands should be excluded from the fields. In the future, advances such as 3-D CT planning, and conformal and stereotactic therapy, should enable more normal tissue to be spared whilst focusing radiation on the tumour itself.

Standard prevention protocols should be developed and adopted by all radiotherapy units. Harris reported that 66% of his patients with ORN had not received a dental assessment before radiotherapy.[121] Jansma *et al.*, in 1992, noted that at least 50% of patients were not screened prior to radiotherapy in seven out of twenty Dutch radiotherapy centres.[136] All patients who are due to undergo radiotherapy to the head and neck should be assessed by a team consisting of an oral and maxillofacial surgeon, an oral hygienist, and, if possible, a restorative dentist. Their dental treatment should be carried out at least 2 weeks prior to radiotherapy and they should be monitored by this team during and following radiotherapy.

If tests can be developed to identify particularly radiosensitive patients, alternative therapies can be employed, either alone or in conjunction with lower doses of radiotherapy in this population. New radioprotective agents which can minimize normal tissue damage, and biochemical agents such as growth factors, which stimulate repair and wound healing, should be tested in randomized controlled prospective studies.

Finally, a satisfactory experimental model of ORN should be developed so that it is possible to objectively assess radiation damage, non-invasive investigation of tissue viability, and therapies.

# References

1. Baker DG. The radiobiological basis for tissue reactions in the oral cavity following therapeutic X-irradiation: a review. *Arch Otolaryngol* 1982; **108**, 21–4.
2. Marx RE, Johnson RP. Studies in the radiobiology of osteoradionecrosis and their clinical significance. *Oral Surg, Oral Med, Oral Pathol* 1987; **64**, 379–91.
3. Hall EJ. *Radiobiology for the Radiologist*, 2nd edn. Philadelphia: Harper & Row, 1978.
4. Sodicoff M, Pratt NE, Sholley MM. Ultrastructural radiation injury of rat parotid gland: a histopathologic dose–response study. *Radiat Res* 1974; **58**, 196–208.
5. Brown LR, Dreizen S, Handler S, *et al.* Effect of radiation-induced xerostomia on human oral microflora. *J Dent Res* 1975; **54**, 740–50.
6. Bras J, de Jonge HK, van Merkesteyn JP. Osteoradionecrosis of the mandible: pathogenesis. *Am J Otolaryngol* 1990; **11**, 244–50.
7. Morton ME. Osteoradionecrosis: a study of the incidence in the North West of England. *Br J Oral Maxillofac Surg* 1986; **24**, 323–31.
8. Wilson GD, McNally NJ, Dische S, *et al.* Cell proliferation in human tumours measured by *in vivo* labelling with bromodeoxyuridine. *Br J Radiol* 1988; **61**, 419–22.
9. Saunders MI, Dische S, Grosch EJ, *et al.* Experience with CHART. *Int J Radiat Oncol Biol Phys* 1991; **21**, 871–8.
10. MacDougall RH, Orr JA, Kerr GR, *et al.* Fast neutron treatment for squamous cell carcinoma of the head and neck: final report of Edinburgh randomised trial. *Br Med J* 1990; **301**, 1241–2.
11. Orton CG, Ellis F. A simplification in the use of the NSD concept on practical radiotherapy. *Br J Radiol* 1973; **46**, 529–37.
12. Fowler JF. The linear-quadratic formula and progress in fractionated radiotherapy. *Br J Radiol* 1989; **62**, 679–84.
13. Archibald D, Lockhart PB, Sonis ST, *et al.* Oral complications of multimodality therapy for advanced squamous cell carcinoma of head and neck. *Oral Surg, Oral Med, Oral Pathol* 1986; **61**, 139–41.
14. Posner MR, Weichselbaum RR, Fitzgerald TJ, *et al.* Treatment complications after sequential combination chemotherapy and radiotherapy with or without surgery in previously untreated squamous cell carcinoma of the head and neck. *Int J Radiat Oncol Biol Phys* 1985; **11**, 1887–93.
15. Marcial VA, Pajak TF, Mohiuddin M, *et al.* Concomitant cisplatin chemotherapy and radiotherapy in advanced mucosal squamous cell carcinoma of the head and neck. Long-term results of the Radiation Therapy Oncology Group study 81–17. *Cancer* 1990; **66**, 1861–8.
16. Tobias JS. What went wrong at Exeter? Many patients over-exposed to radiation but only a few at serious risk. *Br Med J* 1988; **297**, 372–3.
17. Frank RM, Herdly J, Philippe E. Acquired dental defects and salivary gland lesions after irradiation for carcinoma. *J Am Dent Assoc* 1965; **70**, 868–83.
18. Berthrong M. Pathologic changes secondary to radiation. *World J Surg* 1987; **10**, 155–70.
19. Shimanovskaya K, Shiman AD. General data on the effect of ionizing radiation on the skeleton. *Radiation Injury of Bone*. New York, Oxford: Pergamon Press 1983; 1–18.
20. Gotoff SP, Amirokri E, Lieber EJ. Ataxia–telangiectasia. *Am J Dis Child* 1967; **114**, 617–25.
21. Burnet NG, Nyman J, Turesson I, *et al.* Prediction of normal tissue tolerance to radiotherapy from in-vitro cellular radiation sensitivity. *Lancet* 1992; **i**, 1570–1.
22. Jansma J, Vissink A, Spijkervet FK, *et al.* Protocol for the prevention and treat-

ment of oral sequelae resulting from head and neck radiation therapy. *Cancer* 1992; **70**, 2171–80.

23. Spijkervet FKL, Van Saene HKF, Van Saene JJM, *et al.* Effect of selective elimination of oral flora on mucositis in irradiated head and neck cancer patients. *J Surg Oncol* 1991; **46**, 167–73.

24. Joyston-Bechal S. Management of oral complications following radiotherapy. *Dental Update* 1992; **19**, 232–4, 236–8.

25. Miaskowski C. Management of mucositis during therapy. *NCI Monogr* 1990; **9**, 95–8.

26. Barker G, Loftus L, Cuddy P, *et al.* The effects of sucralfate suspension and diphenhydramine syrup plus kaolin-pectin on radiotherapy-induced mucositis. *Oral Surg, Oral Med, Oral Pathol* 1991; **71**, 288–93.

27. Samaranayake LP, Robertson AG, MacFarlane TW, *et al.* The effect of chlorhexidine and benzydamine mouthwashes on mucositis induced by therapeutic irradiation. *Clin Radiol* 1988; **39**, 291–4.

28. Margolin SG, Breneman JC, Denman DL, *et al.* Management of radiation-induced moist skin desquamation using hydrocolloid dressing. *Cancer Nursing* 1990; **13**, 71–80.

29. Stephens LC, Ang KK, Schultheiss TE, *et al.* Target cell and mode of radiation injury in rhesus salivary glands. *Radiother Oncol* 1986; **7**, 165–74.

30. Stephens LC, King GK, Peters LJ, *et al.* Unique radiosensitivity of serous cells in rhesus monkey submandibular glands. *Am J Pathol* 1986; **124**, 479–87.

31. Stephens LC, King GK, Peters LJ, *et al.* Acute and late radiation injury in rhesus monkey parotid glands. Evidence of interphase cell death. *Am J Pathol* 1986; **124**, 469–78.

32. Pyykonen H, Malmstrom M, Oikarinen VJ, *et al.* Late effects of radiation treatment of tongue and floor of mouth cancer on the dentition, saliva secretion, mucous membranes and the lower jaw. *Int J Oral Maxillofac Surg* 1986; **15**, 401–9.

33. Liu RP, Fleming TJ, Toth BB, *et al.* Salivary flow rates in patients with head and neck cancer 0.5 to 25 years after radiotherapy. *Oral Surg, Oral Med, Oral Pathol* 1990; **70**, 724–9.

34. Dreizen S, Brown LR, Daly TE, *et al.* Prevention of xerostomia-related dental caries in irradiated cancer patients. *J Dent Res* 1977; **56**, 99–104.

35. Calman FM, Langdon J. Oral complications of cancer. *Br Med J* 1991; **302**, 485–6.

36. Sullivan MD, Fleming TJ. Oral care for the radiotherapy-treated head and neck cancer patient. *Dental Hygiene* 1986; **March**, 112–14.

37. Horiot JC, Bone MC, Ibrahim E, *et al.* Systematic dental management in head and neck irradiation. *Int J Radiat Oncol Biol Phys* 1981; **7**, 1025–9.

38. Joensuu H, Bostrom P, Makkonen T. Pilocarpine and carbacholine in treatment of radiation-induced xerostomia. *Radiother Oncol* 1993; **26**, 33–7.

39. Greenspan D, Daniels TE. Effectiveness of pilocarpine in postradiation xerostomia. *Cancer* 1987; **59**, 1123–5.

40. Visch LL, 's-Gravenmade EJ, Schaub RMH, *et al.* A double-blind crossover trial of CMC — and mucin-containing saliva substitutes. *Int J Oral Maxillofac Surg* 1986; **15**, 395–400.

41. Epstein JB, McBride BC, Stevenson-Moore P, *et al.* The efficacy of chlorhexidine gel in reduction of *Streptococcus mutans* and *Lactobacillus* species in patients treated with radiation therapy. *Oral Surg, Oral Med, Oral Pathol* 1991; **71**, 172–8.

42. Kusler DL, Rambur BA. Treatment for radiation-induced xerostomia. An innovative remedy. *Cancer Nursing* 1992; **15**, 191–5.

43. Arima R, Shiba R. Radioprotective effect of exogenous glutathione on rat parotid glands. *Int J Radiat Biol* 1992; **61**, 695–702.

44. Anneroth G, Holm LE, Karlsson G. The effect of radiation on teeth. A clinical, histologic and microradiographic study. *Int J Oral Surg* 1985; **14**, 269–74.
45. Beumer J III, Brady FA. Dental management of the irradiated patient. *Int J Oral Surg* 1978; 7, 208–20.
46. Poyton HG. The effects of radiation on teeth. *Oral Surg, Oral Med, Oral Pathol* 1968; **26**, 639–47.
47. Gowgiel JM. Experimental radio-osteonecrosis of the jaws. *J Dent Res* 1960; **39**, 176–97.
48. Nathanson A, Backstrom A. Effects of cobalt-60-irradiation on teeth and jaw bone in the rabbit. *Scand J Plast Reconstr Surg* 1978; **12**, 1–17.
49. Shannon IL, Westcott WB, Starcke EN, et al. Laboratory study of cobalt-60-irradiated human dental enamel. *J Oral Med* 1978; **33**, 23–7.
50. Hutton MF, Patterson SS, Mitchell DF, et al. The effect of cobalt-60 radiation on the dental pulps of monkeys. *Oral Surg* 1974; **38**, 279–86.
51. Carl W, Schaaf NG, Sako K. Oral surgery and the patient who has had radiation therapy for head and neck cancer. *Oral Surg* 1973; **36**, 651–7.
52. Silverman S, Chierici G. Radiation therapy of oral carcinoma. Effects on oral tissues and management of the periodontium. *J Periodontol* 1965; **36**, 478–84.
53. Rohrer MD, Kim Y, Fayos JV. The effect of cobalt-60 irradiation on monkey mandibles. *Oral Surg* 1979; **48**, 424–40.
54. Galler C, Epstein JB, Guze KA, et al. The development of osteoradionecrosis from sites of periodontal disease activity: report of 3 cases. *J Periodontol* 1992; **63**, 310–16.
55. MacLennan WD. Some aspects of the problem of radionecrosis of the jaws. *Proc Roy Soc Med* 1955; **48**, 1017–22.
56. Larson DL, Lindberg RD, Lane E, et al. Major complications of radiotherapy in cancer of the oral cavity and oropharynx. A 10 year retrospective study. *Am J Surg* 1983; **146**, 531–6.
57. Guttenberg SA. Osteoradionecrosis of the jaw. *Am J Surg* 1974; **127**, 326–32.
58. Murray CG, Herson J, Daly TE, et al. Radiation necrosis of the mandible: a 10 year study. Part I. Factors influencing the onset of necrosis. *Int J Radiat Oncol Biol Phys* 1980; **6**, 543–8.
59. Coffin F. The incidence and management of osteoradionecrosis of the jaws following head and neck radiotherapy. *Br J Radiol* 1983; **56**, 851–7.
60. Seto BG, Beumer J, Kagawa T, et al. Analysis of endodontic therapy in patients irradiated for head and neck cancer. *Oral Surg, Oral Med, Oral Pathol* 1985; **60**, 540–5.
61. Bedwinek JM, Shukovsky LJ, Fletcher GH, et al. Osteonecrosis in patients treated with definitive radiotherapy for squamous cell carcinomas of the oral cavity and naso- and oropharynx. *Radiology* 1976; **119**, 665–7.
62. Epstein JB, Rea G, Wong FLW, et al. Osteonecrosis: study of the relationship of dental extractions in patients receiving radiotherapy. *Head Neck Surg* 1987; **10**, 48–54.
63. Beumer J III, Harrison R, Sanders B, et al. Preradiation dental extractions and the incidence of bone necrosis. *Head Neck Surg* 1983; **5**, 514–21.
64. Beumer J III, Harrison R, Sanders B, et al. Postradiation dental extractions: a review of the literature and a report of 72 episodes. *Head Neck Surg* 1983; **6**, 581–6.
65. Murray CG, Herson J, Daly TE, et al. Radiation necrosis of the mandible: a 10 year study. Part II. Dental factors; onset, duration and management of necrosis. *Int J Radiat Oncol Biol Phys* 1980; **6**, 549–53.
66. Amler MH. Time sequence of tissue regeneration in human extraction wounds. *Oral Surg, Oral Med, Oral Pathol* 1969; **27**, 307–18.
67. Shearer HT. Effect of cobalt-60 radiation on extraction healing in the mandible of dogs. *J Oral Surg* 1967; **25**, 115–21.

68. Simpson HE. Healing of extraction wounds. *Br Dent J* 1969; **126**, 550–7.
69. Beumer J III, Curtis T, Harrison RE. Radiation therapy of the oral cavity: sequelae and management, Part 2. *Head Neck Surg* 1979; **1**, 392–408.
70. Rankow RM, Weissman B. Osteoradionecrosis of the mandible. *Ann Otol Rhinol-Laryngol* 1971; **80**, 603–11.
71. McDermott IG, Rosenberg SW. Overdentures for the irradiated patient. *J Prosthet Dent* 1984; **51**, 314–17.
72. Marx RE, Johnson RP, Kline SN. Prevention of osteoradionecrosis: a randomized prospective clinical trial of hyperbaric oxygen versus penicillin. *J Am Dent Assoc* 1985; **111**, 49–54.
73. Maxymiw WG, Wood RE, Liu FF. Postradiation dental extractions without hyperbaric oxygen. *Oral Surg, Oral Med, Oral Pathol* 1991; **72**, 270–4.
74. Daly TE, Drane JB, MacComb WS. Management of problems of the teeth and jaw in patients undergoing irradiation. *Am J Surg* 1972; **124**, 539–42.
75. Engelmeier RL, King GE. Complications of head and neck radiation therapy and their management. *J Prosthet Dent* 1983; **49**, 514–22.
76. King GE, Scheetz J, Jacob RF, *et al.* Electrotherapy and hyperbaric oxygen: promising treatments for postradiation complications. *J Prosthet Dent* 1989; **62**, 331–4.
77. Williams JA Jr, Clarke D, Dennis WA, *et al.* The treatment of pelvic soft tissue radiation necrosis with hyperbaric oxygen. *Am J Obstet Gynecol* 1992; **167**, 412–15.
78. Kindwall EP. Hyperbaric oxygen's effect on radiation necrosis. *Clin Plast Surg* 1993; **20**, 473–83.
79. Dion MW, Hussey DH, Doornbos JF, *et al.* Preliminary results of a pilot study of pentoxifylline in the treatment of late radiation soft tissue necrosis. *Int J Radiat Oncol Biol Phys* 1990; **19**, 401–7.
80. Eppley BL, Connolly DT, Winkelmann T, *et al.* Free bone graft reconstruction of irradiated facial tissue: experimental effects of basic fibroblast growth factor stimulation. *Plast Reconstr Surg* 1991; **88**, 1–11.
81. Rezvani M, Nissan M, Hopewell JW, *et al.* Prevention of X-ray-induced late dermal necrosis in the pig by treatment with multi-wavelength light. *Lasers Surg Med* 1992; **12**, 288–93.
82. Nagorsky MJ. Radiation injury of the temporal bone. *Clin Plast Surg* 1993; **20**, 531–4.
83. Hahn LJ. Osteoradionecrosis of the mandible: clinical observation and treatment in 45 cases. *J Formosan Med Assoc* 1983; **82**, 451–60.
84. Titterington WP. Osteomyelitis and osteoradionecrosis of the jaws. *J Oral Med* 1971; **26**, 7–16.
85. Morrish RB, Chan E, Silverman S Jr, *et al.* Osteonecrosis in patients irradiated for head and neck carcinoma. *Cancer* 1981; **47**, 1980–3.
86. Marx RE. Osteoradionecrosis: a new concept of its pathophysiology. *J Oral Maxillofac Surg* 1983; **41**, 283–8.
87. Friedman RB. Osteoradionecrosis: causes and prevention. [Review]. *NCI Monogr* 1990; **9**, 145–9.
88. Hutchison IL, Cullum ID, Langford JA, *et al.* The investigation of osteoradionecrosis of the mandible by 99mTc-methylene diphosphonate radionuclide bone scans. *Br J Oral Maxillofac Surg* 1990; **28**, 143–9.
89. Marx RE. A new concept in the treatment of osteoradionecrosis. *J Oral Maxillofac Surg* 1983; **41**, 351–7.
90. Epstein JB, Wong FLW, Stevenson-Moore P. Osteoradionecrosis: clinical experience and a proposal for classification. *J Oral Maxillofac Surg* 1987; **45**, 104–10.
91. Rahn AO, Drane JB. Dental aspects of the problems, care and treatment of the irradiated oral cancer patient. *J Am Dent Assoc* 1967; **74**, 957–66.

92. Kluth EV, Jain PR, Stuchell RN, *et al.* A study of factors contributing to the development of osteoradionecrosis of the jaws. *J Prosthet Dent* 1988; **59**, 194–201.
93. Meyer I. Infectious diseases of the jaws. *J Oral Surg* 1970; **28**, 17–26.
94. Parulekar SS, Paonessa DF. Septic osteoradionecrosis of the mandible. *Ann Otol Rhinol Largngol* 1980; **89**, 383–7.
95. Obwegeser HL, Sailer HF. Experience with intraoral resection and immediate reconstruction in cases of radio-osteomyelitis of the mandible. *J Maxillofac Surg* 1978; **6**, 257–65.
96. Pappas GC. Bone changes in osteoradionecrosis. *Oral Surg, Oral Med, Oral Pathol* 1969; **27**, 622–30.
97. Friedlander AH, Mazzarella L, Kisner A. Treatment of osteoradionecrosis by transoral hemimandibulectomy: report of case. *J Oral Surg* 1979; **37**, 504–7.
98. Hart GB, Mainous EG. The treatment of radiation necrosis with hyperbaric oxygen. *Cancer* 1976; **37**, 2580–5.
99. Happonen RP, Viander M, Pelliniemi L, *et al. Actinomyces israelii* in osteoradionecrosis of the jaws. *Oral Surg* 1983; **55**, 580–8.
100. Hutchison IL, Kibbler CC. The significance of micro-organisms in osteoradionecrosis of the mandible. *J Dent Res* 1989; **68**, 575.
101. Hutchison IL, Kibbler CC. The microbiology of mandibular radionecrosis and its implications for management. *Br J Oral Maxillofac Surg* 1991; **29**, 413.
102. Koka VN, Deo R, Lusinchi A, *et al.* Osteoradionecrosis of the mandible: study of 104 cases treated by hemimandibulectomy. *J Laryngol Otol* 1990; **104**, 305–7.
103. Hutchison IL. The surgical management of osteoradionecrosis of the jaws. *Br J Cancer* 1991; **64** (Suppl XV), 13.
104. Stafford N, Waldron J, Davies D, *et al.* Complications following fast neutron therapy for head and neck cancer. *J Laryngol Otol* 1992; **106**, 144–6.
105. Poole TS, Flaxman NA. Use of protective prostheses during radiation therapy. *J Am Dent Assoc* 1986; **112**, 485–8.
106. Levendag PC, Visch LL, Driver N. A simple device to protect against osteoradionecrosis induced by interstitial irradiation. *J Prosthet Dent* 1990; **63**, 665–70.
107. Marunick MT, Leveque F. Osteoradionecrosis related to mastication and parafunction. *Oral Surg, Oral Med, Oral Pathol* 1989; **68**, 582–5.
108. Bradley JC. Age changes in the vascular supply of the mandible. *Br Dent J* 1972; **132**, 142–4.
109. McGregor AD, MacDonald DG. Age changes in the human inferior alveolar artery — a histological study. *Br J Oral Maxillofac Surg* 1989; **27**, 371–4.
110. Spiro RH, Gerold FP, Strong EW. Mandibular 'swing' approach for oral and oropharyngeal tumours. *Head Neck Surg* 1981; **3**, 371–8.
111. Ardran G. Bone destruction not demonstrable by radiography. *Br J Radiol* 1951; **24**, 107–9.
112. Minn H, Aitasalo K, Happonen RP. Detection of cancer recurrence in irradiated mandible using positron emission tomography. *Eur Arch Oto-Rhino-Laryngol* 1993; **250**, 312–15.
113. Cox PH. Abnormalities in skeletal uptake of 99mTc polyphosphate complexes in areas of bone associated with tissues which have been subjected to radiotherapy. *Br J Radiol* 1974; **47**, 851–6.
114. Hutchison IL, Cope M, Delpy DT, *et al.* The investigation of osteoradionecrosis of the mandible by near infrared spectroscopy. *Br J Oral Maxillofac Surg* 1990; **28**, 150–4.
115. Yamashiro M, Amagasa T, Horiuchi J, *et al.* Extensive osteoradionecrosis of the mandible associated with new bone formation. *J Oral Maxillofac Surg* 1987; **45**, 630–3.

116. Hutchison IL, Harris M, Boyde A, *et al.* Can radionecrotic bone resorb? Proceedings of the Bone and Tooth Society, March 1988, Oxford; 15 (unpublished).

117. Dambrain R, Barrelier P. La calcitonine dans l'osteoradionecrose mandibulaire. *Acta Stomatol Belg* 1991; **88**, 123–6.

118. Mansfield MJ, Sanders DW, Heimbach RD, *et al.* Hyperbaric oxygen as an adjunct in the treatment of osteoradionecrosis of the mandible. *J Oral Surg* 1981; **39**, 585–9.

119. McKenzie MR, Wong FL, Epstein JB, *et al.* Hyperbaric oxygen and post-radiation osteonecrosis of the mandible. *Oral Oncol, Eur J Cancer* 1993; **29B**, 201–7.

120. Giebfried JW, Lawson W, Biller HF. Complications of hyperbaric oxygen in the treatment of head and neck disease. *Otolaryngol Head Neck Surg* 1986; **94**, 508–11.

121. Harris M. The conservative management of osteoradionecrosis of the mandible with ultrasound therapy. *Br J Oral Maxillofac Surg* 1992; **30**, 313–18.

122. Barak S, Rosenblum I, Czerniak P, *et al.* Treatment of osteoradionecrosis combined with pathologic fracture and osteomyelitis of the mandible with electromagnetic stimulation. *Int J Oral Maxillofac Surg* 1988; **17**, 253–6.

123. Morton ME, Simpson W. The management of osteoradionecrosis of the jaws. *Br J Oral Maxillofac Surg* 1986; **24**, 332–41.

124. Hahn G, Corgill DA. Conservative treatment of radionecrosis of the mandible. *Oral Surg, Oral Med, Oral Pathol* 1967; **24**, 707–12.

125. Marx RE, Ames JR. The use of hyperbaric oxygen therapy in bony reconstruction of the irradiated and tissue-deficient patient. *J Oral Maxillofac Surg* 1982; **40**, 412–20.

126. Mirante JP, Urken ML, Aviv JE. *et al.* Resistance to osteoradionecrosis in neovascularized bone. *Laryngoscope* 1993; **103**, 1168–73.

127. Baker SR. Management of osteoradionecrosis of the mandible with myocutaneous flaps. *J Surg Oncol* 1983; **24**, 282–9.

128. Pearlman NW, Albin RE, O'Donnell RS. Mandibular reconstruction in irradiated patients utilizing myosseous-cutaneous flaps. *Am J Surg* 1983; **146**, 474–7.

129. Maruyama Y, Urita Y, Ohnishi K. Rib–latissimus dorsi osteomyocutaneous flap in reconstruction of a mandibular defect. *Br J Plast Surg* 1985; **38**, 234–7.

130. Buncke HJ. *Microsurgery: Transplantation — Replantation. An Atlas — Text.* Philadelphia, London: Lea & Febiger, 1991.

131. Berger G, Freeman JL, Briant TD, *et al.* Late post radiation necrosis and fibrosis of the larynx. *J Otolaryngol* 1984; **13**, 160–4.

132. Oppenheimer RW, Krespi YP, Einhorn RK. Management of laryngeal radionecrosis: animal and clinical experience. *Head Neck* 1989; **11**, 252–6.

133. Feldmeier JJ, Heimbach RD, Davolt DA, *et al.* Hyperbaric oxygen as an adjunctive treatment for severe laryngeal necrosis: a report of nine consecutive cases. *Undersea & Hyperbaric Medicine* 1993; **20**, 329–35.

134. Glass JP, Hwang TL, Leavens ME, *et al.* Cerebral radiation necrosis following treatment of extra-cranial malignancies. *Cancer* 1984; **54**, 1966–72.

135. Lee AW, Ng SH, Ho JH, *et al.* Clinical diagnosis of late temporal lobe necrosis following radiation therapy for nasopharyngeal carcinoma. *Cancer* 1988; **61**, 1535–42.

136. Jansma J, Vissink A, Bouma J, *et al.* A survey of prevention and treatment regimens for oral sequelae resulting from head and neck radiotherapy used in Dutch radiotherapy institutes. *Int J Radiat Oncol Biol Phys* 1992; **24**, 359–67.

# 8 Issues in the management of adult soft tissue sarcomas

*Hedy Mameghan and Richard Fisher*

## Introduction

Soft tissue sarcomas constitute an ill-defined, heterogeneous group of tumours representing a variety of histological types and originating from a wide range of sites. Certain tumours included in 'soft tissue sarcomas' are epithelial and some are non-mesodermal in origin; sarcomas within the confines of the dura mater are usually not considered in this group.[1] The soft tissues represent over 50% of body weight yet give rise to only 0.7% of all malignant tumours.[1] The incidence rate of malignant tumours of connective and other soft tissues is about 2.5 cases per 100 000 population;[2] and there are approximately 6000 cases per year reported in the USA.[3] Despite decades of clinical experience and numerous published studies, there is still lack of agreement about the most appropriate way to manage sarcomas arising from soft tissues. A patient presenting with this type of tumour requires expert clinical evaluation and treatment. The multidisciplinary approach to management is generally regarded as the approach offering optimal chance of cure for patients presenting with localized disease and worthwhile palliation in those who are clearly incurable.

In this chapter, Kaposi's sarcoma associated with the acquired immune deficiency syndrome (AIDS) epidemic, Ewing's sarcoma arising in soft tissues and paediatric rhabdomyosarcoma have been excluded. The histopathological types of non-rhabdomyosarcoma soft tissue sarcomas appear to be similar in all age groups, although their relative frequencies may vary.[4] The specific aims of the chapter are to describe recent developments concerning the histopathological typing, grading and staging and to review the current opinions and controversies regarding the management of soft tissue sarcoma. With regard to the last aim we will rely mainly on a review of the results of randomized clinical trials.

# Tumour characteristics

## Histopathology

As in most types of cancer, the histopathological nature of the tumour is one of the most important prognostic factors. Pathologists usually classify sarcomas according to the criteria of Enzinger and Weiss[5] which are based on histogenesis, that is the biological potential of the tissues examined.[1] However, there are difficulties in interpretation with regard to classification, grading and reproducibility of the distinct morphologic entities.

There appears to be no universally accepted grading system. The TNM (tumour, node, metastasis) staging manual,[6] for example, refers to four grades: well-, moderately-, poorly- and un-differentiated. More recently, criteria proposed for grading of tumours include both the histological type and degree of necrosis.[1] This system is becoming widely acceptable and is shown in Table 8.1. Other authors[7] prefer a two-grade system, i.e. low-grade and high-grade, the latter combining intermediate and high grades because Grades 2 and 3 are often not distinguished reliably. Non-uniformity in the use of a grading system has implications in the comparison of results from different retrospective reviews and from different centres participating in multi-institutional randomized studies.[8–11]

Another problem with histopathological diagnosis is its reproducibility between pathologists: discordance rates of between 20% and 34% have been reported.[9,10] Tumour grade appears to be more easily reproducible: 72–83% in one study,[9] 60% in the Scandinavian study[10] and 75% in the study of Coindre et al.[12]

## Staging

The TNM system[6] for sarcomas is relatively straightforward. Tumours are classified according to the size, namely the maximum diameter of the primary tumour (T1 is tumour 5 cm or less; T2 is tumour greater than 5 cm), nodal involvement (N0 or N1) and distant metastases (M0 or M1) according to their presence or absence. Because of the variety of possible sites of involvement, there are no definite guidelines as to how far to pursue the investigation of nodal status. Nodal involvement is determined by clinical examination and imaging and should be histologically verified. The incidence of lymph node involvement is, in general, around 2–3%, but it can be higher in certain histological types (approximately 13% in angiosarcoma and embryonal rhabdomyosarcoma and 16% in epithelioid sarcoma[13]).

As a result of cooperation between the American Joint Committee on Cancer (AJCC) and the Union Internationale Contre le Cancer (UICC), the method of clinical staging, based on the TNM staging system,[6] has become universally accepted. The unusual feature of clinical staging in soft tissue sarcomas is that histological grade (G) of the primary is incorporated in its definition. Table 8.2 shows the currently accepted clinical staging system for soft tissue sarcoma.[6] Essentially, in this system the presence of distant metastasis implies Stage IVB; nodal involvement implies Stage IVA; and thereafter, stage is determined by grade (Grades 1,2, 3–4

**Table 8.1**    Grading of soft tissue sarcoma according to Leyvraz and Costa[1]

| Morphological criteria | Specific types |
| --- | --- |
| *Grade 1* | |
| Histological type or subtype | Lipoma-like liposarcoma<br>Myxoid liposarcoma<br>Epithelial haemangioendothelioma<br>Infantile fibrosarcoma |
| Histological type and location | Deep-seated dermatofibrosarcoma protuberans<br>Subcutaneous myxoid malignant fibrous histiocytoma |
| Histological type, mitoses and differentiation | Malignant haemangiopericytoma, well-differentiated<br>Malignant leiomyosarcoma, well-differentiated<br>Malignant neurofibrosarcoma, well-differentiated<br>Malignant fibrosarcoma, well-differentiated<br>Myxoid chondrosarcoma |
| *Grade 2 or 3* | |
| Histological type and necrosis<br>    G2, necrosis 0–15%<br>    G3, necrosis > 15% | Pleomorphic liposarcoma<br>Round cell liposarcoma<br>Fibrosarcoma<br>Malignant fibrous histiocytoma<br>Malignant haemangiopericytoma<br>Synovial sarcoma<br>Epithelial sarcoma<br>Neurofibrosarcoma<br>Leiomyosarcoma<br>Angiosarcoma<br>Unclassified sarcoma |
| *Grade 3* | |
| Histological type | Alveolar rhabdomyosarcoma<br>Neuroblastoma<br>Extraskeletal Ewing's sarcoma<br>Mesenchymal chondrosarcoma |

correspond to clinical stages I, II and III, respectively); Substages A and B of Stages I, II and III are determined by the T stage.

## Prognostic factors

Many prognostic factors have been reported in the literature for recurrence and for survival. The histological grade appears to be the strongest factor for survival but not for local recurrence in virtually all published reports.

**Table 8.2**   TNM stage definitions for soft tissue sarcoma

| Stage | Grade[a] | T | N | M |
|-------|----------|------|-------|-----|
| IA | G1 | T1 | N0 | M0 |
| IB | G1 | T2 | N0 | M0 |
| IIA | G2 | T1 | N0 | M0 |
| IIB | G2 | T2 | N0 | M0 |
| IIIA | G3 or G4 | T1 | N0 | M0 |
| IIIB | G3 or G4 | T2 | N0 | M0 |
| IVA | Any G | Any T | N1 | M0 |
| IVB | Any G | Any T | Any N | M1 |

[a]Grade, as it appears in the TNM handbook, is the four-grade histopathological system of well-, moderately-, poorly-, un-differentiated. Alternatively, it can be interpreted as the three–grade system as given in Table 8.1 by replacing 'G3 or G4' in Stage III with 'G3' (see Yang *et al.*[3]).

Other prognostic factors are: the degree of necrosis,[10,11,14] cellular DNA content,[14,15] location of the primary tumour (extremity, head and neck, trunk, retroperitoneum), size of the primary tumour (T stage),[16–18] Karnofsky score,[19] positivity of surgical margins,[20,21] age[18] and depth of location of the tumour.[18,22]

## Diagnostic imaging

In addition to history and physical examination, imaging studies are essential to assess the size and extent of local tumour infiltration, as well as presence or absence of nodal and distant metastases. Methods of imaging and staging have evolved in the last 30 years: from whole lung tomography and angiography to computed tomography (CT), magnetic resonance imaging (MRI) and radionuclide imaging. The most accurate non-invasive imaging for primary soft tissue sarcomas appears to be MRI and, to a lesser degree, CT.[23,24] The assessment of distant metastases is best done by MRI, CT and gallium scan,[25] all of which may also be useful for follow-up assessment.

# Management

## Surgery

The primary role of surgery in the management of soft tissue sarcomas has remained unchallenged. Surgery is used (a) to obtain an adequate biopsy for histopathological examination, and (b) to remove as much as possible of the primary tumour. One of the major surgical questions in extremity sarcomas has been whether amputation is necessary or whether limb-sparing surgery (LSS) can be employed. Over the past 10 years there has been a trend towards more frequent use of limb-sparing procedures.

### Surgery of primary tumour

'Shelling out' procedures are universally abhorred because subclinical disease is very often left behind within the compressed periphery, the so-called pseudocapsule. A decreasing risk of local recurrence with increasingly more radical resection (simple excision, wide excision, *en-bloc* resection, compartmental resection and amputation) has been documented.[20] Because of this, simple excision and wide excision are usually not recommended.[20] Radiotherapy is often given after a limb-sparing procedure; this combination appears to produce acceptable local control and preserves function. This course is preferred by some to amputation, in the belief that a better quality of life is obtained at little or no cost to survival.[26-34]

A randomized trial comparing amputation and LSS in adult high-grade extremity soft tissue sarcoma was conducted at the National Cancer Institute[21,35] (see Table 8.3). Between 1975 and 1981, forty-three patients were randomized, in a 1:2 ratio, to receive amputation (sixteen patients) or LSS (twenty-seven patients). There were no local recurrences in the amputation arm and four in the LSS arm ($P = 0.06$). There were no statistically significant differences in disease-free survival (DFS) duration (three versus six recurrences; $P = 0.75$) or overall survival (OS) duration (two versus three deaths; $P = 0.99$). This was a small trial, with limited follow-up (minimum follow-up was 6 months), in which few recurrences and deaths have been observed. The published data are consistent not only with equivalent DFS and OS but also with large, clinically important differences in these quantities. Thus, while there is some evidence that LSS is associated with a higher local recurrence rate, no conclusions can be drawn about DFS or OS.

### Surgery of metastases

In the management of widespread metastases, resection of deposits in lungs and intra-abdominal sites has been shown, in suitably selected patients, to be associated with prolonged survival.[36]

## Chemotherapy

### Adjuvant chemotherapy

The role of adjuvant, postoperative chemotherapy compared with observation has been tested in thirteen randomized clinical trials. Seven trials tested single-agent doxorubicin and six tested multiagent chemotherapy based on doxorubicin. A summary of the designs of these trials is given in Table 8.4. One of these trials is, in fact, two trials (DFCI and MGH) whose data have been combined in reports.[44,45]

The following provides a brief review of each trial, including its particular features and main results. The acronym to be used for each trial is given in parentheses in each case. The trials are presented in chronological order of date of commencement of study.

**Table 8.3** Randomized clinical trials in adult soft tissue sarcoma, other than 'adjuvant chemotherapy versus nil' trials

| Group | Publications | Start of accrual | Median follow-up (years) | No. of patients | Arms | Patients per arm | Results | P-value |
|---|---|---|---|---|---|---|---|---|
| *Surgery* | | | | | | | | |
| NCI | Rosenberg et al.[35] Rosenberg et al.[21] | 1975 | 4.7 | 43 | Amp vs LSS | 16 27 | 5-year DFS: 78% vs 71% 5-year OS: 88% vs 83% | 0.75 0.99 |
| *Chemotherapy* | | | | | | | | |
| EORTC | Pinedo et al.[19] | 1976 | 3.5 | 246 (randomized) 162 (evaluable) | CYVADIC: Simul vs pairs | 125 121 | Overall response: 38% vs 14% Median duration remission: 62 vs 39 wks Median survival (responders): 85 vs 80 wks Median survival (all evaluable): 43 vs 45 wks | 0.001 0.75 0.35 0.062 |
| NCI | Chang et al.[42] | 1981 | 4.4 | 88 | CAM: High dose vs low dose | 41 47 | 5-year DFS: 58% vs 72% 5-year OS: 69% vs 75% | 0.37 0.90 |
| *Radiotherapy* | | | | | | | | |
| NCI | Sindelar et al.[72] | 1980 | 8 | 35 | IORT vs nil | 15 20 | Median OS: 45 vs 52 months Median DFI: 19 vs 38 months Median time to locoregional recurrence: 63 vs 38 months Median time to infield local recurrence: >127 vs 38 months | 0.39 0.58 0.40 < 0.05 |
| MSKCC | Harrison et al.[18] | 1982 | 5.5 | 126 | BRT vs nil | 55 70 | 5-year local control (all patients): 82% vs 67% 5-year local control (high grade): 90% vs 65% 5-year local control (low grade): 76% vs 76% 5-year DSS: 81% vs 80% | 0.049 0.013 NS NS |

Group: NCI = National Cancer Institute; EORTC = European Organization for Research on Treatment of Cancer; MSKCC = Memorial Sloan-Kettering Cancer Center.
Amp = amputation; LSS = limb-sparing surgery; CYVADIC = cyclophosphamide, vincristine, doxorubicin, dacarbazine; CAM = cyclophosphamide, doxorubicin, methotrexate; IORT = intra-operative radiotherapy; BRT = brachytherapy; Simul = simultaneous; vs = versus; DFS = disease-free survival; DFI = disease-free interval; OS = overall survival; DSS = disease-specific survival.

**Table 8.4** Randomized clinical trials of adjuvant chemotherapy in adult soft tissue sarcoma comparing adjuvant chemotherapy with no chemotherapy: details of trial designs

| Group (start year) | Reference | Median follow-up (years) | No. of patients randomized | No. of patients analysed | % Randomized patients excluded | Extremity only? | Grade |
|---|---|---|---|---|---|---|---|
| MDACC (1973) | Lindberg et al.[37] Benjamin et al.[38] | 10.5 | 46 | 43 | 7 | Yes | High |
| GOG (1973) | Omura et al.[39] | 6.5 | 225 | 156 | 31 | No | nr |
| Mayo (1975) | Edmonson et al.[40] | 5.4 | 61[a] | 61 | 0 | No | All |
| NCI/1 (1977) | Rosenberg et al.[41] Chang et al.[42] | 7.1 | 67 | 67 | 0 | Yes | High |
| NCI/2 (1977) | Glenn et al.[43] | 3.0 | 15 | 15 | 0 | No | All |
| DFCI/MGH (1978) | Wilson et al.[44] Antman et al.[45] | >3.8 | 46 | 46 | 0 | No | High |
| ECOG (1978) | Wilson et al.[44] Antman et al.[45] | >4.9 | 47 | 36 | 23 | No | High |
| ISG (1983) | Baker et al.[46] Antman et al.[45] | 1.7 | 92 | 86 | 7 | No | All |
| EORTC (1978) | Bramwell et al.[47] Bramwell et al.[48] | 5.2 | 446 | 317 | 29 | No | All |
| FBB (1980) | Ravaud et al.[49] | 4.4 | 65 | 59 | 9 | No | All |
| SSG (1981) | Alvegard et al.[50] | 3.3 | 240 | 181 | 25 | No | High |
| IORB (1981) | Gherlinzoni et al.[51] Picci et al.[52] Gherlinzoni et al.[53] | 8.8 | 83 | 77 | 7 | Yes | High |
| UCLA (1981) | Eilber et al.[54] Eilber et al.[55] | 2.3 | 119 | 119 | 0 | Yes | High |

[a]Excludes thirteen patients with metastatic presentation.
Groups: MDACC = MD Anderson Cancer Center; GOG: Gynecologic Oncology Group; Mayo = Mayo Clinic; NCI/1 and NCI/2 = National Cancer Institute, Trials 1 and 2; DFCI = Dana-Faber Cancer Institute; MGH = Massachusetts General Hospital; ECOG = Eastern Cooperative Oncology Group; ISG = Intergroup Sarcoma Group; EORTC = European Organization for Research and Treatment of Cancer; FBB = Fondation Bergonie, Bordeaux; SSG = Scandinavian Sarcoma Group; IORB = Instituto

## MD Anderson Cancer Center (MDACC)[37,38]

Forty-seven patients were randomized. The chemotherapy was multiagent VACAR (vincristine, doxorubicin, cyclophosphamide, dactinomycin) or no chemotherapy. The first report, at a median follow-up of 18 months, showed no significant difference in DFS. A later report after a minimum of 10 years' follow-up revealed that DFS favoured the chemotherapy arm ($P = 0.05$), but OS was not significantly different between arms. The effect appeared to be due to reduced local recurrence in the chemotherapy arm.

## Gynaecologic Oncology Group (GOG)[39]

Two hundred and twenty-five patients with FIGO (Fédération Internationale Gynécologique et Obstetrique) Stage I and II uterine sarcomas were randomized. The chemotherapy was doxorubicin (Dx: $60\,mg/m^2$ every 3 weeks for eight cycles). One hundred and fifty-six patients were declared evaluable at minimum follow-up of 24 months. No statistically significant difference in the rates of DFS or OS was found. It was noted that external beam pelvic radiotherapy reduced the rate of vaginal recurrence.

| Local recurrence presentation allowed? | Surgery | Radio-therapy | Preop chemo | Drugs used | Dose intensity of Dx (mg/m²/ wk) | Duration of post-op (chemo (4-week cycles) | Interval from surgery to chemo (weeks) |
|---|---|---|---|---|---|---|---|
| Yes | Rad exc | Yes | No | DxCDmV | 15 | 24 | nr |
| No | Rad exc | Opt | No | Dx | 20 | 6 | 1–4 |
| Yes | Rad exc | No | No | DxCDcDmV | 8 | 12 | <6 |
| Yes | Amp or LSS | If LSS | No | DxCM | 17 | 14 | <3–4 |
| No | Gross res | Yes | No | DxCM | 17 | 14 | 4 |
| Yes | Rad or cons res | If cons res | No | Dx | 22 | 3–5 | nr |
| Yes | Rad or cons res | If cons res | No | Dx | 17 | 7 | nr |
| No | Rad or cons res | If cons res | No | Dx | 17 | 6 | nr |
| Yes | Gross res | Opt | No | DxCDcV | 12 | 8 | 6 (med) |
| No | Rad res | If LSS | No | DxCDcV | 17 | 7 | 1–4 |
| No | Rad exc | If < wide exc | | Dx | 15 | 9 | <6/10 |
| Yes | LSS or Amp | If LSS | If LSS | Dx | 25 | 4.5 | 3d (Amp) |
| Yes | LSS | Preop | Preop | Dx | 22 | 5 | 6 |

Ortopedico Rizzoli, Bologna; UCLA = University of California, Los Angeles.
Surgery: Amp = amputation; LSS = limb-sparing surgery; rad = radical; cons = conservative; res = resection; exc = excision.
Radiotherapy: Opt = optional.
Drugs: C = cyclophosphamide, Dc = dacarbazine, Dm = dactinomycin, Dx = doxorubicin, M = methotrexate, V = vincristine.
Chemo = chemotherapy, Surg = surgery, nr = not recorded.

## Mayo Clinic (Mayo)[40]

Sixty-one patients were randomized. Chemotherapy comprised vincristine, cyclophosphamide and dactinomycin, alternating with vincristine, doxorubicin and darcarbazine (VACAD). The results, at a median follow-up of 5.4 years, showed no significant difference in DFS or OS. It was noted that a rather high proportion of patients (28%) experienced local recurrence which the authors attributed to lack of postoperative radiotherapy.

## National Cancer Institute Trial No. 1 (NCI/1)[42]

Sixty-seven patients with extremity lesions were randomized. Chemotherapy consisted of doxorubicin, cyclophosphamide and high-dose methotrexate (CAM). Median follow-up was 7.1 years. DFS was significantly better in the chemotherapy arm ($P = 0.037$) but OS, whilst longer in the chemotherapy arm, was not significantly different between arms ($P = 0.124$). The study was small and unequal randomization (2:1) was used.

## National Cancer Institute Trial No. 2 (NCI/2)[43]

Fifteen patients with resectable retroperitoneal sarcoma were randomized. Adjuvant chemotherapy consisted of doxorubicin, cyclophosphamide and high-dose methotrexate. The 2-year actuarial DFS and OS rates were inferior in the chemotherapy arm ($P = 0.14$ and $0.06$, respectively). The numbers of patients were too small, however, to allow any conclusions to be drawn.

## Dana-Farber Cancer Institute/Massachusetts General Hospital and Eastern Co-operative Oncology Group (DFCI/MGH and ECOG)[44,45]

There were forty-six patients randomized to either doxorubicin ($90 \, \text{mg/m}^2$ every 3 weeks for five cycles) or controls. Doxorubicin was given postoperatively at DFCI, but at MGH two cycles were given preoperatively and three cycles postoperatively. ECOG randomized forty-seven patients and the dose of doxorubicin was $70 \, \text{mg/m}^2$ for seven cycles versus observation. No significant difference was found between arms with respect to local control, metastasis-free survival, DFS or OS. Subgroup analysis failed to show evidence of a benefit from doxorubicin therapy for either extremity or non-extremity sarcomas.

## Intergroup Sarcoma Group (ISG)[46]

Chemotherapy consisted of doxorubicin ($70 \, \text{mg/m}^2$, with escalation to $90 \, \text{mg/m}^2$, every 3 weeks for six cycles). Although 114 patients were randomized, the results were reported for the first eighty-one patients. In the subgroup of forty-one extremity patients, a trend toward improved DFS for the doxorubicin group was noted ($P = 0.06$) but OS was not significantly different.

## European Organization for Research on Treatment of Cancer (EORTC)[47,48]

This is the largest study with 468 patients randomized and 358 patients eligible. Median follow-up was 44 months. Local recurrence was significantly reduced in the chemotherapy arm ($P = 0.004$) but significance was confined to the non-extremity subgroup ($P = 0.003$) and not to that with limb lesions ($P = 0.38$). There was no significant difference in time to distant metastases ($P = 0.38$) or OS ($P = 0.26$).

## Fondation Bergonie, Bordeaux (FBB)[49]

Fifty-nine patients were randomized. Chemotherapy patients received eight to eleven courses of CYVADIC (cyclophosphamide, vincristine, doxorubicin, dactinomycin) every 3 weeks starting within 4 weeks of surgery. The results showed significant improvement in both DFS and OS. There was some imbalance of histologies and of the proportion of patients with extremity lesions in the two arms. The trial had a small sample size.

## Scandinavian Sarcoma Group (SSG)[50]

Two hundred and forty patients with high-grade extremity sarcomas were randomized to adjuvant doxorubicin ($60 \, \text{mg/m}^2$ every 4 weeks for nine cycles) or control. Over half of them did not complete therapy. At a median follow-up of 40 months, no significant differences were seen with respect to local recurrence, DFS or OS, either for the 181 evaluable or the total 240 randomized.

### *Instituto Ortopedico Rizzoli, Bologna (IORB)*[51-53]

Eighty-three patients with high-grade extremity lesions were randomized. This study is the only one giving a significant result for the use of single-agent doxorubicin. Thirty-three patients were randomized to doxorubicin (75 mg/m$^2$ every 3 weeks for six cycles for a cumulative dose of 450 mg/m$^2$). There was imbalance of risk factors between the arms. Local control, DFS and OS were significantly improved in the doxorubicin group.

### *University of California at Los Angeles (UCLA)*[54,55]

All patients had preoperative intra-arterial doxorubicin (20–30 mg/day continuously for 3 days) and preoperative radiotherapy, and were then randomized to adjuvant doxorubicin (45 mg/m$^2$ daily for 2 days every 4 weeks for five cycles) starting within 6 weeks of surgery versus observation. There was no significant difference in terms of local recurrence, DFS or OS. There was a slightly lower local recurrence rate in patients receiving adjuvant systemic doxorubicin but this did not reach statistical significance.

There is considerable heterogeneity in the design of these trials. The site of involvement was 'extremity only' in four trials and varied in the others (the second NCI trial included only retroperitoneal sarcomas). In nine trials, only high-grade sarcomas were entered. Also, differences occurred in whether locally recurrent presentations were included (six trials), the extent of resection at the time of definitive surgery, whether postoperative radiotherapy was given and whether preoperative chemotherapy was used. In addition, the dosage and timing of chemotherapy, especially that of doxorubicin, were highly variable. The number of patients studied varied considerably between trials but most studies were small: nine of the thirteen trials randomized fewer than 100 patients. The largest trial was the EORTC trial which randomized 446 patients. Four of the trials excluded more than 15% of randomized patients from analysis: the GOG trial (31%), the ECOG trial (23%), the EORTC trial (29%) and the SSG trial (25%).

Table 8.5 summarizes the results of these trials. Three of the thirteen trials, DFCI/MGH, ECOG and ISG trials, used single-agent doxorubicin and have been reported in a combined analysis.[45] They appear in Table 8.5 and in Fig. 8.1 as '3 trials'. There is no uniformity of reporting outcome — rates of distant recurrence or any recurrence (local and distant) and overall or cancer-specific survival. In general, outcomes are under-reported with over-reliance on *P*-values to summarize group comparisons and, worst of all, negative results are incorrectly interpreted. On the latter point, many authors appear to make the mistake of interpreting a *P*-value over 0.10 as indicating that there is no advantage to chemotherapy. A 'negative' trial (*P* > 0.10) can have two possible interpretations: either (a) the chemotherapy had no clinically significant effect or (b) the trial was inconclusive (because the data were consistent with *both* no difference *and* important differences).

**Table 8.5**   Randomized clinical trials in adult soft tissue sarcoma, comparing adjuvant chemotherapy with no chemotherapy: results in terms of 5-year disease-free and overall survival rates

| Group/ref. | Accrual/ last follow-up | Arms | No. analysed per arm | Recurrence-free survival | | | Overall survival | | |
|---|---|---|---|---|---|---|---|---|---|
| | | | | No. recs | Actuarial rate (%) | P | No. deaths | Actuarial rate (%) | P |
| MDACC[38] | 73–78/86 | VACAR | 20 | 9 | 60 | 0.05 | nr | 75 | NS |
| | | Nil | 23 | 15 | 35 | | | 61 | |
| GOG[39] | 73–82/84 | Dx | 75 | 31 | 55 | NS | 30 | 56 | NS |
| | | Nil | 81 | 43 | 44 | | 39 | 46 | |
| Mayo[40] | 75–81/83 | VACAD | 30 | nr | 82 | 0.15 | nr | 90 | 0.55 |
| | | Nil | 31 | | 64[a] | | | 76 | |
| NCI/1[42] | 77–81/86 | CAM | 39 | nr | 75 | 0.037 | nr | 82 | 0.124 |
| | | Nil | 28 | | 54 | | | 60 | |
| NCI/2[43] | 77–81/82 | CAM | 8 | 4 | 51 | 0.14 | 4 | 56 | 0.06 |
| | | Nil | 7 | 1 | 88[b] | | 1 | 89[c] | |
| 3 trials[45] | 78–86/89 | Dx | 80 | 23 | 70 | 0.13 | 25 | 69 | 0.51 |
| | | Nil | 88 | 36 | 58 | | 32 | 60 | |
| EORTC[47] | 78–87/88 | CYVADIC | 150 | 48 | 62 | 0.010 | 33 | 69 | 0.118 |
| | | Nil | 167 | 74 | 48 | | 50 | 60 | |
| FBB[49] | 80–88/90 | CYVADIC | 31 | 5 | 72 | 0.003 | 4 | 87 | 0.002 |
| | | Nil | 28 | 16 | 41[a] | | 13 | 38 | |
| SSG[50] | 81–86/88 | Dx | 93 | nr | 58 | NS | nr | 63 | NS |
| | | Nil | 88 | | 53 | | | 62 | |
| IORB[52] | 81–86/92 | Dx | 33 | 9 | 68 | <0.02 | 3 | 88 | Sig |
| | | Nil | 44 | 24 | 42 | | 13 | 68 | |
| UCLA[55] | 81–84/86 | Dx | 57 | nr | 49 | NS | nr | 80 | NS |
| | | Nil | 62 | | 46[c] | | | 74[d] | |

[a]Metastasis-free rates.
[b]Estimated 2-year rates from fitted exponentials.
[c]At 4 years.
[d]At 3 years.
N.B. DFS = any recurrence, not just metastases (except Mayo, FBB); all *P*-values are two-sided; survival from death from any cause; all rates are actuarial and at 5 years (except NCI/2, UCLA).
NS = not statistically significant; Sig = statistically significant; nr = not recorded.
See text pp. 184–187 for details of each group trial.

When a non-significant *P*-value is obtained, a confidence interval should be used to enable the correct interpretation to be made, either 'no important effect found' or 'result indeterminate'; however, in only one report were confidence intervals provided.[44]

*Summary analysis of adjuvant chemotherapy trials*

We have produced a summary analysis of all the clinical trials (eleven reported analyses from thirteen trials). This is not a proper meta-analysis but we believe it sheds light on the accumulated knowledge from all published trials to date. (See also Zalupski *et al.*[56]) Table 8.5 summarizes 5-year DFS and OS rates from each of the studies. All information in this summary analysis has been obtained from the published reports. The data analysed were 5-year actuarial DFS and 5-year OS rates and their standard errors (SE). Data on local recurrence rates were not reported in enough detail to warrant analysis here.

The actuarial rates were obtained from the text or tables where possible, but otherwise were read off from figures of actuarial curves. The standard errors of these rates were obtained indirectly, using a computer algorithm which incorporated the estimated 5-year rate, the number of patients in the arm, and the lengths of the accrual and follow-up periods; it assumed a uniform rate of accrual and an exponential curve. This calculation, by allowing for incomplete follow-up, produced larger standard errors and wider confidence intervals than if complete follow-up were assumed and the usual binomial standard error had been used. For the Mayo and FBB trials, DFS data were not provided so metastasis-free rates have been used in their place. Rates for the UCLA trial are 4-year (DFS) and 3-year (OS). For the SSG trial, since results were given only for strata defined by whether the surgical procedure was marginal, rates for the arms were calculated as weighted means over these strata. The NCI/2 trial, which showed large differences in favour of observation, was included, despite short follow-up and small size (fifteen patients); rates and standard errors were estimated from fitted exponential curves. The *P*-values in Table 8.5 are all two-sided and are those quoted in the papers. They correspond to comparisons of the overall curves, not just the 5-year rates.

Figure 8.1 presents a graphical summary of these data. It plots the *difference* in actuarial 5-year rates between the chemotherapy and observation arms for each trial together with an approximate 95% confidence interval (95% CI) for each difference. A weighted average difference over all trials, with approximate 95% CI, is also given.[57] The summary weighted mean differences in 5-year rates were (a) for DFS, 13% in favour of adjuvant chemotherapy (95% CI: (7%, 19%)) and (b) for OS, 11% in favour of adjuvant chemotherapy (95% CI: (6%, 17%)).

The weighted overall mean difference in 5-year DFS rates for multiagent chemotherapy was 16% (SE = 5%) and for single-agent chemotherapy was 11% (SE = 4%). There is no statistical evidence that multiagent is more effective than single-agent chemotherapy (*P* = 0.38). The mean difference for extremity-only trials was 17% (SE = 6%) compared with 11% (SE = 3%) for other trials. There is no statistical evidence that chemotherapy is more effective for extremity-only sites than for a range of sites (*P* = 0.38). Results were similar for OS: differences for multiagent versus single-agent chemotherapy were 15% and 9%, respectively (*P* = 0.28) and for

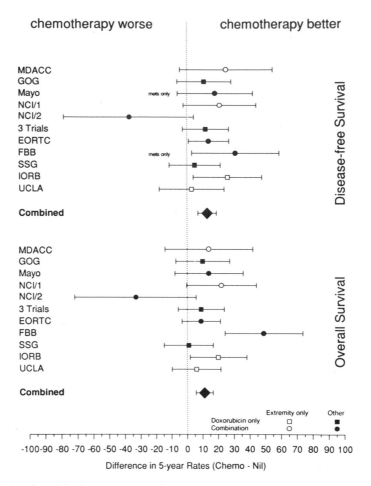

**Fig. 8.1** Graphical summary of the results of all published randomized trials of adjuvant chemotherapy in soft tissue sarcoma. For each trial and for each outcome (DFS and OS) the difference in the 5-year actuarial rates between the chemotherapy arm and the control arm is plotted together with an approximate 95% confidence interval for the difference. Smaller trials, therefore, are represented by wider intervals and larger trials by narrower intervals. Each plotted difference and confidence interval corresponding to 'Combined' represents the weighted average of the corresponding trial difference and its approximate 95% confidence interval. Details of the methodology are given in the text. The term 'mets only' refers to results for metastasis-free survival, used only when DFS (distant and local recurrence) results were not available.

extremity-only versus other trials were 14% and 10% ($P = 0.47$), respectively.

The amount of variation between these trial results, compared with the random variation expected between homogeneous trials (those testing an identical question and with the same design, but allowing for different patient numbers and follow-up periods) can be assessed. The observed variation was not significantly greater for DFS ($P = 0.27$) but was significantly greater for OS ($P = 0.043$) than that expected for homogeneous trials. It appears that the latter result is due mainly to the large observed difference in 5-year survival rates in the FBB trial (87% versus 38%). The relative homogeneity of the results from these trials indicates that claims of significant effects or of non-effects in single trials, and especially for particular subgroups of patients or treatments (e.g. extremity-only patients, or multiagent chemotherapy schedules), should be viewed with some scepticism. An analysis which, statistically, is slightly more sound is that in terms of the 'log odds' of DFS or OS at 5 years (e.g. Zalupski *et al.*[56]). This gave the same conclusions. We have presented this analysis using the difference of rates at 5 years because it is more easily interpretable.

This summary analysis provides a reasonable interpretation of the published information from randomized clinical trials of adjuvant chemotherapy in soft tissue sarcoma. Of necessity, however, it has been based on a number of approximations and assumptions. The question of whether chemotherapy is of benefit in soft tissue sarcoma is therefore not decided, although we believe the evidence from this analysis favours there being a benefit in both DFS and OS.

Most of the trials have not had updates published in the recent past so, potentially, there exist much follow-up data which could be assessed. We believe that there should be a properly conducted meta-analysis of all randomized clinical trials (using original data from all randomized patients from the trial groups and including any unpublished trials) to provide a more reliable consensus opinion of the role of adjuvant chemotherapy.

### Local control

One of the benefits of adjuvant chemotherapy is improved local control. Several trials of multiagent chemotherapy have reported a statistically significant reduction in local recurrence rate: MDACC,[37,38] EORTC,[47,48] NCI/1[42] and FBB.[49] The only trial using multiagent chemotherapy that did not show this effect was from the Mayo Clinic,[40] which omitted radiotherapy and used inadequate chemotherapy.

The effects of adjuvant single-agent doxorubicin are less clear with UCLA[54,55] and IORB[51–53] showing decreased local recurrence following doxorubicin, whilst no such effect was shown with the ECOG[44] trial and insufficient information was provided for the ISG[46] trial.

### Schedule of administration of chemotherapy

A randomized trial was conducted by the EORTC in which two schedules of CYVADIC were compared in patients with advanced progressive adult soft tissue sarcoma: simultaneous administration of the four drugs every 4 weeks versus pairs of drugs alternating every 4 weeks.[19] Two hundred and forty-six patients were randomized, of whom 34% were declared not evaluable. The difference in OS was not statistically significant for the 162 evaluable patients ($P = 0.35$) but almost reached significance when all 246 patients were analysed ($P = 0.062$; the direction of this difference was not given). About half of the inevaluable patients were classified as 'ineligible' presumably as a result of central pathology review. However, the other reasons for inevaluability were early progression, early death, protocol violation, incomplete data and refusal of treatment, which should not be grounds for exclusion from analysis. Consequently, some doubt must be attached to the results of this trial.

The NCI conducted a randomized trial of adjuvant chemotherapy in patients with high-grade soft tissue sarcoma, comparing a high-dose regimen (cyclophosphamide, doxorubicin and methotrexate) with a reduced-dose programme (cyclophosphamide and doxorubicin).[42] There were forty-one patients on the high-dose arm and forty-seven patients on the reduced-dose arm; median follow-up was 4.4 years. The high-dose arm had a lower 5-year DFS rate (58% versus 72%; $P = 0.37$) and a lower 5-year OS rate (69% versus 75%; $P = 0.90$). The authors concluded that 'treatment with reduced cumulative doses of doxorubicin and cyclophosphamide without methotrexate is no different from adjuvant treatment with our high-dose chemotherapy regimen'. Since this is a trial in which the investigators were hoping to prove 'equivalence' of, rather than a difference between, the arms, the use of confidence intervals would have been especially helpful. Our approximate calculations suggest that the data are consistent with an advantage for the high-dose regimen of at most 10% in the 5-year DFS rate and at most 15% in the 5-year OS rate.

### Side-effects of adjuvant chemotherapy

The unwanted effects of chemotherapy (with or without radiotherapy) have been documented in several organ systems such as the cardiovascular system,[58,59] the ovaries,[60] testes[61] and central nervous system.[62]

### Neoadjuvant chemotherapy

It is anticipated that any benefit from adjuvant postoperative chemotherapy will also be produced by neoadjuvant (preoperative) chemotherapy,[63–65] although this approach has not been put to the test in a randomized clinical trial. The trend nowadays seems to be to use initial chemotherapy to reduce the size of the primary tumour and thereby make it more readily resectable. There is one randomized trial of neoadjuvant chemotherapy in progress, conducted by the EORTC.[63] The results are awaited with interest.

## Radiotherapy

Radiotherapy, like surgery, has had a well-established role as a locoregional treatment modality and the two often complement one another. The use of radiotherapy in the management of soft tissue sarcoma has continued to evolve in the last few decades. Surgery alone remains a popular approach and several authors have questioned the need for any treatment other than adequate *en-bloc* resection, such as LSS, of extremity sarcomas when the margins of resection are clear.[22,66,67] Adjuvant external beam radiotherapy can be either preoperative,[68–70] postoperative[29,69] or intraoperative.[71,72] Radiotherapy can also be definitive, that is, administered alone when the lesion is either technically unresectable (because of size or site) or when operation is refused by the patient or is not indicated for medical reasons.[73] Radiotherapy can also be administered as brachytherapy.

## Preoperative radiotherapy

For certain bulky or unresectable tumours, or in situations where limb-sparing treatment is desirable, preoperative radiotherapy has a place.[68-70,74] The radiation field size has been shown to be smaller when preoperative radiotherapy is given compared with the same clinical presentation treated by postoperative radiotherapy.[69]

## Postoperative radiotherapy

For small lesions which have been resected with clear surgical margins, post-operative radiotherapy may be omitted, especially in low-grade sarcomas.[22,66] Local recurrences in low-grade lesions which are amenable to re-excision are best treated by second surgery unless the lesion cannot be excised with clear margins, in which case LSS plus radiotherapy is warranted.

## Brachytherapy

Adjuvant interstitial brachytherapy, close to the time of radical surgery, has been used. In selected cases, it can give additional local control.[7,18,75,76] Ideally, the placement of catheters for the insertion of radioactive material should be planned preoperatively by close collaboration between the surgeon, the radiation oncologist and the radiation physicist. Radioactive iridium ($^{192}$Ir) wire with the calculated activity is then inserted by afterloading, either manually or mechanically, usually 1 week after operation to allow for adequate wound healing.[28] This allows early delivery of a boost dose to the area of maximum risk, which can then be followed by external beam radiotherapy to the entire tumour bed.[77]

A randomized clinical trial of adjuvant brachytherapy in completely resected soft tissue sarcoma, conducted by the Memorial Sloan Kettering Cancer Center, included 126 patients with soft tissue sarcoma of the extremity or superficial trunk, who underwent grossly complete resection with LSS.[18] At the time of operation, patients were randomized to brachytherapy or no further therapy. Following wound healing, $^{192}$Ir wire was used to deliver a tumour dose of 42–45 Gy in 4–6 days in patients in the brachytherapy arm. Follow-up duration was not reported. At 5 years, local control was better in the brachytherapy arm (82%) than control (67%) ($P = 0.049$). This comparison was statistically significant for the high-grade subset of patients ($P = 0.013$) but not the low-grade subset. Distant metastasis rates at 5 years were similar (76%) in both arms, as were 5-year DFS rates (81% versus 80%). The authors concluded that the improved local control did not appear to translate into either decreased distant metastasis or increased disease-specific survival.[18] Because of the small to moderate size of the trial, confidence intervals for 5-year rates, for example, probably include differences of clinical significance. We estimate that the data are consistent with differences of up to 15% in 5-year DFS and OS rates and that it cannot be concluded from these data that brachytherapy does not influence the local recurrence rate for low-grade tumours.

## Intraoperative radiotherapy

The use of intraoperative radiotherapy (IORT) in retroperitoneal sarcomas, compared with that of external beam radiotherapy, has been tested in a randomized trial, conducted at the NCI, with the aim of improving locoregional control and reducing gastrointestinal injury.[72] Forty-eight patients were randomized, prior to surgery, to 20 Gy IORT plus low-dose (35–40 Gy) postoperative external beam radiotherapy versus high-dose (50–55 Gy) postoperative external beam radiotherapy alone. Thirteen patients were declared ineligible because of unresectable or metastatic disease found at laparotomy. This left fifteen eligible patients in the IORT arm and twenty in the control arm. Adjuvant chemotherapy (doxorubicin and cyclophosphamide) was used in the early phase of the study as part of a separate randomization which was later abandoned. Follow-up ranged from 5 to 8 years. The risk of in-field recurrence was significantly lower in the IORT arm (6/15) than in the control (16/20) ($P < 0.05$); there was approximately a 20% difference in 5-year local control rates. Locoregional recurrence rates, however, were not statistically significantly different ($P = 0.40$). Disabling enteritis was greater in the control arm (ten complications in twenty patients) than in the IORT (2/15), but peripheral neuropathy was higher in the IORT (9/15) than in the control arm (1/20). There were no statistically significant differences in DFS ($P = 0.58$) or OS duration ($P = 0.39$); however, the numbers of patients were too small to be able to exclude the possibility that clinically important differences may exist.

## Definitive radiotherapy

Definitive radiotherapy can achieve local cure in selected cases as described above. Ideally, radiosensitization, or some other special approach, should be used to increase the therapeutic ratio. The measures which have been investigated include iododeoxyuridine (IUdR), intra-arterial chemotherapy,[54,55] hyperthermia,[32] fast neutrons[78] and hyperfractionation.[31] The management of aggressive fibromatosis (desmoid tumour) often calls for radiotherapy to unresectable masses.[79–81]

# Prognostic significance of local recurrence

The prognostic significance of local recurrence is an important question in the management of many tumours, and especially so in soft tissue sarcomas. Whether less-radical, limb-sparing surgery, with its attendant increased risk of local recurrence, can be justified instead of amputation, is currently an unresolved question. As indicated above, the only randomized clinical trial addressing this question was too small to provide a definitive answer.

The adverse significance of a local recurrence after a primary definitive surgical procedure has long been recognized.[16,20] Relative risks of death associated with its advent have been reported to be as high as 2.5[82] and

4.5.[83] Such observations have led some authors to conclude that a local recurrence may increase the risk of distant metastasis and hence death and, therefore, that reduction of risk of local recurrence is of paramount importance in management.[82] There is conflicting opinion, however, as to whether local recurrence is in itself a direct cause of death.[82–85]

Some studies have suggested that certain patient subsets, e.g. those receiving LSS, which are associated with a higher risk of local recurrence, do not have an obviously reduced survival duration.[18,72] These authors conclude that avoidance of local recurrence *per se* is not that important for ultimate survival and that LSS is thereby justified.

There is an apparent contradiction between the statements, 'local recurrence is a strong predictor of shorter survival duration' and 'a treatment strategy which is associated with an increased risk of local recurrence is not associated with shorter survival duration'. This apparent contradiction can be resolved by constructing a hypothetical, albeit highly artificial, set of data for which both of the above statements are true. Suppose that grade (low, intermediate, high), say, is the most important determinant of survival, according to Table 8.6, which gives the expected outcome by grade in 100 patients. Suppose, also, that, in a randomized clinical trial comparing

**Table 8.6**   Hypothetical expected survival of 100 patients by grade

|  | Low | Intermediate | High | Total |
|---|---|---|---|---|
| No. surviving | 22 | 20 | 8 | 50 |
| No. dying | 8 | 20 | 22 | 50 |
| (% dying) | (27%) | (50%) | (73%) | (50%) |
| Total | 30 | 40 | 30 | 100 |

amputation with LSS, 100 patients are assigned to each arm and that grade and type of surgery determine risk of local recurrence (l-rec) as follows: among patients treated by amputation, all high-grade tumours recur locally but no others, whereas with patients undergoing LSS all intermediate- and high-grade tumours recur locally and low-grade tumours do not. Expected results from the study, in terms of local recurrence and survival, would be as shown in Table 8.7.

**Table 8.7**   Hypothetical expected local recurrence and survival results

|  | Amputation | | | LSS | | |
|---|---|---|---|---|---|---|
|  | No l-rec | l-rec | Total | No l-rec | l-rec | Total |
| No. surviving | 42 | 8 | 50 | 22 | 28 | 50 |
| No. dying | 28 | 22 | 50 | 8 | 42 | 50 |
| (% dying) | (40%) | (73%) | (50%) | (27%) | (60%) | (50%) |
| Total | 70 | 30 | 100 | 30 | 70 | 100 |

There is a much higher incidence of local recurrence in the LSS arm (70% compared with 30%); however, survival in each arm is identical (50%). For both amputation and LSS, local recurrence is associated with a large increase in the risk of death (over a four-fold increase in the odds of death). For this example, one could say that it does not matter whether local recurrence appears. Local recurrence is acting merely as a manifestation of an underlying prognostic determinant and not as a factor with an independent influence on survival. Analysis could be performed controlling for this underlying determinant, and it would show that local recurrence for a fixed grade is independent of survival. In practice, however, the underlying determinants are unknown, or at best incompletely known, and it is difficult to determine whether the prognostic significance of local recurrence is an independent effect or not.

In passing, it is worth stating that, in a given series, the survival of patients presenting with local recurrence compared with that of patients with primary disease is a different, albeit related, question. These patients, potentially, represent a selected subset of all patients whose tumours recur locally and their survival is compared at different time points in the course of their disease.

It is also worth noting that to test for an association between the occurrence of local failure and subsequent survival duration requires care involving the use of special statistical techniques; the simple comparison of survival curves of patients who fail locally, and those who do not, is statistically invalid as it has an inherent bias in favour of showing longer survival associated with local failure. Valid techniques include 'transient state analysis'[86] or, more generally, the use of time-dependent covariates with Cox's proportional hazards model.[87] The latter technique also allows the effects of other prognostic variables to be simultaneously taken into account. Less efficient, but valid, is the use of a 'landmark' time in the analysis.[16]

As demonstrated above, it should also be remembered that, in the event of showing a significant effect of local failure on survival, only an association has been established and not cause and effect. Thus, certain tumours may have both a tendency to recur locally and an association with shorter survival. Treatments that reduce the local recurrence rate, therefore, may have no impact on survival duration. Barr et al.[84] survey papers which attempt to throw some light on the local recurrence problem. They review the different methodologies that have been used and recommend those most appropriate. These authors point out that to demonstrate an increase in survival duration as a result of reducing the local recurrence rate requires randomized clinical trials which, however, are unlikely to be performed, owing to the large sample sizes required to prove such effects.

## Management of locally recurrent soft tissue sarcoma

For the patient presenting with locally recurrent tumour, careful assessment is required. Assessment includes biopsy confirmation, histological grading and clinical staging to determine whether aggressive treatment would be appropriate in the clinical situation.[88]

# Summary

The management of soft tissue sarcoma for the majority of patients is a multidisciplinary concern. It requires that a radical excision be performed which implies either radical operation alone, if clear margins can be obtained, or conservative wide resection and adjuvant radiotherapy. The total dose of radiation needs to be high and close to the tolerance level of the normal adjacent tissues and special techniques are often needed. There also remains an urgent need to develop more effective drugs with reduced toxicity as systemic therapy. Future generations of oncologists will need to explore how best to integrate surgery, radiotherapy and chemotherapy and to optimize their scheduling.

# References

1. Leyvraz S, Costa J. Histological diagnosis and grading of soft tissue sarcomas. *Semin Surg Oncol* 1988; **4**, 3–6.
2. Coates M, McCredie M, Taylor R. *Cancer in New South Wales. Incidence and Mortality 1991.* New South Wales Cancer Registry, NSW Cancer Council, 1994.
3. Yang JC, Rosenberg SA, Glatstein EJ, *et al.* Sarcomas of soft tissues. In: VT DeVita, S Hellman, SA Rosenberg, eds, *Cancer: Principles & Practice of Oncology*, 4th edn. Philadelphia: JB Lippincott, 1993; 1436–88.
4. Dillon P, Maurer H, Jenkins J, *et al.* A prospective study of nonrhabdomyosarcoma soft tissue sarcomas in the pediatric age group. *J Pediatr Surg* 1992; **27**, 241–4.
5. Enzinger FM, Weiss SW. *Soft Tissue Tumors*, 2nd edn. St Louis: CV Mosby Co, 1988.
6. Beahrs OH, Henson DE, Hutter RVP, *et al.*, eds, *Manual for Staging of Cancer*, 4th edn. Philadelphia: JB Lippincott, 1992; 131–3.
7. Brennan MF, Hilaris B, Shiu MH, *et al.* Local recurrence in adult soft tissue sarcoma: a randomized trial of brachytherapy. *Arch Surg* 1987; **122**, 1289–93.
8. Costa J, Wesley RA, Glatstein E, *et al.* The grading of soft tissue sarcomas: results of a clinicohistopathologic correlation in a series of 163 cases. *Cancer* 1984; **53**, 530–41.
9. Presant CA, Russell WO, Alexander RW, *et al.* Soft-tissue and bone sarcoma histopathology peer review: the frequency of disagreement in diagnosis and the need for second pathology opinions: the Southeastern Cancer Study Group experience. *J Clin Oncol* 1986; **4**, 1658–61.
10. Alvegard TA, Berg NO, for the Scandinavian Sarcoma Group. Histopathology peer review of high-grade soft tissue sarcoma: the Scandinavian Sarcoma Group experience. *J Clin Oncol* 1989; **7**, 1845–52.
11. Jensen OM, Hogh J, Ostgaard SE, *et al.* Histopathological grading of soft tissue tumors. Prognostic significance in a prospective study of 278 consecutive cases. *J Pathol* 1991; **163**, 19–24.
12. Coindre JM, Trojani M, Contesso G, *et al.* Reproducibility of a histopathologic grading system for adult soft tissue sarcoma. *Cancer* 1986; **58**, 306–9.
13. Fong Y, Coit DG, Woodruff JM, *et al.* Lymph node metastasis from soft tissue sarcoma in adults. Analysis of data from a prospective database of 1772 sarcoma patients. *Ann Surg* 1993; **217**, 72–7.
14. Alvegard TA, Berg NO, Baldetorp B, *et al.* Cellular DNA content and prognosis of high-grade soft tissue sarcoma: the Scandinavian Sarcoma Group experience. *J Clin Oncol* 1990; **8**, 538–47.

15. El-Naggar AK, Ayala AG, Abdul-Karim FW, *et al.* Synovial sarcoma: a DNA flow cytometric study. *Cancer* 1990; **65**, 2295–300.
16. Collin CF, Friederich C, Godbolt J, *et al.* Prognostic factors for local recurrence and survival in patients with localised extremity soft tissue sarcoma. *Semin Surg Oncol* 1988; **4**, 30–7.
17. Rooser B, Willen H, Hugoson A, *et al.* Prognostic factors in synovial sarcoma. *Cancer* 1989; **63**, 2182–5.
18. Harrison LB, Franzese F, Gaynor JJ, *et al.* Long-term results of a prospective randomized trial of adjuvant brachytherapy in the management of completely resected soft tissue sarcomas of the extremity and superficial trunk. *Int J Radiat Oncol Biol Phys* 1993; **27**, 259–65.
19. Pinedo HM, Bramwell VHC, Mourisden HT, *et al.* CYVADIC in advanced soft tissue sarcoma: a randomized study comparing two schedules. *Cancer* 1984; **53**, 1825–32.
20. Cantin J, McNeer GP, Chu FC, *et al.* The problem of local recurrence after treatment of soft tissue sarcoma. *Ann Surg* 1968; **168**, 47–83.
21. Rosenberg SA, Tepper J, Glatstein E, *et al.* The treatment of soft-tissue sarcomas of the extremities. Prospective randomized evaluation of (1) limb-sparing surgery plus radiation therapy compared with amputation and (2) the role of adjuvant chemotherapy. *Ann Surg* 1982; **196**, 305–15.
22. Rydholm A, Gustafson P, Rooser B, *et al.* Limb-sparing surgery without radiotherapy based on anatomic location of soft tissue saroma. *J Clin Oncol* 1991; **9**, 1757–65.
23. Demas BE, Heelan RT, Lane J, *et al.* Soft-tissue sarcomas of the extremities: comparison of MR and CT in determining the extent of disease. *Am J Roentgenol* 1988; **150**, 615–20.
24. Bloem JL, Taminiau AHM, Eulderink F, *et al.* Radiologic staging of primary bone sarcoma: MR imaging, scintigraphy, angiography, and CT correlated with pathologic examination. *Radiology* 1988; **169**, 805–10.
25. Southee AE, Kaplan WD, Jochelson MS, *et al.* Gallium imaging in metastatic and recurrent soft-tissue sarcoma. *J Nucl Med* 1992; **33**, 1594–9.
26. Gerson R, Shiu MH, Hajdu SI. Sarcoma of the buttock: a trend toward limb-salvage resection. *J Surg Oncol* 1982; **19**, 238–42.
27. Hilaris BS, Shiu MH, Nori D, *et al.* Limb-sparing therapy for locally advanced soft-tissue sarcomas. *Endocuriether Hypertherm Oncol* 1985; **1**, 17–24.
28. Zelefsky MJ, Nori D, Shiu MH, *et al.* Limb salvage in soft tissue sarcomas involving neurovascular structures using combined surgical resection and brachytherapy. *Int J Radiat Oncol Biol Phys* 1990; **19**, 913–18.
29. Pao WJ, Pilepich MV. Postoperative radiotherapy in the treatment of extremity soft tissue sarcomas. *Int J Radiat Oncol Biol Phys* 1990; **19**, 907–11.
30. Stinson SF, Delaney TF, Greenberg J, *et al.* Acute and long-term effects on limb function of combined modality limb sparing therapy for extremity soft tissue sarcoma. *Int J Radiat Oncol Biol Phys* 1991; **21**, 1493–9.
31. Robinson M, Cassoni A, Harmer C, *et al.* High dose hyperfractionated radiotherapy in the treatment of extremity soft tissue sarcomas. *Radiother Oncol* 1991; **22**, 118–26.
32. Di Filippo F, Giannarelli D, Botti C, *et al.* Hyperthermic antiblastic perfusion for the treatment of soft tissue limb sarcoma. *Ann Oncol* 1992; **3** (Suppl 2), S71–4.
33. Moseley HS. An evaluation of two methods of limb salvage in extremity soft-tissue sarcomas. *Arch Surg* 1992; **127**, 1169–73.
34. Herbert SH, Corn BW, Solin LJ, *et al.* Limb-preserving treatment for soft tissue sarcomas of the extremities. The significance of surgical margins. *Cancer* 1993; **72**, 1230–8.
35. Rosenberg SA, Kent H, Costa J, *et al.* Prospective evaluation of the role of

limb-sparing surgery, radiation therapy and adjuvant chemoimmunotherapy in the treatment of adult soft-tissue sarcomas. *Surgery* 1978; 84, 62–9.

36. Karakousis CP, Blumenson LE, Canavese G, *et al.* Surgery for disseminated abdominal sarcoma. *Am J Surg* 1992; **163**, 560–4.
37. Lindberg RD, Murphy WK, Benjamin RS, *et al.* Adjuvant chemotherapy in the treatment of primary soft tissue sarcomas: a preliminary report. In: *Management of Bone and Soft Tissue Tumors*. MD Anderson Hospital and Tumor Institute. Chicago: Year Book Medical Publishers Inc, 1977; 343–52.
38. Benjamin RS, Terjanian TO, Fenoglio CJ, *et al.* The importance of combination chemotherapy for adjuvant treatment of high-risk patients with soft-tissue sarcomas of the extremities. In: SE Salmon, ed, *Adjuvant Therapy of Cancer V.* New York: Grune & Stratton, 1987; 735–44.
39. Omura GA, Blessing JA, Major F, *et al.* A randomized clinical trial of adjuvant adriamycin in uterine sarcomas: a Gynecologic Oncology Group study. *J Clin Oncol* 1985; **3**, 1240–5.
40. Edmonson JH, Fleming TR, Ivins JC, *et al.* Randomized study of systemic chemotherapy following complete excision of nonosseous sarcomas. *J Clin Oncol* 1984; **2**, 1390–4.
41. Rosenberg SA, Tepper J, Glatstein E, *et al.* Prospective randomized evaluation of adjuvant chemotherapy in adults with soft tissue sarcomas of the extremities. *Cancer* 1983; **52**, 424–34.
42. Chang AE, Kinsella T, Glatstein E, *et al.* Adjuvant chemotherapy for patients with high-grade soft-tissue sarcomas of the extremity. *J Clin Oncol* 1988; **6**, 1491–500.
43. Glenn J, Sindelar WF, Kinsella T, *et al.* Results of multimodality therapy of resectable soft-tissue sarcomas of the retroperitoneum. *Surgery* 1985; **97**, 316–24.
44. Wilson RE, Wood WC, Lerner HL, *et al.* Doxorubicin chemotherapy in the treatment of soft-tissue sarcoma: combined results of two randomized trials. *Arch Surg* 1986; **121**, 1354–9.
45. Antman K, Ryan L, Borden E, *et al.* Pooled results from three randomized adjuvant studies of doxorubicin versus observation in soft tissue sarcoma: 10 year results and review of the literature. In: SE Salmon, ed, *Adjuvant Therapy of Cancer VI.* Philadelphia: WB Saunders, 1990; 529–43.
46. Baker LH. Adjuvant therapy for soft tissue sarcomas. In: JR Ryan, LO Baker, eds, *Recent Concepts in Sarcoma Treatment.* Dordrecht: Kluwer Academic Publishers, 1988; 130–5.
47. Bramwell V, Rouesse J, Steward W, *et al.* European experience of adjuvant chemotherapy for soft tissue sarcoma: interim report of a randomized trial of CYVADIC versus control. In: JR Ryan, LO Baker, eds, *Recent Concepts in Sarcoma Treatment.* Dordrecht, Kluwer Academic Publishers, 1988; 156–63.
48. Bramwell V, Rouesse J, Steward W, *et al.*, for Soft Tissue and Bone Sarcoma Group, Brussels, Belgium. Reduced rate of local recurrence following CYVADIC chemotherapy in localized soft tissue sarcoma: an EORTC randomized trial. *Proc ASCO* 1989; **8**, 320.
49. Ravaud A, Bui NB, Coindre J-M, *et al.* Adjuvant chemotherapy with CYVADIC in high risk soft tissue sarcoma. A randomized prospective trial. In: SE Salmon, ed, *Adjuvant Therapy of Cancer VI.* Philadelphia: WB Saunders, 1990; 556–66.
50. Alvegard TA, Sigurdsson H, Mouridsen H, *et al.*, for the Scandinavian Sarcoma Group. Adjuvant chemotherapy with doxorubicin in high-grade soft tissue sarcoma: a randomized trial of the Scandinavian Sarcoma Group. *J Clin Oncol* 1989; **7**, 1504–13.
51. Gherlinzoni F, Bacci G, Picci P, *et al.* A randomized trial for the treatment of high-grade soft tissue sarcomas of the extremities: preliminary observations. *J Clin Oncol* 1986; **4**, 552–8.

52. Picci P, Bacci G, Gherlinzoni F, *et al.* Results of a randomized trial for the treatment of localized soft tissue tumors of the extremities in adult patients. In: JR Ryan, LO Baker, eds, *Recent Concepts in Sarcoma Treatment.* Dordrecht: Kluwer Academic Publishers, 1988; 144–8.
53. Gherlinzoni F, Picci P, Bacci G, *et al.* Late results of a randomized trial for the treatment of soft tissue sarcomas of the extremities in adult patients. *Proc ASCO* 1993; **12**, 468.
54. Eilber FR, Giuliano AE, Huth JF, *et al.* Adjuvant adriamycin in high-grade extremity soft tissue sarcoma — a randomized prospective trial. *Proc ASCO* 1986; **5**, 125.
55. Eilber FR, Giuliano AE, Huth JF, *et al.* A randomized prospective trial using postoperative adjuvant chemotherapy (adriamycin) in high-grade extremity soft tissue sarcoma. *Am J Clin Oncol* 1988; **11**(1), 39–45.
56. Zalupski MM, Ryan JR, Hussein ME, *et al.* Defining the role of adjuvant chemotherapy for patients with soft tissue sarcoma of the extremities. In: SE Salmon, ed, *Adjuvant Therapy of Cancer VII.* Philadelphia: JB Lippincott Co, 1993; 387–92.
57. Rao CR. *Linear Statistical Inference and its Applications,* 2nd edn. New York: John Wiley & Sons, 1973; 389.
58. Dresdale A, Bonow RO, Wesley R, *et al.* Prospective evaluation of doxorubicin-induced cardiomyopathy resulting from postsurgical adjuvant treatment of patients with soft tissue sarcomas. *Cancer* 1983; **52**, 51–60.
59. Casper ES, Gaynor JJ, Hajdu SI, *et al.* A prospective randomized trial of adjuvant chemotherapy with bolus versus continuous infusion of doxorubicin in patients with high-grade extremity soft tissue sarcoma and an analysis of prognostic factors. *Cancer* 1991; **68**, 1221–9.
60. Shamberger RC, Sherins RJ, Ziegler JL, *et al.* Effects of postoperative adjuvant chemotherapy and radiotherapy on ovarian function in women undergoing treatment for soft tissue sarcoma. *J Natl Cancer Inst* 1981; **67**, 1213–18.
61. Shamberger RC, Sherins RJ, Rosenberg SA. The effects of postoperative adjuvant chemotherapy and radiotherapy in testicular function in men undergoing treatment for soft tissue sarcoma. *Cancer* 1981; **47**, 2368–74.
62. Raney B, Tefft M, Heyn R, *et al.* Ascending myelitis after intensive chemotherapy and radiation therapy in children with cranial parameningeal sarcoma. *Cancer* 1992; **69**, 1498–506.
63. Blackledge G, van Oosterom A, Mouridsen HT, *et al.* on behalf of the EORTC Soft Tissue and Bone Sarcoma Group. The place of chemotherapy in the management of soft tissue sarcoma: experiences of the EORTC Soft Tissue and Bone Sarcoma Group. *Clin Oncol* 1989; **1**, 106–9.
64. Pezzi CM, Pollock RE, Evans HL, *et al.* Preoperative chemotherapy for soft tissue sarcomas of the extremities. *Ann Surg* 1990; **211**, 476–81.
65. Chawla SP, Rosen G, Eilber F, *et al.* Cisplatin and adriamycin as neo-adjuvant and adjuvant chemotherapy in the management of soft tissue sarcomas. In: SE Salmon, ed, *Adjuvant Therapy of Cancer VI.* Philadelphia: WB Saunders, 1990; 567–73.
66. Geer RJ, Woodruff J, Casper ES, *et al.* Management of small soft-tissue sarcoma of the extremity in adults. *Arch Surg* 1992; **127**, 1285–9.
67. Tanabe KK, Pollock RE, Ellis LM, *et al.* Influence of surgical margins on outcome in patients with preoperatively irradiated extremity soft tissue sarcomas. *Cancer* 1994; **73**, 1652–9.
68. Brant TA, Parsons JT, Marcus RB, *et al.* Preoperative irradiation for soft tissue sarcomas of the trunk and extremity in adults. *Int J Radiat Oncol Biol Phys* 1990; **19**, 899–906.
69. Nielsen OS, Cummings B, O'Sullivan B, *et al.* Preoperative and postoperative irradiation of soft tissue sarcomas: effect on radiation field size. *Int J Radiat*

*Oncol Biol Phys* 1991; **21**, 1595–9.
70. Bujko K, Suit HD, Springfield DS, *et al.* Wound healing after preoperative radiation for sarcomas of soft tissues. *Surg Gynecol Obstet* 1993; **176**, 124–34.
71. Tepper JE, Suit HD, Wood WC, *et al.* Radiation therapy of retroperitoneal soft tissue sarcomas. *Int J Radiat Oncol Biol Phys* 1984; **10**, 825–30.
72. Sindelar WF, Kinsella TJ, Chen PW, *et al.* Intraoperative radiotherapy in retroperitoneal sarcomas: final results of a prospective, randomized, clinical trial. *Arch Surg* 1993; **128**, 402–10.
73. Tepper JE, Suit HD. Radiation therapy alone for sarcoma of soft tissue. *Cancer* 1985; **56**, 475–9.
74. Suit HD, Mankin HJ, Wood WC, *et al.* Treatment of the patient with stage M0 soft tissue sarcoma. *J Clin Oncol* 1988; **6**, 854–62.
75. Gemer LS, Trowbridge DR, Neff J, *et al.* Local recurrence of soft tissue sarcoma following brachytherapy. *Int J Radiat Oncol Biol Phys* 1991; **20**, 587–92.
76. Habrand JL, Gerbaulet A, Pejovic MH, *et al.* Twenty years experience of interstitial iridium brachytherapy in the management of soft tissue sarcomas. *Int J Radiat Oncol Biol Phys* 1991; **20**, 405–11.
77. Shiu MH, Hilaris BS, Harrison LB, *et al.* Brachytherapy and function-saving resection of soft tissue sarcoma arising in the limb. *Int J Radiat Oncol Biol Phys* 1991; **21**, 1485–92.
78. Glaholm J, Harmer C. Soft-tissue sarcoma: neutrons versus photons for postoperative irradiation. *Br J Radiol* 1988; **61**, 829–34.
79. Leibel SA, Wara WM, Hill DR, *et al.* Desmoid tumors: local control and patterns of relapse following radiation therapy. *Int J Radiat Oncol Biol Phys* 1983; **9**, 1167–71.
80. Kiel KD, Suit HD. Radiation therapy in the treatment of aggressive fibromatoses (desmoid tumors). *Cancer* 1984; **54**, 2051–5.
81. Marks LB, Suit HD, Rosenberg AE, *et al.* Dermatofibrosarcoma protuberans treated with radiation therapy. *Int J Radiat Oncol Biol Phys* 1989; **17**, 379–84.
82. Emrich LJ, Ruka W, Driscoll DL, *et al.* The effect of local recurrence on survival time in adult high-grade soft tissue sarcomas. *J Clin Epidemiol* 1989; **42**, 105–10.
83. Stotter AT, A'Hern RP, Fisher C, *et al.* The influence of local recurrence of extremity soft tissue sarcoma on metastasis and survival. *Cancer* 1990; **65**, 1119–29.
84. Barr LC, Stotter AT, A'Hern RP. Influence of local recurrence on survival: a controversy reviewed from the perspective of soft tissue sarcoma. *Br J Surg* 1991; **78**, 648–50.
85. Singer S, Antman K, Corson JM, *et al.* Long-term salvageability for patients with locally recurrent soft-tissue sarcomas. *Arch Surg* 1992; **127**, 548–53.
86. Mantel N. Evaluation of response-time data involving transient states: an illustration using heart-transplant data. *J Am Stat Assoc* 1974; **69**, 81–6.
87. Cox DR. Regression models and life tables. *J R Stat Soc B* 1972; **34**, 187–220.
88. Giuliano AE, Eilber FR. The rationale for planned reoperation after unplanned total excision of soft-tissue sarcomas. *J Clin Oncol* 1988; **3**, 1344–8.

# 9 Medulloblastoma — progress and pitfalls

*Patrick R M Thomas*

## Introduction

Of all the childhood brain tumours, medulloblastoma is one of the most studied and, in view of its responsiveness to both radiotherapy and chemotherapy, one of the most rewarding to treat. Nevertheless, although there has been undoubted progress, both in understanding and also in the cure rate, it is clear that success is usually obtained by aggressive treatment programmes that have long term sequelae.

## Early progress

Percival Bailey and Harvey Cushing first distinguished medulloblastoma from other tumours in the posterior fossa[1] and Cushing himself reported the first serious attempt to cure the disease. Despite radical surgery coupled in some cases with local radiotherapy only one patient out of sixty-one lived 3 years. There was a 32% operative mortality.[2]

As the disease was surgically incurable, radiotherapy rapidly became the primary mode of treatment. Early progress was disappointing, mainly because it was not realized that the disease can spread early via the leptomeninges. However, Lampe and McIntyre demonstrated that, by using aggressive systematic radiotherapy (the central nervous system (CNS) was treated in sequence), cures could be obtained.[3] These authors could only find twenty-seven documented 3-year survivors in a search of the literature between 1925 and 1948. In their own personal series, six out of twenty-one (28%) survived.

At Christie Hospital, Manchester, Paterson and Farr showed that by using kilovoltage irradiation and concurrent cranial and spinal fields a 41% 5-year survival rate could be achieved.[4] Forty years ago, therefore, craniospinal irradiation became the mainstay of treatment for medulloblastoma. This is still true today, despite attempts to modify or eliminate it in order to avoid undesirable late sequelae.

The use of telecobalt, and later of linear accelerators, made the disease technically much easier to treat than in the earlier experience. A number of different techniques were developed. Various reviews of single institution experiences have shown improvement in results over a 14-or-more-years period, notably those of Bloom *et al.* at the Royal Marsden Hospital, Surrey (1950–64),[5] Landberg *et al.* at the University Hospital of Lund (1945–75)[6] and Berry *et al.* at the Princess Margaret Hospital, Toronto (1958–78).[7] The Bloom *et al.* series was the first to demonstrate a substantial number of surviving patients (twenty-two of sixty-eight unselected cases — 32%). It was also the first to comment extensively on sequelae, although the subjective analysis presented an optimistic picture with fifteen out of twenty-two classified as 'no disability, active life'.[5]

# Chemotherapy

As chemotherapy developed, it became clear that, compared with other brain tumours, medulloblastoma has favourable characteristics. It is a rapidly dividing radioresponsive tumour and has a high proportion of cells in DNA synthesis. Furthermore, the propensity for leptomeningeal spread allows the effective use of intrathecal medication.[8] Early work suggested that methotrexate given intrathecally was the most active agent.[8,9] Further experience with this drug suggested caution when it is used in an adjuvant setting, particularly if an Ommaya reservoir is employed, as severe CNS toxicity can ensue.[10] The nitrosoureas, platinum compounds and vincristine have demonstrated activity[11] and, using xenografts as a basis for clinical study, so has melphalan.[12]

Adjuvant chemotherapy of medulloblastoma seemed a logical choice as the overall cure rate with craniospinal radiotherapy was approximately 40%. A pilot study at the Royal Marsden Hospital showed 70% 5-year survival in forty children given adjuvant 1-(2-chlorethyl)-3-cyclohexyl-1-nitrosourea (CCNU) and vincristine.[13]

# Randomized trials

Medulloblastoma is not sufficiently common to allow single institutions to perform randomized studies. Thus, all the major experience has come from multi-institutional and, particularly in the case of SIOP (the International Society of Paediatric Oncology), multinational cooperative groups.

## Initial trials (radiotherapy versus radiotherapy plus chemotherapy)

There were three studies initiated which randomized between radiotherapy alone and radiotherapy plus chemotherapy (Table 9.1).

The SIOP-I study and Children's Cancer Group (CCG) studies, as can be seen, were very similar in design, with the exception of the use of prednisone in the North American study. The results of both trials ultimately were disappointing as they failed to demonstrate a clear-cut advantage for patients treated with combined modality therapy.

**Table 9.1** Randomized clinical trials for medulloblastoma following surgery comparing radiotherapy alone with radiotherapy plus chemotherapy

---

*(a)    International Society of Paediatric Oncology (SIOP–I) 1975–79*

| | | |
|---|---|---|
| RT | Posterior fossa | 50–55 Gy |
| | Brain | 34–35 Gy |
| | Spinal | 30–35 Gy |

vs

RT (as above)    +    VCR 1 mg/m$^2$ during RT followed by 6 week cycles CCNU 100 mg/m$^2$, Day 1 VCR 1–5 mg/m$^2$, Days 1, 8 and 15
Chemotherapy for 1 year

*(b)    Children's Cancer Study Group (CCSG) and Radiation Therapy Oncology Group (RTOG) CCG 942, 1975–81*

| | | |
|---|---|---|
| RT | Posterior fossa | 50–55 Gy |
| | Brain | 35–40 Gy |
| | Spine | 35–40 Gy |

vs

RT (as above)    +    VCR 1.5 mg/m$^2$ during RT followed by 6 week cycles CCNU 100 mg/m$^2$, Day 1 VCR 1.5 mg$^2$, Days 1, 8, and 15
Prednisone 40 mg/m$^2$, Days 1–14
Chemotherapy for 1 year

*(c)    Pediatric Oncology Group (POG) POG 7909, 1979–86*

| | | |
|---|---|---|
| RT | Posterior fossa | 54 Gy |
| | Brain | 34 Gy |
| | Spine | 30 Gy |

vs

RT (as above)    followed by 4 week cycles of
Nitrogen mustard 3 mg/m$^2$, Days 1 and 8
+ VCR 1.4 mg/m2, Days 1 and 8
+ Prednisone 40 mg/m$^2$, Days 1–10
+ Procarbazine 50 mg, Day 1, 100 mg, Day 2 and 100 mg/m$^2$, Days 3–10 (MOPP — twelve cycles)

---

RT: radiotherapy. VCR: vincristine. CCNU: 1–(2-chlorethyl)–3-cyclohexyl–1–nitrosourea.

## SIOP-I

In the SIOP-I study (Table 9.1a), opened in 1975, interim analyses were regularly performed. These eventually (1979) showed a difference in disease-free survival in favour of the combined modality arm ($P = 0.005$) and the trial was therefore closed to further accrual, unfortunately limiting the power of the study. The results of the protocol were finally published using data up to 1988 (9 years after the protocol had closed). By this time, the overall significant differences between the two arms had disappeared (Table 9.2).[14] Despite this, however, there were significant differences in the various subgroups. T-stage (Table 9.3)[15] was a highly significant prognostic variable with T3 and T4 tumours doing worse than T1 and T2 tumours ($P < 0.05$). Other significant factors included the extent of surgery (total or subtotal excision vs partial excision or biopsy, $P < 0.05$) and size of participating centre (more than twenty patients entered in study versus less than twenty patients entered, $P < 0.005$). Females did better than males ($P < 0.025$). Combined modality therapy was significantly better for patients with brain stem involvement ($P < 0.005$), T3 and T4 tumours ($P = 0.002$), and in those with partial or subtotal resection ($P < 0.01$).[14]

**Table 9.2**  Results of SIOP–I study

|  | Disease-free survival | |
|---|---|---|
|  | 2-yr (1979) analysis | 5-yr (1988) analysis |
| Radiotherapy alone 145 patients | 71% | 55% |
|  | P = 0.005 | P = 0.07 |
| Radiotherapy and chemotherapy 141 patients | 53% | 42% |

## CCG — initial study

The CCG and Radiation Therapy Oncology Group (RTOG) entered patients onto protocol CCG 942 (Table 9.1b) between 1975 and 1981, and reported the results in 1990 on data available up to 1985.[16]

There were 233 patients classified as having medulloblastoma either by the reviewing or by the institutional pathologist, of which 179 were randomized, found to be eligible, and followed their assigned treatment regimens. The event-free survival at 5 years for all eligible patients was 59% for those treated with combined modality therapy and 50% for those treated with radiotherapy alone. This difference was not significant.

There were, however, statistical differences in favour of the combined modality therapy for those patients with T3 and T4 tumours and advanced M-stage (M1–M4). Other significant non-treatment-related prognostic factors included age of patient (children under 4 years of age fared worst),

**Table 9.3** Operative staging system for cerebellar medulloblastoma

| | |
|---|---|
| T1 | Tumour less than 3 cm in diameter and limited to the classic midline position in the vermis, the roof of the fourth ventricle, and less frequently to the cerebellar hemispheres |
| T2 | Tumour more than 3 cm in diameter, further invading one adjacent structure, or partially filling the fourth ventricle |
| T3a | Tumour further invading two adjacent structures or completely filling the fourth ventricle with extension into the aqueduct of Silvius, foramen of Magendie, or foramen of Luschka, thus producing marked hydrocephalus |
| T3b | Tumour arising from the floor of the fourth ventricle or brain stem and filling the fourth ventricle |
| T4 | Tumour further spreading through the aqueduct of Silvius to involve the third ventricle or midbrain, or tumour extending to the upper cervical cord |
| M0 | No evidence of gross subarachnoid or haematogenous metastases |
| M1 | Microscopic tumour cells in cerebrospinal fluid |
| M2 | Gross nodular seedings demonstrated in cerebellar, cerebral, subarachnoid space or in the third or lateral ventricles |
| M3 | Gross nodular seeding in spinal subarachnoid space |
| M4 | Extraneural metastasis |

Source: Chang *et al.*, *Radiology* 1969; **93**, 1351.[15]

race (black patients did better than whites) and M-stage (M0 patients did significantly better). There was no statistically significant effect of extent of resection and T-stage. Table 9.4 compares the results of the SIOP-I study and CCG 942. It can be seen that the prognostic indicators are dissimilar for the two studies.

## POG — initial study

The Pediatric Oncology Group (POG) study was the only one of the three initial multi-institutional studies to show a statistically significant result in favour of combined modality therapy.[17] There were seventy-one eligible patients randomized between 1979 and 1986 (Table 9.1c). A survival advantage was demonstrated for those patients receiving combined modality therapy ($P = 0.05$) but no overall event-free survival advantages were shown, except in patients of 5 years or older. Non-white patients did significantly better, as in CCG 942. In addition, females had a significantly increased survival over males, as in SIOP-I.

Although this study did show a significant advantage for combined modality treatment, there were relatively few patients entered over a lengthy time span. Toxicity was moderate in the combined modality arm, but there was one treatment-related death and there is potential for secondary malignancy with procarbazine.

**Table 9.4** Comparison of SIOP–I and CCG 942: reported significant factors

|  | SIOP–I | CCG 942 |
| --- | --- | --- |
| Non-treatment related | T-stage<br>Extent of surgery<br>Sex<br>Size of participating centre | M-stage<br>Age at diagnosis<br>Race |
| Treatment related<br>(combined modality<br>better than radiotherapy<br>alone) | T3–T4<br>Brain stem involvement<br>Partial or subtotal resection | M1–M4 |

## Subsequent multimodality trials

The results of the initial trials of radiotherapy alone versus radiotherapy plus chemotherapy unfortunately did not unequivocally establish a role for chemotherapy, nor did they provide overwhelming evidence of prognostic features. Nevertheless, subsequent trials have been designed with patients being divided by tumour extent as low (or standard) risk and high (or increased) risk stage.

### *SIOP-II*

SIOP-II was designed to test the concept of preradiotherapy (neoadjuvant) chemotherapy (procarbazine, vincristine, methotrexate and prednisone); and for patients with poor prognostic feature on SIOP-I (less than complete resection, T3 and T4, M1–4), designated as 'high risk', further chemotherapy was given following radiotherapy. The remaining patients (those with complete resection of T1 and T2 tumours) were designated as 'low risk' and randomized a second time to receive either standard (35 Gy neuraxis, 55 Gy posterior fossa) or reduced dose (25 Gy neuraxis, 55 Gy posterior fossa) radiotherapy (Fig. 9.1).

The protocol registered 446 patients between January 1984 and December 1989. Of those, 364 patients were randomized. No 5-year event-free survival advantage could be demonstrated for those patients receiving preradiotherapy chemotherapy (57.9%, compared with 59.8% for those not receiving it). In addition, no advantage could be demonstrated in those with 'high risk' tumours for preradiotherapy chemotherapy.

One hundred and fifty-three patients designated as 'low risk' were randomized between standard and reduced dose craniospinal irradiation. The

**High risk**

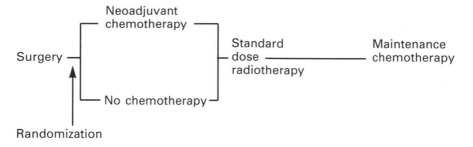

**Low risk**

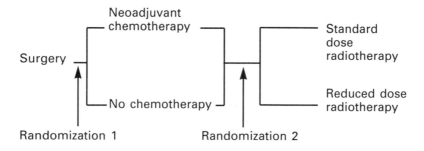

**Fig. 9.1**  SIOP-II schema.

5-year event-free survival rate was 67.6% for those receiving standard and 55.3% for those receiving reduced irradiation ($P = 0.07$). Further breakdown of the results showed that patients receiving preirradiation chemotherapy and reduced dose irradiation fared particularly poorly (41.7% 5-year event-free survival).

In addition, some of the prognostic groups demonstrated in SIOP-I (brain stem involvement, extent of surgical resection) did not retain their significance in SIOP-II, although the presence of central nervous system metastases remained prognostic.[18]

The CCG and POG combined their activities for the low-stage (standard risk) patients in protocol POG 8631/CCG 923. For the high-stage (increased risk) patients, the two groups undertook separate studies.

### POG and CCG high stage

The POG protocol 8695 was a one-arm pilot studying preirradiation chemotherapy with vincristine, cisplatin and cyclophosphamide for 9 weeks, followed by standard dose craniospinal irradiation. Eligibility for the protocol included only those patients with either extensive local lesions (T3–T4 with >1.5 cm$^3$ measurable disease) or neuroimaging evidence of neuraxis dissemination (M2, M3) (Table 9.3). Thirteen of the thirty fully evaluable patients achieved full or partial responses to chemotherapy. The 2-year progressive-free survival was 40%.[19] The CCG study (CCG 921) used the multimodality arm of protocol CCG 942 (Table 9.1b) as the control arm and tested 'eight-in-one' chemotherapy (vincristine, carmustine, procarbazine, hydroxyurea, cisplatin, cystosine arabinoside, cyclophosphamide and prednisone given in 1 day) prior to standard dose craniospinal irradiation. Preliminary results have shown a disadvantage for 'eight-in-one' chemotherapy.[20] In addition, patients with >1.5 $cm^3$ residual postoperative disease had a less favourable outcome.

## POG and CCG low stage

For low-stage disease, the combined POG/CCG study POG 8631 randomized patients following surgery to receive either standard dose radiotherapy (36 Gy to neuraxis with 54 Gy to posterior fossa) or reduced dose radiotherapy (23.4 Gy to neuraxis with 54 Gy to posterior fossa). The rationale for reducing the dose to the neuraxis was based on pilot data from Northwestern University, Illinois.[21] It was felt that reduction of the neuraxis radiotherapy dosage would be likely to reduce the severity of late effects on the central nervous and endocrine systems. Elaborate studies were therefore prospectively performed to evaluate those parameters but it was recognized that the results could not be finally correlated until some years following completion of protocol treatment.

A monitoring committee followed the progress of the study very carefully and, in November 1990, it became apparent that there were an increased number of isolated neuraxis relapses (relapses in the cerebrum or spinal canal with no posterior fossa recurrence) in the reduced-dose-radiotherapy arm. The protocol was therefore closed to further patient entry and an interim analysis was prepared and presented.[22]

Updated results were presented in 1993 and, with a minimum of 3 years on study, the 4-year recurrence-free survival was significantly decreased for patients receiving reduced dose compared with those receiving standard dose irradiation (Table 9.5).[23] The initial observation of a disadvantage for reduced dose neuraxis irradiation was therefore strengthened. Further analysis is planned after the last patient has been on the study for at least 5 years (Novem-

**Table 9.5** Results of POG 8631/CCG 923: percentage 4-year recurrence-free survival

|  | Standard dose radiotherapy ($N$%(SE) = 64) | Reduced dose radiotherapy ($N$%(SE) = 62) | One-sided *P-value* |
|---|---|---|---|
| All relapses | 67.1 (9.9) | 51 (10.3) | 0.02 |
| Isolated neuraxis | 87.7 (7.9) | 72.6 (11.0) | 0.01 |

Source: Thomas *et al. Proceedings of the International Congress of Radiation Oncology*, Kyoto, Japan, June 1993.[23]
SE: standard error.

ber 1995). It is expected that there may well be morerelapses on the standard dose arm by that time. Preliminary neuropsychological data from this protocol have shown, however, that patients treated with standard dose irradiation had significantly increased risk, not only of below-normal intelligence quotients but also of academic achievement.[24]

## Current trials

The previous set of studies had clearly been even more disappointing than the initial trials. The test arms (preirradiation chemotherapy in SIOP-II,[18] low-dose craniospinal irradiation in SIOP-II and POG 8631[22,23] and CCG 921 'eight-in-one' chemotherapy[20]) had all, at least in part, failed. The single protocol that did not have a negative result was an unrandomized pilot study — POG 8695.[19]

### SIOP-III

SIOP-III was designed without stratification into high- and low-risk subsets. It was felt that, as SIOP-II had not confirmed the prognostic factors of SIOP-I, a single randomization was therefore justified. Consequently, the control arm is surgery followed by conventionally delivered craniospinal irradiation (35 Gy) with posterior fossa boost to 55 Gy and the test arm consists of surgery followed by vincristine, carboplatin, etoposide and cyclophosphamide (with mesna uroprotection) followed by identical irradiation. There is at least a 3-month delay before irradiation. This study is still accruing patients and will hopefully show that delaying irradiation by giving chemotherapy is not only safe but beneficial.

The POG and CCG once again both divided their patients into low- and high-stage subgroups and also combined their resources to study low-stage disease. As in second-generation studies, each cooperative group ran separate protocols for patients with high-stage tumours.

### POG and CCG high stage

POG 9031 is the high-stage protocol. This study was designed to test whether the timing of chemotherapy could be important. The schema is presented in Fig. 9.2. As can be seen, the protocol tests preirradiation chemotherapy (cisplatin and VP-16) followed by standard craniospinal radiotherapy and posterior fossa boost, and subsequently vincristine and cyclophosphamide. The 'control' arm is the identical treatment regimen but with irradiation initially followed by the two chemotherapy phases. The study opened in July 1990 and accrual continues at the projected level with 141 eligible patients on study by April 1994. Reported toxicity has been moderate with leucopenia and thrombocytopenia predominating.[25]

The CCG high-stage study (CCG 9931) is a single-arm pilot of neoadjuvant chemotherapy. Figure 9.3 shows the schema of this protocol. All patients receive five courses of chemotherapy alternating between A (cyclophosphamide, cisplatin, etoposide and vincristine) and B (carboplatin and etoposide). Radiotherapy is given using a hyperfractionated

Arm 1:

Pre-irradiation chemotherapy

| Week: | 1 | 4 | 7 |
| Day: | 1 3 4 | 1 3 4 | 1 3 4 |
| | P | P | P |
| | EE | EE | EE |

←3 wks→

Radiotherapy

10
1

**Posterior fossa (53.2 Gy)**
**Whole brain (35.2 Gy)**
**Spine (35.2 Gy)**

1.6 Gy once/day, 5 days/wk with boost to gross spinal seeding

←3 wks→

Post-irradiation chemotherapy

| | 20 24 28 32 36 40 44 48 |
| Days: | 1 + 2 |
| | V Repeat q 4 wks × 7 |
| | C    C |

Arm: 2:

Radiotheraphy as in Arm 1

←3 wks→

Post-irradiation chemotherapy

| | 11 | 14 | 17 |
| Days: 1 3 4 | 1 3 4 | 1 3 4 |
| P | P | P |
| EE | EE | EE |

←3 wks→

Chemotherapy as in Arm 1 above

P = Cisplatin 90 mg/m² IV
E = Etoposide 150 mg/m² IV

V = Vincristine 2 mg/m² IV (max 2 mg dose)
C = Cyclophosphamide 1000 mg/m² IV with Mesna 360 mg/m² IV push
15 min prior to and 3 and 6 hrs following cyclophosphamide

**Fig. 9.2** POG 9031 schema.

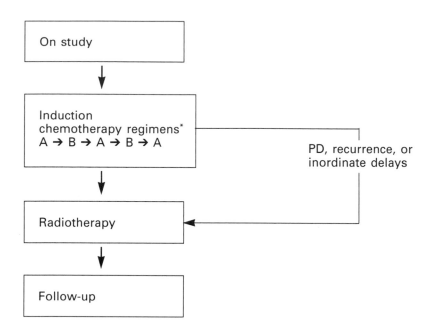

**Fig. 9.3**  CCG 9931 schema. PD = Progressive disease. *See text.

regimen (72 Gy to the posterior fossa and 36 Gy to the craniospinal axis). This protocol has only been recently opened for patient accrual.

### POG and CCG low stage

The POG and CCG combined their resources once again to activate the protocol for low-stage medulloblastoma (POG 9331/CCG 9014). This study had a long gestational period since it was felt that, although standard dose radiotherapy (best arm in the POG 8631) versus standard dose radiotherapy plus chemotherapy was the statistically sound step, it would be seen as regressive by the investigators. It was therefore felt that the test arm should be reduced dose radiotherapy plus chemotherapy, as the results might be equivalent as far as survival and recurrence-free interval are concerned, but there could be less toxicity on the test arm (as had been suggested by POG 8631[24]) although the contribution to the toxicity of chemotherapy remains unknown. The schema for this protocol is presented in Fig. 9.4. In order to be eligible, patients were required to have gross total (or near total) resection of medulloblastoma confined to the posterior fossa without extension into the brain stem. Note that the posterior fossa dosage was increased to 55.8 Gy, as posterior fossa recurrences still occurred with 54 Gy. Cisplatin was added to the chemotherapy regimen because of the highly promising results of Packer *et al.*[26] (see below). In addition, this study investigates prospectively the prognostic significance of ploidy[27] and C-*myc* amplification.[28] The protocol has only recently opened.

| R | REGIMEN A |
|---|---|
| A | 36 Gy to craniospinal axis – 20 fractions – |
| | 1 fraction per day, 19.8 Gy boost to posterior |
| N | fossa – 11 fractions – 1 fraction per day |
| | |
| D | REGIMEN B |
| | |
| O | 23.4 Gy to craniospinal axis – 13 fractions – |
| | 1 fraction per day, 32.4 Gy boost to posterior |
| M | fossa – 18 fractions – 1 fraction per day; |
| | weekly vincristine $(1.5\,mg/m^2)$ during |
| I | irradiation, five 7-week cycles of chemotherapy |
| | consisting of cisplatin $(75\,mg/m^2)$ Day 1 |
| Z | vincristine $(1.5\,mg/m^2)$ Days 1 and 8; |
| | cyclophosphamide $(1000\,mg/m^2)$ Days 22 and 23; |
| E | vincristine $(1.5\,mg/m^2)$ Days 22 and 29. |

**Fig. 9.4** POG 9331/CCG 9014 schema.

# Non-randomized studies

Although the results of randomized studies have been disappointing, much information has been learned from single institutional protocols. Thus, Packer *et al.*, at the Children's Hospital of Philadelphia, reported on forty-two patients, who were considered to have 'poor risk' disease (either T3b/T4, or partial resection/biopsy of tumour, or M1/M3), treated with radiotherapy followed by CCNU, vincristine and cisplatin. Forty of the forty-two patients remained alive with an actuarial 5-year disease-free survival of 92%.[26] As previously mentioned, this directly influenced the choice of regimens for POG 9331/CCG 9014.

With more aggressive treatment protocols, changes in patterns of relapse have been observed. At the Boston Children's Hospital, six (12%) out of fifty patients treated with craniospinal irradiation developed isolated bone metastases. A subsequent cohort of thirty-nine patients were treated with preirradiation vincristine and cisplatin; there were no systemic failures in this group.[29] Posterior fossa failures depended not on adjuvant chemotherapy but on radiotherapy dosage,[27] as had been suggested in earlier series.[13,30]

The dosage of radiotherapy to the neuraxis has remained an issue. Although SIOP-II[18] and POG 8631[22,23] have suggested increased neuraxis failures after reduced dose craniospinal axis irradiation (in the SIOP study this included patients who had received chemotherapy), the potential for reduced long-term toxicity has maintained the interest. The University of California, San Francisco, studied thirty-nine children treated with 24–26 Gy to the spinal axis (54 Gy to posterior fossa) with procarbazine and hydroxyurea. They found that there was a 5-year actuarial survival of 83% in the 'good risk' (>75% resected, T1–T3, M0) group and 58% in the 'poor risk' patients. The predominant site of failure was the posterior fossa with only three out of twenty-two failures classified as isolated neuraxis.[31] This suggests that further studies of reduced dose craniospinal irradiation plus chemotherapy are indicated.

## Medulloblastoma in infants

The effects of craniospinal irradiation on infants are devastating due to the incomplete myelination. Thus, attempts to delay and reduce radiotherapy have been justified. At MD Anderson Hospital, Van Eys *et al.* treated all patients with infant brain tumours with MOPP (mechlorethamine, vincristine (oncovin), procarbazine, prednisone).[32] Eight out of twelve infants with medulloblastoma were alive without evidence of disease at a median of 7 years from diagnosis.[33]

The POG study reported a 2-year disease-free survival of 34% (± 8%) for sixty-two patients under 3 years of age with medulloblastoma, with 70% for those with complete resection. Treatment consisted of two courses of cyclophosphamide and vincristine, with one course of etoposide and cisplatin, repeated for 12–24 months.[34]

The CCG studied eight-in-one chemotherapy in children under 2 years of age. The 3-year progression-free survival was 22% (30% for those who were classified as M0 at diagnosis).[35]

Although these results are encouraging and show that craniospinal irradiation may be delayed, it is clear that the majority of patients will need this modality. At St Jude Children's Research Hospital, a group of thirteen patients, who either had residual disease at completion of chemotherapy (two patients) or had progressive disease, were treated with craniospinal radiotherapy. Three of these remain alive 48–104 months postdiagnosis but they have neurodevelopmental defects.[36]

## Late effects of treatment

Although it is clear that a substantial proportion of the medulloblastoma patients can be cured, there are a number of serious late effects. In a classic paper, Probert and Parker reported measurements of the sitting heights of irradiated children and found that the most damage occurred during periods of growth (if radiotherapy was given at <6 years of age or at puberty) and with doses greater than 35 Gy.[37] Recent results from the Children's Hospital of Philadelphia suggest that effects on bone growth velocity may be worsened by the addition of chemotherapy (vincristine, CCNU ± cisplatin) with 37 Gy to the spine and 42 Gy to the pituitary.[38]

There has been much interest in neuropsychological effects of treatment for brain tumours. Interviews with 342 adults who had been treated for central nervous system tumours before the age of 20 demonstrated that they had suffered a poor-quality life with unemployment, disability and emotional problems, which were significantly higher than in 479 matched siblings.[39]

At the Children's Hospital of Philadelphia, forty-three consecutive survivors were studied, a median of 4.5 years after diagnosis. Although the average full-scale IQ was 97, specific learning disorders, memory and fine motor disabilities were founded in over half of the patients.[40] However, in a review article, Duffner and Cohen conclude that evaluation of patients treated in prospective studies has not revealed the frequency of mental retardation that had been expected from earlier reports. There is, however, a noticeable decline in IQ by 2 years following treatment, with most patients developing learning disabilities and attention deficit disorders.[41]

Current studies have been designed to include prospective evaluation of neuropsychological, endocrine and skeletal parameters. As far as possible, patients are evaluated prior to treatment. As mentioned, the preliminary data of Mulhern have shown differences based on treatment regimen.[24] In the next few years, much information should become available from the various completed and currently accruing clinical trials.

## Conclusions

In the past 15 years, since the prospectively randomized clinical trials have been in operation, we have learned much about medulloblastoma and the results and unwanted effects of its treatment. Unfortunately, this knowledge has not as yet been translated into major progress from the point of view of relapse and overall cure rate.

Clearly 'standard' dose irradiation (36 Gy neuraxis, 54 Gy posterior fossa) remains the gold standard for patients with low-stage disease (the term 'good risk' is unfortunate as it implies a good result, which is not certain). Although reduction in neuraxis dose may reduce late effects, two studies have shown that it is associated with increased number of relapses. It remains to be seen whether lower dose neuraxis radiotherapy (23.4 Gy) plus chemotherapy is as effective and less toxic than standard (36 Gy) craniospinal irradiation.

For high-stage disease, radiotherapy plus chemotherapy appears to be established. The current data suggest that regimens containing cisplatin (or platinum analogues) should be further explored. It is to be hoped that eventually less toxic regimens can be designed for this group of patients.

## References

1. Bailey P, Cushing H. Medulloblastoma cerebelli, common type of mid-cerebellar glioma of childhood. *Arch Neurol Psychiatr* 1925; **14**, 192–224.
2. Cushing H. Experiences with cerebellar medulloblastoma: critical review. *Acta Pathol Microbiol Scand* 1930; **7**, 1–86.
3. Lampe I, McIntyre RS. Experiences in radiation therapy of medulloblastoma of the cerebellum. *Am J Roentgenol Radiat Ther Nucl Med* 1954; **71**, 659–68.
4. Paterson E, Farr RF. Cerebellar medulloblastoma treatment of irradiation of whole central nervous system. *Acta Radiol* 1953; **39**, 323–36.
5. Bloom HJG, Wallace ENK, Henk JM. The treatment and prognosis of medulloblastoma in children. *Am J Roentgenol Radiat Ther Nucl Med* 1969; **105**, 43–62.
6. Landberg TG, Lindgren ML, Cavallin-Stahl EK, *et al.* Improvements in the radiotherapy of medulloblastoma. *Cancer* 1980; **45**, 670–8.

7. Berry MP, Jenkin RDT, Keen CW, *et al*. Radiation treatment for medulloblastoma – A 21 year review. *J Neurosurg* 1981; **55**, 43–51.
8. Shapiro WR. Chemotherapy of childhood brain tumors. *Cancer* 1975; **35**, 965–72.
9. Newton WA, Sayers MD, Samuels LD. Intrathecal methotrexate therapy for brain tumors in children. *Cancer Chemother Rep* 1968; **52**, 257–61.
10. Thomas PRM, Duffner PK, Cohen ME, *et al*. Multimodality therapy for medulloblastoma. *Cancer* 1980; **45**, 666–9.
11. Friedman HS, Oakes WS. The chemotherapy of posterior fossa tumors in childhood. *J Neurooncol* 1987; **5**, 216–29.
12. Friedman HS, Schold SC, Mahaley MS, *et al*. Phase II treatment of medulloblastoma and pinealoblastoma with melphalan: clinical therapy based on experimental models of human medulloblastoma. *J Clin Oncol* 1989; 7, 904–11.
13. Bloom HJG. Intracranial tumours: response and resistance to therapeutic endeavors. *Int J Radiat Oncol Biol Phys* 1982; **8**, 1083–113.
14. Tait DM, Thornton-Jones H, Bloom HJG, *et al*. Adjuvant chemotherapy for medulloblastoma: the first multi-centre control trial of the International Society of Paediatric Oncology (SIOP-I). *Eur J Cancer* 1990; **26**, 464–9.
15. Chang CH, Housepian EM, Herbert C. An operative staging system and a megavoltage radiotherapeutic technique for cerebellar medulloblastomas. *Radiology* 1969; **93**, 1351–9.
16. Evans AE, Jenkins RDT, Sposto R, *et al*. The treatment of medulloblastoma. Results of a prospective randomized trial of radiation therapy with or without CCNU, vincristine, and prednisone. *J Neurosurg* 1990; **72**, 572–82.
17. Krischer JP, Ragab AH, Kun L, *et al*. Nitrogen mustard, vincristine, procarbazine and prednisone as adjuvant chemotherapy in medulloblastoma. A Pediatric Oncology Group Study. *J Neurosurg* 1991; **74**, 905–9.
18. Bailey CC, Gnekow A, Wellek S, *et al*. Prospective randomized trial of chemotherapy given before radiotherapy in childhood medulloblastoma. *International Society of Paediatric Oncology (SIOP) and the German Society of Paediatric Oncology (GPO) SIOP II* (in press).
19. Mosijczuk AD, Nigro MA, Thomas PRM, *et al*. Preradiation chemotherapy in advanced medulloblastoma. A Pediatric Oncology Group pilot study. *Cancer* 1993; **72**, 2755–62.
20. Boyelt J, Zeltzer P, Finlay J, *et al*. Progression-free survival (PFS) and risk factors for primative neuroectodermal tumours (PNET) of the posterior fossa (PF) (medulloblastoma) in children. Report of the Children's Cancer Group (CCG) randomized trial CCG-921. *Proc ASCO* 1995; **14**, 147.
21. Tomita T, McLone DG. Medulloblastoma in childhood: results of radical resection and low dose neuroaxis therapy. *J Neurosurg* 1986; **64**, 238–42.
22. Deutsch M, Thomas PRM, Boyett JM, *et al*. A Children's Cancer Study Group (CCSG) and Pediatric Oncology Group (POG) randomized study of standard vs reduced neuraxis irradiation. *Proc ASCO* 1991; **10**, 124 (Abstract).
23. Thomas PRM, Deutsch M, Krischer JP, *et al*. Further evidence of superiority of standard dose compared with reduced dose irradiation in low stage medulloblastoma. *Proceedings of the International Congress of Radiation Oncology*, Kyoto, Japan, June 1993; 253 (02–4).
24. Mulhern RK, personal communication.
25. POG 9031, unpublished data.
26. Packer RJ, Sutton LN, Goldwein JW, *et al*. Improved survival with the use of adjuvant chemotherapy in the treatment of medulloblastoma. *J Neurosurg* 1991; **74**, 433–40.
27. Yasue M, Tomita T, Englehard H, *et al*. Prognostic importance of DNA ploidy in medulloblastoma of childhood. *J Neurosurg* 1989; **70**, 385–91.
28. Bigner SH, Friedman HS, Vogelstein B, *et al*. Amplification of the c-*Myc* gene

in medulloblastoma cell lines and xenografts. *Cancer Res* 1990; **50**, 2347–50.

29. Tarbell NJ, Loeffler JS, Silver B, *et al*. The change in patterns of relapse in medulloblastoma. *Cancer* 1991; **68**, 1600–4.

30. Silverman CL, Simpson JR. Cerebellar medulloblastoma: the importance of posterior fossa dose to survival and patterns of failure. *Int J Radiat Oncol Biol Phys* 1982; **8**, 2023–7.

31. Halberg FE, Wara WM, Fippin LF, *et al*. Low dose craniospinal radiotherapy for medulloblastoma. *Int J Radiat Oncol Biol Phys* 1991; **20**, 651–4.

32. Van Eys J, Cangir A, Coody D. MOPP regimen as primary chemotherapy for brain tumors in infants. *J Neurooncol* 1985; **3**, 237–43.

33. Ater JL, Needle MN. Progress and expectations in the treatment of childhood brain tumors. *Cancer Bull* 1992; **44**, 490–5.

34. Duffner PK, Horowitz M, Krischer J, *et al*. Postoperative chemotherapy and delayed radiation in children less than two years of age with malignant brain tumors. *N Engl J Med* 1993; **328**, 1725–31.

35. Geyer JR, Zeltzer PM, Boyett JM, *et al*. Survival of infants with primitive neuroectodermal tumors or malignant ependymomas of the CNS treated with eight drugs in 1 day: a report from the Children's Cancer Group. *J Clin Oncol* 1994; **12**, 1607–15.

36. Gajjas A, Mulhern RK, Heideman RL, *et al*. Medulloblastoma in very young children. Outcome of definitive craniospinal irradiation following incomplete response to chemotherapy. *J Clin Oncol* 1994; **12**, 1212–16.

37. Probert JC, Parker BR. The effect of radiation therapy on bone growth. *Radiology* 1975; **114**, 115–62.

38. Olshan JS, Gubernick J, Packer RJ, *et al*. The effects of adjuvant chemotherapy on growth in children with medulloblastoma. *Cancer* 1992; **70**, 2013–17.

39. Mostow EN, Byrne J, Connelly RR, *et al*. Quality of life in long-term survivors of CNS tumors of childhood and adolescence. *J Clin Oncol* 1991; **9**, 592–9.

40. Packer RJ, Sposto R, Atkins TE, *et al*. Quality of life in children with primitive neuroectodermal tumors (medulloblastoma) of the posterior fossa. *Pediatr Neurosci* 1987; **13**, 169–75.

41. Duffner PK, Cohen ME. Changes in the approach to central nervous system tumors in childhood. *Pediatr Clin North Am* 1992; **39**, 859–77.

# 10 The role of radiotherapy in the management of neuroblastoma

*Mark N Gaze*

## Neuroblastoma: an overview

### Introduction

Neuroblastoma is an embryonal tumour of the sympathetic nervous system. In his 1910 paper 'Neurocytoma or neuroblastoma, a kind of tumour not normally recognised', Homer Wright[1] gave a name and a unified identity to a group of syndromes previously thought to be separate. His detailed description of the characteristic rosette arrangement of cells and the demonstration of the tumour's neural origin by specific staining enabled neuroblastoma to be regarded, despite its heterogeneous features, as a single clinicopathological entity.

### Incidence

Neuroblastoma is the most common extracranial solid tumour of childhood, and accounts for about 7–8% of all paediatric malignant disease.[2] It is also the most common infant malignancy, becoming less frequent in each succeeding year. About half the cases occur under the age of 3 years. Neuroblastoma in adult life is well recognized but very rare. The sex ratio is about equal.

### Clinical features

A few asymptomatic patients are found to have neuroblastoma, either unexpectedly during a routine examination or as a result of a screening programme, but most present with symptoms. These may be caused directly by either the primary tumour or metastases, or by excess catecholamine production, or they may be the general, non-specific symptoms of disseminated malignancy.

Because of the embryological development of the sympathetic nervous system from the neural crest, neuroblastoma may develop at any site from the skull base to the pelvis. Most (62%) occur in the abdomen (including the adrenal gland and other retroperitoneal sites). Less frequently, neuroblastoma may arise in the thorax (14%), pelvis (5%) or other sites such as the neck.[3-9]

Neuroblastoma spreads by invasion and destruction of adjacent structures as well as by lymphatic and haematogenous metastasis. Tumours may extend through the neural foramina of the spine ('dumb-bell' tumours) and cause spinal cord compression and scoliosis.

The most common sites for blood-borne dissemination are the liver and the skeleton. Hepatic metastases, often massive, are more common in infants under the age of 6 months, perhaps as a result of transplacental metastasis in the case of congenital neuroblastoma.[10] Hepatic metastasis is also a particular feature of the International Neuroblastoma Staging System (INSS) Stage 4S disease.[11] Skeletal metastases, which are of grave prognostic significance, must be clearly differentiated from involvement of the bone marrow alone, which, in the case of INSS Stage 4S disease, is compatible with a high cure rate. Pulmonary and cerebral metastases are not common; metastases in a wide variety of other sites are occasionally seen.

## Pathology

Histologically, neuroblastoma is one of the 'small, round, blue cell tumours of childhood', a group which also includes lymphoma, rhabdomyosarcoma and Ewing's sarcoma. It is a highly cellular tumour, with homogeneous masses of small, round or occasionally ovoid cells with scanty cytoplasm and darkly staining nuclei. In up to half of neuroblastoma cases, typical rosettes are visible. These may contain a tangle of fibrillary material with a neuritic origin. The number of mitotic figures varies considerably from one case to the next. Typically, there is only a sparse vascular connective tissue stroma. Sometimes cells showing early neuroblastic differentiation are found. These cells have larger nuclei and more clearly defined cytoplasm and form less densely cellular groups set in a fine fibrillary stroma.

Immunohistochemical techniques are used to distinguish neuroblastoma from other tumours. Antigens expressed include neural cell adhesion molecule,[12] neurone-specific enolase,[13] neurofilament proteins[14] and the ganglioside $G_{D2}$.[15] As none of these is wholly specific for neuroblastoma, it is best if a panel of antibodies is used for diagnosis.[16]

## Biochemistry

Neuroblastoma shares with the postganglionic nerves of the sympathetic nervous system and the chromaffin cells of the adrenal medulla, the ability to synthesize and release the catecholamines adrenaline (epinephrine), noradrenaline (norepinephrine) and dopamine. In addition, neuroblastoma cells possess a mechanism for the reuptake of catecholamines whose physiological functions are to terminate the neurotransmitter action of nor-adrenaline and the hormonal action of adrenaline. This mechanism is exploited therapeutically in the targeted radiotherapy of neuroblastoma by *meta*-iodobenzylguanidine (*m*IBG).

The principal catecholamine metabolites, valuable tumour markers in the diagnosis and surveillance of patients with neuroblastoma, can be detected and quantified in urine. They are 4-hydroxy-3-methoxymandelic acid (HMMA, more commonly known as vanillylmandelic acid or VMA), produced from adrenaline and noradrenaline, and 2-hydroxy-3-methoxyphenyl-acetic acid (HMPA, commonly known as homovanillic acid, HVA) from dopamine.

Urinary catecholamine metabolites may be used for the screening of asymptomatic infants for neuroblastoma. Unfortunately, as screening programmes have not led to a reduction in mortality rate from neuroblastoma, their implementation cannot be recommended.[17]

## Molecular genetics

Although the cause of neuroblastoma is unknown, occasional reports of familial cases of neuroblastoma suggest that there may be a genetic basis, at least in some instances.[18-20] Chromosomal anomalies, principally affecting chromosomes 1 and 17, are often found in tumour cells,[21] but identifiable constitutional aberrations are unusual.[22,23] It is possible that individuals with one constitutional chromosomal abnormality are at risk of developing malignancy if a second critical area of genetic material is damaged.[24]

The most common abnormality on chromosome 1 is a deletion of the distal region of the short arm, suggesting that loss of a tumour suppressor gene (or genes) may be responsible. Detailed molecular analysis of this chromosomal region has shown the deletion breakpoint to vary, usually being located at 1p31 or 1p32,[25] but sometimes as far distal as 1p36.[26,27] Loss of heterozygosity in this region is often associated with poor prognostic factors such as advanced stage and N-*myc* amplification,[28] although it is not necessarily, by itself, associated with a worse outcome.[29] *In-situ* DNA hybridization with a probe specific for the short arm of the chromosome has shown a relationship between chromosome 1 abnormalities and advanced stage at presentation.[30]

Amplification of the oncogene N-*myc*, located on chromosome 2 at 2p23–24, is one of the more powerful prognostic indicators in neuroblastoma.[31] It is found in between one-quarter and one-third of patients, more commonly in association with advanced disease. A relationship has been found in cell lines between N-*myc* amplification and sensitivity to treatment.[32] Although N-*myc* amplification was traditionally assessed by Southern blotting analysis, the polymerase chain reaction has proved to be a rapid and sensitive alternative technique.[33]

## Diagnosis

The gold standard for the diagnosis of neuroblastoma is examination of tumour tissue by histopathology and immunohistochemistry. However, as initial surgery is not indicated in patients with advanced disease who require systemic therapy, international criteria have been established which permit a reliable diagnosis to be made without a biopsy.[34] A diagnosis of neuroblastoma is established if bone marrow contains unequivocal tumour cells (e.g. syncytia or clusters of cells positive on immunocytology) and urine contains increased urinary catecholamine metabolites. This may be defined by urinary VMA and/or HVA levels greater than three standard deviations above the mean per milligram creatinine for the age of the patient. Both the VMA and HVA levels should be measured. Normalization per milligram of creatinine makes a timed collection unnecessary and avoids potential false negatives due to dilute urine.

## Staging

Tumour stage is one of the more important prognostic factors in neuroblastoma; a reliable and widely accepted staging system is therefore necessary. Until recently, many different classifications were in use. These have now been replaced by the International Neuroblastoma Staging System (INSS) set out in Table 10.1.[34,35]

## Treatment policies

### Early disease

Localized tumours, Stage 1 and Stage 2a, are usually amenable to surgery with curative intent. Adjuvant treatment with radiotherapy or chemotherapy is not indicated, even if there is microscopic residual disease.[36,37] Careful follow-up is necessary as local recurrence or distant metastasis may occur rarely.

### More advanced operable disease

Treatment of patients with lymph node involvement, that is Stage 2b and some Stage 3 cases, is again principally surgical. The need for adjuvant treatment depends on age. In infants younger than 6 months, chemotherapy is controversial.[21] In older children, chemotherapy is definitely warranted, using a schedule such as 'OPEC', which comprises vincristine (oncovin), cisplatin, etoposide and cyclophosphamide.[38] Irradiation of the tumour bed to eradicate residual disease is controversial, and is discussed fully below.

### Stage 4S disease

Patients with Stage 4S disease have a good prognosis. If the disease is not causing distressing or life-threatening symptoms, it is possible to follow a policy of observation in the hope of spontaneous regression. If there is embarrassing hepatomegaly, chemotherapy may be used, perhaps followed by excision of the primary tumour. Alternatively, irradiation may precipitate regression.

**Table 10.1**   The International Neuroblastoma Staging System (INSS)[34,35]

| | |
|---|---|
| Stage 1 | Localized tumour[a] with complete gross excision, with or without microscopic residual disease; representative ipsilateral lymph nodes negative for tumour microscopically (nodes attached to and removed with the primary tumour may be positive) |
| Stage 2A | Localized tumour with incomplete gross excision; representative ipsilateral non-adherent lymph nodes negative for tumour microscopically |
| Stage 2B | Localized tumour, with or without complete gross excision, with ipsilateral non-adherent lymph nodes positive for tumour Enlarged contralateral lymph nodes must be negative microscopically |
| Stage 3 | Unresectable tumour infiltrating across the midline,[b] with or without regional lymph node involvement; or localized unilateral tumour with contralateral regional lymph node involvement; or midline tumour with bilateral extension by infiltration (unresectable) or by lymph node involvement |
| Stage 4 | Any primary tumour with dissemination to distant lymph nodes, bone, bone marrow, liver, skin and/or other organs (except as defined in Stage 4S) |
| Stage 4S | Localized primary tumour (as defined for Stage 1, 2A or 2B), with dissemination limited to skin, liver and/or bone marrow[c] (limited to infants less than 1 year of age) |

[a]  Multifocal primary tumours (e.g. bilateral adrenal primary tumours) should be staged according to the greatest extent of disease, as defined above, and followed by a subscript 'M' (e.g. 3M).

[b]  The midline is defined as the vertebral column. Tumours originating on one side and 'crossing the midline' must infiltrate to or beyond the opposite side of the vertebral column.

[c]  Marrow involvement in Stage 4S should be minimal, i.e. less than 10% of total nucleated cells identified as malignant on bone marrow biopsy or on marrow aspirate. More extensive marrow involvement would be considered to be Stage 4. The *m*IBG scan (if done) should be negative in the marrow.

### Inoperable disease

Patients with advanced disease, that is those with Stage 4 or inoperable Stage 3 disease, should receive initial chemotherapy with OPEC or a similar schedule. Dose intensification strategies, designed to achieve a greater degree of cytoreduction and to circumvent the development of resistant clones by using a larger number of non-cross-resistant drugs in higher doses over a shorter period, are feasible but have not yet proved significantly superior to OPEC.[39–41] If chemotherapy has rendered the Stage 3 tumour operable, it should be removed. In Stage 4 patients, surgery to remove residual primary tumour should also be considered if there has been a complete remission at metastatic sites.

### Megatherapy

Intensive treatment protocols, referred to as 'megatherapy', which combine high dose chemotherapy and/or total body irradiation with autologous bone marrow transplantation, have been developed with the aim of improving the outlook in advanced disease. The rationale for this approach is simple. If the small burden of occult residual disease in patients apparently in complete remission — yet destined to relapse — can be eradicated, then the patient is cured. As these residual cells, having survived induction chemotherapy, may well be drug-resistant, alternative ways to kill cells are required. Higher than conventional doses of chemotherapy may be effective in cells which are resistant to usual levels, as they can by-pass inadequate membrane transport and saturate detoxification pathways and DNA repair mechanisms. Further cell kill can also be achieved by irradiation, which needs to be to the whole body to cover occult disseminated disease.

Bone marrow transplantation, or, more recently, peripheral blood stem cell reinfusion, is used to circumvent myelosuppression, which is the first dose-limiting toxicity both for most chemotherapeutic agents and for total body irradiation. In this way, drug doses three- to ten-fold greater than are conventional may be used. Many different cytotoxic drugs have been used in megatherapy regimens, but as high dose melphalan in a randomized trial has been proved to improve survival, its place in future protocols is assured.[42,43]

## Prognosis

The survival of children with neuroblastoma has improved over recent years, largely because of the development of effective chemotherapy. For example, the 5-year survival rate of patients diagnosed in 1971–3 is 15% and for 1983–5 is 43%.[44]

Age at diagnosis is the single most important prognostic factor, with those older than 1 year faring worse. Five-year survival figures for children diagnosed in 1983–5 are: for those aged less than 1 year, 77%; aged 1 year, 39%; aged 2 years, 28%; and from 3 to 9 years, less than 25%.[44] After age comes stage: the outlook for patients with INSS Stages 1 and 4S is much better than in those with more advanced disease. Location of the tumour is also important: patients with mediastinal tumours do better than those with tumours in the adrenal or other retroperitoneal sites. Histology is relevant, as signs of differentiation predict a more favourable outcome.[45] Finally, genetic factors such as N-*myc* amplification and 1p deletion correlate with a poor prognosis.[46]

# Radiobiology

## Radiosensitivity of neuroblastoma cell lines

Because of the rarity and heterogeneous nature of neuroblastoma, laboratory studies of its radiobiology using cell lines have proved easier than clinical studies. The settings of such experimental investigations are necessarily artificial, and care must be taken before extrapolating laboratory results to the clinical situation. Nonetheless, there is good evidence that cell lines retain the radiosensitivities of their parent tumour type. For example, one analysis of published data of sixty-four cell lines derived from tumours of low, intermediate or high clinical radiosensitivity showed a correlation between the radiobiological parameters and the clinical group, although there was some overlap.[47]

Experimental data on the response to irradiation of a cell line can be fitted into a radiobiological model, usually either the linear-quadratic or the multitarget model, to yield various indices of radiosensitivity. Although no single parameter can be used to describe the shape of the cell survival curve, there is one which gives a useful indication of the radiosensitivity of a cell line, regardless of which model best fits the data. This is the surviving fraction at 2 Gy, or $SF_2$, which describes the initial slope of the cell survival curve and has been found to discriminate well between sensitive and resistant lines.[48] With the recognition of the value of $SF_2$ as an indicator of radiosensitivity, and the realization that an observed value is preferable to a parameter calculated from a model, there is now less debate about the relative merits of the multitarget and linear-quadratic models.

The radiation response, obtained by clonogenic assay, of five neuroblastoma cell lines is reviewed by Steel and Wheldon.[49] Values for $SF_2$ range from 0.085 to 0.37, with a median of 0.13. These indicate that neuroblastoma is indeed sensitive by comparison with tumours such as osteosarcoma (median $SF_2$: 0.37) and glioma (median $SF_2$: 0.69). Data from spheroid regrowth experiments also indicate the radiosensitivity of neuroblastoma. The $D_0$ values for four cell lines are 0.81, 0.9, 1.04 and 1.3.[50,51]

## Fractionation and dose-rate effects

Response to a single dose is, however, not necessarily of clinical relevance as radiotherapy is usually fractionated. The principal reason for this is to allow normal tissues to recover from sublethal damage, and increase the therapeutic ratio. If the tumour also recovers to the same extent, the advantage conferred by fractionation is lost. The ability of tumour cells to accumulate and repair sublethal damage can be investigated by split-dose experiments. Using a total dose of 4 Gy, Deacon *et al.* demonstrated that HX138 cells plated in agar are able to repair a modest amount of damage within 3 hrs.[52] With a time interval of 6 hrs, Schwachöfer *et al.* likewise demonstrated a modest repair ability in NB-100 cells grown as spheroids, but only at total doses greater than 6 Gy.[53] Also using spheroids, Wheldon *et al.* were unable to show any sparing effect of fractionation with a 6-hr interval at total doses up to 3.5 Gy in the cell line NB1-G.[54] Taken together, these experiments suggest that at the fraction sizes conventionally used in paediatric radiotherapy, significant sublethal damage repair between fractions is unlikely.

A dose sparing effect similar to that seen with fractionation can occur when dose rates lower than conventional rates exceeding 1 Gy/min are used. This is particularly relevant in targeted radiotherapy where the total dose is delivered at low dose rate over a period of days. Studies on two neuroblastoma cell lines at dose rates from 0.2 Gy/min down to 0.0025 Gy/min have been reported.[55] At dose rates lower than 0.02 Gy/min, HX138 shows only a small degree of sparing, while HX142 shows an even smaller effect.

Until recently, it was believed that repair capacity was the major determinant of cellular radiosensitivity, and therefore that the observed sensitivity of neuroblastoma was due to deficiencies in the repair process.[56,57] However, the data above indicating some element of repair between fractions and at low dose rate, coupled with the measurement of DNA double-strand breaks using neutral filter elution, have suggested that the level of damage initially induced in DNA by ionizing radiation may be an additional factor.[58]

## Hypoxia

Many years ago, tumour hypoxia was suggested as a possible cause of clinical radioresistance following the observations that human tumours contain hypoxic cells and that cells irradiated in the absence of oxygen are relatively resistant. The same features have also been identified in neuroblastoma. Spheroids of NB1-G larger than about 300 μm have necrotic cores and NB-100 spheroids have low oxygen tension centrally.[59] An oxygen enhancement ratio of 1.5 *in vitro* and 2.0 *in vivo* has been shown for the neuroblastoma line HX138.[52] The significance of these findings to clinical radiotherapy in the case of neuroblastoma is not clear but, as various therapeutic strategies aimed at overcoming hypoxia in other tumours have not proved beneficial, it seems unlikely that hypoxia is as important as once was thought.

# External beam radiotherapy

## Clinical radiosensitivity

The general perception of paediatric radiotherapists is that neuroblastoma is a radiosensitive tumour.[60] Radiotherapy to the liver may be used as an alternative to chemotherapy in Stage 4S patients with hepatomegaly. Lateral-opposed portals are used to spare the kidneys and vertebrae, as in such young children the adverse effects of irradiation are more marked. Doses as low as 4.5 Gy in three fractions may be sufficient to precipitate regression, though it is not believed that this dose kills all clonogenic cells. For neuroblastoma at other sites in infants, courses of 18–20 Gy given in 1.2–1.4 Gy fractions are appropriate. In older children, 25–35 Gy in daily fractions of 1.5–1.8 Gy may be given, perhaps boosting bulk disease up to 40 Gy. The use of a lower total dose and smaller fraction sizes in infants is partly due to the better prognosis of neuroblastoma in this age group, and partly to the desire to avoid late normal-tissue damage, to which younger children are more susceptible. There are, however, some doubts about the efficacy of normal-tissue sparing by small fraction size in very young children.[49]

## Dose–response relationships and age

These dose/fractionation schedules are not the result of randomized trials, but have been empirically derived, based on clinical experience gained over decades.

An analysis of seventy-six patients irradiated after surgery for limited disease gives a clear indication of the relevance of age to the dose needed to achieve local control.[61] Under the age of 12 months, local control occurred in all patients receiving 15 Gy, but one failure occurred among five patients given a lower dose. No local failures were seen among children aged 1 and 2 years; the lowest dose given in this group was 14.4 Gy. Two 3-year-olds failed with doses under 30 Gy, and two older chilen, one aged 11 the other 16, developed local failure at doses of 40 Gy and 45 Gy.

Radiotherapy failed to achieve local control in four of eleven Stage III patients.[62] Three of these, all over 1 year old, received doses less than 16 Gy, another indication that tumours in older children require higher doses.

## Postoperative radiotherapy

The precise role of postoperative radiotherapy remains unclear. In a retrospective review of patients with Children's Cancer Study Group (CCSG: USA) Stage II disease, no significant benefit was seen in irradiated patients.[63]

In a Pediatric Oncology Group (POG: USA) randomized trial, designed to evaluate the place of radiotherapy in addition to chemotherapy in patients over 1 year of age found to have nodal disease at resection of the primary tumour, the dose used was age related. A total of 24 Gy in sixteen daily fractions was used in those aged from 12 to 24 months, whereas older children received 30 Gy in twenty fractions over 4 weeks.[64] Of twenty-nine eligible patients randomized to chemotherapy alone, thirteen achieved complete remission and nine are disease-free after therapy. Twenty-two of thirty-three eligible patients treated with radiotherapy in addition to chemotherapy achieved complete remission, and nineteen have no evidence of disease on follow-up. The significantly improved local control and survival rates seen in irradiated patients confirm the clinical radiosensitivity of neuroblastoma. The chemotherapy schedule used in this study was less intensive than that now considered standard, and it remains possible that results with more intensive chemotherapy might be as good as those in the combined-modality arm of the trial. This question is currently being addressed by further trials.

## Total body irradiation

Total body irradiation (TBI) has been widely used as part of 'megatherapy' with marrow transplantation in the treatment of neuroblastoma. Although the maximum tolerable radiation dose is relatively low, about 14 Gy when fractionated, significant cell killing may occur as neuroblastoma, like leukaemia where the value of TBI was first demonstrated, is a radiosensitive tumour.

There are conflicting data about the place of TBI. One indication of its value is the report of a 20% progression-free survival at 2 years in a group of relapsed patients treated with megatherapy including TBI, which was achieved in none of the patients receiving megatherapy without TBI.[65] In another study of patients given megatherapy during complete or partial remission, no advantage was shown at 2 years for those receiving TBI compared with those who were not.[40,66] Because of this uncertainty, and in view of the possible adverse effects of irradiation in children, the efficacy of TBI in megatherapy schedules requires prospective evaluation.

The European Bone Marrow Transplantation Group (EBMTG) experience, typical of other published series, indicates the current place of megatherapy. A review of 439 procedures, of which 385 were consolidation of initial therapy and fifty after relapse or progression, allows some conclusions to be drawn.[67] Of those treated for consolidation of first-line therapy, 40% are alive without progression at 2 years. This survival rate is unaffected by whether or not (a) TBI was used, (b) marrow purging was undertaken, (c) residual disease was present and (d) also by whether one or two transplants were given. Two-year survival does not equal cure, however, and the five-year survival is less than 20%. Megatherapy is of no value in patients with resistant relapses. None in this category is alive and progression free at 2 years compared with 30% of those treated for a sensitive relapse. The treatment-related mortality in this series was 11% when the indication was consolidation of initial treatment and 18% when used for relapses, and was higher when TBI was used.

## Palliative radiotherapy

In the care of terminally ill children with recurrent or refractory neuroblastoma, external beam radiotherapy can be valuable. It is most widely used for the relief of pain from bone metastases. A single 8-Gy fraction usually results in a rapid and lasting benefit. In some cases, however, symptoms may recur at the same site, in which case retreatment can be considered. A fractionated regimen, such as 20 Gy in five daily treatments, may be considered preferable in some circumstances, such as for the relief of spinal cord compression, or if there is extensive orbital disease.

# Targeted radiotherapy

## Principles of targeted radiotherapy

Targeted radiotherapy is a new and still largely experimental therapeutic strategy designed to overcome the twin constraints of conventional radiotherapy. These are tumour dissemination beyond the treated area when small fields are used, and normal-tissue tolerance, which may limit the achievable dose to subcurative levels, when using wide-field irradiation. Targeted radiotherapy involves the use of radionuclides which preferentially localize in or around tumour deposits. Biological differences between normal and malignant cells are exploited to achieve the required differential distribution. Following the development of monoclonal antibodies,[68] targeted radiotherapy or 'radioimmunotherapy' was evaluated in many diseases, including neuroblastoma. The antibodies UJ13A[69,70] and 3F8[71] have been used in patients with neuroblastoma, but the clinical results are disappointing.

## *m*IBG

One of the principal limitations of antibodies as targeting agents is the size of the immunoglobulin molecule, which often precludes good penetration of the tumour.[72] Low molecular weight compounds that are processed by metabolic pathways offer an exciting alternative to antibodies. The pharmaceutical *m*IBG (*meta*-iodobenzylguanidine), an analogue of the adrenergic neurone blocking drugs guanethidine and bretylium, is the best example (Fig. 10.1). *m*IBG is taken up into cells of sympathetic nervous origin, such as neuroblastoma cells, by an active transport process named Uptake one[73] which involves the noradrenaline (epinephrine) transporter molecule.[74] When labelled with a suitable radionuclide, most often [131]I, *m*IBG can be used for both scintigraphy and treatment of neuroblastoma and related tumours.

[131]I-*m*IBG was first used for the treatment of neuroblastoma[75] following the demonstration that it could, like phaeochromocytoma, be imaged by this radiopharmaceutical. Subsequently, its use has been widespread, but, because of the rarity of neuroblastoma, only limited numbers of patients were treated at any one centre.

A conference was held in Rome in September 1986 to bring together the pioneers of *m*IBG therapy for neuroblastoma. As none at that time had experience of more than eighteen patients, and most fewer than ten, the data from nine groups have been pooled.[76-84] A total of seventy-five patients, of whom seventy-two had primarily refractory or relapsed disease, underwent [131]I-*m*IBG treatment. An objective response or disease stabilization was seen in forty-four (59%) of this group. Only four had complete

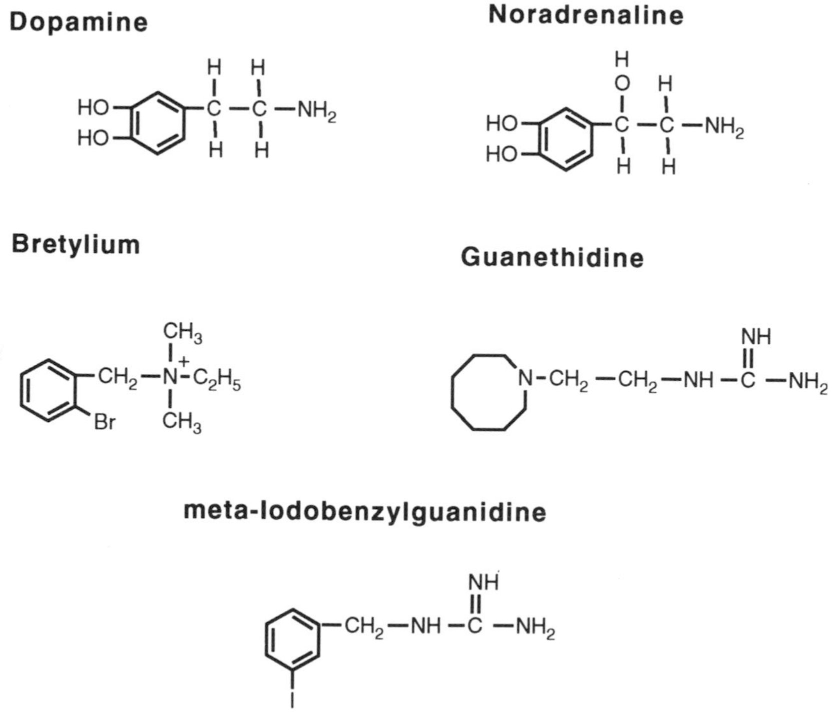

**Fig. 10.1**  Structural relationships between catecholamines, adrenergic neurone blocking drugs and *meta*-iodobenzylguanidine.

remissions, twenty-eight had partial remissions and twelve had disease stabilization. [131]I-*m*IBG was given as consolidation therapy to two patients in remission after chemotherapy,[82] and one 10-month-old baby with Stage 3 disease received [131]I-*m*IBG as primary treatment at presentation.[83] A complete response was seen in this case, and a later report indicates that the child remained well with no other treatment 18 months after diagnosis.[85]

Data from such a portmanteau series as this must be interpreted cautiously, as the patient population was heterogeneous with regard to extent of disease and prior treatment, [131]I-*m*IBG administration and dosimetry were not standardized, and the international criteria for response assessment[34] had not yet been formulated. Despite this caveat, the results show that some benefit may be expected in a heavily pretreated group of patients for whom conventional therapy offers little else.

The principal side-effect reported by participants at the 1986 Rome conference was myelosuppression, particularly thrombocytopenia, which was especially marked in cases with extensive bone marrow involvement or following megatherapy with autologous bone marrow transplantation. While no toxicity was encountered in four of sixteen neuroblastoma patients treated with [131]I-*m*IBG, thrombocytopenia was noted in four patients, leukopenia in one and general myelosuppression in five.[86] Similar findings are reported in a detailed assessment of haematological toxicity.[87] Autologous transplantation after marrow-ablative *m*IBG treatment has been used in an attempt to overcome the haematological problems associated with *m*IBG in pretreated patients.[88]

More recently, larger series of neuroblastoma patients have been reported which show varying response rates to [131]I-*m*IBG therapy. Of thirty-one heavily pretreated children with relapsed or refractory disease, two patients had complete and three partial responses (an overall response rate of only 16%), while fifteen had mixed responses or stable disease and ten progressed.[89] In a series of fifty similar patients treated in Amsterdam, seven patients had complete and twenty-two had partial responses: an overall response rate of 58%.[90] Results of the UK CCSG Phase I/II study are intermediate between those of the Italian and Dutch series, with a response rate of 30% (confidence limits 10–50%).[91] This study involving eight British centres included twenty-five patients with advanced, recurrent or resistant disease. It was designed to develop both a reproducible standard protocol for *m*IBG administration and a reliable dosimetric system, and to correlate toxicity with the whole body radiation dose received. In addition, uniform and conventional assessments of the effectiveness and toxicity of [131]I-*m*IBG were used. While many patients showed no objective tumour reduction, pain relief is often dramatic, making non-curative treatment worthwhile.[92]

In the early clinical studies outlined above, [131]I-*m*IBG has clearly demonstrated its potential as a valuable palliative treatment for neuroblastoma. It is impressive to see any complete responses in patients at the end of conventional therapy. The use of [131]I-*m*IBG at an earlier stage in the illness, where its chances of success might be greater, are now being explored. Two approaches have been suggested. These are use at presentation prior to conventional treatment and use as consolidation therapy after remission induction.

In Amsterdam, newly diagnosed Stage 3 or Stage 4 patients are given at least two courses of $^{131}$I-*m*IBG after one course of chemotherapy. This is given for logistic reasons as it takes time to arrange the facilities necessary for $^{131}$I-*m*IBG treatment. The results in four patients have been reported.[90] In each case, there was a complete response at metastatic sites and a considerable reduction in the size of the primary tumour, which was in all cases converted by surgery into a complete response. The *m*IBG treatment is followed by a short, intensive chemotherapy protocol and autologous bone marrow transplantation. It is too early to give long-term results.

In the alternative strategies $^{131}$I-*m*IBG is given, following intensive remission induction chemotherapy, as part of the megatherapy consolidation with autologous bone marrow transplantation, with the aim of eradicating minimal residual disease. At the Royal Marsden Hospital, Surrey, the consolidation entails high dose melphalan, $^{131}$I-*m*IBG and transplantation.[93] An approach which incorporates TBI, described below, is being evaluated in Glasgow.[94] In both centres, only a few patients have been treated — sufficient to confirm the feasibility, but not the efficacy, of this approach.

Several strategies have been suggested to enhance the therapeutic ratio of *m*IBG therapy by modulation of its pharmacokinetics to improve the target to non-target ratio. Following the demonstration that the calcium antagonist nifedipine could suppress noradrenaline secretion by a phaeochromocytoma,[95] this drug has been tested clinically for its ability to modify *m*IBG kinetics.[96] In one of eight patients with metastatic phaeochromocytoma, tumour uptake was enhanced by a factor of 1.5 and retention time was prolonged, although no changes in plasma *m*IBG levels were noted. The beneficial effect in this patient was confirmed when the study was repeated 9 months later. An effect was also seen in two other patients: in one, the tumour uptake was increased by nifedipine but the half-life was unaffected; in the other, the half-life was prolonged by nifedipine although tumour uptake remained the same. In an alternative approach, the use of intravenous hydration to produce an accelerated diuresis led to a more rapid clearance of *m*IBG from normal tissues, without affecting the tumour concentration.[97] In this way, the target to non-target ratio is increased.

The development of carrier-free (no carrier added) *m*IBG offers another opportunity to enhance the tumour to normal-tissue ratio of this drug.[98]

# Combined external beam and targeted radiotherapy

## Rationale

In conventional cancer therapy, smaller tumours are easier to eradicate than larger ones, largely because they contain fewer clonogenic cells. By contrast, micrometastases smaller than about 1 mm diameter are predicted to be more difficult to cure with $^{131}$I-*m*IBG therapy.[99,100] This is because radionuclide disintegration energy is absorbed inefficiently in microtumours whose diameter is less than the mean range of the $^{131}$I β-particles, which is about 600 μm. This hypothesis has recently been supported by experimental evidence using neuroblastoma spheroids.[101] Targeted radionuclide therapy using $^{131}$I-*m*IBG is most likely to cure tumours of about 2 mm diameter.[100] The likelihood of cure is reduced below this optimal size by the physical characteristics of $^{131}$I β-particles, and above this size by the greater number of clonogenic cells.

The use of $^{131}$I-*m*IBG, in combination with other treatments which are effective outside its optimal size range, is predicted to overcome this limitation.[102] The efficacy of TBI is limited by the maximum dose which can be tolerated. Tumours up to about 1 mm diameter are likely to be cured by TBI, whereas larger deposits will contain too many clonogenic cells for eradication. Tumour masses greater than about 1 cm may be revealed by modern imaging techniques, and can be treated by localized, high dose external beam radiotherapy.

Figure 10.2 shows the relationship between tumour size and the number of clonogenic cells killed, assuming typical values for the radiosensitivity of

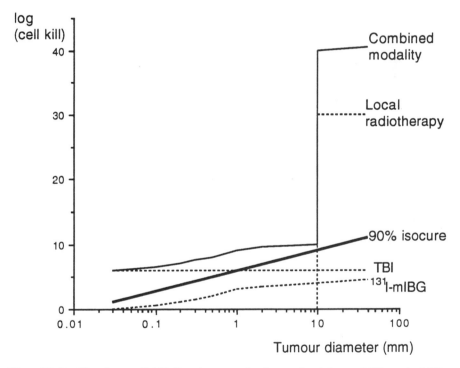

**Fig. 10.2** The log cell kill (i.e. log survival) required for a 90% probability of cure for neuroblastoma tumours of different sizes is shown by the straight, thick line, assuming typical parameters for neuroblastoma cells. For tumours of a particular size, a value of log cell kill which falls above this line is likely to be curative, whereas cure is unlikely if the value falls below the line. Dotted lines show the log cell kills achieved with TBI alone (limited, and therefore likely to be ineffective for tumours greater than 1 mm diameter), $^{131}$I-*m*IBG alone (less effective in tumours less than 2 mm diameter), and local radiotherapy alone (restricted to detectable tumours greater than about 1 cm diameter). The continuous line shows the calculated log cell kill for combined modality therapy. As this is above the 90% isocure line at all tumour sizes, a high likelihood of cure is achieved.

neuroblastoma.[102] TBI to a total dose of 14 Gy is predicted to achieve a log cell kill of 6, which is likely to eradicate micrometastases of less than 1 mm diameter. Tumour deposits greater than 1 cm diameter will be sterilized if they are detected by imaging and treated by local radiotherapy. Tumour deposits of intermediate size, which are too large for cure by TBI and too small to be detected by imaging, may therefore lead to failure of treatment using a combination of TBI and local radiotherapy. [131]I-*m*IBG, with its optimum cure size measured in millimetres, used in addition to TBI and local radiotherapy, may increase the chance of eradicating all tumour deposits and, thus make cure of the patient more likely.

## Clinical experience

In a pilot study of multimodality megatherapy, five patients — four boys and one girl, aged from three to eleven years — with Stage 4 neuroblastoma were treated with multimodality megatherapy following initial chemotherapy and surgery.[94] Ideally, scintigraphy had shown that the tumour took up [131]I-*m*IBG, but patients in whom this investigation had not been performed, or in whom it was negative at a time when they had no bulk disease, were also considered eligible. This was because most patients with neuroblastoma do exhibit uptake of [131]I-*m*IBG, and its use, even in a patient without uptake, would still exert a therapeutic effect through the non-specific whole body irradiation it caused, and so would not be 'wasted'. [131]I-*m*IBG estimated to give a whole body absorbed radiation dose of about 2 Gy[103] was administered on Day 0. Whole body retention of [131]I (necessary for whole body dosimetry) was determined by monitoring the dose rate at 1.25 m from the patient. Scintigraphy was carried out on Days 2, 5 and 9 for whole body dosimetry and to determine sites of [131]I-*m*IBG accumulation. On Day 10, melphalan, 140 mg/m$^2$, was administered. On Days 12–15, TBI, 12.6 Gy in seven fractions — maximum lung dose — was given. Marrow was then reinfused and supportive care was given, as required, until engraftment.

As tumours larger than a centimetre or so diameter are unlikely to be sterilized by the radiation doses achievable with either TBI or [131]I-*m*IBG,[102] localized external beam radiotherapy was also given to the residual abdominal tumour mass in one patient, following haematological recovery. Her tumour received 5.20 Gy from [131]I-*m*IBG, 12.10 Gy from TBI and 23.40 Gy local radiotherapy in thirteen fractions over 17 days, resulting in a total tumour dose of 40.70 Gy. Additional radiotherapy was not given to the mass detected in another patient as this showed exceptionally high [131]I-*m*IBG uptake, and the calculated total radiation dose, 58 Gy, was deemed adequate.

The combined treatment was generally well tolerated despite marked haematological toxicity. In all patients, including those in clinical remission and the patient in whom [131]I-*m*IBG scintigraphy was negative, areas of disease were shown by scanning, following [131]I-*m*IBG administration. In two patients with measurable disease, calculated tumour doses of 44 Gy and 5.2 Gy were delivered by the *m*IBG component, in addition to that received from TBI.

Given that conventional megatherapy for neuroblastoma carries a mortality rate greater than 10%,[67] this experience indicates that multi-modality megatherapy is safe, and that the inevitable acute toxicity is tolerable, given full supportive care. Further follow-up is necessary before late morbidity can be assessed. It is not possible to evaluate the efficacy of this strategy in such a small number of patients, and more patients must be studied.

Clearly, when treatments are combined, the relative proportions of each are important. Mathematical studies suggest that killing of neuroblastoma deposits will be greatest when the whole body dose from the targeted component is 4 Gy, rather than the 2 Gy that we have used.[104] Dose escalation of $^{131}$I-*m*IBG should therefore be attempted, with corresponding reduction of the TBI component.

# Conclusions

The modern management of neuroblastoma requires the combined expertise of a multidisciplinary team, including radiologists and pathologists, as well as paediatricians, radiotherapists, oncologists and surgeons. Radiation is an active agent but its place in neuroblastoma management remains a matter for further investigation. Targeted radiotherapy with $^{131}$I-*m*IBG, in conjunction with chemotherapy and perhaps TBI, offers hope for improving the outlook for patients with advanced disease. Nonetheless, targeted radiotherapy continues to be an experimental strategy and further studies are in progress. Clinicians are urged, wherever possible, to enrol eligible patients in appropriate national and international trials.

# Note added in proof

The UKCCSG has just started a pilot study of $^{131}$I-*m*IBG as the first treatment in patients with advanced neuroblastoma. If this confirms the feasibility of combining up-front $^{131}$I-*m*IBG and standard chemotherapy it is hoped to move on to a randomized Phase III clinical trial to test the efficacy of this approach.

# References

1. Homer Wright J. Neurocytoma or neuroblastoma, a kind of tumour not normally recognised. *J Exp Med* 1910; **12**, 556–61.
2. Office of Population Censuses and Surveys. *Childhood Cancer in Britain, Incidence, Survival and Mortality.* London: HMSO, 1982.
3. Stowens D. Neuroblastoma and related tumours. *Arch Pathol* 1957; **63**, 451–9.
4. Bodian M. Neuroblastoma. *Pediatr Clin North Am* 1959; **6**, 449–72.
5. Gross RE, Farber S, Martin LW. Neuroblastoma sympatheticum: a study and report of 217 cases. *Pediatrics* 1959; **23**, 1179–91.
6. Fortner J, Nicastri A, Murphy ML. Neuroblastoma: natural history and results of treating 133 cases. *Ann Surg* 1968; **167**, 132–42.
7. de Lorimier AA, Bragg KU, Linden G. Neuroblastoma in childhood. *Am J*

*Dis Child* 1969; **118,** 441–50.

8.  Stella JG, Schweisguth O, Schlienger M. Neuroblastoma: a study of 144 cases treated at the Institut Gustave-Roussy over a period of 7 years. *Am J Roentgenol* 1970; **108,** 324–32.

9.  Kinnier Wilson LM, Draper GJ. Neuroblastoma, its natural history and prognosis: a study of 487 cases. *Br Med J* 1974; **302,** 301–7.

10. Wieberdink J. Foetal haemic metastasis: an explanation of the 'Pepper-type' of metastasis in adrenal neuroblastoma. *Br J Cancer* 1957; **11,** 378–83.

11. Evans AE, D'Angio GJ, Randolph J. A proposed staging for children with neuroblastoma. Children's Cancer Study Group A. *Cancer* 1971; **27,** 374–8.

12. Allan PM, Garson JA, Harper EI, *et al.* Biological characterisation and clinical applications of a monoclonal antibody recognising an antigen restricted to neuroectodermal tissues. *Int J Cancer* 1983; **31,** 591–8.

13. Dhillon AP, Rode J, Leathem A. Neurone specific enolase: an aid to the diagnosis of melanoma and neuroblastoma. *Histopathology* 1982; **6,** 81–92.

14. Carlei F, Polak JM, Ceccamea A, *et al.* Neuronal and glial markers in tumours of neuroblastic origin. *Virchows Archiv A (Pathol Anat)* 1984; **404,** 313–324.

15. Cheung N-KV, Saarinen UM, Neely JE, *et al.* Monoclonal antibodies to a glycolipid antigen on human neuroblastoma cells. *Cancer Res* 1985; **45,** 2642–9.

16. Kemshead JT, Fritschy J, Goldman A, *et al.* Use of panels of monoclonal antibodies in the differential diagnosis of neuroblastoma and lymphoblastic disorders. *Lancet* 1983; **i,** 12–15.

17. Murphy SB, Cohn SL, Craft AW, *et al.* Do children benefit from mass screening for neuroblastoma? Consensus statement from the American Cancer Society workshop on neuroblastoma screening. *Lancet* 1991; **337,** 344–6.

18. Chatten J, Voorhess ML. Familial neuroblastoma: report of a kindred with multiple disorders, including neuroblastomas in four siblings. *N Engl J Med* 1967; **277,** 1230–6.

19. Hecht F, Hecht BK, Northrup JC, *et al.* Genetics of neuroblastoma: long-range studies. *Cancer Genet Cytogenet* 1982; **7,** 227–30.

20. Kuschner BH, Gilbert F, Helson L. Familial neuroblastoma. *Cancer* 1986; **57,** 1887–93.

21. Ninane J. Neuroblastoma. In: PN Plowman, CR Pinkerton, eds, *Paediatric Oncology: Clinical Practice and Controversies.* London: Chapman and Hall, 1991; 351–77.

22. Sanger WG, Howe J, Fordyce R, *et al.* Inherited partial trisomy #15 complicated by neuroblastoma. *Cancer Genet Cytogenet* 1984; **11,** 153–9.

23. Michalski AJ, Cowell JK. Constructing a physical map around a constitutional t(1;13)(q22;q12) breakpoint in a patient with a ganglioneuroblastoma. In: AE Evans, JL Biedler, GM Brodeur, *et al.,* eds, *Advances in Neuroblastoma Research 4.* New York: Wiley-Liss, 1994; 79–85.

24. Knudson AG, Meadows AT. Developmental genetics of neuroblastoma. *J Natl Cancer Inst* 1976; **57,** 675–82.

25. Hunt JD, Tereba A. Molecular evaluation of abnormalities of the short arm of chromosome 1 in neuroblastoma. *Genes Chromosom Cancer* 1990; **2,** 137–46.

26. Martinsson T, Weith A, Cziepluch C, *et al.* Chromosome 1 deletions in human neuroblastomas: generation and fine mapping of microclones from distal 1p region. *Genes Chromosom Cancer* 1989; **1,** 67–78.

27. White PS, Fujimori M, Marshall HN, *et al.* Characterisation of the region of consistent deletion within 1p36 in neuroblastomas. In: AE Evans, JL Biedler, GM Brodeur, *et al.,* eds, *Advances in Neuroblastoma Research 4.* New York: Wiley-Liss, 1994; 3–9.

28. Fong C, White PS, Peterson K, *et al.* Loss of heterozygosity for chromosomes 1 or 14 defines subsets of advanced neuroblastomas. *Cancer Res* 1992; **52,** 1780–5.

29. Michon J, Delattre O, Zucker JM, *et al.* Prospective evaluation of Nmyc amplification and deletion of the short arm of chromosome 1 in neuroblastoma tumours. In: AE Evans, JL Biedler, GM Brodeur, *et al.*, eds, *Advances in Neuroblastoma Research 4.* New York: Wiley-Liss, 1994; 11–17.

30. Christiansen H, Schestag J, Bielke W, *et al.* Chromosome 1 interphase-cytogenetics in 32 primary neuroblastomas of different clinical stages. In: AE Evans, GJ D'Angio, AG Knudson, *et al.*, eds, *Advances in Neuroblastoma Research, 3.* New York: Wiley-Liss, 1991; 99–105.

31. Seeger RC, Brodeur GM, Sather H, *et al.* Association of multiple copies of the N-myc oncogene with rapid progression of neuroblastomas. *N Engl J Med* 1985; **313**, 1111–16.

32. Livingstone A, Mairs RJ, Russell J, *et al.* N-myc gene copy number in neuroblastoma cell lines and resistance to experimental treatment. *Eur J Cancer* 1994; **30A**, 382–9.

33. Norris MD, Haber M, Gilbert J, *et al.* N-myc gene amplification in neuroblastoma determined by the polymerase chain reaction. In: AE Evans, JL Biedler, GM Brodeur, *et al.*, eds, *Advances in Neuroblastoma Research 4.* New York: Wiley-Liss, 1994; 27–33.

34. Brodeur GM, Seeger RC, Barrett A, *et al.* International criteria for diagnosis, staging and response to treatment in patients with neuroblastoma. *J Clin Oncol* 1988; **6**, 1874–81.

35. Brodeur GM, Pritchard J, Berthold F, *et al.* Revisions of the international criteria for neuroblastoma diagnosis, staging and response to treatment. In: AE Evans, JL Biedler, GM Brodeur, *et al.*, eds, *Advances in Neuroblastoma Research 4.* New York: Wiley-Liss, 1994; 363–9.

36. Ninane J, Pritchard J, Morris Jones PH, *et al.* Stage II neuroblastoma: adverse prognostic significance of lymph node involvement. *Arch Dis Childhood* 1982; **57**, 438–42.

37. Hayes F, Green A, Hustu O, *et al.* Surgicopathologic staging of neuroblastoma: prognostic significance of regional lymph node metastases. *J Pediatr* 1983; **102**, 59–62.

38. Shafford EA, Rogers DW, Pritchard J. Advanced neuroblastoma: improved response rate using a multiagent regimen (OPEC) including sequential cisplatin and VM-26. *J Clin Oncol* 1984; **2**, 742–7.

39. Bernard JL, Philip T, Zucker JM, *et al.* Sequential cisplatin/VM-26 and vincristine/cyclophosphamide/doxorubicin in metastatic neuroblastoma: an effective alternating non-cross-resistant regimen? *J Clin Oncol* 1987; **5**, 1952–9.

40. Hartmann O, Benhamou E, Beaujean F, *et al.* Repeated high-dose chemotherapy followed by purged autologous bone marrow transplantation as consolidation therapy in metastatic neuroblastoma. *J Clin Oncol* 1987; **5**, 1205–11.

41. Pinkerton CR, Zucker JM, Hartmann O, *et al.*, on behalf of the European Neuroblastoma Study Group. Short duration, high dose, alternating chemotherapy in metastatic neuroblastoma. (ENSG 3C induction regimen). *Br J Cancer* 1990; **62**, 319–23.

42. Pritchard J, McElwain TJ, Graham-Pole J. High dose melphalan with autologous marrow for treatment of advanced neuroblastoma. *Br J Cancer* 1982; **45**, 86–94.

43. Pritchard J, Germond S, Jones D, *et al.* Is high dose melphalan of value in treatment of advanced neuroblastoma? Preliminary results of a randomised trial by the European Neuroblastoma Study Group. *Proc ASCO* 1986; **5**, 205 (Abstract).

44. Stiller CA, Bunch KJ. Trends in survival for childhood cancer in Britain diagnosed 1971–85. *Br J Cancer* 1990; **62**, 806–15.

45. Shimada H, Chatten J, Newton WA, *et al.* Histopathologic prognostic factors in neuroblastic tumors: definition of subtypes of ganglioneuroblastoma and an

age linked classification of neuroblastomas. *J Natl Cancer Inst* 1984; **73**, 405–13.

46.  Brodeur GM, Seeger RC, Schwab M, *et al.* Amplification of N-*myc* in untreated human neuroblastomas correlates with advanced disease stage. *Science* 1984; **244**, 1121–4.

47.  Fertil B, Malaise EP. Intrinsic radiosensitivity of human cell lines is correlated with radioresponsiveness of human tumors: analysis of 101 published survival curves. *Int J Radiat Oncol Biol Phys* 1985; **11**, 1699–707.

48.  Deacon J, Peckham MJ, Steel GG. The radioresponsiveness of human tumours and the initial slope of the cell survival curve. *Radiother Oncol* 1984; **2**, 317–23.

49.  Steel GG, Wheldon TE. The radiation biology of paediatric tumours. In: PN Plowman, CR Pinkerton, eds, *Paediatric Oncology: Clinical Practice and Controversies.* London: Chapman and Hall, 1991; 73–86.

50.  Wheldon TE, Livingstone A, Wilson L, *et al.* The radiosensitivity of human neuroblastoma cells estimated from regrowth curves of multicellular tumour spheroids. *Br J Radiol* 1985; **58**, 661–4.

51.  Schwachöfer JHM, Crooijmans RPMA, van Gasteren JJM, *et al.* Radiosensitivity of different human tumour cell lines grown as multicellular spheroids determined from growth curves and survival data. *Int J Radiat Oncol Biol Phys* 1989; **17**, 1015–20.

52.  Deacon JM, Wilson PA, Peckham MJ. The radiobiology of human neuroblastoma. *Radiother Oncol* 1985; **3**, 201–9.

53.  Schwachöfer JHM, Crooijmans RPMA, van Gasteren JJM, *et al.* Repair of sublethal damage in two human tumour cell lines grown as multicellular spheroids. *Int J Radiat Oncol Biol Phys* 1989; **17**, 591–5.

54.  Wheldon TE, Wilson L, Livingstone A, *et al.* Radiation studies on multicellular tumour spheroids derived from human neuroblastoma: absence of sparing effect of dose fractionation. *Eur J Cancer Clin Oncol* 1986; **22**, 563–6.

55.  Holmes A, McMillan TJ, Peacock JH, *et al.* The radiation dose-rate effect in two human neuroblastoma cell lines. *Br J Cancer* 1990; **62**, 791–5.

56.  Schwachöfer JHM, Crooijmans RPMA, Borm GF, *et al.* Repair of radiation induced damage in two human tumour cell lines grown as spheroids and monolayers. *Strahlenther Onkol* 1990; **166** , 753–60.

57.  Schwachöfer JHM, Crooijmans RPMA, Hoogenhout H, *et al.* Differences in repair of radiation induced damage in two human tumour cell lines as measured by cell survival and alkaline DNA unwinding. *Strahlenther Onkol* 1991; **167**, 35–40.

58.  McMillan TJ, Eady JJ, Holmes A, *et al.* The radiosensitivity of human neuroblastoma: a cellular and molecular study. *Int J Radiat Biol* 1989; **56**, 651–6.

59.  Schwachöfer JHM, Acker H, Crooijmans RPMA, *et al.* Oxygen tensions in two human tumour cell lines grown and irradiated as multicellular spheroids. *Anticancer Res* 1991; **11**, 273–80.

60.  Plowman PN. Tumours in children. In: HF Hope-Stone, ed, *Radiotherapy in Clinical Practice.* London: Butterworths, 1986; 238–57.

61.  Jacobson GM, Sause WT, O'Brien RT. Dose response analysis of pediatric neuroblastoma to megavoltage radiation. *Am J Clin Oncol* 1984; **7**, 693–7.

62.  Halperin EC, Cox EB. Radiation therapy in the management of neuroblastoma: the Duke University Medical Center Experience 1967–1984. *Int J Radiat Oncol Biol Phys* 1986; **12**, 1829–937.

63.  Matthay KK, Sather HN, Seeger RC, *et al.* Excellent outcome of stage II neuroblastoma is independent of residual disease and radiation therapy. *J Clin Oncol* 1989; **7**, 236–44.

64.  Castleberry RP, Kun LE, Schuster JJ, *et al.* Radiotherapy improves the outlook for patients older than 1 year with Pediatric Oncology Group Stage C

neuroblastoma. *J Clin Oncol* 1991; **9**, 789–95.

65. Philip P, Pinkerton R. Neuroblastoma. In: I McGrath, ed, *New Directions in Cancer Treatment*. Berlin: UICC Springer-Verlag, 1989; 605–11.

66. Philip T, Bernard JL, Zucker JM, et al. High-dose chemotherapy with bone marrow transplantation as consolidation treatment in neuroblastoma: an unselected group of Stage IV patients over 1 year of age. *J Clin Oncol* 1987; **5**, 266–71.

67. Ladenstein R, Philip T. Megatherapy and immunotherapy in paediatric solid tumours. In: PN Plowman, CR Pinkerton, eds, *Paediatric Oncology: Clinical Practice and Controversies*. London: Chapman and Hall, 1991; 460–94.

68. Köhler G, Milstein C. Continuous cultures of fused cells secreting antibody of predefined specificity. *Nature* 1975; **256**, 495–7.

69. Lashford LS, Clarke J, Gordon I, et al. A comparative study of the biodistribution of *meta*-iodobenzyl guanidine (*m*IBG) and the monoclonal antibody UJ13A in patients and animal models. In: AE Evans, GJ D'Angio, eds, *Advances in Neuroblastoma Research* 2. New York: Alan R Liss, 1988; 643–54.

70. Kemshead JT, Lashford LS, Jones DH et al. Diagnosis and therapy of neuroectodermally associated tumours using targeted radiation. *Dev Neurosci* 1987; **9**, 69–83.

71. Cheung N-KV, Yeh SDJ, Gulati S, et al. [131]I-3F8: clinical applications of imaging studies and therapeutic applications. In: AE Evans, GJ D'Angio, AG Knudson, et al., eds, *Advances in Neuroblastoma Research 3*. New York: Wiley-Liss, 1991; 409–15.

72. Mairs RJ, Angerson W, Gaze MN, et al. Differential penetration of alternative targeting agents into human neuroblastoma spheroids. *Br J Cancer* 1991; **63**, 404–9.

73. Mairs RJ, Gaze MN, Barrett A. The uptake and retention of metaiodobenzyl guanidine by the neuroblastoma cell line NB1-G. *Br J Cancer* 1991; **64**, 293–5.

74. Pacholczyk T, Blakely RD, Amara SG. Expression cloning of a cocaine- and antidepressant-sensitive human noradrenaline transporter. *Nature* 1991; **350**, 350–4.

75. Lumbroso J, Hartmann O, Lemerle J, et al. Scintigraphic detection of neuroblastoma using [131]I and [123]I labelled meta-iodobenzylguanidine. *Eur J Nucl Med* 1985; **11**, A16 (Abstract).

76. Beierwaltes WH. Treatment of neuroblastoma with [131]I-mIBG — dosimetric problems and perspectives. *Med Pediatr Oncol* 1987; **15**, 188–91.

77. Bestagno M, Guerra P, Puricelli GP, et al. Treatment of neuroblastoma with 131-I meta-iodobenzylguanidine: the experience of an Italian study group. *Med Pediatr Oncol* 1987; **15**, 203–4.

78. Cottino F, Mussa GC, Madon E, et al. [131]I-meta-iodobenzylguanidine treatment in neuroblastoma: report of two cases. *Med Pediatr Oncol* 1987; **15**, 216–19.

79. Fischer M, Wehinger H, Kraus C, et al. Treatment of neuroblastoma with [131]I-meta-iodobenzylguanidine: experience of the Munster/Kassel group. *Med Pediatr Oncol* 1987; **15**, 196–8.

80. Hartmann O, Lumbruso J, Lemerle J, et al. Therapeutic use of [131]I-meta iodobenzylguanidine (mIBG) in neuroblastoma: a phase II study in nine patients. *Med Pediatr Oncol* 1987; **15**, 205–11.

81. Sanguinetti M. Considerations on [131]I meta-iodobenzylguanidine therapy of six children with neuroblastoma. *Med Pediatr Oncol* 1987; **15**, 212–15.

82. Treuner J, Klingebiel T, Bruchelt G, et al. Treatment of neuroblastoma with metaiodobenzylguanidine: results and side effects. *Med Pediatr Oncol* 1987; **15**, 199–202.

83. Troncone L, Riccardi R, Montemaggi P, et al. Treatment of neuroblastoma with [131]I-meta-iodobenzylguanidine. *Med Pediatr Oncol* 1987; **15**, 220–3.

84.  Voûte PA, Hoefnagel CA, de Kraker J, *et al.* Radionuclide therapy of neural crest tumors. *Med Pediatr Oncol* 1987; **15**, 192–5.

85.  Mastrangelo R, Troncone L, Lasorella A, *et al.* [131]I-meta-iodobenzylguanidine in the treatment of neuroblastoma at diagnosis. *Am J Pediatr Haematol/Oncol* 1989; **11**, 28–31.

86.  Hoefnagel CA, Voûte PA, de Kraker J, *et al.* Radionuclide diagnosis and therapy of neural crest tumours using iodine-131 metaiodobenzylguanidine. *J Nucl Med* 1987; **28**, 308–14.

87.  Sisson JC, Hutchinson RJ, Carey JE, *et al.* Toxicity from treatment of neuroblastoma with [131]I-meta iodobenzylguanidine. *Eur J Nucl Med* 1988; **14**, 337–40.

88.  Klingebiel T, Treuner J, Ehninger G, *et al.* [[131]I]-meta-iodobenzylguanidine in the treatment of metastatic neuroblastoma: clinical pharmacological and dosimetric aspects. *Cancer Chemother Pharmacol* 1989; **25**, 143–8.

89.  Garaventa A, Guerra P, Arrighini A, *et al.* Treatment of advanced neuroblastoma with I-131 meta-iodobenzylguanidine. *Cancer* 1991; **67**, 922–8.

90.  Voûte PA, Hoefnagel CA, de Kraker J, *et al.* Results of treatment with [131]I-meta-iodobenzylguanidine in patients with neuroblastoma. Future prospects of zetotherapy. In: AE Evans, GJ D'Angio, AG Knudson, *et al.*, eds, *Advances in Neuroblastoma Research 3.* New York: Wiley-Liss, 1991; 439–5.

91.  Lewis IJ, Lashford LS, Fielding S, *et al.* A phase I/II study of [131]I mIBG in chemo-resistant neuroblastoma. In: AE Evans, GJ D'Angio, AG Knudson, *et al.*, eds, *Advances in Neuroblastoma Research 3.* New York: Wiley-Liss, 1991; 463–9.

92.  Gerrard M, Eden OB, Merrick MV. Imaging and treatment of disseminated neuroblastoma with [131]I-meta iodobenzylguanidine. *Br J Radiol* 1987; **60**; 393–5.

93.  Corbett R, Pinkerton R, Tait D, *et al.* [131]I-mIBG and high-dose chemotherapy with bone marrow rescue in advanced neuroblastoma. *J Nucl Biol Med* 1991; **35**, 228–31.

94.  Gaze MN, Wheldon TE, O'Donoghue JA, *et al.* Multi-modality megatherapy with [[131]I]-meta-iodobenzylguanidine, high dose melphalan and total body irradiation with bone marrow rescue: feasibility study of a new strategy for advanced neuroblastoma. *Eur J Cancer* 1995; **31A**, 252–6.

95.  Serfas D, Shobak DM, Lorell BH. Phaeochromocytoma and hypertrophic cardiomyopathy: apparent suppression of symptoms and noradrenaline secretion by calcium channel blockade. *Lancet* 1983; **ii**, 711–13.

96.  Blake GM, Lewington VJ, Fleming JS, *et al.* Modification by nifedipine of [131]I-meta-iodobenzylguanidine kinetics in malignant phaeochromocytoma. *Eur J Nucl Med* 1988; **14**, 345–8.

97.  Darte L, Tennvall J. Enhanced therapeutic tumour dose of [131]I-mIBG by accelerated diuresis. *Eur J Nuclear Med* 1988; **14**, 512–14.

98.  Mairs RJ, Gaze MN, Watson DG, *et al.* Carrier-free [131]I-meta-iodobenzylguanidine: comparison of production from meta-diazobenzylguanidine and from meta-trimethylsilylbenzylguanidine. *Nucl Med Commun* 1994; **15**, 268–74.

99.  O'Donoghue JA, Wheldon TE, Babich JW, *et al.* Implications of the uptake of [131]I-radiolabelled meta-iodobenzylguanidine (mIBG) for the targeted radiotherapy of neuroblastoma. *Br J Radiol* 1991; **64**, 428–34.

100. Wheldon TE, O'Donoghue JA, Barrett A, *et al.* The curability of tumours of differing size by targeted radiotherapy using [131]I or [90]Y. *Radiother Oncol* 1991; **21**, 91–9.

101. Gaze MN, Mairs RJ, Boyack SM, *et al.* [131]I-meta-iodobenzylguanidine therapy in neuroblastoma spheroids of different sizes. *Br J Cancer* 1992; **66**, 1048–52.

102. Wheldon TE, Amin AE, O'Donoghue JA, *et al.* Radiocurability of dissemi-
    nated malignant disease by external beam irradiation and targeted radionu-
    clide therapy. In: AA Epenetos, ed, *Monoclonal Antibodies 2: Applications in
    Clinical Oncology.* London: Chapman and Hall, 1993; 245–53.
103. Lashford LS, Moyes J, Ott R, *et al.* The biodistribution and pharmacokinet-
    ics of meta-iodobenzylguanidine in childhood neuroblastoma. *Eur J Nucl Med*
    1988; **13**, 574–7.
104. O'Donoghue JA. Optimal scheduling of biologically targeted radiotherapy and
    total body irradiation with bone marrow rescue for the treatment of systemic
    malignant disease. *Int J Radiat Oncol Biol Phys* 1991; **21**, 1587–94.

# 11 Hodgkin's disease: current management techniques and results

*Nancy Price Mendenhall and James W Lynch Jr*

## Epidemiology and aetiology

Approximately 7900 new cases of Hodgkin's disease (HD) occur in the United States each year.[1] Half of the cases occur in patients between the ages of 15 and 30 years. The disease is rare before age 5 and uncommon over age 70. The overall male:female ratio is 1.2:1, but there is a strong male predominance before adolescence.[2]

The cause of HD is unknown. Occasionally, clusters of cases have been identified, suggesting the possibility of a common environmental factor as an aetiological component prior to a latency period.[3-13] Epstein–Barr virus (EBV) is known to be associated with other malignancies, such as endemic Burkitt's lymphoma and undifferentiated nasopharyngeal carcinoma.[14] New molecular techniques that are capable of identifying sequences of EBV genome incorporated into the DNA of human cells have demonstrated evidence of prior EBV infection in most patients with HD.[15-17] One of the EBV genes identified in the Reed–Sternberg cells is a gene coding for latent membrane protein (LMP), believed to be responsible for inducing cell transformation and thus carrying the potential for being an aetiological agent in HD.[16,18] Some theories propose that HD is a rare consequence of a latent infection with EBV, developing in the setting of a host response to subsequent antigenic stimulation.[19]

## Pathology

The diagnosis of HD is based on the finding of Reed–Sternberg cells in the midst of an appropriate inflammatory background of eosinophils, plasma cells, and normal lymphocytes. The lineage of the Reed–Sternberg cell is in question, although it is believed to be of the monocyte line. There are four basic histological subtypes characterized by an increasing number of Reed–Sternberg cells and a decreasing number of normal-appearing inflammatory cells: lymphocyte predominant, nodular sclerosis, mixed cellularity, and lymphocyte depleted. The diagnosis of HD is usually easy for the haematopathologist, but even expert haematopathologists frequently disagree as to the histological subtype. Although treatment is not predicated on histological subtype, patterns of presentation correlate with subtype. Most patients with large mediastinal masses have the nodular-sclerosis subtype. The mixed-cellularity subtype is most frequently associated with subclinical disease in the abdomen (identified at laparotomy) and, in some series, with recurrence of the disease in pelvic lymph nodes.[20] A high proportion of patients with limited peripheral disease have lymphocyte-predominant HD.

Immunophenotyping and flow cytometry are important tools for excluding other lymphoid malignancies from the differential diagnosis, although neither technique will definitively identify HD, which has a heterogeneous phenotype. A subset of the lymphocyte-predominant histological subtype has an immunophenotype consistent with B-lymphocytes.[16,21,22]

# Patterns of involvement and spread

HD is a disease of the lymph nodes and usually remains within lymph nodes, with extranodal extension occurring only in the presence of bulky disease. Some lymph node groups are much more likely to be affected than others. When a single nodal site is involved (Stage I), it is in the low neck or supraclavicular area in approximately 70% of cases, the mediastinum in 10%, the axillae in 10%, and the inguinal and femoral nodes in the remaining 10% of cases. When more than one but fewer than five sites are involved, the pattern of involvement is almost exclusively that of contiguous nodal groups. One apparent exception is the common involvement of the low neck or supraclavicular nodes and the spleen and/or upper abdominal (coeliac, porta hepatic, splenic hilar, and upper para-aortic) nodes; the lower neck and upper abdominal nodes are directly related through the thoracic duct. Preauricular nodes may be involved in the presence of bulky upper neck nodes. Epitrochlear, popliteal, occipital, mesenteric, internal iliac, and presacral nodes are rarely involved in HD, even in advanced stages.

Extranodal involvement most commonly comprises direct extension to the lung from adjacent mediastinal masses; pulmonary nodules, usually associated with large mediastinal masses or hilar adenopathy; or liver, bone, or bone marrow involvement, usually associated with extensive involvement of the spleen. Central nervous system involvement is extremely rare, even in advanced disease; however, direct extension into bone and the spinal canal occurs with bulky disease, usually in the lower neck area. Involvement of Waldeyer's ring is rare, even in the presence of bulky upper neck adenopathy, and makes the diagnosis suspect.

# Diagnosis and staging

## Biopsy technique

Lymph nodes involved by HD are usually non-tender, firm but not rock-hard, rubbery, and plump. The history may be confusing because adenopathy in HD may wax and wane. Most patients have had a trial of antibiotic therapy before biopsy. The differential diagnosis in children and young adults with adenopathy includes infection, particularly cat-scratch fever and EBV, inflammatory processes such as sarcoidosis, and other malignancies such as non-Hodgkin's lymphoma, leukaemia, lymphoepithelioma, and rhabdomyosarcoma, as well as HD. When biopsy is performed, it is preferable to remove the largest, most clinically suspicious node rather than a smaller, more superficial node as there are often enlarged, but histologically normal, nodes associated with HD. The entire lymph node should be removed, if possible, because some processes are focal, and knowledge of the pattern of involvement within the lymph node may be useful to the pathologist. The histology must be reviewed by an expert haematopathologist, because HD may be confused with benign processes and non-Hodgkin's lymphoma. If HD or non-Hodgkin's lymphoma is suspected, biopsy material should always be sent for flow cytometry and immunophenotyping, in addition to histological study. Biopsy rather than needle aspiration should be the method of choice for *initial* diagnosis of HD, because the pathological criteria are highly dependent on nodal architecture and the background cellularity, as well as the presence of Reed–Sternberg cells.

## Staging system

The Ann Arbor staging system is used for staging of the tumour (Table 11.1).[23] A useful modification is the distinction between Stage $III_1$ disease, which includes only involvement of the upper abdomen (the spleen, splenic hilar, coeliac, and porta hepatic nodes), and $III_2$ disease, which includes lower abdominal involvement (para-aortic and pelvic nodes).[24] A further refinement, distinguishing between para-aortic adenopathy ($III_2$) and pelvic adenopathy ($III_3$), has prognostic significance with certain treatment approaches.[25] In all stages, spleen involvement is indicated by the postsubscript S and extranodal extension by the postsubscript E.

All patients are also classified as to whether constitutional symptoms are present; if one or more of these symptoms is present, a postscript B is added to the stage, and, if not, a postscript A is added. The constitutional symptoms are strictly defined as unexplained weight loss of greater than 10% of normal body weight in a period of no more than 6 months before diagnosis, fever greater than 101°F, and night sweats. Other symptoms noted to occur in patients with HD, but not classified as B symptoms, include pruritus and alcohol-induced pain. The pruritus is frequently generalized and severe, and may be the reason the patient seeks medical attention. Alcohol-induced pain is rare, but striking when present; it is usually localized to sites of disease and may be the first indication of disease recurrence.

**Table 11.1** Staging system[23]

| Stage | Description |
|-------|-------------|
| I | Involvement of single lymph node region (I) or localized involvement of a single extralymphatic organ or site ($I_E$) |
| II | Involvement of two or more lymph node regions on the same side of the diaphragm (II) or localized involvement of a single associated extralymphatic organ or site and lymph nodes on the same side of the diaphragm ($II_E$). Note: the number of lymph node regions involved may be indicated by a subscript (e.g. $II_3$) |
| III | Involvement of lymph node regions on both sides of the diaphragm (III), which may also be accompanied by localized involvement of an associated extralymphatic organ or site ($III_E$), by involvement of the spleen ($III_S$), or both ($III_{E+S}$) |
| IV | Disseminated (multifocal) involvement of one or more extralymphatic organs, with or without associated lymph node involvement, or isolated extralymphatic organ involvement with distant (non-regional) nodal involvement |

## Staging evaluation

A thorough history is obtained with emphasis on the presence of B symptoms, other constitutional symptoms, general performance status, and symptoms indicative of sites of disease such as cough, shortness of breath, chest pain, back pain, and bone pain. The past medical history is explored for evidence of prior infection, specifically mononucleosis and a history of warts.[26] In children, the remaining growth potential is assessed based on age, parental stature, and Tanner stage.

A thorough physical examination is performed, documenting abnormalities in Waldeyer's ring, the condition of the teeth, the presence and size of any abnormal lymph nodes in all potential node-bearing sites, and the status of the liver and spleen. A routine cardiopulmonary examination is performed, and the axial skeleton is percussed to elicit any bony tenderness.

Routine laboratory studies include complete blood cell count, platelet count, sedimentation rate, liver-function studies, renal profile, and baseline thyroid-function studies.

Routine imaging studies include chest roentgenogram and computed tomography (CT) of the chest, abdomen, and pelvis.

Lymphangiography has been a standard part of the staging evaluation, because of its capacity to identify filling defects and architectural changes indicative of HD in normal-sized lymph nodes that would not be apparent on CT. Lymphangiograms are technically difficult to perform, however, and difficult for the inexperienced radiologist to interpret, and therefore have been used less universally than in the past. In addition, studies comparing the accuracy of CT and lymphangiograms in HD show only small, if any, significant advantages for lymphangiograms.[27–31] Lymphangiograms do aid in treatment planning for patients receiving pelvic irradiation[32] and in follow-up for the early detection of pelvic lymph node recurrences.

Additional imaging studies that are useful in certain settings include magnetic resonance imaging (MRI) in the chest to delineate hilar adenopathy and pericardial extension; gallium scanning, particularly in assessing response to treatment and detecting recurrence; and MRI in the abdomen to distinguish unfilled bowel and vessels from retroperitoneal, porta hepatic, and coeliac adenopathy.

Despite the use of modern abdominal imaging techniques, the inaccuracy of clinical staging is 25–45% (Table 11.2).[33–36] Laparotomy for pathologic staging has been a standard component in staging HD patients. This procedure includes removal of the spleen, multiple wedge and needle biopsies of the liver, and multiple biopsies of abdominal and pelvic lymph nodes. Because chemotherapy is effective in eliminating subclinical disease, and there is added expense and morbidity with surgical staging, the role of laparotomy is in question. One major complication arising from laparotomy is an increased risk of infection, specifically from encapsulated organisms such as *Pneumococcus*, leading to pneumonia, sepsis, and meningitis. The rate of such infections, even before the development of prophylactic presplenectomy vaccination with Pneumovax 23 (Merck Sharp & Dohme), was quite low, estimated at 5–10% (Table 11.3).[20,37–44] Since the routine administration of Pneumovax before splenectomy and prophylactic antibiotic therapy after splenectomy, most major institutions treating children with HD report an infectious mortality rate of less than 1%.[37] Other complications include routine postoperative complications and a long-term risk of a small bowel obstruction, which occurs in 5–10% of patients and occasionally requires a second surgical procedure.[35,37]

The main advantage of laparotomy is knowledge of the presence and extent of abdominal and pelvic disease, which may influence the radiation treatment volume and the amount of chemotherapy delivered. Additional advantages of laparotomy include an opportunity for oophoropexy in female patients and, because the spleen is removed, a significant decrease in the amount of lung and kidney irradiated. Larger volumes of these organs are necessarily exposed to radiation when the spleen must be irradiated. The primary use of laparotomy today is for selection of patients who are candidates for treatment with radiotherapy alone.

# Treatment modalities

## Radiotherapy (RT)

### Treatment volume

Treatment was initially given only to the site of involvement, but early attention to the patterns of failure after localized treatment showed that most failures occurred outside the irradiated volume in adjacent nodal sites, leading to the concept of 'complementary field' or adjacent nodal area irradiation to eliminate subclinical disease.[45] Standard radiation treatment volumes commonly employed include the following:

**Table 11.2**  Incidence of stage change with laparotomy

| Institution, accrual dates | No. of patients | Age range (years) | Patients with stage change at laparotomy | | |
|---|---|---|---|---|---|
| | | | Up-staged | Down-staged | Total changed (%) |
| Children's Hospital of Western Ontario, 1970–86[33] | 39 | ≤ 18 | 5 | 12 | 17 (44) |
| Stanford University Medical Center, 1970–83[34] | 53 | ≤ 14 | 14 | 7 | 21 (40) |
| Joint Center for Radiation Therapy, 1969–86[35] | 692 | 3–73 | 24% | 42% | 190 (27) |
| Pediatric Oncology Group, 1986–91[36] | 203[a] | ≤ 21 | 52 | 4 | 56 (28) |

[a]Only twenty-two patients were Stage III or IV before laparotomy.

**Table 11.3**  Risk of serious infection after splenectomy for HD[37]

| Institution, date of report | No. of patients | Patients with serious infection (%) | Patients dead from infection (%) |
|---|---|---|---|
| Collected series, 1972[38] | 1170 | 16 (<1) | 6 (<1) |
| Baltimore Cancer Research Center, 1975[39] | 92 | 6 (<7) | 3 (3) |
| Children's Cancer Study Group, 1976[40] | 200 | 18 (9) | 8 (4) |
| Stanford University Medical Center, 1982[41] | 146 | 16 (11) | <4 (<3) |
| Intergroup Hodgkin's Disease in Childhood Study, 1984[42] | 234 | 4 (1.7) | 0 (0) |
| University of Chicago, 1985[43] | 239 | 2 (<1) | 1 (<1) |
| Bologna, 1986[44] | 342 | 5 (1.8) | 3 (1) |
| Joint Center for Radiation Therapy, 1988[20] | 315 | 8 (2) | 2 (<1) |
| University of Florida, 1992[37] | 133 | 9 (7) | 1 (<1) |

- *Involved-field irradiation* includes the entire nodal area (not just the particular node).
- *Extended-field irradiation* includes the involved nodal area and the clinically uninvolved contiguous nodal areas at risk for subclinical disease.[46]
- *Mantle-field irradiation* includes the neck, supraclavicular, infraclavicular, axillary, mediastinal, hilar, and inferior mediastinal lymph nodes. This field is extended to include the entire cardiac silhouette and half or all the lung parenchyma, when indicated.
- *Total nodal irradiation* treats all nodal areas usually involved in HD, including mantle, spleen (if present), and para-aortic, pelvic, inguinal, and femoral lymph node fields.
- *Subtotal or modified total nodal irradiation* is identical to total nodal irradiation except that it does not include the pelvic, inguinal, and femoral lymph nodes.
- *Inverted-Y irradiation* treats the femoral, inguinal, pelvic, and para-aortic nodes.

In patients with disease in the neck, a small preauricular field is usually added; it is rarely necessary to add a Waldeyer's ring field (which treats not only preauricular, postauricular, occipital, and submental nodes, but also the lymphoid tissue in the tonsil, base of tongue, and nasopharynx).

In patients with advanced abdominal disease, the liver is often treated if there is documented liver or spleen involvement. It is rarely necessary to irradiate the entire abdomen, as mesenteric nodes are only rarely involved.

### Dose

Early studies demonstrated increased control rates in HD with doses of 25 Gy or higher.[45] In early studies, the relationship between tumour control and radiation dose was described as either linear[46] or a sigmoid curve.[47] Recent retrospective studies have failed to demonstrate increased control rates with doses above 30 Gy, providing additional evidence for a sigmoidal dose–response relationship in HD.[48–50] At the University of Florida, doses of 35 Gy for clinically evident disease and 25–30 Gy for subclinical disease are provided when radiotherapy is used alone.

When radiotherapy is used in conjunction with chemotherapy, the doses of radiation may be reduced. When a complete response is achieved with six cycles of chemotherapy, a dose of 15–25 Gy is sufficient in children.[34,51–55] Response to chemotherapy is predictive of the likelihood of local control. If less than a complete response is achieved with chemotherapy, it is unclear whether the dose of radiation can be reduced, so standard doses (30–35 Gy for clinically evident disease and 25–30 Gy for subclinical disease) are recommended.

### Technique

The treatment technique for HD is difficult and varies even among centres with extensive experience in the management of HD. Appropriate treatment techniques are described in other sources.[46,56,57] The national Patterns of Care study demonstrated that the likelihood of relapse or death in patients treated with radiation therapy for HD varies with the institution, and that relapse and death rates, which are associated with inadequate field margins, are significantly higher in community practices than in academic institutions.[48] Therefore, if radiotherapy is used in a patient with HD, it should be delivered by an experienced physician.

## Chemotherapy (CT)

### Historical perspective

The early development of chemotherapy for HD remains the paradigm for application of scientific observation to the design of treatment for patients with cancer. For most practising oncologists, thinking of advanced HD as an invariably incurable malignancy seems inconceivable, yet this was the truth only 30 years ago. In 1964, VT DeVita and others at the National Cancer Institute (NCI) in Bethesda, Maryland, began a programme of combination chemotherapy based on evidence from multiple disciplines. First, certain classes of drugs, namely Vinca alkaloids, a derivative of mustard gas, and procarbazine (a methylhydrazine derivative), were known to possess *in-vitro* antineoplastic activity for lymphoma cell lines. Second, the ability of these drugs to kill tumour cells *in vitro* was directly related to the total dose, and eradication of populations of tumour cells was possible with repeated administration of the agent. Third, combinations of these agents were more effective than single agents. Finally, each of the compounds had been noted to induce tumour shrinkage when given to human patients with HD. On this basis, investigators designed and administered the first combination chemotherapy regimen, MOPP (mechlorethamine, vincristine, procarbazine, prednisone), to patients with advanced HD.[58-60] Subsequent trials, first at the NCI and then throughout the rest of the world, have transformed our thinking about HD specifically, and cancer in general. In fact, this early work not only remains the model for developmental therapeutics for curable malignancies, but also formed the very foundation of the discipline of medical oncology.

### Theoretical considerations

The development of this new type of treatment was guided by a new set of principles, some based on scientific observation and others based on tumour biology and in need of confirmation by empirical observation. As the pool of active agents has expanded, the number of possible combinations of drugs has increased exponentially; the newer combinations may be more effective on average and will probably be associated with fewer late complications. However, the six principles developed for the design and delivery of MOPP still guide us today.[60]

1. Use of multiple drugs that are known not to be cross-resistant.
2. Use of these agents in their maximally tolerated doses according to their optimal schedule of administration.
3. Choice of agents with as little overlapping organ toxicity as possible.
4. Administration in a cyclic manner to allow time for patient recovery.
5. Adherence to a rigid schedule of administration whenever possible, but

with modifications of either dose or timing according to a sliding scale based largely on myelosuppression.

6. Empirical delivery of two cycles of chemotherapy beyond achievement of complete response as determined by physical examination, radiographs, and pathological evaluation.

All current efforts to improve chemotherapy for HD stem from one of these original ideas. For example, the development of new drug combinations relies on the principles of avoiding cross-resistance and overlapping toxicity. The use of autologous bone marrow or stem cell rescue and haematopoietic growth factors is a way to increase the maximally tolerated dose. Experiments with infusional regimens instead of high dose bolus therapy in many institutions, including the University of Florida, are attempts to determine the best route or schedule of administration. Finally, even investigations aimed at defining specific genetic lesions that may be suitable for molecular documentation of minimal residual disease are, in essence, a search for more sophisticated means of defining a complete response.

## Evolution of chemotherapy and current treatment recommendations

With the reported success of the MOPP programme, numerous modifications of MOPP were developed, including ChlVPP (chlorambucil, vinblastine, procarbazine, prednisone), MVPP (mechlorethamine, vinblastine, procarbazine, prednisone), BCVPP carmustine (BCNU), cyclophosphamide, vinblastine, procarbazine, prednisone), and LOPP (chlorambucil, vincristine, procarbazine, prednisone).[61] BCVPP was shown to be superior to MOPP in an Eastern Cooperative Oncology Group (ECOG) trial, but this study altered the dosing schedule of MOPP, thereby potentially compromising its efficacy. It has also been noted that nitrosoureas are associated with an alarming incidence of late bone marrow complications. The initial results obtained at the NCI with MOPP have not been replicated in other institutions.[62-64] A variety of factors may have contributed to this discrepancy.

1. Patients treated at the NCI may have had a better performance status.
2. The administration of MOPP chemotherapy outside the NCI may be associated with dose reductions (such as 'capping' vincristine doses) or poor dosing schedules for procarbazine.
3. Patient compliance is an important component of the MOPP programme, which calls for 14 days of oral procarbazine and prednisone, and may be less reliable in certain clinical settings outside the NCI.

Despite the many difficulties with MOPP, and the many alternative regimens, MOPP is still the most frequently used alkylating-agent-based regimen.

At the Milan Cancer Institute in Italy, a novel chemotherapy programme based entirely on new drugs (relative to MOPP) was developed in the early 1970s. This regimen, ABVD (doxorubicin, bleomycin, vinblastine, and dacarbazine (DTIC)) was noted to be effective in patients who relapsed after MOPP treatment, and has been studied extensively both as salvage and primary therapy, either alone or in combination with other regimens.[62,63,65-69] In 1992, the results of a prospective randomized trial were reported, comparing three different treatments for advanced HD:[70] twelve cycles of MOPP alternating with ABVD, compared with six to eight cycles of MOPP or ABVD. It had long been argued by those who examined tumour biology that alternating non-cross-resistant chemotherapies early in the treatment of cancer might result in a higher cure rate by killing tumour cells prior to their developing resistance to all of the agents being used. This trial demonstrated the MOPP-alone arm to be inferior. More importantly, it demonstrated that 12 months of therapy with alternating treatment was no better than 6–8 months of standard ABVD, with disease-free survival at 5 years of 60–65%. Hence, shorter duration chemotherapy is as effective, no doubt less toxic, and therefore probably preferable.

The best results reported, to date, from any single institution and for any single regimen are from the group at Vancouver, British Columbia, using the hybrid regimen of MOPP–ABV.[71] Rather than alternating full cycles of MOPP and ABVD, this combination combines one half cycle of MOPP with the most active agents from ABVD, eliminating dacarbazine because of its questionable efficacy and its tendency to increase acute toxicity (nausea, vomiting, and flu-like syndrome). Also, the dose of doxorubicin is increased from 25 mg/m$^2$ to 35 mg/m$^2$. In their series, most recently updated in 1988, seventy-four of seventy-six evaluable patients experienced a complete response, sixty-four with chemotherapy alone and ten with the addition of involved-field radiotherapy. Among the seventy-four patients scored as complete responders, sixty-seven were alive and disease-free with a median follow-up of 46 months (range, 29–71 months), for a disease-free survival of 85% for all evaluable patients. A randomized trial comparing this regimen with sequential MOPP and ABVD has been completed and is awaiting sufficient follow-up for final reporting.[72]

In summary, approximately 55–75% of patients with HD will be cured with combination chemotherapy. The development of chemotherapy for advanced HD has largely been responsible for transforming a universally fatal disease into one that physicians approach with guarded optimism. The MOPP–ABV regimen may be the best treatment described, to date, because of its excellent therapeutic efficacy in Phase II and III trials and its presumably lower risk of long-term sequelae. New approaches are being developed with the goal of reducing toxicity in first-line therapy and exploiting potential pharmacological advantages of constant infusion therapy and high dose chemotherapy with peripheral blood progenitor cells and autologous bone marrow rescue in patients who relapse.[73]

## Combined modality therapy (CMT)

The pattern of failure after treatment with chemotherapy alone is primarily in nodal areas[74,75] known to be involved, whereas failures after radiotherapy are usually outside radiation portals, either in unirradiated contiguous nodal areas or at the margin of the radiation field where the extent of tumour may be underestimated or the dose of radiation may be low. The striking difference in patterns of failure after chemotherapy and irradiation suggests a rationale for combined modality therapy. Additionally, it is clear that major toxicities of treatment are dose related and that the doses of both radiotherapy and chemotherapy can be reduced in combined modality regimens.

# Management approaches and results

Paradoxically, the very success achieved in HD therapy has made the management of this disease one of the most complex and difficult in oncology. For any given presentation of the disease, many valid treatment choices exist that result in acceptable survival rates. In addition, successful second-line therapy is possible after some initial treatment approaches.

The very high cure rate in a population primarily composed of teenagers and young adults means that quality of life and treatment sequelae must also be considered in evaluating therapeutic choices. Each therapeutic modality carries its own set of potential toxicities, and all of the major toxicities appear to be dose related. Thus, the final choice of therapy in a given patient is a complex one that involves consideration of not only the probability of survival and freedom from disease relapse, but also the likelihood of various toxicities that may limit an otherwise normal life.

Clearly, patients with extensive disease require more therapy than those with minimal disease. In fact, previously untreated patients may be grouped into three risk groups that correlate with the amount of therapy needed. The low-risk group includes Stage I and II patients who lack specific poor prognostic factors such as bulky disease in the mediastinum or elsewhere, B symptoms, and more than four sites of involvement. The intermediate group includes those Stage I and II patients who have poor prognostic factors and Stage $IIIA_1$ patients with minimal or no splenic involvement. The high-risk group includes patients with Stage $IIIA_2$, IIIB, and IV disease. In addition, a heterogeneous group of patients require treatment for recurrent disease.

## Low risk

The results achieved in Stage I and II HD with radiation therapy alone, at a number of institutions, are shown in Table 11.4[20,76-82] The results appear to vary somewhat as certain institutions have included only asymptomatic patients, only laparotomy-staged patients, or only Stage I patients. However, most institutions report a freedom-from-relapse rate of at least 75% in all Stage I and II patients, a disease-free survival of at least 85%, and an overall survival at more than 10 years of at least 75%, with much higher figures when patients with B symptoms and large mediastinal masses are excluded.

A variety of factors which predict a relatively poor prognosis with radiation therapy alone within Stage I and II HD patients have been identified, including large mediastinal masses, large tumour bulk, more than three or four sites of involvement, B symptoms, and elevated erythrocyte sedimentation rate.[20,50,76,80,81,83-86] Most of these factors reflect tumour volume, extent of disease, and tumour biology; the particular factors identified vary to some extent among reports, partly because not all of these factors can be assessed in each data set. The three factors most important for predicting a poor prognosis with radiation therapy alone in Stage I and II patients treated at the University of Florida were tumour dimension greater than 6 cm, B symptoms, and more than four sites of involvement. Patients without these poor prognostic factors had relapse-free and cause-specific survival rates after radiation therapy alone of 84–95%, whereas patients with one or more of these factors had relapse-free and cause-specific survival rates of only 53% and 75%, respectively, after radiation therapy.[81] It would appear that, for patients with Stage I and II disease, without any poor prognostic factors, radiation therapy alone is adequate. It is important to note, however, that the majority of the experience in the US in early-stage patients has been in laparotomy-staged patients (see Table 11.4).

**Table 11.4** Results of treatment with radiation alone[a] for Stage I and II Hodgkin's disease

| Investigator | No. of patients | Stage | % Survival (years) | |
| --- | --- | --- | --- | --- |
| | | | Relapse-free | Absolute |
| University of Minnesota[76] | 20 | P IA–B | 100 (5 y) | 92 (5 y) |
| | 58 | P IIA | 79 (5 y) | 92 (5 y) |
| | 7 | P IIB | 67 (5 y) | 57 (5 y) |
| University of Chicago[77] | 28 | P I–IIA, B | 83 (10 y) | 83 (10 y) |
| University of Rochester[78] | 40 | P IA | 92 (10 y) | 91 (10 y) |
| | 44 | P IIA | 48 (10 y) | 83 (10 y) |
| Joint Center for Radiation Therapy, Boston, MA[79] | 315 | P IA, IIA | 82 (14 y) | 93 (14 y) |
| Stanford[80] | 109 | P I–IIA, B | 77 (10 y) | 84 (10 y) |
| University of Florida[81,b] | 120 | CP I–IIA, B | 75 (10 y) | 77 (10 y) |
| St Bartholomew's[82] | 90 | CP IA, B | 78 (15 y) | 75 (15 y) |

[a]Modified total nodal irradiation or total nodal irradiation in the majority of cases.
[b]University of Florida, data 1964–86; analysis 8/91.
P: pathologic stage; C: clinical stage.

An interesting question raised by two recent prospective trials[74,75,87] is whether chemotherapy alone would achieve as good a result in early-stage HD as radiation therapy alone. The results of these two trials are shown in Table 11.5. Both trials randomized laporotomy-staged patients to receive either mantle and para-aortic irradiation or six cycles of MOPP chemotherapy (mechlorethamine, vincristine, procarbazine, prednisone). The NCI study[87] included patients with large mediastinal masses, B symptoms, and Stage IIIA$_1$ disease; the Italian study[75] included only asymptomatic, Stage I and II patients. In the NCI study, there was a significant advantage in disease-free and overall survival in patients treated with chemotherapy when patients with large mediastinal masses and Stage III disease were included. No significant difference was found, however, in either disease- free or overall survival when patients with large mediastinal masses and Stage IIIA$_1$ disease were excluded. In the Italian study, there was no difference in freedom

**Table 11.5**   Results of prospective randomized trials comparing chemotherapy alone in early stage Hodgkin's disease

| Investigator | Stage | No. of patients | Treatment regimen | Rate of CR (%) | % Survival (years) | | | |
| --- | --- | --- | --- | --- | --- | --- | --- | --- |
| | | | | | Relapse-free (patients with CR) | P-value | Absolute | P-value |
| Universities of Rome and Florence[75] | P I–IIA | 45 | MPA | 100 | 70 (8 y) | n.d. | 93 (8 y) | <0.001 |
| | | 44 | MOPP × 6 | 91 | 71 (8 y) | | 56 (8 y) | |
| NCI[87] | P I–IIA–B | 51 | MPA | 96 | 67[a] | 0.009 | 85 (10 y)[a] | n.d |
| | | 54 | MOPP × 6 | 96 | 82[a] | | 90 (10 y)[a] | |

[a]Excluding patients with peripheral IA and IIIA$_1$ disease or massive mediastinal disease.
CR: complete response; P: pathologic stage; MPA: mantle and para-aortic irradiation; MOPP: mechlorethamine, vincristine, procarbazine, prednisone; n.d.: no difference.

from relapse at 8 years between the treatment arms, but there was a significant survival advantage for those patients treated with irradiation. Although the frequency of relapse was similar in the two treatment groups, the survival probability was higher for patients who relapsed after radiation than for those who relapsed after chemotherapy (85% vs 15%, $P = 0.02$).[75] In addition, significantly more toxicity was recorded for patients treated with chemotherapy, so the conclusion of the Italian study was that radiation therapy alone was the treatment of choice in early-stage HD.

## Intermediate risk

The relatively low relapse-free survival in Stage I and II patients with poor prognostic factors warrants placement of this subset of Stage I and II patients into an intermediate-risk group that may benefit from slightly more aggressive therapy. When Stage I and II patients with one or more of these poor prognostic factors were treated initially, at the University of Florida, with combined modality therapy (usually two to three cycles of chemotherapy followed by standard radiotherapy), the relapse-free survival rate was significantly better (81% vs 53%, $P = 0.02$), although cause-specific survival was the same (78% vs 75%, $P = 0.68$).[81]

In selected series of patients with large mediastinal masses, excellent results are reported with radiation therapy alone, after very careful evaluation of the extent of disease and meticulous treatment technique by experienced radiation oncologists.[76,88] Most series, however, demonstrate relatively high relapse rates in patients with large mediastinal masses treated with radiation therapy alone, and significantly better freedom-from-relapse rates with the use of combined modality therapy.[84,89]

Excellent results have also been reported in selected Stage III patients (those $IIIA_1$ patients with little or no splenic disease) treated with radiation therapy alone, with comprehensive treatment volumes and careful technique,[54,90,91] but relapse rates are usually relatively high with radiotherapy alone in all but a very small subset of Stage III patients, and are significantly improved in patients managed with combined modality therapy.[92]

Several institutions, including MD Anderson Hospital, have reported excellent results with the use of limited (two to three cycles) chemotherapy prior to standard radiotherapy in both Stage I and II patients with poor prognostic factors and in Stage III disease, as shown in Table 11.6.[93–96] The advantages of this approach are that most major toxicities of chemotherapy are very strongly dose related and much less probable after two cycles of chemotherapy than after six, and that relapse (and exposure to salvage chemotherapy) is much less likely after this approach than with radiotherapy alone.

## High risk

Patients with Stage $IIIA_1$ with extensive splenic involvement, $IIIA_2$, IIIB, and IV disease have been managed with chemotherapy alone or combined modality therapy. Salvage rates are poor after treatment failure in patients with advanced disease at presentation, so maximum efforts to achieve the highest relapse-free survival rates are justified. Whether the addition of radiation

**Table 11.6** Results of combined modality therapy with two to three cycles of chemotherapy in intermediate-risk patients

| Investigator | Stage | No. of patients | Treatment regimen | % Survival (years) | |
|---|---|---|---|---|---|
| | | | | Relapse-free | Absolute (cause-specific) |
| MDAH[96] | I–IIA, B | 24 | MOPP × 2 + RT | 79　(4 y) | 100　(4 y) |
| MDAH[93] | IIIA | 197 | MOPP × 2 + MTNI/TNI | 79–86　(10 y) | 66　(10 y) |
| | IIIB | | MOPP × 2 + MTNI/TNI | 79–85　(10 y) | 57　(10 y) |
| Hôpital St Louis[95] | II–IIIA | 53 | MOPP × 3 + RT | 88　(5 y) | 86　(8 y) |
| | II–IIIB | | MOPP × 6 + RT | 91　(5 y) | 89　(8 y) |
| SWOG[94] | IIIA, B | 53 | MOPP-bleo × 3 + TNI | ~85　(5 y) | 89　(5 y) |

MOPP: mechlorethamine, vincristine, procarbazine, prednisone; RT: radiotherapy; MTNI: modified total nodal irradiation; TNI: total node irradiation; bleo: bleomycin; MDAH: MD Anderson Hospital, Houston, TX; SWOG: Southwest Oncology Group.

therapy is beneficial to all patients with high-risk disease is unknown.

Approximately 70–80% of patients will attain a complete remission with chemotherapy alone, and approximately 70% of the complete remissions will be durable, for relapse-free survival rates of 50–60%. Some investigators have found that ABVD or alternating and hybrid ABVD–MOPP regimens appear to be more effective than MOPP, BCVPP, MVPP, or COPP (cyclophosphamide, vincristine, procarbazine, prednisone).[63,69,70,97–100]

Although good results are reported with chemotherapy alone,[61,63,64,70,97,101–105] a substantial number of patients relapse, usually in nodal sites that were known to be involved at original presentation, suggesting a possible benefit of involved-field radiotherapy (which, in these patients, frequently means extensive radiation fields). Patients with bulky sites of involvement appear to be at a particularly high risk of relapse if treated with chemotherapy alone.[87,104,106,107] The results of several prospective randomized trials[94,103,108,109] that have attempted to address this question are shown in Table 11.7. Most of the studies show differences (statistically significant or trends) for either relapse-free or overall survival in favour of the addition of radiation therapy.

## Recurrent and refractory HD

Recurrent HD implies a remanifestation of the disease after demonstrated response to treatment and apparent disease control. Refractory HD implies disease that progresses despite therapy or within 6 months of completion of therapy. The management of recurrent and refractory disease depends heavily on the extent of disease (both at initial presentation and relapse), prior therapy (both the particular drugs and the amount), and responsiveness to prior therapy (both the completeness and duration of response). These factors help determine the patient's prognosis and which treatment modalities are likely to be effective. Although patients with recurrent and refractory HD are a heterogeneous group because of the factors listed above, they can be grouped into three categories for the purpose of predicting prognosis and selecting salvage treatment: first relapse after initial treatment with radiotherapy alone, first relapse after treatment with chemotherapy or combined modality therapy, and relapse after two or more chemotherapy regimens or refractory disease.

### *Recurrent disease*

*First relapse after RT for early-stage disease*

Patients treated initially with RT alone for early-stage disease constitute the group with the best prognosis. With combination chemotherapy (usually six cycles), with or without consolidative irradiation, the relapse-free survival at 4–10 years is 50–60%.[110–113]

Within this group of patients, the most important prognostic variable is probably extent of disease at the time of recurrence.[111] Other factors that may be important include age[112] and initial stage of disease.[110] In a retrospective study from Stanford,[111] it was noted that in patients with either B symptoms or more extensive disease than Relapse Stage I (RS I, using the

**Table 11.7** Results of treatment of advanced Hodgkin's disease in prospective randomized trials comparing chemotherapy alone with combined modality therapy

| Investigator | No. of patients | Stage | Treatment regimen | % Survival (years) | | | |
| --- | --- | --- | --- | --- | --- | --- | --- |
| | | | | Freedom from relapse or relapse-free survival | P-value | Absolute | P-value |
| Stanford[108] | 22 | III–IV | PAVe/ABVD | 67 (3 y) | | 77 (3 y) | |
| | 16 | | PAVe/TNI | 85 (3 y) | 0.17 | 100 (3 y) | 0.11 |
| SWOG[94] | 64 | III | MOPP–bleo × 10 | ~65 (5 y) | | 87 (5 y) | |
| | 53 | IIINS[a] | MOPP–bleo × 3 + TNI | ~85 (5 y) | 0.16 | 89 (5 y) | n.d. |
| | 35 | | MOPP–bleo × 10 | ~75 (5 y) | | n.d. | |
| | 31 | | MOPP–bleo × 3 + TNI | ~85 (5 y) | 0.05 | n.d. | |
| SEG[103] | 15 | IIB–IV | BCVPP | n.d. | | 67 (5 y)[b] | |
| | 15 | | BCVPP + RT | n.d. | | 100 (5 y)[b] | 0.05 |
| SWOG[109] | 278 | III–IV | MOP-BAP | 68 (67)[c] | 0.09 (0.002)[c] | 79 | |
| | | | MOP-BAP + IF RT | 79 (85)[c] | | 86 | 0.14 |

[a]Nodular sclerosis histology subset, eligible for study.
[b]Determinate survival.
[c]Numbers in parentheses refer to subset of patients who actually received assigned treatment.
PAVe: procarbazine, melphalan, vinblastine; ABVD: doxorubicin, bleomycin, vinblastine, dacarbazine; TNI: total nodal irradiation; MOPP: mechlorethamine, vincristine, procarbazine, prednisone; bleo: bleomycin; BCVPP: carmustine (BCNU); cyclophosphamide, vinblastine, procarbazine, prednisone; RT: radiotherapy; MOP-BAP: mechlorethamine, vincristine, prednisone, bleomycin, doxorubicin, procarbazine; IF: involved field radiotherapy; SWOG: Southwest Oncology Group; SEG: Southeastern Oncology Group.

Ann Arbor system) at relapse, CMT produced better relapse-free and overall survival rates than chemotherapy alone. One study concluded that ABVD was the best chemotherapy regimen for salvage after RT failure.[114] One factor that *does not* negatively affect the patient's chance at a second complete remission or durable response is prior RT or extent of RT, either for early-stage disease[110,111,113] or more advanced disease.[115]

### First relapse after CT or CMT

*Second-line chemotherapy*   The second group of patients with recurrent disease are those with relapse after one first-line CT regimen. In most of the published data, the initial treatment has been MOPP, with or without RT. The most popular treatment option in this group of patients has been a non-cross-resistant CT regimen, with or without RT. Complete responses are usually achieved in 35–60% of patients; in 40–50% of complete responders the responses are durable. However, the overall relapse-free survival rate (disease-free, freedom from secondary disease progression, event-free, etc.) after second-line CT is usually less than 20% at 5 years.[116–122] The most important factor for predicting a second remission is duration of first remission (<12 months).

*RT for salvage*   In patients with a relapse after treatment with CT alone, whose recurrent disease is confined to nodal sites, good results have been achieved with RT alone in *selected* patients.[123–125] Aggressive radiation treatment volumes (total nodal irradiation, with or without lung and liver irradiation, as indicated) are required, however.

### Failure after two or more CT regimens

A third group of patients with a particularly poor prognosis are those with relapse after treatment with two or more CT regimens. The results with third-line standard CT regimens are generally poor, with complete responses usually in the range of 15–20% and relapse-free survivals of 5–15% at 18 months.[126–130]

Another option for this group is high dose chemotherapy with bone marrow transplantation. Several good reviews of this subject are available.[131–136]

It appears that approximately half of patients will attain a complete response and approximately half of the complete responses will be durable (lasting more than 2 years).[137–145] Follow-up is inadequate to assess 5-year results. Prognostic factors thus far identified for patients undergoing bone marrow transplant (BMT) include chemosensitive disease and extent of disease present at the time of BMT, refractory versus recurrent disease, the number of previous regimens, and patient performance status.[136,138,139,141]

It appears that patients will have the best chance of durable response if they enter BMT in complete remission. The vast majority of failures after BMT occur in prior sites of disease, rarely in the bone marrow. The patterns of failure have led some investigators to conclude that inadequate pre-transplant conditioning is the primary cause of treatment failure.[143] The patterns of failure also suggest that RT could be an effective part of such regimens. The long-term sequelae of BMT are unknown. At present, BMT is probably the treatment of choice for selected patients with poor-risk recurrences or refractory HD. However, it should only be performed as part of a well-designed clinical investigation.

Several alternative treatments are currently under investigation, including radioisotope-labelled monoclonal antibodies,[146,147] hyperthermia,[148] and immunotherapy.[149] These approaches should be employed only in the setting of a clinical trial, after all options for standard therapy are exhausted.

# Complications of treatment

## Radiotherapy

Complications of radiotherapy are related to total dose, dose per treatment, the volume of tissue treated, tolerance of the normal tissues in the treatment volume, and age of the patient. Commonly recognized complications of radiotherapy (with the standard doses and techniques currently employed) include a 25–50% rate of subsequent thyroid dysfunction,[150] an increased risk of dental problems unless good dental hygiene is maintained, a 1–2% rate of both acute and late pulmonary and cardiac problems, a 1% rate of abdominal complications, a probable increase in secondary malignancy rate, and musculoskeletal hypoplasia in small children treated with standard doses of radiation (35–40 Gy).

Most complications associated with irradiation are related to the mantle treatment volume. The major acute pulmonary complication of radiotherapy is pneumonitis, usually seen after hemilung or whole lung irradiation in patients with clinical evidence of pulmonary involvement or a high risk of subclinical pulmonary or pleural involvement in the presence of large mediastinal or hilar disease. Occasionally, pneumonitis is associated with the cessation of steroids when chemotherapy is given after irradiation. In patients with bulky mediastinal disease given standard radiotherapy and elective lung irradiation, the risk of pneumonitis is of the order of 10–15%.[151] The risk of pneumonitis can be decreased with the use of a thin lung transmission block or split-course treatment, techniques that alter the dose per treatment and the overall time during which the radiation is delivered.[57,152,153] Management in symptomatic patients should be immediate and aggressive, with steroids, observation in the hospital, and supportive therapy, because this complication can be fatal. The steroid dosage should be 60–100 mg of prednisone per day with a very slow taper beginning only after resolution of all symptoms and protracted over several months. If the patient has received chemotherapy, other sources for pneumonia should be ruled out by appropriate diagnostic evaluation after steroids have been administered. Pulmonary fibrosis may occur, but is usually confined to the apices of the lung and paratracheal parenchyma and rarely results in impairment of pulmonary function.[154]

With optimal treatment technique and dose, the risk of cardiac dysfunction is low.[155,156] Acute pericarditis occurs 6 weeks to 1 year after irradiation; the risk is related to treatment technique (delivery of most of the dose through an anterior portal), dose per fraction, total dose, and volume of heart irradiated.[152,157,158] Pericardial effusions are often asymptomatic and resolve without therapy; if the patient is symptomatic, steroids may be administered and the effusion tapped. Constrictive pericarditis can occur in subsequent years of follow-up and is probably related to the same factors as acute pericarditis. Paracentesis should be reserved either for treatment of tamponade or as a diagnostic test to rule out other causes when indicated. Surgical intervention should only be used when conservative measures have failed. Other cardiac events such as myocardial infarction appear to be increased in successfully treated patients and may be related to acceleration of atherosclerotic plaque formation in the coronary vessels within the treatment field. However, many of the patients in whom cardiac events have been observed have other risk factors including Type IV hyperlipidaemia, history of smoking, familial history of cardiac disease, obesity, hypertension, and diabetes. All patients with HD should be counselled against smoking and screened periodically for hyperlipidaemia and hypertension.

An additional complication rarely observed is transverse myelitis, which in most cases is related to suboptimal radiotherapy technique in matching fields. A more frequent neurological side-effect of mantle irradiation is Lhermitte's syndrome, a transient effect probably related to damage and regeneration of myelin. With Lhermitte's syndrome, the patient reports a shock-like sensation radiating down the legs, usually precipitated by walking, jogging, or simple flexion of the cervical spine. Lhermitte's syndrome usually appears within 6 weeks to 3 months of irradiation and may last from several weeks to more than 6 months. It occurs in about 20% of patients receiving mantle irradiation and does not herald any permanent neurologic sequelae.

Thyroid dysfunction after mantle irradiation is most often hypothyroidism, but hyperthyroidism has been reported. Thyroid function studies are performed routinely after radiotherapy, usually at yearly intervals in the asymptomatic patient, and thyroid hormone replacement is instituted on development of abnormal thyroid function studies, before symptoms develop.

Prophylactic daily fluoride applications and regular dental care prevent dental complications in most patients; the risk of xerostomia or subsequent dental problems is very low unless a Waldeyer's ring field was treated.

The most frequent abdominal complication after radiotherapy for HD is bowel adhesion, which is rare in patients who have not had abdominal surgery (e.g. staging laparotomy). With doses of 35 Gy or less, and daily doses of no more than 2 Gy, the risk is 1% or less.[159] No significant risk of renal, liver, or intrinsic bowel complications has been noted. An increase in total or daily dose will increase the complication rate.[157]

Permanent gonadal injury, secondary to radiation, can be avoided in most male patients with special testicular shielding during irradiation. Without special testicular shielding, the oligospermia rate is at least 50% after pelvic irradiation.[160] In male patients receiving greater than 40 Gy to the pelvic nodes after laparotomy, a small incidence of hydrocele has also been noted.

The ovaries are less sensitive to scattered irradiation than the testicles, but require special protection if the pelvic nodes are irradiated. Protection of the ovaries is much more difficult than testicular shielding. An oophoropexy can be performed at laparotomy; if laparotomy was not performed, or if the ovaries have migrated after laparotomy, they can be transfixed through a laparoscopy procedure.[161] Even with oophoropexy and careful shielding, the ovaries receive a substantial amount of scattered irradiation and are at some risk for temporary or permanent ablation with pelvic irradiation. The only cases of ovarian failure observed in the Stanford series were associated with more than three cycles of MOPP chemotherapy and pelvic irradiation with no ovarian shielding or suboptimal ovarian shielding.[160] The success in preserving ovarian function when pelvic irradiation is administered varies[162] and is highly technique dependent.

In addition to the complications listed above, which can occur in patients of all ages, paediatric patients treated for HD are also at risk for impaired development of bone and soft tissues within the field of irradiation. Doses in excess of 40 Gy also place the child at risk for significant subsequent fibrosis and possible arm or leg oedema. Musculoskeletal hypoplasia is clearly related to the dose administered and to the age and developmental status of the child at the time of treatment. Doses of 25 Gy or less in adolescents, 20 Gy in 6-year-old to 10-year-old children, and 15 Gy in children less than 6 years old cause no significant hypoplasia.[34]

Second malignancies are noted in survivors of HD. In one paediatric series, the probability of developing any second malignancy was 2% at 5 years, 5% at 10 years and 9% at 15 years, and most second solid malignancies occurred in previously irradiated fields.[163] Two second malignancies of particular concern are breast and lung cancers. With the apparent overall rise in the incidence of breast cancer in the US, it is difficult to determine the degree of increased risk conferred on the HD survivor by radiotherapy. However, many of the subsequent breast cancers have been bilateral and medial in location — the part of the breast usually included in previous radiation portals. The true incidence of second malignancy will not be realized until large cohorts of children cured of HD pass through the sixth to eighth decades of life, when most adult malignancies appear. The vast majority of lung cancers observed in HD survivors have occurred in smokers. All HD survivors should be counselled on the risks of second malignancy, and the necessity of avoiding other carcinogenic factors (smoking); and they should be considered for aggressive surveillance programmes.

## Chemotherapy

The rate of fatal sepsis with modern administration of chemotherapy is about 1%. Chemotherapy regimens, such as MOPP, that are based on alkylating agents carry three major toxicities of concern: acute leukaemias, myelodysplastic syndromes, or other second malignancies; sterility; and neuropathy. The major risks of the antibiotic-based regimens such as ABVD are cardiac[164] and pulmonary.[156]

Acute leukaemia has been linked to the alkylating agents in MOPP and occurs in approximately 6% of children receiving six cycles of MOPP[34] and involved-field radiotherapy. Data on adults suggest that the risk is clearly related to the dose of alkylating agent and possibly to age, stage, and splenectomy.[163,165-174] Whether the addition of irradiation to an alkylating-agent-based chemotherapy regimen increases the leukaemia risk is unclear, but most studies addressing this issue have not demonstrated a significant increase due to irradiation; in addition, leukaemias are seen only rarely after radiotherapy alone. Most often, leukaemia occurs between 2 and 8 years after exposure to the alkylating agent, but later occurrence of leukaemia is occasionally reported.

The rate of male sterility after six cycles of MOPP[160] or other alkylating agents[162] approaches 100%. Occasionally, the azoospermia is transient, as a few men have recovered normal sperm counts more than 10 years after chemotherapy.[113,160] The male sterility risk is dose related and is only about 50% after two cycles of MOPP.[175] The high risk of sterility with six cycles of MOPP applies to male patients both before and after puberty.[160] Peripheral neuropathy is a common, but usually transient, side-effect related to vincristine.

In twenty asymptomatic children treated with six cycles of alternating ABVD–MOPP and low dose (15–25 Gy) involved-field radiotherapy, a comparison of pretreatment and post-treatment pulmonary function studies showed that more than 50% of children had a reduced or abnormal carbon monoxide diffusing capacity, and 40% had restrictive or obstruction changes in lung volume and spirometry; the clinical significance of these findings is unknown.[156] The abnormalities in pulmonary function were observed after bleomycin doses as low as 36 units/m$^2$ (the equivalent of one dose). On cardiac nuclear gated angiograms, 14% of patients had a low resting ejection fraction or decreased response to exercise. Twenty-one per cent had abnormal results on thyroid function studies. The authors concluded that the risks of thyroid and cardiac dysfunction were low, but the pulmonary risks were high and warranted close attention.

# New directions

The challenges in HD are to develop less toxic, but equally efficacious, treatment approaches in early- and intermediate-stage disease and to develop more effective treatment regimens for patients with advanced and recurrent disease.

In the past two decades, significant progress has come from the recognition that most toxicity is dose related and that, with the use of combined modality therapy, the doses of both radiation and chemotherapy agents can be reduced significantly without reducing efficacy.

Significant progress in reducing treatment failure has also been made through combining different chemotherapy regimens and radiotherapy, and by providing better supportive care for the acute effects of therapy. Future directions include the search for better and less toxic agents,[176] development of better methods of controlling and delivering treatment, attempts to understand the causes of treatment failure, and efforts to address these causes with specific therapies.

# References

1. Boring CC, Squires TS, Tong T. Cancer statistics, 1993. *CA* 1993; **43**, 7–26.
2. Kung F. Hodgkin's disease in children 4 years of age or younger. *Cancer* 1991; 67, 1428–30.

3.  Schwartz RS, Callen JP, Silva J Jr. A cluster of Hodgkin's disease in a small community: evidence for environmental factors. *Am J Epidemiol* 1978; **108**, 19–25.
4.  Dörken H. Hodgkin's disease: an epidemiological study on 140 children — urban/rural relation, profession of parents, domestic animal contact. *Arch Geschwulstforsch* 1975; **45**, 283–98.
5.  Corbett S, O'Neill BJ. A cluster of cases of lymphoma in an underground colliery. *Med J Aust* 1988; **149**, 178–9, 181–2, 184–5.
6.  Alexander FE, Ricketts TJ, McKinney PA, *et al.* Community lifestyle characteristics and incidence of Hodgkin's disease in young people. *Int J Cancer* 1991; **48**, 10–14.
7.  Glaser SL. Cluster investigations: spatial clustering of Hodgkin's disease in the San Francisco Bay area. *Am J Epidemiol* 1990; **132** (Suppl 1), S167–77.
8.  Ross A, Davis S. Point pattern analysis of the spatial proximity of residences prior to diagnosis of persons with Hodgkin's disease. *Am J Epidemiol* 1990; **132** (Supp 1), S53–62.
9.  Abramson JH, Goldblum N, Avitzur M, *et al.* Clustering of Hodgkin's disease in Israel: a case–control study. *Int J Epidemiol* 1980; **9**, 137–44.
10. Hamadeh RR, Armenian HK, Zurayk HC. A study of clustering of cases of leukemia, Hodgkin's disease and other lymphomas in Bahrain. *Trop Geogr Med* 1981; **33**, 42–9.
11. Buehler SLK. The epidemiology of Hodgkin's disease in Newfoundland. *Diss Abstr Int (Sci)* 1983; **44**, 1792–B.
12. Mangoud A, Hillier VF, Leck I, *et al.* Space–time interaction in Hodgkin's disease in Greater Manchester. *J Epidemiol Community Health* 1985; **39**, 58–62.
13. Greenberg RS, Grufferman S, Cole P. An evaluation of space–time clustering in Hodgkin's disease. *J Chronic Dis* 1983; **36**, 257–62.
14. Gaffey MJ, Weiss LM. Viral oncogenesis: Epstein–Barr virus. *Am J Otolaryngol* 1990; **11**, 375–81.
15. Knecht H, Odermatt BF, Bachmann E, *et al.* Frequent detection of Epstein–Barr virus DNA by the polymerase chain reaction in lymph node biopsies from patients with Hodgkin's disease without genomic evidence of B- or T-cell clonality. *Blood* 1991; **78**, 760–7.
16. Pallesen G, Hamilton-Dutoit SJ, Rowe M, *et al.* Expression of Epstein–Barr virus latent gene products in tumour cells of Hodgkin's disease. *Lancet* 1991; **337**, 320–2.
17. Samoszuk M, Ravel J. Frequent detection of Epstein–Barr viral deoxyribonucleic acid and absence of cytomegalovirus deoxyribonucleic acid in Hodgkin's disease and acquired immunodeficiency syndrome-related Hodgkin's disease. *Lab Invest* 1991; **65**, 631–6.
18. Herbst H, Dallenbach F, Hummel M, *et al.* Epstein–Barr virus latent membrane protein expression in Hodgkin and Reed Sternberg cells. *Proc Natl Acad Sci USA* 1991; **88**, 4766–70.
19. Mueller N. An epidemiologist's view of the new molecular biology findings in Hodgkin's disease. *Ann Oncol* 1991; **2** (Suppl 2), 23–8.
20. Mauch P, Tarbell N, Weinstein H, *et al.* Stage IA and IIA supradiaphragmatic Hodgkin's disease: prognostic factors in surgically staged patients treated with mantle and para-aortic irradiation. *J Clin Oncol* 1988; **6**, 1576–83.
21. Jarrett RF, Gallagher A, Jones DB, *et al.* Detection of Epstein–Barr virus genomes in Hodgkin's disease: relation to age. *J Clin Pathol* 1991; **44**, 844–8.
22. Weiss LM. Epstein–Barr virus and Hodgkin's disease. A correlative in situ hybridization and polymerase chain reaction study. *Am J Pathol* 1991; **139**, 1259–65.
23. American Joint Committee on Cancer. *Manual for Staging of Cancer*, 3rd edn. Philadelphia: JB Lippincott, 1988; 255–7.

24. Desser RK, Golomb HM, Ultmann JE, *et al.* Prognostic classification of Hodgkin disease in pathologic stage III, based on anatomic considerations. *Blood* 1977; **49**, 883–93.

25. Rodgers RW, Fuller LM, Hagemeister FB, *et al.* Reassessment of prognostic factors in stage IIIA and IIIB Hodgkin's disease treated with MOPP and radiotherapy. *Cancer* 1981; **47**, 2196–203.

26. Mauch PM, Weinstein H, Botnick L, *et al.* An evaluation of long-term survival and treatment complications in children with Hodgkin's disease. *Cancer* 1983; **51**, 925–32.

27. Castellino RA, Hoppe RT, Blank N, *et al.* Computed tomography, lymphography, and staging laparotomy: correlations in initial staging of Hodgkin disease. *Am J Roentgenol* 1984; **143**, 37–41.

28. Jonsson K, Karp W, Landberg T, *et al.* Radiologic evaluation of subdiaphragmatic spread of Hodgkin's disease. *Acta Radiol Diag* 1983; **24**, 153–9.

29. Magnusson A, Hagberg H, Hemmingsson A, *et al.* Computed tomography, ultrasound and lymphography in the diagnosis of malignant lymphoma. *Acta Radiol Diag* 1982; **23**, 29–35.

30. Mansfield CM, Fabian C, Jones S, *et al.* Comparison of lymphangiography and computed tomography scanning in evaluating abdominal disease in stages III and IV Hodgkin's disease. A Southwest Oncology Group study. *Cancer* 1990; **66**, 2295–9.

31. Sombeck MD, Mendenhall NP, Kaude JV, *et al.* Correlation of lymphangiography, computed tomography, and laparotomy in the staging of Hodgkin's disease. *Int J Radiat Oncol Biol Phys* 1993; **25**, 425–9.

32. Mendenhall NP, Holland KW, Sombeck MD. The role of lymphangiography in designing fields for elective pelvic node irradiation in Hodgkin's disease. *Int J Radiat Oncol Biol Phys* 1994; **30**, 993–5.

33. Schneeberger AL, Girvan DP. Staging laparotomy for Hodgkin's disease in children. *J Pediatr Surg* 1988; **23**, 714–17.

34. Donaldson SS, Link MP. Combined modality treatment with low-dose radiation and MOPP chemotherapy for children with Hodgkin's disease. *J Clin Oncol* 1987; **5**, 742–9.

35. Mauch P, Larson D, Osteen R, *et al.* Prognostic factors for positive surgical staging in patients with Hodgkin's disease. *J Clin Oncol* 1990; **8**, 257–65.

36. Mendenhall NP, Cantor AB, Williams JL, *et al.* With modern imaging techniques, is staging laparotomy necessary in pediatric Hodgkin's disease? A Pediatric Oncology Group study. *J Clin Oncol* 1993; **11**, 2218–25.

37. Jockovich M, Mendenhall NP, Sombeck MD, *et al.* Long-term complications of laparotomy in Hodgkin's disease. *Int J Radiat Oncol Biol Phys* 1994; **219**, 615–24.

38. Desser RK, Ultmann JE. Risk of severe infection in patients with Hodgkin's disease or lymphoma after diagnostic laparotomy and splenectomy. *Ann Intern Med* 1972; **77**, 143–6.

39. Schimpff SC, O'Connell MJ, Greene WH, *et al.* Infections in 92 splenectomized patients with Hodgkin's disease. A clinical review. *Am J Med* 1975; **59**, 695–701.

40. Chilcote RR, Baehner RL, Hammond D. Investigators and Special Studies Committee of the Children's Cancer Study Group. Septicemia and meningitis in children splenectomized for Hodgkin's disease. *N Engl J Med* 1976; **295**, 798–800.

41. Donaldson SS, Kaplan HS. Complications of treatment of Hodgkin's disease in children. *Cancer Treat Rep* 1982; **66**, 977–89.

42. Hays DM, Ternberg JL, Chen TT, *et al.* Complications related to 234 staging laparotomies performed in the Intergroup Hodgkin's Disease in Childhood Study. *Surgery* 1984; **96**, 471–8.

43.  Cornbleet MA, Vitolo U, Ultmann JE, *et al.* Pathologic stages IA and IIA Hodgkin's disease: results of treatment with radiotherapy alone (1968–1980). *J Clin Oncol* 1985; **3**, 758–68.

44.  Baccarani M, Fiacchini M, Galieni P, *et al.* Meningitis and septicaemia in adults splenectomized for Hodgkin's disease. *Scand J Haematol* 1986; **36**, 492–8.

45.  Peters MV. Prophylactic treatment of adjacent areas in Hodgkin's disease. *Cancer Res* 1966; **26**, 1232–43.

46.  Kaplan HS. *Hodgkin's Disease*, 2nd edn, Cambridge, MA: Harvard University Press, 1980.

47.  Fletcher GH, Shukovsky LJ. The interplay of radiocurability and tolerance in the irradiation of human cancers. *J Radiol Electrol* 1975; **56**, 383–400.

48.  Hanks GE, Kinzie JJ, White RL, *et al.* Patterns of Care outcome studies. Results of the national practice in Hodgkin's disease. *Cancer* 1983; **51**, 569–73.

49.  Schewe KL, Reavis J, Kun LE, *et al.* Total dose, fraction size, and tumor volume in the local control of Hodgkin's disease. *Int J Radiat Oncol Biol Phys* 1988; **15**, 25–8.

50.  Thar TL, Million RR, Hausner RJ, *et al.* Hodgkin's disease, stages I and II. Relationship of recurrence to size of disease, radiation dose, and number of sites involved. *Cancer* 1979; **43**, 1101–5.

51.  Behrendt H, Van Bunningen BNFM, Van Leeuwen EF. Treatment of Hodgkin's disease in children with or without radiotherapy. *Cancer* 1987; **59**, 1870–3.

52.  Dionet C, Oberlin O, Habrand JL, *et al.* Initial chemotherapy and low-dose radiation in limited fields in childhood Hodgkin's disease: results of a joint cooperative study by the French Society of Pediatric Oncology (SFOP) and Hôpital Saint-Louis, Paris. *Int J Radiat Oncol Biol Phys* 1988; **15**, 341–6.

53.  Jenkin D, Chan H, Freedman M, *et al.* Hodgkin's disease in children: treatment results with MOPP and low-dose, extended-field irradiation. *Cancer Treat Rep* 1982; **66**, 949–59.

54.  Prosnitz LR, Cooper D, Cox EB, *et al.* Treatment selection for stage IIIA Hodgkin's disease patients. *Int J Radiat Oncol Biol Phys* 1985; **11**, 1431–7.

55.  Prosnitz LR, Farber LR, Kapp DS, *et al.* Combined modality therapy for advanced Hodgkin's disease: 15-year follow-up data. *J Clin Oncol* 1988; **6**, 603–12.

56.  Million RR. The lymphomatous diseases (Introduction; Hodgkin's disease; Non-Hodgkin's lymphoma). In: GH Fletcher, ed, *Textbook of Radiotherapy*, 2nd edn, Philadelphia: Lea & Febiger, 1973; 498–526.

57.  Mendenhall NP. Hodgkin's disease. In: JR Cassady, ed, *Radiation Therapy in Pediatric Oncology*. Berlin: Springer-Verlag, 1994; 151–74.

58.  DeVita VT Jr, Serpick A. Combination chemotherapy in the treatment of advanced Hodgkin's disease. *Proc Am Assoc Cancer Res* 1967; **8**, 13 (Abstract).

59.  DeVita VT Jr, Serpick AA, Carbone PP. Combination chemotherapy in the treatment of advanced Hodgkin's disease. *Ann Intern Med* 1970; **73**, 881–95.

60.  DeVita VT Jr, Simon RM, Hubbard SM, *et al.* Curability of advanced Hodgkin's disease with chemotherapy: long-term follow-up of MOPP-treated patients at the National Cancer Institute. *Ann Intern Med* 1980; **92**, 587–95.

61.  Bakemeier RT, Anderson JR, Costello W, *et al.* BCVPP chemotherapy for advanced Hodgkin's disease: evidence for greater duration of complete remission, greater survival, and less toxicity than with a MOPP regimen. Results of the Eastern Cooperative Oncology Group study. *Ann Intern Med* 1984; **101**, 447–56.

62.  Bonadonna G, Zucali R, Monfardini S, *et al.* Combination chemotherapy of Hodgkin's disease with Adriamycin, bleomycin, vinblastine, and imidazole carboxamide versus MOPP. *Cancer* 1975; **36**, 252–9.

63. Bonadonna G, Valagussa P, Santoro A. Alternating non-cross-resistant combination chemotherapy or MOPP in stage IV Hodgkin's disease. A report of 8-year results. *Ann Intern Med* 1986; **104**, 739–46.

64. Hancock BW, Vaughan Hudson G, Vaughan Hudson B, *et al*. British National Lymphoma Investigation randomized study of MOPP (mustine, Oncovin, procarbazine, prednisolone) against LOPP (Leukeran substituted for mustine) in advanced Hodgkin's disease — long term results. *Br J Cancer* 1991; **63**, 579–82.

65. Sutcliffe SB, Wrigley PFM, Stansfield AG, *et al*. Adriamycin, bleomycin, vinblastine and imidazole carboxymide (ABVD) therapy for advanced Hodgkin's disease resistant to mustine, vinblastine, procarbazine and prednisolone (MVPP). *Cancer Chemother Pharmacol* 1979; **2**, 209–13.

66. Harker WG, Kushian P, Rosenberg SA. Combination chemotherapy for advanced Hodgkin's disease after failure of MOPP, ABVD and B-CAVe. *Ann Intern Med* 1984; **101**, 440–6.

67. Papa G, Mandelli F, Anselmo AP, *et al*. Treatment of MOPP-resistant Hodgkin's disease with Adriamycin, bleomycin, vinblastine and dacarbazine (ABVD). *Eur J Cancer Clin Oncol* 1982; **18**, 803–6.

68. Piga A, Ambrosetti A, Todeschini G, *et al*. Doxorubicin, bleomycin, vinblastine and dacarbazine (ABVD) salvage of mechlorethamine, vincristine, prednisone, and procarbazine (MOPP)-resistant advanced Hodgkin's disease. *Cancer Treat Rep* 1984; **68**, 947–51.

69. Santoro A, Bonadonna G, Valagussa P, *et al*. Long-term results of combined chemotherapy–radiotherapy approach in Hodgkin's disease: superiority of ABVD plus radiotherapy versus MOPP plus radiotherapy. *J Clin Oncol* 1987; **5**, 27–37.

70. Canellos GP, Anderson JR, Propert KJ, *et al*. Chemotherapy of advanced Hodgkin's disease with MOPP, ABVD, or MOPP alternating with ABVD. *N Engl J Med* 1992; **327**, 1478–84.

71. Klimo P, Connors JM. An update on the Vancouver experience in the management of advanced Hodgkin's disease treated with the MOPP/ABV hybrid program. *Semin Hematol* 1988; **25** (2) (Suppl 2), 34–40.

72. Glick J, Tsiatis A, Schilsky R, *et al*. A randomized phase III trial of MOPP/ABV hybrid vs. sequential MOPP–ABVD in advanced Hodgkin's disease: preliminary results of the intergroup trial. *Proc Am Soc Clin Oncol* 1991; **10**, 271 (Abstract).

73. Mowat R, Lynch JW, Miller AM, *et al*. A pilot study of continuous infusion etoposide and bolus cyclophosphamide with autologous bone marrow transplantation for relapsed lymphoma. (Unpublished).

74. Cimino G, Biti GP, Anselmo AP, et al. MOPP chemotherapy versus extended-field radiotherapy in the management of pathological stages I–IIA Hodgkin's disease. *J Clin Oncol* 1989; 7, 732–7.

75. Biti GP, Cimino G, Cartoni C, *et al*. Extended-field radiotherapy is superior to MOPP chemotherapy for the treatment of pathologic stage I–IIA Hodgkin's disease: eight year update on an Italian prospective randomized study. *J Clin Oncol* 1992; **10**, 378–82.

76. Lee CKK, Aeppli DM, Bloomfield CD, *et al*. Hodgkin's disease: a reassessment of prognostic factors following modification of radiotherapy. *Int J Radiat Oncol Biol Phys* 1987; **13**, 983–91.

77. Farah R, Ultmann J, Griem M, *et al*. Extended mantle radiation therapy for pathologic stage I and II Hodgkin's disease. *J Clin Oncol* 1988; **6**, 1047–52.

78. Zagars G, Rubin P. Laparotomy-staged IA versus IIA Hodgkin's disease: a comparative study with evaluation of prognostic factors for stage IIA disease. *Cancer* 1985; **56**, 864–73.

79. Mauch P, Tarbell N, Weinstein H, *et al*. Stage IA and IIA supradiaphragmatic

Hodgkin's disease: prognostic factors in surgically staged patients treated with mantle and paraaortic irradiation. *J Clin Oncol* 1988; **6**, 1576–83.

80. Hoppe RT, Coleman CN, Cox RS, *et al*. The management of stage I–II Hodgkin's disease with irradiation alone or combined modality therapy: the Stanford experience. *Blood* 1982; **59**, 455–65.

81. Mendenhall NP, Cantor AB, Barré DM, *et al* The role of prognostic factors in treatment selection for early-stage Hodgkin's disease. *Am J Clin Oncol* 1994; **17**, 189–95.

82. Ganesan TS, Wrigley PFM, Murray PA, *et al*. Radiotherapy for stage I Hodgkin's disease: 20 years experience at St. Bartholomew's Hospital. *Br J Cancer* 1990; **62**, 314–18.

83. Henry-Amar M, Friedman S, Hayat M, *et al*. Erythrocyte sedimentation rate predicts early relapse and survival in early-stage Hodgkin disease. *Ann Intern Med* 1991; **114**, 361–5.

84. Schomberg PJ, Evans RG, O'Connell MJ, *et al*. Prognostic significance of mediastinal mass in adult Hodgkin's disease. *Cancer* 1984; **53**, 324–8.

85. Specht L, Nordentoft AM, Cold S, *et al*. Tumor burden as the most important prognostic factor in early stage Hodgkin's disease. Relations to other prognostic factors and implications for choice of treatment. *Cancer* 1988; **61**, 1719–27.

86. Tubiana M, Henry-Amar M, van der Werf-Messing B, *et al*. A multivariate analysis of prognostic factors in early stage Hodgkin's disease. *Int J Radiat Oncol Biol Phys* 1985; **11**, 23–30.

87. Longo DL, Glatstein E, Duffey PL, *et al*. Radiation therapy versus combination chemotherapy in the treatment of early-stage Hodgkin's disease: seven-year results of a prospective randomized trial. *J Clin Oncol* 1991; **9**, 906–17.

88. Behar RA, Hoppe RT. Radiation therapy in the management of bulky mediastinal Hodgkin's disease. *Cancer* 1990; **66**, 75–9.

89. Levitt SH, Lee CKK. Dilemmas and decisions. *Int J Radiat Oncol Biol Phys* 1990; **18**, 485–8.

90. Lee CKK, Bloomfield CD, Levitt SH. Liver irradiation in stage IIIA Hodgkin's disease patients with splenic involvement. *Am J Clin Oncol* 1984; **7**, 149–57.

91. Hoppe RT, Rosenberg SA, Kaplan HS, *et al*. Prognostic factors in pathological stage IIIA Hodgkin's disease. *Cancer* 1980; **46**, 1240–6.

92. Mauch P, Goffman T, Rosenthal DS, *et al*. Stage III Hodgkin's disease: improved survival with combined modality therapy as compared with radiation therapy alone. *J Clin Oncol* 1985; **3**, 1166–73.

93. Hagemeister FB, Fuller LM, Velasquez WS, *et al*. Two cycles of MOPP and radiotherapy: effective treatment for stage IIIA and IIIB Hodgkin's disease. *Ann Oncol* 1991; **2**, 25–31.

94. Grozea PN, DePersio EJ, Coltman CA, *et al*. Chemotherapy alone versus combined modality therapy for stage III Hodgkin's disease: a five-year follow-up of a Southwest Oncology Group study (SWOG-7518) USA. In: F Cavalli, G Bonadonna, M Rozencweig, eds, *Malignant Lymphomas and Hodgkin's Disease: Experimental and Therapeutic Advances*, Proceedings of the Second International Conference on Malignant Lymphomas, Lugano, Switzerland, 13–16 June 1984. Boston, MA: Martinus Nijhoff Publishing, 1985; 345–61.

95. Ferme C, Teiller F, D'Agay MF, *et al*. Surgical restaging after 3 to 6 courses of MOPP chemotherapy in Hodgkin's disease. In: F Cavalli, G Bonadonna, M Rozencweig, eds, *Malignant Lymphomas and Hodgkin's Disease: Experimental and Therapeutic Advances*, Proceedings of the Second International Conference on Malignant Lymphomas, Lugano, Switzerland, 13–16 June 1984. Boston, MA: Martinus Nijhoff Publishing, 1985; 363–9.

96. Fuller LM, Hagemeister FB, North LC, *et al*. The adjuvant role of two cycles of MOPP and low-dose lung irradiation in stage IA through IIB Hodgkin's

disease: preliminary results. *Int J Radiat Oncol Biol Phys* 1988; **14**, 683–92.

97.  Valagussa P, Santoro A, Boracchi P, *et al.* 9-year results of two randomized studies with MOPP and ABVD in Hodgkin's disease (HD): multiple regression analysis. *Proc Am Soc Clin Oncol* 1989; **8**, 250.

98.  Glick J, Tsiatis A, Chen M, *et al.* Improved survival with MOPP–ABVD compared to BCVPP ± radiotherapy (RT) for advanced Hodgkin's disease: 6-year ECOG results. *Blood* 1990; **76**, 350a.

99.  Koza I, Bohunicky L, Mocikova K, *et al.* Comparison of two non-cross-resistant combinations (ABVD/LOPP) with COPP plus bleomycin in the treatment of advanced Hodgkin's disease. *Neoplasma* 1991; **38**, 583–93.

100. Radford J, Ganesan T, Crowther D, *et al.* MVPP versus a 7 drug hybrid regimen for Hodgkin's disease (HD): initial results of a randomized trial at two specialist centres. *Br J Cancer* 1991; **63**(9) Abstract 12.

101. Frei E III, Luce JK, Gamble JF, *et al.* Combination chemotherapy in advanced Hodgkin's disease: induction and maintenance of remission. *Ann Intern Med* 1973; **79**, 376–82.

102. Jones SE, Coltman CA Jr, Grozea PN, *et al.* Conclusions from clinical trials of the Southwest Oncology Group. *Cancer Treat Rep* 1982; **66**, 847–53.

103. Brizel DM, Winer EP, Prosnitz LR, *et al.* Improved survival in advanced Hodgkin's disease with the use of combined modality therapy. *Int J Radiat Oncol Biol Phys* 1990; **19**, 535–42.

104. Bonadonna G, Valagussa P, Santoro A. Prognosis of bulky Hodgkin's disease treated with chemotherapy alone or combined with radiotherapy. *Cancer Surv* 1985; **4**, 439–58.

105. Longo DL, Young RC, Wesley M, *et al.* Twenty years of MOPP therapy for Hodgkin's disease. *J Clin Oncol* 1986; **4**, 1295–306.

106. Longo DL, Russo A, Duffey PL, *et al.* Treatment of advanced-stage massive mediastinal Hodgkin's disease: the case for combined modality treatment. *J Clin Oncol* 1991; **9**, 227–35.

107. Bennett CJ Jr, Mendenhall NP, Lynch JW Jr. Is combined modality therapy necessary for advanced Hodgkin's disease? *Int J Radiat Oncol Biol Phys* (in press).

108. Rosenberg SA, Kaplan HS. The evolution and summary results of the Stanford randomized clinical trials of the management of Hodgkin's disease: 1962–1984. *Int J Radiat Oncol Biol Phys* 1985; **11**, 5–22.

109. Fabian C, Mansfield CM, Dahlberg S, *et al.* Low-dose involved field radiation after chemotherapy in advanced Hodgkin disease: a Southwest Oncology Group randomized study. *Ann Intern Med* 1994; **120**, 903–12.

110. Mauch P, Ryback ME, Rosenthal D, *et al.* The influence of initial pathologic stage on the survival of patients who relapse from Hodgkin's disease. *Blood* 1980; **56**, 892–7.

111. Roach M III, Brophy N, Cox R, *et al.* Prognostic factors for patients relapsing after radiotherapy for early-stage Hodgkin's disease. *J Clin Oncol* 1990; **8**, 623–9.

112. Vinciguerra V, Propert KJ, Coleman M, *et al.* Alternating cycles of combination chemotherapy for patients with recurrent Hodgkin's disease following radiotherapy. A prospectively randomized study by the Cancer and Leukemia Group B. *J Clin Oncol* 1986; **4**, 838–46.

113. Mendenhall NP, Taylor BW Jr, Marcus RB Jr, *et al.* The impact of pelvic recurrence and elective pelvic irradiation on survival and treatment morbidity in early-stage Hodgkin's disease. *Int J Radiat Oncol Biol Phys* 1991; **21**, 1157–65.

114. Santoro A, Viviani S, Villarreal CJ, *et al.* Salvage chemotherapy in Hodgkin's disease irradiation failures: superiority of doxorubicin-containing regimens over MOPP. *Cancer Treat Rep* 1986; **70**, 343–8.

115. Cooper MR, Pajak TF, Gottlieb AJ, et al. The effects of prior radiation therapy and age on the frequency and duration of complete remission among various four-drug treatments for advanced Hodgkin's disease. *J Clin Oncol* 1984; **2**, 748–55.

116. Brusamolino E, Castelli G, Pagnucco G, et al. CAV chemotherapy (CCNU, melphalan, etoposide) as salvage treatment for relapsing or resistant Hodgkin's disease. *Hematology* 1990; **75**, 340–5.

117. Fisher RI, DeVita VT, Hubbard SP, et al. Prolonged disease-free survival in Hodgkin's disease with MOPP reinduction after first relapse. *Ann Intern Med* 1979; **90**, 761–3.

118. Harker WG, Kushlan P, Rosenberg SA. Combination chemotherapy for advanced Hodgkin's disease after failure of MOPP: ABVD and B-CAVe. *Ann Intern Med* 1984; **101**, 440–6.

119. Perren TJ, Selby PJ, Milan S, et al. Etoposide and Adriamycin containing combination chemotherapy (HOPE-Bleo) for relapsed Hodgkin's disease. *Br J Cancer* 1990; **61**, 919–23.

120. Santoro A, Bonfante V, Bonadonna G. Salvage chemotherapy with ABVD in MOPP-resistant Hodgkin's disease. *Ann Intern Med* 1982; **96**, 139–43.

121. Tannir N, Hagemeister F, Velasquez W, et al. Long-term follow-up with ABDIC salvage chemotherapy of MOPP-resistant Hodgkin's disease. *J Clin Oncol* 1983; **1**, 432–9.

122. Longo DL, Duffey PL, Young RC, et al. Conventional-dose salvage combination chemotherapy in patients relapsing with Hodgkin's disease after combination chemotherapy. *J Clin Oncol* 1992; **10**, 210–18.

123. Fox KA, Lippman SM, Cassady JR, et al. Radiation therapy salvage of Hodgkin's disease following chemotherapy failure. *J Clin Oncol* 1987; **5**, 38–45.

124. Mauch P, Tarbell N, Skarin A, et al. Wide-field radiation therapy alone or with chemotherapy for Hodgkin's disease in relapse from combination chemotherapy. *J Clin Oncol* 1987; **5**, 544–9.

125. Roach M III, Kapp DS, Rosenberg SA, et al. Radiotherapy with curative intent: an option in selected patients relapsing after chemotherapy for advanced Hodgkin's disease. *J Clin Oncol* 1987; **5**, 550–5.

126. Hagemeister FB, Tannir N, McLaughlin P, et al. MIME chemotherapy (methyl-GAG, ifosfamide, methotrexate, etoposide) as treatment for recurrent Hodgkin's disease. *J Clin Oncol* 1987; **5**, 556–61.

127. Ryback ME, McCarroll K, Kaplan RJ, et al. Phase II trial of etoposide and cis-diaminodichloro-platinum in patients with refractory and relapsed Hodgkin's disease: Cancer and Leukemia Group B (CALGB) study 8353. *Med Pediatr Oncol* 1990; **18**, 177–80.

128. Santoro A, Viviani S, Bonfante V, et al. CEP in Hodgkin's disease (HD) resistant to MOPP and ABVD. *Proc Am Soc Clin Oncol* 1987; **6**, 199.

129. Schulman P, McCarroll K, Cooper MR, et al. Phase II study of MOPLACE chemotherapy for patients with previously treated Hodgkin's disease: a CALGB study. *Med Pediatr Oncol* 1990; **18**, 482–6.

130. Tseng A Jr, Jacobs C, Coleman CN, et al. Third-line chemotherapy for resistant Hodgkin's disease with lomustine, etoposide, and methotrexate. *Cancer Treat Rep* 1987; **71**, 475–8.

131. Ahmed T. Autologous marrow transplantation for Hodgkin's disease. Current techniques and prospects. *Cancer Invest* 1990; **8**, 99–106.

132. Armitage JO, Barnett MJ, Carella AM, et al. Bone marrow transplantation in the treatment of Hodgkin's lymphoma: problems, remaining challenges, and future prospects. *Recent Results Cancer Res* 1989; **117**, 246–53.

133. Buzaid AC, Lippman SM, Miller TP. Salvage therapy of advanced Hodgkin's disease. Critical appraisal of curative potential [published erratum appears in *Am J Med* 1987; **83** (6): All]. *Am J Med* 1987; **83**, 523–32.

134. Canellos GP, Nadler L, Takvorian T. Autologous bone marrow transplantation in the treatment of malignant lymphoma and Hodgkin's disease. *Semin Hematol* 1988; **25**(2) (Suppl 2), 58–65.
135. Williams SF, Bitran JD. The role of high-dose therapy and autologous bone marrow reinfusion in the treatment of Hodgkin's disease. *Hematol Oncol Clin North Am* 1989; **3**, 319–30.
136. Vose JM, Bierman PJ, Armitage JO. Hodgkin's disease: the role of bone marrow transplantation. *Semin Oncol* 1990; **6**, 749–57.
137. Broun ER, Tricot G, Akard L, *et al*. Treatment of refractory lymphoma with high dose cytarabine cyclophosphamide and with either TBI or VP-16 followed by autologous bone marrow transplantation. *Bone Marrow Transplant* 1990; **5**, 341–4.
138. Carella AM, Congiu AM, Gaozza E, *et al*. High-dose chemotherapy with autologous bone marrow transplantation in 50 advanced resistant Hodgkin's disease patients: an Italian Study Group report. *J Clin Oncol* 1988; **6**, 1411–16.
139. Gribben JG, Linch DC, Singer CRJ, *et al*. Successful treatment of refractory Hodgkin's disease by high-dose combination chemotherapy and autologous bone marrow transplantation. *Blood* 1989; **73**, 340–4.
140. Hurd DD, Haake RJ, Lasky LC. Treatment of refractory and relapsed Hodgkin's disease: intensive chemotherapy and autologous bone marrow or peripheral blood stem cell support. *Med Pediatr Oncol* 1990; **18**, 447–53.
141. Jones RJ, Piantodosi S, Mann RB, *et al*. High-dose cytotoxic therapy and bone marrow transplantation for relapsed Hodgkin's disease. *J Clin Oncol* 1990; **8**, 527–37.
142. Kessinger A, Bierman PJ, Vose JM, *et al*. High-dose cyclophosphamide, carmustine, and etoposide followed by autologous peripheral stem cell transplantation for patients with relapsed Hodgkin's disease. *Blood* 1991; **77**, 2322–5.
143. Phillips GL, Wolff SN, Herzig RH. Treatment of progressive Hodgkin's disease with intensive chemotherapy and autologous bone marrow transplantation. *Blood* 1989; **73**, 2086–92.
144. Spinolo JA, Jagannath S, Dicke KA, *et al*. High-dose combination chemotherapy with cyclophosphamide, carmustine, etoposide, and autologous bone marrow transplantation in 60 patients with relapsed Hodgkin's disease: the M.D. Anderson experience. *Recent Results Cancer Res* 1989; **117**, 233–8.
145. Yahalom J, Gulati S. Autologous bone marrow transplantation for refractory or relapsed Hodgkin's disease: the Memorial Sloan-Kettering Cancer Center experience using high-dose chemotherapy with or without hyperfractionated accelerated total lymphoid irradiation. *Ann Oncol* 1991; **2** (Suppl 2), 67–71.
146. Vriesendorp HM, Herpst JM, Leichner PK, *et al*. Polyclonal $^{90}$yttrium labeled antiferritin for refractory Hodgkin's disease. *Int J Radiat Oncol Biol Phys* 1989; **17**, 815–21.
147. Lenhard RE Jr, Order SE, Spunberg JJ, *et al*. Isotopic immunoglobulin: a new systematic therapy for advanced Hodgkin's disease. *J Clin Oncol* 1985; **3**, 1296–300.
148. Holt JA. Alternative therapy for recurrent Hodgkin's disease: radiotherapy combined with hyperthermia by electromagnetic radiation to create complete remission in 11 patients without morbidity. *Br J Radiol* 1980; **53** (635), 1061–7.
149. Rybak ME, McCarroll K, Bernard S, *et al*. Interferon therapy of relapsed and refractory Hodgkin's disease: Cancer and Leukemia Group B study 8652. *J Biol Response Mod* 1990; **9**, 1–4.
150. Hancock SL, Cox RS, McDougall IR. Thyroid diseases after treatment of Hodgkin's disease. *N Engl J Med* 1991; **325**, 599–605.
151. Tarbell NJ, Thompson L, Mauch P. Thoracic irradiation in Hodgkin's disease:

disease control and long-term complications. *Int J Radiat Oncol Biol Phys* 1990; **18**, 275–81.

152. Carmel RJ, Kaplan HS. Mantle irradiation in Hodgkin's disease: an analysis of technique, tumor eradication, and complications. *Cancer* 1976; **37**, 2813–25.
153. Thar TL, Million RR. Complications of radiation treatment of Hodgkin's disease. *Semin Oncol* 1980; **7**, 174–83.
154. Smith LM, Mendenhall NP, Cicale MJ, *et al.* Results of a prospective study evaluating the effects of mantle irradiation on pulmonary function. *Int J Radiat Oncol Biol Phys* 1989; **16**, 79–84.
155. Green DM, Gingell RL, Pearce J, *et al.* The effect of mediastinal irradiation on cardiac function of patients treated during childhood and adolescence for Hodgkin's disease. *J Clin Oncol* 1987; **5**, 239–45.
156. Mefferd JM, Donaldson SS, Link MP. Pediatric Hodgkin's disease: pulmonary, cardiac, and thyroid function following combined modality therapy. *Int J Radiat Oncol Biol Phys* 1989; **16**, 679–85.
157. Cosset JM, Henry-Amar M, Girinski T, *et al.* Late toxicity of radiotherapy in Hodgkin's disease. The role of fraction size. *Acta Oncol* 1988; **27**, 123–9.
158. Cosset JM, Henry-Amar M, Pellae-Cosset B, *et al.* Pericarditis and myocardial infarctions after Hodgkin's disease therapy. *Int J Radiat Oncol Biol Phys* 1991; **21**, 447–9.
159. Coia LR, Hanks GE. Complications from large field intermediate dose infradiaphragmatic radiation: an analysis of the Patterns of Care outcome studies for Hodgkin's disease and seminoma. *Int J Radiat Oncol Biol Phys* 1988; **15**, 29–35.
160. Ortin TTS, Shostak CA, Donaldson SS. Gonadal status and reproductive function following treatment for Hodgkin's disease in childhood: the Stanford experience. *Int J Radiat Oncol Biol Phys* 1990; **19**, 873–80.
161. Williams RS, Mendenhall NP. Laparoscopic oophoropexy for preservation of ovarian function before pelvic node irradiation. *Obstet Gynecol* 1992; **80**, 541–3.
162. Brämswig JH, Heimes U, Heiermann E, *et al.* Postpubertal gonadal function in 138 patients treated for Hodgkin's disease (HD) during childhood and adolescence. *Proc Am Soc Clin Oncol* 1989; **8**, 279 (Abstract 1088).
163. Meadows AT, Obringer AC, Marrero O, *et al.* Second malignant neoplasms following childhood Hodgkin's disease: treatment and splenectomy as risk factors. *Med Pediatr Oncol* 1989; **17**, 477–84.
164. Lipschultz SE, Colan SD, Gelber RD, *et al.* Late cardiac effects of doxorubicin therapy for acute lymphoblastic leukemia in childhood. *N Engl J Med* 1991; **324**, 808–15.
165. Andrieu JM, Ifrah N, Payen C, *et al.* Increased risk of secondary acute non-lymphocytic leukemia after extended-field radiation therapy combined with MOPP chemotherapy for Hodgkin's disease. *J Clin Oncol* 1990; **8**, 1148–59.
166. Baccarani M, Bosi A, Papa G. Second malignancy in patients treated for Hodgkin's disease. *Cancer* 1980; **46**, 1735–40.
167. Boivin JF, Hutchison GB. Leukemia and other cancers after radiotherapy and chemotherapy for Hodgkin's disease. *J Natl Cancer Inst* 1981; **67**, 751–60.
168. Coleman CN. Secondary neoplasms in patients treated for cancer: etiology and perspective. *Radiat Res* 1982; **92**, 188–200.
169. Coltman CA Jr, Dixon DO. Second malignancies complicating Hodgkin's disease: a Southwest Oncology Group 10-year followup. *Cancer Treat Rep* 1982; **66**, 1023–33.
170. Glicksman AS, Pajak TF, Gottlieb A, *et al.* Second malignant neoplasms in patients successfully treated for Hodgkin's disease: a Cancer and Leukemia Group B study. *Cancer Treat Rep* 1982; **66**, 1035–44.
171. Henry-Amar M, Pellae-Cosset B, Bayle-Weisgerber C, *et al.* Risk of secondary acute leukemia and preleukemia after Hodgkin's disease: the Institut Gustave-

Roussy experience. *Recent Results Cancer Res* 1989; **117**, 270–83.

172. Pedersen-Bjergaard J. Incidence of acute nonlymphocytic leukemia, preleukemia, and acute myeloproliferative syndrome up to 10 years after treatment of Hodgkin's disease. *N Engl J Med* 1982; **307**, 965–71.

173. Kaldor JM, Day NE, Clarke EA, *et al.* Leukemia following Hodgkin's disease. *N Engl J Med* 1990; **322**, 7–13.

174. Mendenhall NP, Shuster JJ, Million RR. The impact of stage and treatment modality on the likelihood of second malignancies and hematopoietic disorders in Hodgkin's disease. *Radiother Oncol* 1989; **14**, 219–29.

175. Da Cunha MF, Meistrich ML, Fuller LM, *et al.* Recovery of spermatogenesis after treatment for Hodgkin's disease: limiting dose of MOPP chemotherapy. *J Clin Oncol* 1984; **2**, 571–7.

176. Horning SJ, Hoppe RT, Hancock SL, *et al.* Vinblastine, bleomycin, and methotrexate: an effective adjuvant in favorable Hodgkin's disease. *J Clin Oncol* 1988; **6**, 1822–31.

# 12 Clinical strategies for adult non-Hodgkin's lymphoma

*James D Bridges and Eli Glatstein*

## Introduction

The non-Hodgkin's lymphomas (NHL) are a heterogeneous group of malignant neoplasms arising primarily in lymph nodes but with cases having been reported in almost all organ systems. The most commonly reported sites of presentation outside lymph nodes include the gastrointestinal tract, Waldeyer's ring, orbit, brain, thyroid gland, paranasal sinuses, testes, oral cavity and bone.[1]

Treatment of NHL is extremely diverse and driven mainly by the fact that the natural history and response to therapy vary with the specific histopathological subtype and extent of disease. Although certain treatment approaches have gained relatively wide acceptance, such as use of radiation therapy in the treatment of early-stage low-grade lymphomas and chemotherapy in advanced-stage intermediate- and high-grade lymphomas, many controversies continue to exist. Such controversial areas include the role of chemotherapy in the early-stage low-grade lymphomas, the role of radiation therapy as an adjuvant to chemotherapy in early-stage intermediate-grade lymphomas, aggressive versus watch-and-wait therapy in advanced-stage low-grade lymphomas, and the role of bone marrow transplant in NHL.

## Epidemiology

In the United States, NHL represents the sixth most commonly diagnosed malignancy and the sixth most common cause of cancer death. It is estimated by the American Cancer Society (ACS) that, in 1995, 50 900 new cases of NHL will be diagnosed and 22 700 deaths will be attributed to NHL. This represents almost 4% of the newly diagnosed invasive cancers in the United States, excluding basal and squamous cell skin cancer and in-situ bladder cancer.[2] The median age at diagnosis of adult onset disease is reported in most series to be between 50 and 65 years of age, with a male to female predominance of approximately 1.3:1. Over the last decade there has been an increase in the incidence of NHL with the major but not total component of the increase being secondary to the human immunodeficiency virus (HIV) epidemic.[3]

# Natural history

Although the prognosis of patients with NHL varies significantly with the specific histological subtypes and extent of disease, some generalizations can be made. Many authors make comparisons with Hodgkin's disease when addressing the natural history. Specifically, as a group, NHL have a remarkable propensity to spread beyond the lymphatic system with increased instances noted in Waldeyer's ring, gastrointestinal tract, bone marrow and central nervous system (CNS). Patients with NHL tend to be several decades older than those with Hodgkin's but, in contrast, are less likely to have systemic symptoms (B symptoms) (10–15% versus 30–35%). While the majority of patients with Hodgkin's present with localized disease (60–70% Stage I and II), the large majority of patients with NHL present with more advanced disease (Stage III and IV). In patients with nodular histology, less than 20% will present with pathological Stage I and II disease, whereas in the diffuse histology 30–50% will present with early-stage disease, 5–15% of those presenting with Stage I disease.[4-7] Even though a large portion of patients present with advanced-stage disease, median survival is still relatively long — measured in excess of 5–7 years.[8] Specifically, low-grade follicular lymphomas can have a very indolent course with many years of waxing and waning adenopathy, and, in some cases, long-term spontaneous remissions have been reported.[9,10] In contrast, the diffuse/aggressive/high-grade lymphomas, when diagnosed in advanced stages with extranodal organ involvement, demonstrate an aggressive and rapidly fatal clinical course without medical intervention.

# Diagnostic work-up

The pretreatment evaluation of patients with NHL is listed in Table 12.1. Areas of controversy still include the need for lymphangiogram, the role of gallium scanning and the need for staging laparotomy. Lymphangiogram in practical terms is becoming less widely used because of its labour intensiveness and the growing lack of trained radiologists experienced in its interpretation. Although CT (computed tomography) is better at assessing upper abdominal/mesenteric disease, the lymphangiogram remains the most sensitive test for evaluating retroperitoneal lymph node involvement. The only

**Table 12.1**   Recommended evaluation for non-Hodgkin's lymphoma

---

*Required*
Biopsy with haematopathologist review
History with exploration of 'B' symptoms (fever, night sweats, weight loss)
Physical examination with particular interest to node bearing regions,
  Waldeyer's ring/nasopharynx/oral cavity (laryngoscopy recommended)
Bilateral iliac crest bone marrow biopsies
Radiological studies to include:
 PA/LAT chest X-ray
 CT scan of abdomen and pelvis
 Bipedal lymphangiogram if CT scan of abdomen is negative
Laboratory studies to include CBC, ESR, BUN, creatinine, uric acid, UA,
  liver function to include LDH, serum alkaline phosphatase

*Required/indicated in certain situations*
Aspiration and cytology of existing effusions
Staging laparotomy if results would alter therapy/outcome
Bone scan if bone pain present with negative plain X-rays
Upper GI series with small bowel follow-through if clinically indicated
  (Waldeyer's ring involvement)
CT scan of brain with neurological symptoms
CT scan of chest and neck, if involved
Pretreatment T3, T4, TSH if neck radiation to be used

*Optional/complementary*
Gallium scan
Percutaneous/peritoneoscopy directed liver biopsy

---

PA/LAT: posteroanterior and lateral chest X-ray; CBC: complete blood count; ESR: erythrocyte sedimentation rate; BUN: blood urea nitrogen; UA: urinalysis; LDH: lactate dehydrogenase; TSH: thyroid-stimulating hormone.

criterion of abnormality for CT is size; the lymphangiogram also gives important information on nodal architecture itself. We feel that the abdominal CT scan should be conducted first, and if identification of periaortic nodal involvement would alter the course of treatment the lymphangiogram should then be done.

The gallium scan is positive in a large percentage of NHL patients, depending on the histological subtype. However, due to the low specificity there is a question as to whether this study should be done as part of the initial staging work-up. The gallium scan is best used to follow patients who originally have an uptaking tumour to assess for residual or recurrent disease. Some authors recommend the use of the gallium scan in intermediate/high-grade histologies with a bulky tumour mass, where the potential for a residual mass after chemotherapy might be expected.[11,12] Such patients who continue to have gallium-positive masses after chemotherapy have a poor prognosis and should then be considered for consolidation radiation therapy or other experimental therapies.[13] Personally, we do not routinely recommend gallium scanning because of the high rate of false positive and false negative interpretations.

The staging laparotomy, although still widely used in Hodgkin's disease, is much less used in NHL. The reasons for its less frequent use include the following:

1. the patient population is older, resulting in increased morbidity with staging laparotomy;
2. a high percentage of patients are found to have advanced-stage disease by less invasive procedures, and findings of the staging laparotomy would therefore not alter therapy (which usually involves chemotherapy or a watch-and-wait approach);
3. clinical Stage I and II indolent lymphoma patients who are treated with involved-field radiation therapy are treated with at least a 30% chance of occult disease in the abdomen. However, treating these clinically staged I and II indolent lymphoma patients with involved-field or extended-field radiation results in minimal long-term toxicity and a chance for cure in some. In addition, even if they had been upstaged by laparotomy to Stage III or IV, a watch-and-wait approach with palliative radiation to involved sites can be considered appropriate therapy.

# Staging

The Ann Arbor Staging System (Table 12.2) used for Hodgkin's disease is also the most widely used staging system used for adult-onset non-Hodgkin's lymphoma. A modification to the Ann Arbor Staging System[14] has been proposed and includes the use of a subscript 'x' to denote bulky disease, which is defined as the following:

1. nodal mass greater than 10 cm in the abdomen; or
2. a mass in the chest with a width greater than one-third the thoracic width at the T5–T6 interspace measured on an upright posteroanterior (PA) chest X-ray.

**Table 12.2**  Ann Arbor staging classification[a]

| | |
|---|---|
| Stage I | Involvement of a single lymph node region (I) or a single extra-lymphatic organ or site ($I_E$) |
| Stage II | Involvement of two or more lymph node regions on the same side of the diaphragm (II) or localized involvement of an extralymphatic organ or site and one or more lymph node regions on the same side of the diaphragm ($II_E$) |
| Stage III | Involvement of lymph node regions on both sides of the diaphragm (III), which may also be accompanied by involvement of the spleen ($III_S$) or by localized involvement of an extralymphatic organ or site ($III_E$), or both ($III_{SE}$) |
| Stage IV | Diffuse or disseminated involvement of one or more extralymphatic organs or tissues, with or without associated lymph node involvement |

[a]The absence or presence of fever, night sweats, or loss of 10% or more body weight is denoted in all cases by the suffix A or B, respectively.

In addition, a Stage III$_1$ was proposed to denote involvement of porta hepatic, coeliac and splenic disease as minimal Stage III disease. Because of the heterogeneous nature of NHL, the staging system is not as prognostically accurate as in Hodgkin's disease. In the NHL there is little long-term survival difference between Stage II, III, IV of nodular histology and little difference in overall survival between Stage III and IV diffuse histologies.

# Pathological classification

Almost no other aspect of NHL has had as much controversy or different viewpoints as have the histological classification systems. At least six different systems have been used throughout the world, each with its own particular problem areas. The Working Formulation (Table 12.3) described in 1982 now serves as a translator between the other six major classification systems.[15] It compares and equates the different systems based on morphology, clinical features, and prognosis. Just as no other system has been an end-all answer, it also contains problems as well as omissions of histological subtypes that have been identified since its inception. Although excellent (95% probability) at differentiating the indolent patterns (one of

**Table 12.3**    Working formulation of non-Hodgkin's lymphoma

*Low grade*
A    Small lymphocytic
        Consistent with chronic lymphocytic leukaemia

B    Follicular, predominantly small cleaved cell
        Diffuse areas, sclerosis

C    Follicular mixed, small cleaved and large cell
        Diffuse areas, sclerosis

*Intermediate grade*
D    Follicular, predominantly large cell
        Diffuse areas, sclerosis

E    Diffuse small cleaved cell

F    Diffuse mixed, small and large cell
        Sclerosis, epithelioid cell component

G    Diffuse large cell
        Cleaved, non-cleaved, sclerosis

*High grade*
H    Large cell, immunoblastic
        Plasmacytoid, clear cell, polymorphous, epithelioid cell component

I    Lymphoblastic lymphoma
        Convoluted cell, non-convoluted cell

J    Malignant lymphoma small non-cleaved cell
        Burkitt's lymphoma, follicular areas

the major prognostic factors in predicting natural history and planning treatment), several studies have shown considerable variation in the reproducibility of the histological subtypes between different pathologists and the same pathologist evaluating the slides on separate occasions.[16,17]

Even with its limitations, the Working Formulation offers a system which can be used as a common language, particularly among oncologists and pathologists who are not yet engendered to one of the other classification systems. Its use can facilitate interpretation of clinical results and clinical trials by using a commonly accepted terminology. It is therefore the system (with minor modifications) that will be used throughout the remainder of this chapter.

# Treatment of non-Hodgkin's lymphoma

The treatment of NHL is influenced primarily by the histological classification, the stage of disease at presentation and the associated natural history. Various authors have described modifications to the Working Formulation in order to arrange more accurately histological subtypes into groups to which common treatment approaches can be applied. Some authors have directly used the groupings of the Working Formulation (low, intermediate, and high grade); others have divided them into indolent, aggressive, and highly aggressive groups while still others have used a more simplistic approach of favourable and unfavourable groupings.[18-21] Based on current treatment practices, it appears most consistent to group NHL into three groups based on both the untreated natural history and the currently accepted treatment practices and observed responses of the specific histological subtypes.

This approach (with minor modification), described by authors from the US National Cancer Institute (NCI)[21] and shown in Table 12.4, is a modification of the Working Formulation with the addition of diffuse intermediately differentiated lymphoma (mantle zone or DIDL) and diffuse small cleaved (DSC) cell lymphoma to the low-grade or indolent group, the addition of immunoblastic lymphoma (IBL) to the intermediate or aggressive group, and the addition of adult T-cell leukaemia–lymphoma to the high-grade or highly aggressive group. Further discussion of therapy in this chapter will use the groupings as shown in Table 12.4 and concentrate on the treatment of the adult NHL patient.

## Treatment of early-stage low-grade/indolent lymphomas (SL, FSC, FM, DSC, DIDL)

Localized low-grade/indolent lymphomas (Stage I or contiguous Stage II) are rare presentations consisting of only 10–20% of NHL. They may be successfully treated using involved-field or extended-field radiation therapy. Most of the data on which the above statement is made are based on results of studies looking mainly at follicular small cleaved cell (FSC) and follicular mixed lymphoma (FML). Data on the rarer histologies (DSC, DIDL, SL (small lymphocytic)) has typically been obtained from looking at larger series of the more common histological subtypes and extracting data on the

**Table 12.4**    Histological grouping for treatment purposes

---

*Low grade/indolent*
Small lymphocytic (SL)
Follicular predominately small cleaved (FSC)
Follicular mixed small cleaved and large cell (FM)
Diffuse small cleaved (DSC)[a]
Diffuse intermediately differentiated lymphoma (mantle zone) (DIDL)[b]

*Intermediate grade/aggressive*
Follicular predominately large cell (FLC)
Diffuse mixed small cleaved and large cell (DM)
Diffuse large cell (DLC)
Large cell immunoblastic lymphoma (IBL)[c]

*High grade/highly aggressive*
Diffuse small non-cleaved cell (Burkitt's lymphoma)
Diffuse small non-cleaved cell (non-Burkitt's lymphoma)
Lymphoblastic lymphoma (LL)
Adult T-cell leukaemia–lymphoma[b]

---

[a]Working Formulation intermediate grade with an indolent natural history.
[b]Histology not included in Working Formulation.
[c]Working Formulation high-grade lymphoma with intermediate-grade natural history.

rarer histological subtypes found in these series. No clear evidence exists that the treatment of these rarer histologies (DSC, DIDL, SL) should be any different from that of the other low-grade lymphomas.

A number of series[22–28] report the efficacy of radiation therapy in both the pathologically and clinically staged patients, with some series showing an apparent plateauing of the disease-free survival curves with follow-up beyond 5 years.

In the Princess Margaret experience,[22] overall survival of 190 clinical Stage I and II indolent lymphoma patients treated with curative radiotherapy was 58% at 12 years with a relapse-free survival of 53% at 12 years. In addition, in a select group of 'good prognosis patients' (aged less than 70, small or medium bulk disease) the 12-year actuarial survival rate was 92% and the relapse-free survival rate was 73%.

In the United States NCI experience,[23] which retrospectively reviewed fifty-four patients with Stage I and II low-grade lymphoma treated with radiotherapy, the overall survival and disease free survival rates at 10 years were 69% and 48%, respectively. No relapses occurred in patients with Stage I disease after 6 years, thus supporting the concept of long-term survival (cure) after radiotherapy in indolent lymphomas.

In the Stanford University series,[24] 124 patients with Stage I and II indolent lymphomas treated with radiotherapy had 5-, 10-, and 15-year actuarial survivals of 84%, 68%, and 42%, with 5- and 10-year freedom from relapse of 62% and 54%, respectively. In addition, a plateau in the freedom-from-relapse curve was seen after 5 years at approximately 50%, again supporting the idea of potential cure in early-stage indolent lymphomas.

The addition of chemotherapy to radiation therapy for the early-stage low-grade NHL remains controversial. Five prospectively randomized trials[29-33] have evaluated the addition of multiagent chemotherapy following radiation therapy. Four studies have evaluated the addition of CVP chemotherapy (cyclophosphamide, vincristine, prednisone) while a fifth evaluated the addition of CHOP chemotherapy (cyclophosphamide, doxorubicin, vincristine, prednisone). These studies included Stage I and Stage II patients with both low- and intermediate-grade histologies. All five studies have revealed statistically improved relapse-free survival rates (range with chemotherapy and radiation of 71–90% versus range with radiation alone of 46–54%) with only one showing a significant improvement in overall survival.[31] However, when the low-grade histologies are evaluated separately, only one of the studies[32] continues to show a significant improvement in relapse-free survival (54% versus 71%) and none of them show a significant improvement in overall survival. One must be cautioned that these series contained small numbers of patients with low-grade NHL, making the power of these studies less than desirable. Given the lack of a clear proven benefit of the addition of chemotherapy in well-conducted randomized trials containing primarily indolent lymphoma patients, the current standard of care for most Stage I or contiguous Stage II low-grade/indolent NHL should continue to be locoregional radiation therapy. In general, an involved-field approach is recommended, where the involved nodal group plus the next adjacent nodal groups are treated. Doses to the uninvolved nodal groups are approximately 30 Gy and sites of involvement may be boosted to 36–40 Gy.

## Treatment of advanced-stage low-grade/indolent lymphomas (SL, FSC, FM, DSC, DIDL)

Optimal therapy for the advanced Stage III and IV low-grade NHL remains controversial. This controversy exists because, although prolonged survival can be achieved, no currently available therapy clearly offers a proven 'cure' in these patients. After years of randomized, non-randomized, retrospective and prospective studies using all conventional treatment modalities and combinations, the following generalities can be made:

1. Response rates range from 50% to 90%.
2. Median survivals range from approximately 8 to 12 years.
3. Durations of responses are similar and almost independent of treatment modality (median duration usually 20–36 months).
4. Few if any plateaus in survival curves are seen, supporting the idea that cure is not yet possible in the advanced-stage low-grade NHL.

Current therapy options include single-agent chemotherapy[34-37] (chlorambucil or cyclophosphamide), radiation therapy (total lymphoid irradiation (TLI)[38,39] or total central lymphatic irradiation (TCL) for Stage III disease),[40,41] combination chemotherapy without[42] or with radiation[35,43] and deferred therapy with careful observation in asymptomatic patients.[44,45]

Single-agent chemotherapy has resulted in response rates in the range of 35–69% but with long-term durable remissions being very few.[34-37] The addition of multiagent chemotherapy has appeared to improve the response rate to the range of 50–90% in this group of patients but, as can be seen, there is overlap with the results of single-agent chemotherapy and, in at least one randomized trial, single-agent chemotherapy fared no worse than multiagent chemotherapy.

Hoppe *et al.*[35] reported the results of a randomized trial comparing single-agent chemotherapy (chlorambucil or cyclophosphamide) versus CVP chemotherapy versus total body irradiation (TBI). There was no difference in the results between these groups with regard to response, relapse-free survival or overall survival. Anderson *et al.*[46,47] treated a group of patients with either CVP or C-MOPP (cyclophosphamide, vincristine, prednisone, procarbazine) and reported a complete response rate of 67% but relapse-free survival was only 25% of the complete responders at 6 years, with no plateauing of the relapse-free survival curve. Although some authors argue that the chemotherapy used in these series was suboptimal because it did not contain doxorubicin, a recently reported study from the Southwest Oncology Group (SWOG)[42] does not reveal any improvement using CHOP chemotherapy over CVP or single-agent chemotherapy in advanced-stage indolent NHL; doxorubicin as a single agent is not especially effective and its cardiotoxicity probably precludes it as a routine agent for these generally elderly patients. In the above report, Dana *et al.*[42] reviewed the results of 415 Stage III and IV patients treated with CHOP chemotherapy on SWOG randomized protocols between 1972 and 1983. The complete response rate was 64% and, with a median follow-up of 12.8 years, the median survival was 6.9 years and no definite survival curve plateau was seen. These authors concluded that doxorubicin-containing chemotherapy (CHOP) did not prolong the median survival in this group of patients when compared with less aggressive treatment programmes (chlorambucil or CVP).

The 'curative role' of radiation therapy alone in the advanced-stage low-grade group is now limited to use in the Stage III patient. Although whole body irradiation[48,49] alone has been used in both stage III and IV patients with good response rates, relapses were frequent and long-term relapse-free survivors were few. In Stage III patients, several authors have reported promising results of total lymphoid irradiation (TLI) or total central lymphatic irradiation (TCL).[8,39,40,41] Jacobs *et al.*[41] reported the results of thirty-four patients with Stage III disease treated with TCL (Waldeyer's ring, mantle, abdomen and pelvis). With a median follow-up of 9.7 years, they reported life table overall, disease-free and cause-specific survivals at 15 years of 28%, 40% and 46%, respectively. Only one relapse was observed after 9 years of follow-up. These authors concluded that TCL is generally superior to single-agent chemotherapy, combination chemotherapy or biological response modifiers, and is less toxic than and as good as combined chemotherapy and irradiation. Paryani *et al.*[39] reported on sixty-one patients with Stage III follicular lymphomas treated with TLI, with and without chemotherapy (forty-eight patients TLI only, thirteen patients combined modality therapy). With a median follow-up of 9.6 years, actuarial survivals at 5, 10 and 15 years were 78%, 50% and 37%, respectively, with a freedom from relapse at 5 and 10 years of 60% and 40%. In a prospective randomized trial of sixteen of these patients comparing TLI (eight patients) versus TLI plus CVP (eight patients), no significant difference in survival or freedom from relapse was noted between the two groups. In addition, these authors identified a subgroup of good prognosis patients (with no B symptoms, fewer than five sites of disease, and maximum tumour size <10 cm) who had an excellent prognosis with 15-year survival and freedom from relapse of 100% and 88%, respectively. In view of these results, it can be concluded that in favourable Stage III disease radiation alone may be a potentially curative modality and that it may not be justifiable to withhold radiation in all asymptomatic patients with Stage III indolent lymphomas.

McLaughlin *et al.*[43] have reported results on Stage III follicular lymphoma patients treated with combined chemotherapy (CHOP–bleomycin) and radiation therapy similar to TCL. With a median follow-up of 7 years, the 5-year survival rate and relapse-free survival rate were 75% and 52%, respectively. These results appeared no better than those with TCL or TLI as reported by Jacobs *et al.*[41] and Paryani *et al.*[39] and raise questions as to the need to add chemotherapy to radiation therapy in Stage III patients with indolent lymphomas who undergo immediate therapy.

The need for immediate therapy in any asymptomatic Stage III or IV low-grade NHL patient remains one of the biggest controversies in treating NHL. The 'watch-and-wait' approach has been evaluated by several authors. Horning and Rosenberg[44] evaluated eighty-three (74% Stage IV) advanced-stage low-grade NHL patients who were initially managed without therapy. With a median follow-up of 4.2 years, actuarial survival rates at 5, 10, and 15 years were 82%, 73% and 40%, respectively, with a median actuarial survival of 11 years. The median time to requiring therapy for the entire group was 3 years, with the median time for the three histological subgroups (FM, FSC, SL) differing significantly at 16.5, 48.0, and 72.0 months, respectively. When this group was compared with seventy-three Stage III and IV low-grade NHL patients, initially asymptomatic and judged eligible for no treatment but who were initially treated, no difference in survival between these groups was seen.

Young *et al.*[45] reported the results of a prospective randomized study conducted at the NCI, comparing no initial therapy with very aggressive combined modality therapy using ProMACE–MOPP flexitherapy (prednisone, methotrexate, doxorubicin, cyclophosphamide, etoposide, mechlorethamine, vincristine, procarbazine, prednisone) followed by low dose TLI (24 Gy). In this study, the 'watch-and-wait' group were allowed to undergo small-field low dose palliative radiation therapy, but if chemotherapy was required for systemic symptoms or histological conversion they were crossed to the aggressive ProMACE–MOPP regimen. Forty-one patients on the 'watch-and-wait' arm and forty-three patients on the aggressive arm were evaluated. At presentation fifteen patients were felt to require initial systemic therapy and were treated in accordance with the combined modality arm of the protocol. At the time of this report twenty-three of forty-one patients (56%) were still on the watch-and-wait arm not requiring crossover, with a median time to crossover of 34 months. Forty-three per cent of those crossing over achieved a complete response (CR). Of the seventy-three randomized patients initially undergoing aggressive therapy, 78% achieved a CR. In the fifteen patients not randomized but receiving initial chemotherapy, the CR rate was 50%. The overall survival (75%) at 5 years was equal in both the randomized groups and the initially treated group.

In addition, a 51% disease-free survival at 4 years was seen in the randomized initially treated group. The CR rate for all initially treated patients (forty-three randomized and fifteen treated due to symptoms) was 71%.

From this series, the following observations are made:

1. Both the CR rate (71%) and the overall survival at 5 years (75%) are no different from results of other reported series with less aggressive therapy.
2. The relapse-free survival of 51% at 4 years (medium duration 45+ months) is better than most other series using less aggressive therapy. A much longer follow-up will be needed to determine if this improved disease-free survival will result in a plateau of the survival curves.
3. The risk of myelodysplasia/leukaemia was significant (five patients) and was sufficient to preclude such therapy from being a standard recommendation.

In summary, the approach to therapy in the advanced-stage low-grade NHL should be enrolment in clinical trials to help resolve the related controversies. Off protocol, our recommended approach is that of 'watchful waiting' in asymptomatic patients. However, two subgroups of asymptomatic patients exist where initial therapy may be indicated:

1. patients with favourable Stage III disease (no 'B' symptoms, fewer than five individual sites, maximum tumour size 10 cm) can be considered for TLI or TCL, with or without chemotherapy, with hope of long-term disease-free survival; and
2. patients with FML may be considered due to the reported early requirement for crossover (16.2 months).[44]

When crossover is required, or if the patient requires therapy at presentation, the aggressiveness of therapy should be based on the extent of disease, toxicities of therapy, performance status of the patient, and need for a rapid response. At this point, the goal of therapy is palliation of symptoms and not necessarily a complete elimination of all known disease. The least toxic and time-consuming therapy that will accomplish this goal is presently considered optimal.

### Treatment of early-stage intermediate-grade/aggressive lymphomas (FLC, DM, DLC, IBL)

Traditionally, radiation therapy has been the primary treatment of choice for this group of lymphomas. However, with advances in multiagent chemotherapy, the standard of care has now evolved to multiagent chemotherapy, with or without radiation therapy.

Excellent results have been reported in pathological Stage I intermediate-grade NHL using radiation therapy only.[50–56] In the University of Chicago series[55] of thirty-six patients with pathological Stage I and II diffuse histiocytic lymphoma with a 7-year median follow-up, the 10-year actuarial relapse-free survival for Stage I patients was 91%, in stark contrast to a 10-year actuarial relapse-free survival of 35% in pathological Stage II patients. However, the results of clinical Stage I patients have been less impressive using radiation therapy only, with long-term relapse-free survivals in the range of 60–70%.[57] When clinical Stage II patients are treated with radiation therapy alone the results are even worse, with relapse-free survival rates less than 50%.[27,29,58]

With the addition of adjuvant chemotherapy following locoregional radiation, many authors have reported a benefit[29,30,31,33,59] while others have not.[51] In a recently reported randomized trial of radiation therapy followed with or without CHOP chemotherapy in clinical Stage I and II NHL, a significant improvement in relapse-free survival was seen in the intermediate-grade histologies, in favour of the combined modality approach.[33] Specifically, the 7-year actuarial relapse-free survival for the intermediate-grade group was 86% for radiation followed by CHOP chemotherapy and 20% for radiation therapy alone ($P = 0.004$). The corresponding actuarial survival rates were 92% and 47%, respectively ($P = 0.08$).

Motivated by advances in the use of multiagent doxorubicin-containing chemotherapy in advanced-stage intermediate-grade NHL, several authors reported excellent results with chemotherapy alone or chemotherapy followed by locoregional radiation in the early-stage intermediate-grade lymphomas.[60–63] The desire to initiate chemotherapy early in the treatment scheme, prior to radiation, has been motivated by the observation of rapid systemic failure seen in many patients treated with radiotherapy only. The results of these earlier series have been further confirmed by additional series using chemotherapy initially, followed with or without radiation therapy, where 5-year relapse-free survivals range from 82 to 100% and overall survival rates range from 80 to 90%.[64–68]

Jones *et al.*[66] reported the combined Arizona and Vancouver experience of CHOP-based chemotherapy, with or without the use of local radiation therapy, in 142 clinical Stage I and II intermediate-grade NHL patients. Virtually all patients in the Vancouver series were treated with three cycles of CHOP followed by involved-field radiation therapy, whereas in the Arizona group radiation therapy was given at the physician's discretion. The complete response rate was 99%, and with a median follow-up of 4.4 years the actuarial 5-year relapse-free survival and overall survival rates were 82% and 80%, respectively. When relapse-free survival was compared between those receiving combined modality therapy and those receiving chemotherapy alone, no significant difference was seen. However, when radiation therapy was used, fewer cycles of chemotherapy were used and a trend toward improvement in relapse-free survival was noted. Tondini *et al.*[67] reported the results of 183 clinical Stage I and II patients treated with CHOP chemotherapy followed by extended-field radiation therapy. The CR rate was 98%, and with a median follow-up of 4.2 years the 5-year relapse-free survival and overall survival rates were both 83%.

Longo *et al.*[65] (and recently updated by Sullivan *et al.*[68]) reported the NCI experience of sixty-two clinical Stage I intermediate-grade patients treated with ProMACE–MOPP followed by involved-field radiation therapy. They reported a CR rate of 97%, and with a 7.4-year median follow-up the 10-year actuarial relapse-free survival was 95%, with a 10-year actuarial overall survival of 87%.

It is the results of such studies which have made combined modality therapy, with or without radiation therapy, the current standard of care in the treatment of early-stage intermediate-grade lymphoma. However, two questions remain to be answered:

1. the importance of adding radiation to chemotherapy;

2. the optimal number of cycles of chemotherapy with or without radiation therapy.

Currently, clinical trials are underway that should help to define the optimal treatment approach in early-stage intermediate-grade NHL. The Southwest Oncology Group (SWOG) is currently randomizing these patients between eight cycles of CHOP chemotherapy versus three cycles of CHOP chemotherapy followed by involved-field radiation therapy. The Eastern Cooperative Oncology Group (ECOG) is randomizing these patients between eight cycles of CHOP, with or without involved-field radiation therapy. Until the results are known, it appears most appropriate to continue to treat the intermediate-grade clinical Stage I and II NHL patients with three to eight cycles of CHOP-like chemotherapy followed by involved-field radiation therapy to a dose of approximately 40 Gy.

## Treatment of advanced-stage intermediate-grade/aggressive lymphomas (FLC, DM, DLC, IBL)

The treatment of choice of advanced-stage intermediate-grade NHL is clearly combination chemotherapy. Currently, the use of multiagent chemotherapy in this group of patients results in an approximately 50% long-term survival rate. As to the best chemotherapy regimen, there still remains much debate with dose intensification using such regimens as ProMACE–cytaBOM (cytaBOM: cytarabine, bleomycin, vincristine, methotrexate), m-BACOD, and MACOP-B being favoured by some investigators[69] while less intensive regimens such as CHOP are preferred by others. A recently reported SWOG randomized trial[70] compared CHOP, m-BACOD, MACOP-B, and ProMACE-cytaBOM and found no difference in disease-free or overall survival. This report confirms that CHOP chemotherapy still remains the standard of comparison.

Radiation therapy in this group of patients is usually reserved for consolidation of residual tumour masses seen at the completion of chemotherapy, consolidation of sites of bulk disease (>10 cm) seen at the start chemotherapy and for the treatment for symptomatic local problems. Although some patients may theoretically benefit from the use of consolidative radiation therapy, no randomized trials have yet addressed this issue. Shipp et al.[71] in a review from the Dana-Farber Cancer Institute found that advanced-stage patients do not consistently relapse in sites of prior bulk disease. They contend that consolidative radiotherapy would have little impact on the ultimate outcome in these patients.

## Treatment of high-grade/highly aggressive lymphomas (LL, diffuse small non-cleaved cell (Burkitt's/non-Burkitt's), adult-T-cell)

These rare and extremely aggressive subtypes of NHL are treated with multiagent chemotherapy which in many cases is patterned after the treatment of acute lymphocytic leukaemia (ALL), including maintenance therapy. Lymphoblastic lymphoma (LL), which often occurs in young patients with associated large mediastinal masses, bone marrow and CNS involvement, is best treated with regimens similar to that used in ALL.[72-74] Diffuse small non-cleaved cell lymphomas (Burkitt's and non-Burkitt's) are also treated with multiagent chemotherapy using regimens similar to those used in advanced-stage intermediate-grade lymphomas and for poor prognosis patient regimens similar to those used in lymphoblastic lymphoma.[75-77] Adult T-cell lymphoma is a highly aggressive form of lymphoma, which although responsive to standard lymphoma chemotherapy is rarely curable, and treatment morbidity is extremely high secondary to the associated immunodeficiency seen in these patients

## Treatment of human immunodeficiency virus (HIV)-related lymphomas

In the US since 1985, the increase of NHL has increased at the same rate as the reported cases of acquired immune deficiency syndrome (AIDS). Currently, 3.3% of the 200 000 documented AIDS patients reported to the Centers of Disease Control (CDC) have been associated with a diagnosis of NHL. The majority of these cases are intermediate- or high-grade lymphomas and patients generally present with more advanced-stage disease, more frequently have extranodal involvement, have a more aggressive course, and are less responsive to chemotherapy. The most commonly used treatment regimens include multiagent chemotherapy such as CHOP and m-BACOD, as used in advanced-stage intermediate-grade NHL. In addition, since CNS relapses are common, many investigators include prophylactic CNS chemotherapy[78,79] as well as the use of colony-stimulating factors.[80] Such regimens routinely require dose reductions and delays in therapy. The role of radiation therapy in HIV-related lymphoma has been limited to palliation or for use in certain specific 'localized' sites such as primary CNS lymphoma.

## Treatment of specific localized sites

In general, most extranodal sites of NHL are treated based on histological subtypes and extent of disease. However, several sites require modified approaches of treatment regimens due to differences in observed treatment successes or limitation of treatment approaches due to normal-tissue tolerances.

## Gastrointestinal tract lymphoma

The gastrointestinal (GI) tract is the most common site of extranodal NHL. Gastric lymphoma accounts for approximately 50–60% of the GI tract lymphomas. Historically, surgery with total or partial gastrectomy has been the most commonly used treatment modality, with or without postoperative chemotherapy or radiotherapy. Five-year disease-free survival rates are in the range of 40–70%.[81-83] Much controversy continues as to the role of radiation and chemotherapy in this disease, either as an adjuvant to surgery or as sole treatment.[84] Concern has been raised in the past about the risk of gastric perforation if radiation therapy and chemotherapy are used without surgery. Maor et al.[85] from MD Anderson Cancer Center treated thirty-four patients without gastrectomy using CHOP-bleomycin and locoregional radiation. None of these patients developed perforation, gastric ulcer or haemorrhage. In addition, the 5-year disease-free survival and overall survival rates were 62% and 73%, respectively, which compare favourably with results of surgical series. In the surviving patients twenty-four of twenty-six (92%) did not have stomach resections and retained good stomach function. Since this approach allows organ preservation and avoids the potential morbidities of gastrectomy such as malabsorption and dumping syndromes, combined modality therapy with chemotherapy and radiation may be the preferred treatment in many patients. In our opinion, surgical resection is indicated for presentations of severe GI bleeding, but little evidence of benefit is seen from its routine use in all GI lymphoma patients. Randomized trials are needed to answer this question fully.

## Primary central nervous system lymphoma

Primary CNS lymphoma is a particularly virulent form of extranodal lymphoma. Although radiation therapy has significantly improved the overall outcome compared with surgery (improvement in median survival from 5 to 15 months), local recurrence rates remain high (60–70%) even when high dose radiation therapy is used. Recent reports using combined modality therapy have been promising. DeAngelis et al.[86] reported on thirty-one patients treated using preradiation systemic methotrexate, intrathecal methotrexate, whole brain irradiation (40 Gy with 14 Gy boost) and post-irradiation systemic cytarabine (ARA-C). They report a median time to CNS recurrence of 41 months and a median survival of 42.5 months. These results are considerably better than those of most series using radiation therapy only. The Radiation Therapy Oncology Group (RTOG)[87] treated patients using whole brain irradiation to 40 Gy with a 20 Gy boost and reported a median survival of 12 months and a 2-year survival of 28%. Currently, the best results reported are a small series from the University of Oregon (Neuwelt et al.[88]) using chemotherapy after altering the blood–brain barrier; an estimated median survival of 44.5 months is reported. Given the difficulty of maintaining local control in this setting, high dose radiation therapy should continue to be part of the treatment regimen of CNS lymphoma.

## Thyroid gland lymphomas

Primary lymphoma of the thyroid gland is extremely rare and accounts for less than 2% of extranodal lymphomas. It is most commonly seen in elderly females and is usually of intermediate-grade histology. Historically, surgery had been the most common form of treatment, given the difficulty of preoperatively distinguishing lymphoma from carcinoma or thyroiditis. With the advent of thyroid biopsy and fine needle aspiration (FNA), and the effectiveness of radiation in lymphomas, surgery became less important as a treatment modality and radiotherapy emerged as the primary treatment modality. Several recent series[89,90] have shown improvement in both local control and distant relapse rates when combined modality therapy is used.

It appears that, as in other intermediate-grade histologies, chemotherapy or combined modality may be superior to radiation therapy alone. An exception to this may be in small-volume Stage $IA_E$ patients, where radiation therapy alone has been shown to be extremely effective.[91,92]

## Orbital lymphoma

Primary orbital lymphoma can be successfully treated by radiation therapy with excellent results.[93] The majority of these cases represent low-grade lymphomas where radiotherapy is usually the sole form of treatment. In the intermediate-grade tumours, chemotherapy has been added by some investigators but the number of patients reported in the literature is small. One is therefore left to extrapolate results from other sites when considering the addition of chemotherapy to the treatment regimens. Detailed treatment planning and lens shielding should be employed, when possible, to minimize the potential for long-term morbidity.[93,94] Most series report excellent control rates (greater than 90%) with doses in the range of 24–35 Gy for all histological subtypes while other authors recommend doses of 35–40 Gy for the higher-grade orbital lymphomas.[95]

## Testicular lymphoma

Lymphoma of the testis is the most common testicular neoplasm in males of age 60 and older. It is typically an intermediate- or high-grade lymphoma, has a tendency to be bilateral and is associated with CNS and Waldeyer's ring involvement.[96] Historically, treatment included orchiectomy followed by scrotal and regional nodal irradiation. This approach resulted in excellent locoregional control but distant dissemination was common. As in other intermediate- and high-grade lymphomas, the addition of multiagent chemotherapy has resulted in a significant improvement in outcome.[97] Currently, the best results are obtained with orchiectomy and multiagent chemotherapy.

## Primary bone lymphoma

Primary bone lymphoma represents a rare form of extranodal NHL and comprises less than 1% of all non-Hodgkin's lymphomas. Like many of the other extranodal sites of lymphoma, intermediate-grade histologies are most common. Although the roles of chemotherapy and radiotherapy have yet to be completely defined, it appears that, in most series, radiotherapy alone is associated with a 50% rate of distant relapse, supporting the need for systemic treatment. While most studies show a clear benefit of adding chemotherapy to radiotherapy, others do not.[98,99] Only a Phase III randomized, controlled clinical trial will determine whether chemotherapy plus radiotherapy is superior to either alone. Until such a trial is completed, combined modality therapy with radiation therapy doses of 45–55 Gy to the involved bone is recommended, especially if a weight-bearing location is involved.

# Future directions and protocols

Due to the poor long-term outcome seen in certain subgroups of NHL, the importance of completion of clinical trials is paramount. The NCI Physicians Data Query (PDQ) currently lists over 150 active protocols available, to which NHL patients can be enrolled. These include approximately sixty-three Phase I, seventy-five Phase II, and seventeen Phase III protocols. Thirty-four of these protocols include radiation therapy in the treatment plan. Areas addressed by these protocols include:

1. optimum number of cycles of CHOP chemotherapy in Stage I and II intermediate-grade lymphomas;
2. role of radiation therapy in Stage I and II intermediate-grade lymphomas;
3. role of radiation and α-interferon in Stage III and IV indolent lymphomas;
4. optimal treatment of CNS lymphoma;
5. optimal treatment of gastric lymphoma;
6. role of autologous bone marrow transplant in both *de novo* and relapsed NHL.

Given the exquisite sensitivity of NHL to radiation and the excellent local control rates, radiation therapy should continue to play a role in the treatment of these patients. It will only be with the completion of these clinical trials that the optimal role of radiation therapy in NHL will be completely identified.

# References

1. Cox JD. Lymphomas and leukemia. In: WT Moss, JD Cox, eds, *Radiation Oncology, Rationale, Technique, Results*. St Louis: CV Mosby Co, 1989; 667.
2. Ellingo PA, Tong T, Bolden S, *et al.* Cancer statistics. *CA–A Cancer Journal for Clinicians* 1995; **45**, 8–30.
3. Ries LAG, Hankey BF, Miller BA, *et al.* Cancer statistics review, 1973–1988. *NIH Pub No 91–2789*. Bethesda, MD: National Cancer Institute, 1991.
4. Castellani R, Bonadonna G, Spinelli P, *et al.* Sequential pathologic staging of untreated non-Hodgkin's lymphomas by laparoscopy and laparotomy combined with marrow biopsy. *Cancer*. 1977; **40**, 2322–8.
5. Chabner BA, Johnson RE, Young RC, *et al.* Sequential nonsurgical and surgical staging of non-Hodgkin's lymphoma. *Ann Intern Med* 1976; **85**, 149–54.
6. Goffinet DR, Castellino RA, Kim H, *et al.* Staging laparotomies in unselected previously untreated patients with non-Hodgkin's lymphomas. *Cancer* 1973; **32**, 672–81.
7. The Non-Hodgkin's Lymphoma Pathologic Classification Project: National Cancer Institute sponsored study of classifications of non-Hodgkin's lymphomas: summary and description of a formulation for clinical usage. *Cancer* 1982; **49**, 2112–35.
8. Jones SE, Fuks Z, Bull M, *et al.* Non-Hodgkin's lymphomas. V. Results of radiotherapy. *Cancer* 1973; **32**, 682.
9. Portlock CS, Rosenberg SA. No initial therapy for stage III and IV non-

Hodgkin's lymphomas of favorable histologic types. *Ann Intern Med* 1979; **90**, 10–13.

10. Krikorian JG, Portlock CS, Cooney DP, *et al.* Spontaneous regression of non-Hodgkin's lymphomas. A report of nine cases. *Cancer Res* 1980; **46**, 2093–9.

11. Longo DL, DeVita VT, Jaffe ES, *et al.* Lymphocytic lymphomas. In: VT DeVita, S Hellman, SA Rosenberg, eds, *Cancer Principles and Practice of Oncology*, 4th edn. Philadelphia: JB Lippincott Co, 1993; 1889.

12. Longo DL, Schilsky RL, Blei L, *et al.* Gallium-67 scanning has limited usefulness in staging patients with non-Hodgkin's lymphoma. *Am J Med* 1980; **68**, 695–700.

13. Kaplan WD, Jochelson MS, Herman TS, *et al.* Gallium-67 imaging: a predictor of residual tumor viability and clinical outcome in patients with diffuse large-cell lymphoma. *J Clin Oncol* 1990; **8**, 1966–70.

14. Lister TA, Crowther D, Sutcliffe SB, *et al.* Report of a committee convened to discuss the evaluation and staging of patients with Hodgkin's disease: Cotswold meeting. *J Clin Oncol* 1989; **7**, 1630–6.

15. The Non-Hodgkin's Lymphoma Pathological Classification Project. National Cancer Institute sponsored study of classification of non-Hodgkin's lymphomas: summary and description of a working formulation for clinical usage. *Cancer* 1982; **49**, 2112–35.

16. NCI Non-Hodgkin's Classification Project Writing Committee. Classification of non-Hodgkin's lymphomas: reproducibility of major classification systems. *Cancer* 1985; **55**, 91–5.

17. Dick F, Van Lier S, Banks P, *et al.* Use of the working formulation for non-Hodgkin's lymphoma in epidemiologic studies: agreement between reported diagnoses and a panel of experienced pathologists. *J Natl Cancer Inst* 1987; **78**, 1137–44.

18. Jones RJ, Seifter EJ, Ambunder RF. Non-Hodgkin's lymphoma. In: JE Niederhuber, ed, *Current Therapy in Oncology*. St Louis: Mosby-Year Book, 1993; 564–70.

19. Portlock CS. The management of favorable histology non-Hodgkin's lymphomas. In: SK Carter, E Glatstein, RB Livingston, eds, *Principles of Cancer Treatment*. New York: McGraw-Hill, 1982; 819–23.

20. Coltman CA. Management of unfavorable histology non-Hodgkin's lymphoma. In: SK Carter, E Glatstein, RB Livingston, eds, *Principles of Cancer Treatment*. New York: McGraw-Hill, 1982; 824–31.

21. Longo DL, DeVita VT, Jaffe ES, *et al.* Lymphocytic lymphomas. In: VT DeVita, S Hellman, SA Rosenberg, eds, *Cancer Principles and Practice of Oncology*, 4th edn. Philadelphia: JB Lippincott Co, 1993; 1874.

22. Gospodarowicz MK, Bush RS, Brown TC. Prognostic factors in nodular lymphomas: a multivariate analysis based on the Princess Margaret experience. *Int J Radiat Oncol Biol Phys* 1984; **10**, 489–97.

23. Lawrence TS, Urba WJ, Steinberg SM, *et al.* Retrospective analysis of stage I and II indolent lymphomas at the National Cancer Institute. *Int J Radiat Oncol Biol Phys* 1988; **14**, 417–24.

24. Paryani SB, Hoppe RT, Cox RS, *et al.* Analysis of non-Hodgkin's lymphoma with nodular and favorable histologies, stages I and II. *Cancer* 1983; **52**, 2300–7.

25. Gomez GA, Barcos M, Kismamsetty RM, *et al.* Treatment of early-stages I and II nodular, poorly differentiated lymphocytic lymphoma. *Am J Clin Oncol* 1986; 9, 40–44.

26. Richards MA, Gregory WM, Hall PA, *et al.* Management of localized non-Hodgkin's lymphoma: the experience at St. Bartholomew's Hospital 1972–1985. *Hematol Oncol* 1989; **7**, 1–18.

27. Chen MG, Prosnitz LR, Gonzales-Serva A, *et al.* Results of radiotherapy in control of stage I and II non-Hodgkin's lymphomas. *Cancer* 1979; **43**, 1245–54.

28. McLaughlin P, Fuller L, Velasquez WS, *et al*. Stage I–II follicular lymphoma: treatment results in 76 patients. *Cancer* 1986; **58**, 1596–1601.
29. Nissen NI, Ersboll J, Hansen HS, *et al*. A randomized study of radiotherapy versus radiotherapy plus chemotherapy in stage I–II non-Hodgkin's lymphomas. *Cancer* 1983; **52**, 1–7.
30. Landberg TG, Hakansson LG, Moller TR, *et al*. CVP–remission–maintenance in stage I or II non-Hodgkin's lymphomas: preliminary results of a randomized study. *Cancer* 1979; **44**, 831–8.
31. Monfardini S, Banfi A, Bonadonna G, *et al*. Improved five-year survival after combined radiotherapy–chemotherapy for stage I–II non-Hodgkin's lymphoma. *Int J Radiat Oncol Biol Phys* 1980; **6**, 125–34.
32. Carde P, Burgers JMV, van Glabbeke M, *et al*. Combined radiotherapy–chemotherapy for early stages non-Hodgkin's lymphomas: the 1975–1980 EORTC controlled lymphoma trial. *Radiother Oncol* 1984; **2**, 301–12.
33. Yahalom J, Varsos G, Fuks Z, *et al*. Adjuvant cyclophosphamide, doxorubicin, vincristine, and prednisone chemotherapy after radiation therapy in stage I low-grade and intermediate-grade non-Hodgkin's lymphoma. *Cancer* 1993; **71**, 2342–50.
34. Portlock CS, Rosenberg SA, Glatstein E, *et al*. Treatment of advanced non-Hodgkin's lymphomas with favorable histologies: preliminary results of a prospective trial. *Blood* 1976; **47**, 747–56.
35. Hoppe RT, Kushlan P, Kaplan HS, *et al*. The treatment of advanced stage favorable histology non-Hodgkin's lymphoma: a preliminary report of a randomized trial comparing single agent chemotherapy, combination chemotherapy, and whole body irradiation. *Blood* 1981; **58**, 592–98.
36. Kennedy BJ, Bloomfield CD, Kiang DT, *et al*. Combination versus successive single agent chemotherapy in lymphocytic lymphoma. *Cancer* 1978; **41**, 23–8.
37. Jones SE, Rosenberg SA, Kaplan HS, *et al*. Non-Hodgkin's lymphomas II. Single agent chemotherapy. *Cancer* 1972; **30**, 31–8.
38. Glatstein E, Fuks Z, Goffinet DR, *et al*. Non-Hodgkin's lymphomas of stage III extent. Is total lymphoid irradiation appropriate treatment? *Cancer* 1976; **37**, 2806–12.
39. Paryani SB, Hoppe RT, Cox RS, *et al*. The role of radiation therapy in the management of stage III follicular lymphomas. *J Clin Oncol* 1984; **2**, 841–8.
40. Cox JD, Komaki R, Kun LE, *et al*. Stage III nodular lymphoreticular tumors (non-Hodgkin's lymphoma): results of central lymphatic irradiation. *Cancer* 1981; **47**, 2247–52.
41. Jacobs JP, Murray KJ, Schultz CJ, *et al*. Central lymphatic irradiation for stage III nodular malignant lymphoma: long term results. *J Clin Oncol* 1993; **11**, 233–8.
42. Dana BW, Dahlberg S, Nathuiani BN, *et al*. Long-term follow-up of patients with low-grade malignant lymphomas treated with doxorubicin-based chemotherapy or chemoimmunotherapy. *J Clin Oncol* 1993; **11**, 644–51.
43. McLaughlin P, Fuller LM, Velasquez WS, *et al*. Stage III follicular lymphoma: durable remissions with a combined chemotherapy–radiotherapy regimen. *J Clin Oncol* 1987; **5**, 867–74.
44. Horning SJ, Rosenberg SA. The natural history of initially untreated low-grade non-Hodgkin's lymphomas. *N Engl J Med* 1984; **311**, 1471–5.
45. Young RC, Longo DL, Glatstein E, *et al*. The treatment of indolent lymphomas: watchful waiting v. aggressive combined modality treatment. *Semin Hematol* 1988; **25**, 11–16.
46. Anderson T, Bender RA, Fisher RI, *et al*. Combination chemotherapy in non-Hodgkin's lymphoma: results of long-term follow up. *Cancer Treat Rep* 1977; **6**, 1057–66.

47. Anderson KC, Skarin AT, Rosenthal DS, *et al.* Combination chemotherapy for advanced non-Hodgkin's lymphomas other than diffuse histiocytic or undifferentiated histologies. *Cancer* 1984; **68**, 1343–50.
48. Carabell SC, Chaffey JT, Rosenthal DS, *et al.* Results of total body irradiation in the treatment of advanced non-Hodgkin's lymphomas. *Cancer* 1979; **43**, 994–1000.
49. Choi NC, Timothy AR, Kaufman SD, *et al.* Low dose fractionated whole body irradiation in the treatment of advanced non-Hodgkin's lymphoma. *Cancer* 1979; **43**, 1636–42.
50. Bitran JD, Kinzie J, Sweet DL, *et al.* Survival of patients with localized histiocytic lymphomas. *Cancer* 1977; **39**, 342–46.
51. Glatstein E, Donaldson SS, Rosenberg SA, *et al.* Combined modality therapy in malignant lymphomas. Cancer Treat Rep. 1977; **61**, 1199–1207.
52. Levitt SH, Bloomfield CD, Frizzera G, *et al.* Curative radiotherapy for localized diffuse histiocytic lymphoma. *Cancer Treat Rep* 1980; **64**, 175–7.
53. Sweet DL, Kinzie J, Gaike ME, *et al.* Survival of patients with localized diffuse histiocytic lymphoma. *Blood* 1981; **58**, 1218–23.
54. Vokes EE, Ultmann JE, Golomb HM, *et al.* Long-term survival of patients with localized diffuse histiocytic lymphoma. *J Clin Oncol* 1985; **3**, 1309–17.
55. Hallahan DE, Farah R, Vokes EE, *et al.* The patterns of failure in patients with pathological stage I and II diffuse histiocytic lymphoma treated with radiation therapy alone. *Int J Radiat Oncol Biol Phys* 1989; **17**, 767–71.
56. Toonkel LM, Fuller LM, Gamble JF, *et al.* Laparotomy stage I and II non-Hodgkin's lymphomas: preliminary results of radiotherapy and adjunctive chemotherapy. *Cancer* 1980; **45**, 249–60.
57. National Cancer Institute. *Physicians Data Query (PDQ) on Treatment of Non-Hodgkin's Lymphoma.* Bethesda, MD: NCI, 1994.
58. Kaminski MS, Coleman CN, Colby TV, *et al.* Factors predicting survival in adults with stage I and II large-cell lymphoma treated with primary radiation therapy. *Ann Intern Med* 1986; **104**, 747–56.
59. Mauch P, Leonard R, Skarin A, *et al.* Improved survival following combined radiation therapy and chemotherapy for unfavorable prognosis stage I–II non-Hodgkin's lymphomas. *J Clin Oncol* 1985; **3**, 1301–8.
60. Miller TP, Jones SE. Chemotherapy of localized histiocytic lymphoma. *Lancet* 1979; **1**, 1358–60.
61. Cabanillas F. Chemotherapy as definitive treatment of stage I–II large cell and diffuse mixed lymphomas. *Hematol Oncol* 1985; **3**, 25.
62. Miller TP, Jones SE. Initial chemotherapy for clinically localized lymphomas of unfavorable histology. *Blood* 1983; **62**, 413–18.
63. Prestidge BR, Horning SJ, Hoppe RT. Combined modality therapy for stage I–II large cell lymphoma. *Int J Radiat Oncol Biol Phys* 1988; **15**, 633–9.
64. Connors JM, Klimo P, Fairey RN, *et al.* Brief chemotherapy and involved field radiation therapy for limited-staged histologically aggressive lymphomas. *Ann Intern Med* 1987; **107**, 25–30.
65. Longo DL, Glatstein E, Duffey PL, *et al.* Treatment of localized aggressive lymphomas with combination chemotherapy followed by involved-field radiation therapy. *J Clin Oncol* 1989; **7**, 1295–1302.
66. Jones SE, Miller TP, Connors JM. Long-term follow-up and analysis for prognostic factors for patients with limited-stage diffuse large-cell lymphomas treated with initial chemotherapy with or without adjuvant radiotherapy. *J Clin Oncol* 1989; **7**, 1186–91.
67. Tondini C, Zanini M, Lombardi F, *et al.* Combined modality treatment with primary CHOP chemotherapy followed by locoregional irradiation in stage I or II histologically aggressive non-Hodgkin's lymphomas. *J Clin Oncol* 1993; **11**, 720–5.

68. Sullivan FJ, Hann SM, Johnstone PA, *et al.* Radiation therapy in the National Cancer Institute combined modality trial of localized aggressive non-Hodgkin's lymphoma: what constitutes the involved field? *J Clin Oncol* (submitted).

69. Longo DL, DeVita VT, Jaffe ES, *et al.* Lymphocytic lymphomas. In: VT Devita, S Hellman, SA Rosenberg, eds, *Cancer Principles and Practice of Oncology,* 4th edn. Philadelphia: JB Lippincott Co, 1993; 1905–12.

70. Fisher RI, Gaynor ER, Dahlberg S, *et al.* Comparison of standard regimen (CHOP) with three intensive chemotherapy regimens for advanced non-Hodgkin's lymphoma. *N Engl J Med* 1993; **328**, 1002–6.

71. Shipp MA, Klatt MM, Beaw Y, *et al.* Patterns of relapse in large-cell lymphoma patients with bulk disease: implications for the use of radiation therapy. *J Clin Oncol* 1989; **7**, 613–18.

72. Wollner N, Wachtel AE, Exelby PR, *et al.* Improved prognosis in children with intra-abdominal non-Hodgkin's lymphoma following $LSA_2-L_2$ protocol chemotherapy. *Cancer* 1980; **45**, 3034–9.

73. Weinstein HJ, Cassady JR, Levey R, *et al.* Long-term results of the APO protocol (vincristine, doxorubicin and prednisone) for the treatment of mediastinal lymphoblastic lymphoma. *J Clin Oncol* 1983; **1**, 537–44.

74. Coleman CN, Picozzi VJ Jr, Cox RS, *et al.* Treatment of lymphoblastic lymphoma in adults. *J Clin Oncol* 1986; **4**, 1628–36.

75. Magrath IT, Janus C, Edwards BK, *et al.* An effective therapy in both undifferentiated (including Burkitt's) lymphomas and lymphoblastic lymphomas in children and young adults. *Blood* 1984; **63**, 1102–8.

76. Straus DJ, Wong GY, Liu J, *et al.* Small non-cleaved cell lymphoma (undifferentiated lymphoma, Burkitt's type) in American adults: results with treatment designed for acute lymphoblastic leukemia. *Am J Med* 1991; **90**, 328–37.

77. McMaster ML, Greer JP, Greco FA, *et al.* Effective treatment of small non-cleaved cell lymphoma with high-intensity, brief duration chemotherapy. *J Clin Oncol* 1991; **9**, 941–6.

78. Gill PS, Levin AM, Krailo M, *et al.* Aids-related malignant lymphoma: results of prospective treatment trials. *J Clin Oncol* 1987; **5**, 1322–8.

79. Levine AM, Wernz JC, Kaplan L, *et al.* Low-dose chemotherapy with central nervous system prophylaxis and zidovudine maintenance in AIDS-related lymphoma: a prospective multi-institutional trial. *JAMA* 1991; **266**, 84–8.

80. Walsh C. Colony-stimulating factors in the treatment of HIV-associated non-Hodgkin's lymphoma. *Oncol* 1989; **3**, 79–86.

81. Shimm DS, Dosoretz DE, Anderson T, *et al.* Primary gastric lymphoma: an analysis with emphasis on prognostic factors and radiation therapy. *Cancer* 1983; **52**, 2044–8.

82. Shiu MH, Nisce LZ, Pinna A, *et al.* Recent results of multimodal therapy of gastric lymphoma. *Cancer* 1986; **58**, 1389–99.

83. Mittal B, Wasserman TH, Griffith RC. Non-Hodgkin's lymphoma of the stomach. *Am J Gastroenterol* 1983; **78**, 781–7.

84. Ricci JL, Turnbull ADM. Spontaneous gastroduodenal perforation in cancer patients receiving cytotoxic therapy. *J Surg Oncol* 1989; **41**, 219–21.

85. Maor MH, Velasquez WS, Fuller LM, *et al.* Stomach conservation in stage IE and IIE gastric non-Hodgkin's lymphoma. *J Clin Oncol* 1990; **8**, 266–71.

86. DeAngelis LM, Yaholom J, Thaler HT, *et al.* Combined modality therapy for primary CNS lymphoma. *J Clin Oncol* 1992; **10**, 635–43.

87. Nelson DF, Martz KL, Bonner H, *et al.* Non-Hodgkin's lymphoma of the brain: can high dose, large volume radiation therapy improve survival? Report on a prospective trial by the Radiation Therapy Group (RTOG): RTOG 8315. *Int J Radiat Oncol Biol Physics* 1992; **23**, 9–17.

88. Neuwelt EA, Goldman DI, Suellen AD, *et al.* Primary CNS lymphoma treated with osmotic blood–brain barrier disruption: prolonged survival and preserva-

tion of cognitive function. *J Clin Oncol* 1991; **9**, 1580–90.

89. Doria R, Jekel JF, Cooper DL. Non-Hodgkin's lymphoma of the thyroid gland: prognostic factors and treatment outcome. The Princess Margaret Hospital Lymphoma Group. *Int J Radiat Oncol Biol Phys* 1993; **27**, 599–604.

90. Vigliotti A, Kong JS, Fuller LM. Thyroid lymphoma. The case for combined modality therapy. *Cancer* 1994; **73**, 200–6.

91. Vigliotti A, Kong JS, Fuller LM, *et al.* Thyroid lymphomas stages IE and IIE: comparative results for radiotherapy only, combination chemotherapy only, and multimodality treatment. *Int J Radiat Oncol Biol Phys* 1986; **12**, 1807–12.

92. Logue JP, Hale RJ, Stewart AL, *et al.* Primary malignant lymphoma of the thyroid: a clinicopathological analysis. *Int J Radiat Oncol Biol Phys* 1992; **22**, 929–33.

93. Smitt MC, Donaldson SS, *et al.* Radiotherapy is successful treatment for orbital lymphoma. *Int J Radiat Oncol Biol Phys* 1993; **26**, 59–66.

94. Harisiadis L, Misisco DJ, Schell MC, *et al.* Irradiation of bilateral orbital lymphoma: a non-coplanar technique with case reports. *Radiat Oncol* 1987; **8**, 123–8.

95. Minehan KJ, Martenson JA, Garrity JA, *et al.* Local control and complications after radiation therapy for primary orbital lymphoma: a case for low-dose treatment. *Int J Radiat Oncol Biol Phys* 1991; **20**, 791–6.

96. Buskirks SJ, Richard GE, Banks PM, *et al.* Primary lymphoma of testis. *Int J Radiat Oncol Biol Phys* 1982; **8**, 1699–703.

97. Connors JM, Klimo P, Voss N, *et al.* Testicular lymphoma: improved outcome with brief early chemotherapy. *J Clin Oncol* 1988; **6**, 776–81.

98. Barr J, Burkes R, Bell R, *et al.* Primary non-Hodgkin's lymphoma of bone. *Cancer* 1994; **73**, 1194–9.

99. Fairbanks RK, Banner JA, Carrie YI, *et al.* Treatment of Stage IE primary lymphoma of bone. *Int J Radiat Oncol Biol Phys* 1994; **28**, 363–72.

# 13 Current management of multiple myeloma

*Catherine D Williams and Jeffrey S Tobias*

## Introduction

Multiple myeloma is an uncontrolled, malignant proliferation of plasma cells in the bone marrow. The formation of plasma cell tumours causes bone destruction, marrow failure, production of a monoclonal immunoglobulin (or light chain) and suppression of normal immunoglobulin synthesis. A small proportion of patients will have a single bone lesion (solitary plasmacytoma); however, the majority will have more widespread disease. The disease may remain asymptomatic and stable for months or years before it progresses to the symptomatic stage. Multiple myeloma accounts for about 1% of all malignancies and the annual incidence worldwide is approximately 4 per 100 000 of the population. There is a clear male predisposition and it is twice as common in blacks than in whites.[1] It occurs predominantly in the elderly; the mean age at diagnosis is 65 years and, although the disease can occur in those much younger, onset before the age of 40 years is very uncommon.[2]

The sensitivity of multiple myeloma to radiation has long been recognized[3] and, until the 1950s, radiotherapy was the only treatment available. Towards the end of that decade, chemotherapy was introduced as an alternative treatment and proved to be more effective. As a result, radiotherapy took second place and was used mainly for the palliation of painful sites.[4] However, despite nearly 40 years of systemic drug treatment, the prognosis has changed little since its introduction, with less than 10% of patients living beyond 10 years after diagnosis and no suggestion of a plateau of long survivors.[5] Recently, attention has turned to alternative systemic therapies, such as hemibody irradiation and total body irradiation, combined with chemotherapy and bone marrow transplantation. Local radiotherapy remains of particular importance in providing pain relief and for the management of complications such as fracture or spinal cord compression.

## Solitary plasmacytoma of bone

About 5% of patients with myeloma will have a single, painful bone lesion due to a monoclonal cell infiltrate, with further studies showing no evidence of bone marrow plasmacytosis. This solitary lesion, known as a plasmacytoma, may involve any bone but most commonly arises in the vertebrae, occurring in this site in approximately one-third of patients. Myeloma protein (M-protein) is found in the serum and/or urine in about 50% of patients.[6]

The treatment of choice for this condition is local radiotherapy, using external beam radiotherapy with cobalt-60 or a linear accelerator. Treatment fields should encompass all defined disease and include a margin of normal tissue. The dose of radiation required may vary but, though lower doses may be sufficient, most centres recommend 40 and 55 Gy to achieve the best chance of cure.[6,7] Nearly all patients will be relieved of pain, and local tumour recurrence is less than 10%. The myeloma protein disappears in 25–50% of evaluable patients,[8] possibly indicating that the disease has been completely eradicated. About one-third of patients will remain disease-free for more than 10 years; the others will eventually develop multiple myeloma, the median time for this being 2–3 years. The median overall survival of patients with a solitary plasmacytoma exceeds 10 years, with 10–20% of patients dying from other, unrelated, causes. In several studies, non-secretory disease and persistent myeloma protein after treatment have been found to be adverse prognostic factors.[8,9] There is no convincing evidence that adjuvant chemotherapy improves the prognosis; however, α-interferon may be worth considering after radiotherapy in light of recent studies.[10]

## Multiple myeloma

### Diagnosis and when to treat

The first and most important step in the management of multiple myeloma is to be sure of the diagnosis. The disease must be distinguished from a monoclonal gammopathy of unknown significance (MGUS), as the latter condition does not require any treatment. MGUS is defined as an isolated serum monoclonal protein of < 30 g/l with < 10% plasma cells in the marrow. There are no other signs or symptoms of multiple myeloma present, such as anaemia, renal failure or hypercalcaemia, though a small proportion of patients have Bence-Jones proteinuria. In one series, 22% of patients with MGUS went on to develop multiple myeloma at a median time of 9.6 years after recognition of the M-protein.[11] Although these patients do not require treatment, indefinite follow-up is essential to recognize if multiple myeloma, macroglobulinaemia, amyloidosis or a related disorder develops.

Smouldering multiple myeloma (SMM) is typically characterized by a serum M-protein level of > 30 g/l and > 10% plasma cells in the bone marrow (Fig. 13.1). There is, however, no anaemia, renal insufficiency or lytic lesions and all ancillary tests are negative. Treatment of SMM is usually inappropriate[12] as alkylating agents can lead to myelodysplasia or secondary leukaemias. If these patients are entered into clinical trials of chemotherapy or bone marrow transplantation they must be stratified separately, as their very long survival may skew the results of the study.[13] However, once again, they must be carefully followed up for disease progression to multiple myeloma, which will require treatment. Diagnostic criteria for MGUS, SMM and multiple myeloma are outlined in Table 13.1.

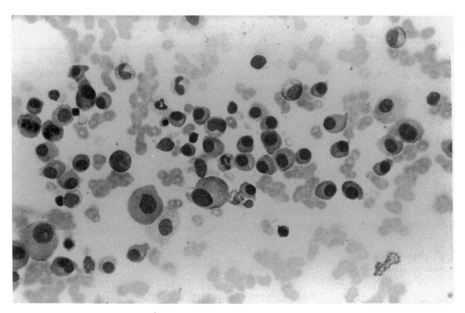

**Fig. 13.1** Bone marrow aspirate from a patient with multiple myeloma showing marked infiltration with plasma cells, characterized by a large, eccentric nucleus.

## Staging

A clinical staging system for multiple myeloma was devised by Durie and Salmon[14] by analysing data on seventy-one patients and relating clinical features with myeloma cell mass (myeloma cells $\times$ $10^{12}/m^2$ of body surface area). Response to chemotherapy and survival in these patients showed a significant correlation with measured myeloma cell burden. The staging system is shown in Table 13.2 and divides patients into three stages, with tumour burden and prognosis worsening the higher the stage. Placing patients into a staging category at diagnosis may assist in deciding which treatment is appropriate and is also useful for both recruiting patients and analysing data in clinical trials.

**Table 13.1** Diagnostic criteria for MGUS, SMM and multiple myeloma

*MGUS*
Serum monoclonal protein < 30 g/l
Less than 10% plasma cells in the bone marrow and no aggregates on
  trephine biopsy
No anaemia, renal failure or hypercalcaemia
Ancillary tests negative: Bone lesions absent on radiographic bone survey
                         Bone marrow plasma cell labelling index < 0.8
                         Normal β2 microglobulin level
                         Urinary light chain < 500 mg/24 hrs

*SMM*
Serum monoclonal protein > 30 g/l
Greater than 10% plasma cells in the bone marrow or aggregates on
  trephine biopsy
No anaemia, renal failure or hypercalcaemia
Ancillary tests negative: Bone lesions absent on radiographic bone survey
                         Bone marrow plasma cell labelling index < 0.8
                         Normal β2 microglobulin level
                         Urinary light chain < 500 mg/24 hrs

*Multiple myeloma*
M-protein present in serum or urine (usually > 30 g/l)
Greater than 10% plasma cells in the bone marrow or aggregates on
  trephine biopsy (or histological proof of a plasmacytoma)
One or more ancillary findings (must not be attributable to another cause):
                         Anaemia
                         Renal failure
                         Lytic lesions (on X-ray, computed tomography or
                         magnetic resonance imaging) or severe osteoporosis
                         Hypercalcaemia
                         Raised β 2 microglobulin level
                         Plasma cell labelling index > 0.8

## Prognostic factors

Determination of prognostic factors in individual patients has become
increasingly important in recent years, as selected patients may now have
the option of high dose therapy and bone marrow transplantation. Also,
proper recognition of these factors allows patients being entered into clinical trials to be stratified. The Durie–Salmon staging system [14] remains the
main prognostic indicator for patients with multiple myeloma, due to its
simplicity and easy application to all patients. Serum β2 microglobulin and
plasma cell labelling index (PCLI) are also now recognized as two of the
most significant independent indicators;[15,16] at least one of these should be
measured in all patients at diagnosis. Both the Durie–Salmon staging system and the β2 microglobulin relate to tumour burden, whereas the PCLI
does not. Serum markers such as C-reactive protein have been thought to
be useful as markers of high-risk disease[17] but this has recently been dis-
puted.[16] Other serum markers, such as lactate dehydrogenase,[18] may also
identify poor prognostic groups. Immunoglobulin isotype does not appear

**Table 13.2**   Myeloma staging system

| Stage | Criteria | Measured myeloma cell mass (cells × 10$^{12}$/m$^2$) |
|---|---|---|
| I | *All* of the following:<br>1. Haemoglobin > 10 g/dl<br>2. Serum calcium value normal (≤ 3.0 mmol/l)<br>3. Normal bone structure on X-ray or<br>   solitary bone plasmacytoma only<br>4. Low M-component production rates:<br>   a. IgG value < 50 g/l<br>   b. IgA value < 30 g/l<br>   c. Urinary light-chain M-component<br>      on immunofixation < 4 g/24 hrs | 0.6<br>(Low) |
| II | Fitting neither Stage I nor Stage III | 0.6–1.20<br>(Intermediate) |
| III | One or more of the following:<br>1. Haemoglobin < 8.5 g/dl<br>2. Serum calcium value > 3.0 mmol/l<br>3. Advanced lytic bone lesions (Scale 3)<br>4. High M-component production rates:<br>   a. IgG value > 70 g/l<br>   b. IgA value > 50 g/l<br>   c. Urinary light-chain M-component<br>      on immunofixation > 12 g/24 hrs | > 1.20<br>(High) |

*Subclassification*

A = Relatively normal renal function (serum creatinine < 180 μmol/l)
B = Abnormal renal function (serum creatinine ≥ 180 μmol/l)

to make any difference in patients receiving standard dose chemotherapy; however, those with an IgG isotype do appear to have better results with high dose therapy and bone marrow transplantation.[19] Evaluation of these factors has now enabled good separation of particularly good and poor prognostic groups but there remains a large intermediate group of patients for whom the outcome is less clear. It is hoped that the introduction of new biological techniques will allow the measurement of IL6, the central growth factor in multiple myeloma, and also the IL6 receptor (IL6R) which is expressed on the cell surface of myeloma cells but not on normal plasma cells. These parameters may further delineate prognostic groups.

## Symptomatic treatment

Patients presenting with newly diagnosed myeloma frequently have severe symptoms related to their disease, such as bone pain, paraplegia, hypercalcaemia, renal failure, infections, anaemia and thrombocytopenia. These need prompt, effective treatment in order to make the patient more comfortable and allow initiation of systemic treatment for the disease as soon as possible, and also because these disorders can, in themselves, be life threatening.

### Localized radiation therapy for bone pain/paraplegia

Radiotherapy plays a particularly important role in the treatment of bone pain and paraplegia. Severe bone pain at a particular focal site is the major presenting feature in over 60% of patients with multiple myeloma, or often develops during the early months of chemotherapy in spite of improvements in other respects. Generalized bone pain may also not resolve for months with standard drug treatments. Pain is usually at the site of osteolytic lesions and demineralization produced by the stimulation of osteoclasts by an activating factor released from neoplastic myeloma cells (Fig. 13.2a,b).

The treatment of choice in these cases is localized irradiation, which is given to relieve pain or for the management of complications such as fracture or spinal cord compression. For pain relief, a dose of 8 Gy, administered in a single fraction, is usually employed,[20] although smaller doses may be sufficient. Following fractionated courses, pain relief (complete or partial) is achieved in just over 90% of patients with myeloma by the time the course of radiotherapy is completed (delivering 15–20 Gy in fractions of 2–3 Gy or 30–35 Gy in ten to fifteen fractions). There is no difference in rapidity of onset or duration of pain relief between a single fraction of 8 Gy and a fractionated course.[4] Irradiation of a fracture (or impending fraction) of a long bone should be delivered either before, or after, surgical fixation. Prophylactic fixation is recommended for impending fracture as this is often followed by more rapid mobilization than if a fracture had already occurred. The most important factor for neurological recovery in cases of spinal cord compression is rapid diagnosis and treatment. High dose dexamethasone should be commenced on clinical suspicion, and irradiation given as soon as urgent magnetic resonance imaging (MRI) or myelography has confirmed the diagnosis, or as soon as possible after surgical decompression. Fractionated radiotherapy, using doses of 25–30 Gy in 1–2 weeks, is generally preferred due to the risk of radiation-induced oedema following large single fractions.

### Renal failure

Renal dysfunction is present at diagnosis in about 50% of patients with multiple myeloma. It is often due to a combination of factors such as dehydration, hypercalcaemia, hyperuricaemia and light-chain deposition causing tubular damage. Until recently, there was a high fatality rate among these patients as shown in the third Medical Research Council (MRC) trial.[21] Seventy per cent of the patients who presented with a serum urea of > 15 mmol/l had died within 100 days. This mortality rate has now been greatly reduced by simple measures such as vigorous rehydration and the treatment of hypercalcaemia before, and during, intensive chemotherapy. This was shown in the fourth MRC trial[22] when patients whose serum urea was still > 15 mmol/l or serum creatinine was > 200 µmol/l after 48 hrs of

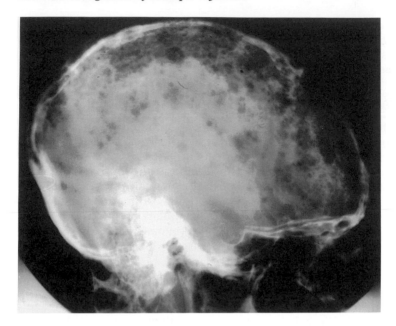

a

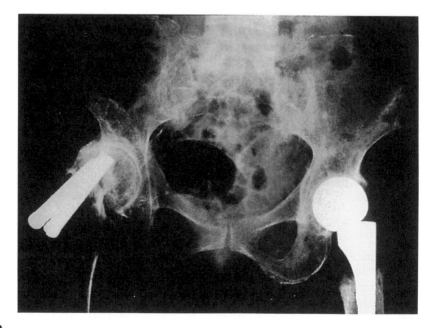

b

**Fig. 13.2**   Lytic bone lesions in multiple myeloma. (a) Lateral X-ray of the skull of a patient with multiple myeloma showing the classic 'pepperpot' appearance. (b) Pelvic X-ray in advanced-stage myeloma showing marked demineralization, lytic lesions and evidence of previous fractures.

hydration therapy continued to receive 3 litres of fluid daily for at least 3 months. Following this, the fatality in the first 100 days fell to 40%, while the serum creatinine returned to normal in one-third of the survivors. Treatment for hypercalcaemia should also be administered, if necessary, and allopurinol, in reduced doses for renal failure, should be given for hyperuricaemia, if indicated.

## Hypercalcaemia

About 30% of patients present with acute hypercalcaemia (serum calcium > 2.75 mmol/l) and a further 30% will develop it during the course of the disease. Symptoms include anorexia, nausea and vomiting, polydipsia, polyuria, abdominal pain and constipation. Eventually mental confusion and drowsiness may develop. Renal failure may be precipitated by the deposition of calcium salts in the renal parenchyma. Urgent treatment is required in all cases, and supervised intravenous hydration combined with a loop diuretic, such as frusemide, will be effective in most patients. Steroids, such as prednisolone, can be added at 30 mg daily and may correct the hypercalcaemia by blocking the activation of osteoclasts. In addition, diphosphonates are increasingly used in the treatment of acute hypercalcaemia. These agents are pyrophosphate analogues which depress the activity of osteoclasts, reducing bone resorption. Using intravenous diphosphonate therapy, the serum calcium levels usually fall to normal limits within 2–4 days in the majority of patients,[23,24] though they may rise again within 10–14 days of treatment, in which case maintenance therapy with oral diphosphonates may become necessary.

## Infection

Patients with multiple myeloma are particularly prone to infection as they usually have an immune paresis, secondary to the high levels of serum M-protein. They may also be neutropenic if their bone marrow is heavily infiltrated with plasma cells. At diagnosis, any signs of infection should be sought and treated promptly with the appropriate antibiotics, given intravenously if necessary. Within the first year of treatment, approximately 20% of patients will suffer from pneumonia, which may be fatal, particularly in elderly patients. It is advisable for patients to keep their own supply of amoxycillin or cotrimoxazole.

## Anaemia and thrombocytopenia

Bone marrow failure due to infiltration of plasma cells may be present at diagnosis and is often exacerbated during the early stages of treatment by chemotherapy. This often results in anaemia, which may require red cell transfusions, and in thrombocytopenia. Platelet transfusions are rarely required but may be necessary if there are any signs of bleeding, if an invasive procedure is planned, or prophylactically, if the platelet count drops below $20 \times 10^9/l$. Non-steroidal anti-inflammatory drugs, including aspirin, should be avoided in any patient who is thrombocytopenic.

## Chemotherapy

Chemotherapy is the mainstay of treatment for multiple myeloma, though the choice of agents and the doses employed have become increasingly controversial in the last 10 years. As approximately 50% of patients with multiple myeloma are over 65 years of age, aggressive treatments were initially not favoured and, as a result, oral melphalan (L-PAM), combined with prednisolone (MP), was introduced in the 1960s.[25] However, the fact that 30–40% of patients remained refractory to this treatment, and the growing realization that there were many younger patients with the disease who might tolerate more intensive therapy, led to the introduction of combination chemotherapy in the 1980s. However, the superiority of these newer regimens is still not clear, despite many clinical trials and meta-analyses,[26] and their benefit over MP remains controversial.

### *Melphalan and prednisolone*

The combination of melphalan, an alkylating agent, and prednisolone was introduced over 20 years ago and remains the 'gold standard' for management of patients with multiple myeloma.[27] It is certainly the initial treatment of choice for elderly patients and for patients unable to tolerate combination chemotherapy. Melphalan is administered at $8 \, mg/m^2$ on Days 1–4 inclusive, and prednisolone at 1–1.5 mg/kg, also on Days 1–4. Both drugs are given orally and a pulse schedule is used, repeating the treatment every 4–6 weeks, depending on blood counts. The variability of absorption of melphalan is a major concern of this treatment and sequential dose escalation (in 20% increments) may be employed to produce at least some myelosuppression.[28] Recently, a European study has suggested that resistance may be explained by intrinsic differences in cell sensitivity, rather than absorption, by showing similar drug-induced white cell and platelet count reduction in both responding and non-responding patients.[29] Renal failure influences both the toxicity and effectiveness of melphalan, so careful monitoring of blood counts and biochemistry is recommended in patients with renal dysfunction. General dose reduction is not necessary due to the individual variations in absorption. A fluid intake of at least 3 l/day is essential for all patients taking the drug.[22]

Response to treatment can be categorized according to various parameters. A reduction in the myeloma protein of 50% is considered a good clinical response[30] and will be seen in about 50–60% of newly diagnosed patients.[26] Of these responders, approximately two-thirds (i.e. 40% of all patients) will achieve a partial remission (PR), defined as at least a 75% reduction in the production of serum myeloma protein, a 95% reduction in Bence-Jones proteinuria, and a reduction of bone marrow infiltration to less than 5% plasma cells. A small group of patients (about 3% of all those treated) will achieve complete remission (CR), defined as complete disappearance of the M-protein and Bence-Jones proteinuria, and a normal bone marrow biopsy.[31] Evaluation of response to therapy should be carried out at 3 months to identify those patients who remain resistant to treatment. This must include measurement of serum immunoglobulins (by immunofixation) and urinary Bence-Jones protein, and bone marrow examination.

Failure of response at this stage is an indication to start alternative therapy.

In most responding patients the disease will reach a 'plateau' after an initial improvement, despite continued treatment. This usually occurs within the first year but the optimal duration of treatment thereafter remains unclear. Several studies show that indefinite maintenance therapy until relapse offers no survival advantage,[28,32] but does increase the risk of developing secondary leukaemias. It is now generally recommended that induction therapy should continue for 12–18 months, with treatment either stopping at the time of reaching plateau or continuing for up to 6 months beyond this time. All patients stopping therapy must be monitored carefully for possibility of relapse. Serum and urinary myeloma proteins, bone marrow examination and a skeletal survey should be repeated at this time. The patient should then be seen and reviewed regularly. Relapse may occur in 10–15% of patients without an increase in the myeloma protein[33] and may only be revealed by an increase in number or size of bony lesions. In addition, relapse may develop in extramedullary sites. Serial measurement of the serum $\beta$ 2 microglobulin can be useful as it may increase significantly either before, or at the time of, clinical relapse.

The median duration of remission (or 'plateau') is approximately 2 years, and median overall survival is approximately 3 years. Less than 10% of patients live longer than 10 years after diagnosis.[34] This compares to a mean survival of 7.1 months 40 years ago, before the introduction of chemotherapy, although other factors such as early diagnosis (one-third of patients are now diagnosed on routine serum protein electrophoresis before any evidence of clinical symptoms)[35] and improved supportive care have also influenced survival. Factors which influence response and survival are discussed above (see section, 'Prognostic factors').

### Combination chemotherapy

Combination chemotherapy was introduced in the early 1970s, as the combined use of non-cross-resistant drugs was presumed to be more effective than a single agent.[36,37] Since that time, several chemotherapeutic regimens have been tried in the treatment of multiple myeloma. Unfortunately, the advantages offered by these new regimens over standard melphalan and prednisolone therapy have been extremely difficult to assess for several reasons. First, there has been a failure to run randomized trials of sufficient size and, second, patients entered into these trials are very heterogeneous, with some more likely to benefit from chemotherapy than others. Stratification of patients within trials by prognostic factors has rarely been performed. As a result, response and survival data have been varied, with combination chemotherapy being shown to be superior to MP in inducing remission in virtually all studies, but no improvement in survival in the majority of trials.[38–44] A meta-analysis of eighteen trials which compared the results of combination chemotherapy to MP found no difference in overall efficacy, with survival as the endpoint between the two treatments.[26] Nonetheless, it is important to note that two of the largest studies conducted, which incorporate combinations of alkylating agents plus an anthracycline, both show significant survival benefits over melphalan therapy (see Table 13.3). The Southwest Oncology Group (SWOG) study[45] compared

**Table 13.3** Results of combination chemotherapy compared with melphalan and prednisolone

| Study | Regimen | Control | P-value (if known) |
|---|---|---|---|
| SWOG[45] | VMCP–VBAP | MP | |
| Overall response | 53% | 32% | |
| Overall survival (at 8 years) | 20% | 10% | |
| Median survival (months) | 42 | 23 | $P = 0.021$ |
| MRC[46] | ABCM | M | |
| Overall response | 61% | 49% | $P = 0.004$ |
| Overall survival (at 5 years) | 24% | 17% | |
| Median survival (months) | 32 | 24 | $P = 0.0003$ |
| Samson *et al.*[47] | VAD | M7 | |
| Overall response | 84% | 57% | $P < 0.05$ |
| Overall survival (at 2 years) | 75% | 50% | $P =$ Not significant |
| Median survival (months) | 44 | 24 | $P < 0.05$ |

M: melphalan in any dose schedule (usually given intermittently); M7: melphalan given in a specific dose schedule defined by the MRC.

the results of vincristine, melphalan, cyclophosphamide and prednisolone (VMCP) alternating with vincristine, BCNU (1-3-bis(2-chloroethyl)-l-nitrosourea, or carmustine), doxorubicin and prednisolone (VBAP) with the results of vincristine, cyclophosphamide and prednisolone (VCP) by means of a randomized trial. Four hundred and forty previously untreated patients were recruited and the two treatment groups balanced for major prognostic factors. The patients receiving the VMCP–VBAP had a median survival of 48 months — a significant difference compared with the 29 months survival in the VCP-treated group and 23 months in a comparable group of patients treated with MP in a previous study. The fifth MRC trial[46] compared intermittent melphalan (M7) with ABCM (doxorubicin, BCNU, cyclophosphamide, melphalan) as first-line treatment. Levels of $\beta2$ microglobulin at presentation were used as a prognostic factor to stratify patients. Overall, survival was longer in the group receiving ABCM ($P = 0.0003$). The 75% median and 25% survivals were, respectively, 7, 24 and 42 months with M7, and 10, 32 and 56 months with ABCM. Plateau was achieved by 61% of the patients given ABCM and 49% of those given M7 ($P = 0.004$).

Newer regimens using vincristine and doxorubicin as an infusion over several days, followed by high dose steroids, have been introduced in the last 5 years as both primary and relapse therapy for myeloma.[47,48] VAD (vincristine, doxorubicin, dexamethasone) can be given at full dose even in the presence of renal failure and has been reported as achieving a response in over 80% of patients. Similarly, VAMP (vincristine, doxorubicin, methylprednisolone), either alone or combined with cyclophosphamide (C-VAMP), also offers a high level of both overall and complete response. However, the responses are not lasting with any of these regimens and, hence, in an effort to improve survival, they are now being used by some centres in combination with myeloablative therapy and bone marrow transplantation.

### Choice of chemotherapy

The choice of induction chemotherapy remains controversial and will vary between treatment centres and even individual physicians. Overall, melphalan and prednisolone is still considered the standard therapy as it is easy to administer and less expensive. Combination chemotherapy such as ABCM is generally the preferred treatment in young patients (i.e. < 65 years) with MP being used in older patients or those unable to tolerate intravenous therapy. Recent results imply that MP may be superior for patients with an intrinsically good prognosis and inferior for those patients with a poor prognosis.[26] VAD or C-VAMP regimens are the treatment of choice in patients with renal failure, as no dose-reduction is necessary and excretion of the drugs is predominantly non-renal. Similarly, these regimens are now widely used in patients resistant to previous chemotherapy and in younger patients who may proceed to high dose chemotherapy and bone marrow transplantation.

## Double hemibody irradiation

Multiple myeloma is a disease in which the sensitivity to radiation has long been recognized, so the suggestion that systemic irradiation may be of value in its treatment is not unreasonable. This was first postulated in the early 1970s, with the suggestion that division of total body irradiation (TBI) into two doses, 4–6 weeks apart, would allow recovery of irradiated marrow.[49] This technique is known as double hemibody irradiation (DHBI).

Techniques vary, but patients generally receive radiation therapy initially to either their upper or lower hemibody fields, as indicated by their site of maximum pain. The second HBI is administered approximately 6–12 weeks after the first, when the blood count is showing signs of bone marrow recovery. A neutrophil count of $> 1 \times 10^9/l$ and platelet count of $> 100 \times 10^9/l$ are suitable levels at which to consider giving the second dose. The upper-body field is generally positioned from the lower border of the mandible, with the head fully extended, to the umbilicus. It may be extended to include the skull with shielding of the eyes and mouth, but the toxicity of the technique will be correspondingly greater. If the skull is not included, however, there may be a risk of isolated disease progression at this site.[50] The lower field is from the umbilicus to the mid-calf. In our practice, irradiation is administered from a slow cobalt source at a dose of 0.25 Gy/min using an anteroposterior field arrangement at a source–skin distance (SSD) of 200 cm. The optimal dose of HBI is controversial, as higher doses increase the risk of radiation pneumonitis but lower doses may be less effective. The standard dose is 7.5 Gy to the upper hemibody and 10 Gy to the lower hemibody, with separate skull fields which deliver a midplane dose of 3 Gy daily for 3 days. Some centres use fractionated HBI, particularly in patients who have received previous intensive chemotherapy and may be at risk of radiation pneumonitis.[51] This, however, may lead to the patient receiving a lower equivalent dose. Dose reductions may be necessary if the patient is neutropenic and/or thrombocytopenic, and patients treated at a higher dose rate (e.g. by linear accelerator) should also have a dose reduction of approximately 25%.

Side-effects of HBI include nausea and vomiting, which occur in up to 50% of patients during the 48 hrs after treatment, though appropriate pre-medication with antiemetics may help. Loss of taste may occur, which can last for up to 3 weeks, and also dryness of the mouth, which can last for 3 months. Transient alopecia is usual when the skull is treated. Diarrhoea, vaginitis and/or dermatitis of the thigh may occur following lower HBI. As already mentioned, leucopenia and thrombocytopenia are common and are often more severe when the marrow is heavily infiltrated. Approximately 30% of patients require platelet transfusions post-DHBI, and over 60% require red cell transfusions.[52,53] Mean time to achieve a total white cell count of $1 \times 10^9/l$ and a platelet count of $100 \times 10^9/l$ is about 3 months.[53] The most serious side-effect of upper-body HBI is radiation pneumonitis, which can be fatal. It usually occurs within 1–6 months after treatment and presents with cough and dyspnoea. Some cases respond to oral steroids. The risk of developing pneumonitis is increased by previous radiation to the lungs or mediastinum[54] and by previous drug treatment. The risks of developing pneumonitis are almost zero at doses up to 7.5 Gy, 3% with a dose of 8 Gy (single doses), increasing rapidly to 50% at 9.3 Gy,[55] thus giving further strength to the argument that single-fraction treatments should be kept below 8 Gy.

The most widely acknowledged result of HBI is rapid relief of bone pain, occasionally within 24–48 hrs[56] and regularly within 7 days.[52,57] It has also been reported to reduce the serum M-protein, Bence-Jones proteinuria, degree of hypercalcaemia and the level of marrow infiltration with myeloma cells.[52,58] Survival data from different studies are difficult to compare as patient characteristics and previous treatments received will vary. Several studies have found it to be beneficial to some patients, particularly those with drug-resistant disease, with response rates varying from 20%[51] to 100%.[59] Survival of over 19 months in some patients has been reported,[52,59] with patients having Stage I or II disease doing better than those with Stage III. In a recent study at our own centre, assessing the role of DHBI in fifty-five patients with relapsed or primary chemoresistant disease, the overall and progression-free survivals were 11 and 8 months, respectively.[53] Other studies investigating the role of HBI as consolidation therapy (after primary exposure to chemotherapy) have found little benefit from HBI compared with consolidation chemotherapy, with the side-effects being more severe.[51,60] Maintenance therapy post-HBI with α-interferon has shown no survival advantage.[53,61] Hence, the place of HBI in the treatment of multiple myeloma still remains controversial. As a 'consolidation' treatment it has not proved successful; however, its use in patients with chemoresistant disease, especially following relapse, appears to be of value and warrants further investigation.

## Myeloablative therapy

As already discussed, the survival of patients with multiple myeloma remains poor, despite an improved response rate with new combination chemotherapy regimens. As a result, there has been an increasing interest in high dose myeloablative therapy supported with either autologous or allogeneic bone marrow transplantation or, more recently, peripheral blood stem cells. Obviously, only younger patients with adequate cardiac and renal function would be eligible for transplantation and it is therefore not suitable for the majority of patients with multiple myeloma. Several studies have now been reported but results are difficult to compare due to the heterogeneity of both the disease with regard to stages and remission status at transplant and also the conditioning regimens used. Results of some of these studies are shown in Table 13.4. The efficacy of high dose therapy and transplant compared to treatment by chemotherapy alone remains unclear as there has not been, to date, any fully reported randomized study.

### The role of total body irradiation (TBI)

TBI was first described as a systemic therapy for multiple myeloma in 1956.[62] Low doses (approximately 2 Gy) were used and found to be well tolerated, and also to provide effective pain relief. With the development of bone marrow transplantation over the last decade, the combination of TBI with high dose chemotherapy can now be used in the treatment of multiple myeloma. Doses employed vary from 8 to 12 Gy and are usually combined with either intravenous high dose melphalan or cyclophosphamide. TBI can be given as either a single dose or fractionated over several days. Whether TBI–chemotherapy combinations are a more effective conditioning regimen than high dose chemotherapy alone remains controversial; however, several studies have shown an improved response rate with TBI in refractory patients.[63,64] Also, recent data show good response rates and survival durations in patients in early-phase disease.[65]

Side-effects of treatment include interstitial pneumonitis which occurs in up to 13% of matched and 47% of mismatched patients undergoing allogeneic BMT.[66] Incidence is lower with fractionated rather than single-dose irradiation regimens. Other side-effects of TBI include hypothyroidism, infertility and development of cataracts, all of which must be monitored for many years following treatment.

### Allogeneic bone marrow transplant (BMT)

Allogeneic bone marrow transplantation may, for the first time, present a possible cure in multiple myeloma as it allows high dose therapy combined with the reinfusion of bone marrow free of myeloma cells. It is, however, only available to a small select group of patients — those who are under 50 years of age with an HLA-matched sibling — making up about 4% of all patients with multiple myeloma. Several large studies have been reported

**Table 13.4**   Results of bone marrow transplant and peripheral blood stem cell transplant in multiple myeloma

| Study | Disease status at transplantation | No. of patients | Regimen | No. of patients | Outcome CR[a] | PFS |
|---|---|---|---|---|---|---|
| *Allogeneic bone marrow transplantation* | | | | | | |
| Gahrton et al.[67] | Responsive | 57 | Chemo + TBI | 81 | 58% | 31% at 3 yrs |
| | Resistant | 33 | Chemotherapy | 9 | | |
| Bensinger et al.[69] | Responsive | 10 | BU/CY | 20 | 80% | 32% at 17 months |
| | Resistant | 10 | | | | |
| *Autologous bone marrow transplantation* | | | | | | Overall survival |
| Jagannath et al.[19] | Responsive | 34 | Chemo + TBI | 55 | 27% | 82% at 48 months |
| | Resistant | 21 | | | | |
| Attal et al.[75] | Newly diagnosed | 35 | Chemo + TBI | 35 | 43% | 81% at 42 months |
| Cunningham et al.[77] | Newly diagnosed | 53 | Melphalan | 53 | 75% | 63% at 54 months |
| *Peripheral stem cell transplantation* | | | | | | |
| Fermand et al.[85] | Responsive | 19 | Chemo + TBI | 63 | 20% | 69% at 36 months |
| | Resistant | 44 | | | | |

[a] Percentage of *assessable* patients in complete remission (CR).
PFS: progression-free survival; BU/CY: busulphan/cyclophosphamide; TBI: total body irradiation.

over the last 5 years.[67-69] The procedure-related mortality ranges from 30%[67] up to 65%[68] in patients with resistant disease. A European Bone Marrow Transplant (EBMT) Registry study[67] looked at results from ninety patients undergoing allogeneic BMT from HLA-matched siblings, with more than 80% receiving TBI–chemotherapy conditioning. The CR rate was 43% and overall survival at 5 years was 40%. The median duration of relapse-free survival among patients who were in CR after transplantation was 48 months. Two post-transplantation factors pedicted better long-term survival: complete remission after engraftment and Grade I graft versus host disease, rather than Grades II, III or IV. A study from Seattle[69] looked at twenty patients who underwent allogeneic BMT with busulphan/cyclophosphamide conditioning. Eighty per cent of assessable patients achieved CR, which was sustained in 35%. Both these studies found that survival was better in patients with chemosensitive disease. Of particular note in these studies is the suggestion of a plateau in disease-free survival for patients who have survived 3 years from transplant. However, current analysis of EBMT data shows that the latest relapse, to date, has occurred 4 years post-transplant[70] and longer follow-up is therefore needed to judge whether these patients are cured. A recent update is now available.[103]

## Autologous BMT (ABMT)

Studies done at the Royal Marsden Hospital, Surrey, in the early 1980s showed that high dose melphalan (80–140 mg/m$^2$) can be used to achieve rapid and marked tumour cytoreduction in multiple myeloma.[71,72] This work, using melphalan (140 mg/m$^2$) alone, without BMT, has been recently updated with long-term follow-up on sixty-three patients.[73] Median duration of response was 18 months and no difference was seen between those patients achieving CR and those in PR. Overall median survival is 47 months with 35% of patients expected to be alive at 9 years after diagnosis. However, only six patients remain free from disease progression.

By the mid-1980s further studies were being performed looking at dose escalation of chemotherapy or combining it with total body irradiation. Studies from the MD Anderson Hospital[63,74] showed that mortality from these myeloablative conditioning regimens was reduced by autologous transplantation but that there was no evidence of durable remission in the majority of patients. More recently, several studies have evaluated the role of ABMT as consolidation following initial induction chemotherapy. Attal *et al.*[75] looked at the outcome of thirty-five patients treated with VAD or VMCP chemotherapy who went onto ABMT using melphalan (140 mg/m$^2$) and TBI (8.5 Gy) conditioning. A remission was achieved in 83% of the patients (CR in 43%), and at 33 months post-ABMT there was a 53% probability of progression-free survival. Similar results have been obtained at University College Hospital, London, where twenty-three patients underwent ABMT using TBI–melphalan conditioning.[76] Remission was achieved in 75% of patients and there was a 50% progression-free survival at a median follow-up time of 17 months. The Royal Marsden Hospital recently reported results on fifty-three patients,[77] updated from a previous study,[31] who received high dose melphalan (200 mg/m$^2$) plus methylprednisolone, 1.5 mg daily for 5 days, with ABMT after cytoreductive therapy. Seventy-five per cent of patients achieved CR post-ABMT and there was one treatment-related death. The estimated probability of survival at 54 months is 63%.

To date, there has been only one prospective randomized trial comparing ABMT with chemotherapy in myeloma, and only preliminary results are currently available.[65] Attal et al.[104] have recruited 200 patients with newly diagnosed multiple myeloma, of whom half have been treated with conventional chemotherapy (VMCP–BVAP) and the others with two courses of the same chemotherapy followed by ABMT (melphalan 140 mg/m$^2$, TBI 8 Gy). The prognostic factors of the two groups were comparable. In the first 100 patients, the response rate for those receiving ABMT was significantly higher than for those treated with conventional chemotherapy only: 24.5% of patients in the first group achieved CR compared with 2% in the latter group. Similarly, the probability of progression-free survival of the ABMT group is significantly better: 67% at 30 months compared with 10% in the chemotherapy-only arm. A further analysis of the study is due shortly.

A recent non-randomized study by Alexanian et al. looked at results in forty-nine patients with late-stage disease who had received at least 1 year of prior chemotherapy, and compared them with similar patients who did not receive intensive treatment for socioeconomic reasons.[78] Pre-ABMT, twenty-three patients had resistant relapse despite treatment with VAD chemotherapy, fifteen patients had prolonged primary resistance (> 1 year), and eleven patients were in late remission following successful treatment with VAD. All received TBI–chemotherapy conditioning. Of the twenty-three patients with resistant relapse, 61% had a response to ABMT, but the median remission time was only 3 months. Of the fifteen patients with primary resistance, six responded but none achieved CR. Median remission was 17 months in these patients. Only four of the eleven patients in late remission achieved CR and there has been disease recurrence within 2 years in nearly all these patients. Overall, survival was not improved compared with that of the control patients in all three groups.

Prognostic factors for outcome of transplant have been examined in several studies. A low β2 microglobulin level at diagnosis has been found to be favourable for response to transplant,[75] as have haemoglobin levels of > 10 g/dl and early stage disease at diagnosis for survival.[73,77] Several parameters have been reported to have an unfavourable impact on duration of response: resistant relapse at time of ABMT, high pre-ABMT β2 microglobulin values and non-IgG isotype.[76,79] Duration of response has been found to be signficantly longer for patients achieving CR than for those who do not.[31,75,77] The use of purged bone marrow has been examined and appears to make little difference to outcome.[80,81]

Overall, ABMT appears to be relatively safe in patients up to 65 years of age, with a transplant-related mortality of between 5% and 10%. However, there is, to date, no evidence of a disease-free plateau or long-term survivors. Preliminary data show that ABMT may be more effective than chemotherapy alone but this needs to be reassessed at a longer follow-up, and further prospective studies undertaken. It is now becoming apparent that it is not helpful for patients in the late stages of myeloma and should therefore be reserved for patients early in the disease who are either initially refractory or in a remission that is likely to be short.

## Peripheral blood stem cell transplantation (PBSCT)

Recently, peripheral blood stem cell (PBSC) autografts for multiple myeloma have increasingly been carried out as they appear to confer several advantages over bone marrow transplantation. They allow patients who have considerable bone marrow infiltration with plasma cells to be harvested, since it is thought that the PBSC harvest product is only minimally contaminated with myeloma cells. There is, however, some evidence that this may not be the case, with several *in-vitro* studies[82,83] showing cells belonging to the myeloma clone present in peripheral blood, including following high dose chemotherapy. To overcome this, there is now the option for specific selection of CD34+ stem cells using immunoaffinity columns, resulting in 'positive purging' of the harvest product.

Initial studies were carried out at the Arkansas Cancer Research Center[84] where seventy-five patients aged less than 70 years underwent PBSCT and ABMT. Cyclophosphamide (6 g/m²) and granulocyte colony stimulting factor (GCSF) were used for mobilization of PBSC and this was found to be impaired when prior treatment exposure was longer than 12 months. Median haematological recovery was 15 days and there was one transplant-related death. The overall response rate was 68% with a 12-month event-free survival of 85%. A recent study from Paris[85] assessed the role of PBSCT using TBI and chemotherapy conditioning in sixty-three patients. There were seven toxic deaths but, in most patients, sustained haemopoietic recovery occurred within 15 days. Twenty per cent of patients achieved CR post-transplant and the median overall and event free survivals were 59 months and 43 months, respectively. Preliminary results of PBSCT in multiple myeloma using CD34+ cells have been reported by Schiller *et al.*[86] Nine patients with advanced, chemoresponsive disease were harvested after priming with cyclophosphamide (2.5 mg/m²), prednisolone and GCSF. CD34+ progenitor cells were purified from the leukopheresis product using a cellular immunoabsorption method, with purity of collection ranging from 50% to 91%. Immunoglobulin gene primers showed no evidence of tumour contamination of the CD34+ autograft. Mean times to granulocyte ($> 500/\mu$ l) and platelet ($> 20\,000/\mu$ l) recovery were 13 and 12 days, respectively. No data are currently available for survival of these patients.

Conclusions regarding PBSCT that can be drawn from these early studies are that both neutrophil and platelet recovery times post-transplant appear quicker, and transplant-related mortality is less than with ABMT. Overall and event-free survival is comparable to ABMT, and may prove, especially with CD34+ transplants, to be even better. However, trials comparing this procedure with conventional chemotherapy are currently underway, and results of these will need to be considered before PBSCT is used more extensively as an established part of consolidation therapy for myeloma.

## α -Interferon

Interferon is a biological therapeutic agent with antitumoural activity in both experimental systems and humans. Among the tentative mechanisms of actions of α-interferon *in vivo* in multiple myeloma are a direct cytotoxic effect on myeloma cells,[87] a decrease in monoclonal immunoglobulin production,[88] and an inhibition of the growth-promoting effect of IL6.[89] Interferon can be used in both induction treatment of multiple myeloma and as maintenance therapy.

### Induction therapy

α-Interferon has been evaluated as an induction agent as both a single agent and also combined with other chemotherapy. Several studies have shown it to have a good clinical effect as a single agent (at a dose of 3 megaunits, three times a week), with response rates between 14% and 50% in previously untreated patients.[90,91] Three studies have reported increased responsiveness in IgA isotypes[90,92,93] but this has not been confirmed by other investigators. Despite these results, the overall clinical effect of interferon has not been found to be superior to conventional chemotherapy with regard to response frequency and duration, or overall survival.

Further studies looking at the efficacy of interferon combined with cytotoxic chemotherapy have been reported recently. Two of these compare α-interferon with melphalan and prednisolone[94,95] and one with cyclophosphamide.[96] Although two of these trials showed an overall increased remission rate with interferon,[94,96] none of them showed any difference in median duration of response or overall survival. However, a significant survival advantage was observed in one study[94] in those patients with IgA and Bence-Jones myeloma who were treated with combined interferon and melphalan–prednisone.

### Maintenance therapy

The rationale for the use of α-interferon as maintenance therapy in multiple myeloma lies in the recognition that it causes 'accumulation' of myeloma cells in plateau phase (i.e. G0 phase of the cell cycle) and, hence, markedly reduces their capacity for self-renewal. The first study to look at this came from Italy. Mandelli et al.[10] looked at 101 patients with multiple myeloma who had responded to 12-monthly courses of induction chemotherapy. The median duration of response (from diagnosis) was 26 months in the patients given interferon and 14 months in untreated patients ($P = 0.0002$), whereas median duration of survival was not significantly different at 52 and 39 months in the treated and untreated groups, respectively. This significant increase in duration of plateau phase with interferon treatment has also been seen in another study,[97] but was not found in several others.[98,99] This prolongation of remission duration is not necessarily translated into longer overall survival with recent updated analysis of the Italian study[10] and other trials,[98,99] including a recent prospective study from the Southwestern Oncology Group,[100] showing no survival benefit.

The optimal dose of interferon still needs to be established but current recommended doses vary between 3 and 5 Mu (megaunits), three times a week, subcutaneously. It is generally well tolerated although side-effects, which are often self-limiting, include a mild influenza-like syndrome, headache, and mild thrombocytopenia and neutropenia. Blood counts must therefore be reviewed regularly in patients receiving interferon. Duration of treatment is controversial with some practitioners stopping after 12–18 months if there is no sign of myeloma progression, while others continue therapy indefinitely until evidence of disease relapse.

### Post-bone-marrow-transplant therapy

The effect of maintenance interferon post-BMT is now of special interest, in view of the increasing number of patients undergoing this procedure for multiple myeloma combined with the evidence that interferon may be active against residual disease. One non-randomized study evaluated the survival of patients undergoing ABMT with melphalan (140 mg/m$^2$) and TBI (8 Gy) conditioning, followed by maintenance interferon.[101] α-Interferon was started at a dose of 3 Mu/m$^2$ when neutrophil counts had reached 0.5 × 10$^9$/l and platelets over 50 × 10$^9$/l. At a median follow-up time of 15 months, projected probability of remaining progression-free survival at 18 months was 80% for all patients, 100% for patients in CR and 60% for patients in PR. A further, more recent study also found similar results.[75] How durable these remissions will be, and whether post-transplant interferon maintenance delays rather than prevents relapse, remains to be seen, as longer follow-up is needed.

# Future prospects

Multiple myeloma remains an incurable condition, despite great interest and effort in developing more effective therapies. There are, however, two major avenues that may be pursued and have an impact on prognosis:

1. optimization of current treatment strategies; and
2. therapies based upon a clearer understanding of the pathophysiological basis of the condition.

Further high-intensity combination chemotherapy regimens may be developed, with the possibility of peripheral blood stem cell support to counteract prolonged neutropenia. Multidrug resistance, characterized by the expression of a *p*-glycoprotein on the cell surface which is encoded for by the *mdr-1* gene, is found in the majority of patients with chemoresistant myeloma. Ways of overcoming this phenomenon, such as the use of calcium channel blockers, e.g. verapamil, and the development of new agents, may enable chemoresistant disease to be treated more effectively. Bone marrow and peripheral blood stem cell transplantation, with high dose chemotherapy–radiotherapy, is also an area where advances are being made. Improved mobilization techniques and supportive treatment will allow an increasing number of patients to undergo these procedures. Purging techniques of the harvest product are continuing to be developed, resulting in improved purity and efficiency of target cell selection. Minimal residual disease detectable in stem cell harvest collections, and in patients following both autologous and allogeneic transplantation, can now be evaluated using molecular biology techniques, looking at patient specific immunoglobulin heavy-chain gene rearrangement with the polymerase chain reaction (PCR). This will allow assessment of disease modulation by biological agents, such as α-interferon, and may also elucidate disease development and progression.

Determining the pathophysiological basis of multiple myeloma will require new insights into the nature of the malignant clone. Characterization of myeloma cells by molecular and cellular biology techniques may reveal novel strategies for diagnosis and treatment. The identification of specific patterns of immunophenotype, adhesion molecule and oncogene expression may well have clinical relevance in terms of the modulation of the malignant clone. Indeed, the identification of specific gene deletions and mutations, such as the recently described mutation in the tumour suppressor gene *p53*,[102] will define targets for new strategies in the future, such as gene therapy.

# References

1. Michaeli J, Durie BGM. Plasma cell disorders. In: W Kelley, ed, *Textbook of Internal Medicine*. Philadelphia: JB Lippincott, 1991; 1087–96.
2. Hewell GM, Alexanian R. Myeloma in young persons. *Ann Intern Med* 1976; **84**, 441–3.
3. Medinger FG, Craver LF. Total body irradiation. *Am J Roentgenol* 1942; **48**, 651–71.
4. Rowell NP, Tobias JS. The role of radiotherapy in the management of multiple myeloma. *Blood Rev* 1991; **5**, 84–9.
5. Kyle RA. Long-term survival in multiple myeloma. *N Engl J Med* 1983; **308**, 314–16.
6. Frassica DA, Frassica FJ, Schray MF, *et al.* Solitary plasmacytoma of bone: Mayo Clinic experience. *Int J Radiat Oncol Biol Phys* 1989; **16**, 43–8.
7. Greenberg P, Parker RG, Fu YS, *et al.* The treatment of solitary plasmacytoma of bone and extramedullary plasmacytoma. *Am J Clin Oncol* 1987; **10**, 199–204.
8. Dimopoulos MA, Goldstein J, Fuller L, *et al.* Curability of solitary bone plasmacytoma. *J Clin Oncol* 1992; **10**, 587–90.
9. Wollersheim HC, Holdrinet RS, Haanen C. Clinical course and survival in 16 patients with localized plasmacytoma. *Scand J Haematol* 1984; **32**, 423–8.
10. Mandelli F, Avvisati G, Amadori S, *et al.* Maintenance treatment with recombinant interferon alfa-2b in patients with multiple myeloma responding to conventional induction chemotherapy. *N Engl J Med* 1990; **322**, 1430–4.
11. Kyle RA. Monoclonal gammopathy of undetermined significance and smoldering multiple myeloma. *Eur J Haematol Suppl* 1989; **51**, 70–5.
12. Kyle RA, Greipp PR. Smoldering multiple myeloma. *N Engl J Med* 1980; **302**, 1347–9.
13. Oken M, Greipp PR, Kay NE, *et al.* Multiple myeloma. In: JR McArthur, ed, *Hematology — 1993*, Education Program, American Society of Haematology. University of Washington School of Medicine and Stanford University, 1993.
14. Durie BGM, Salmon SE. Clinical staging system for multiple myeloma. Correlation of measured myeloma cell mass with presenting clinical features, response to treatment and survival. *Cancer* 1975; **36**, 842–54.
15. Greipp PR, Katzmann JA, O'Fallon WM, *et al.* Value of beta-2 microglobulin level and plasma cell labeling indices as prognostic factors in patients with newly diagnosed myeloma. *Blood* 1988; **72**, 219–23.
16. Greipp PR, Katzmann JA, O'Fallon WM, *et al.* Value of β2 microglobulin level and plasma cell labelling indices as prognostic factors in patients with newly

diagnosed myeloma. *Blood* 1988; **72**, 219–23.

17. Bataille R, Boccadoro M, Klein B, *et al.* C-reactive protein and beta-2 microglobulin produce a simple and powerful myeloma staging system. *Blood* 1992; **80**, 733–7.

18. Barlogie B, Smallwood L, Smith T, *et al.* High serum levels of lactate dehydrogenase identify a high grade lymphoma-like myeloma. *Ann Intern Med* 1989; **110**, 521–5.

19. Jagannath S, Barlogie B, Dicke K, *et al.* Autologous bone marrow transplantation in multiple myeloma: identification of prognostic factors. *Blood* 1990; **76**, 1860–6.

20. Price P, Hoskin PJ, Easton D, *et al.* Prospective randomised trial of single and multifraction radiotherapy schedules in the treatment of painful bony metastases. *Radiother Oncol* 1986; **6**, 247–55.

21. Medical Research Council. Prognostic features in the third myelomatosis trial. *Br J Cancer* 1980; **42**, 831–40.

22. Medical Research Council Working Party in Leukaemia in Adults. Analysis and management of renal failure in the fourth MRC myelomatosis trial. *Br Med J* 1980; **288**, 1411–16.

23. Paterson AD, Kanis JA, Cameron EC, *et al.* The use of dichloromethylene diphosphanate for the management of hypercalcaemia in multiple myeloma. *Br J Haematol* 1983; **54**, 121–32.

24. Kanis JA, McCloskey EV, Paterson AHG. Use of diphosphanates in hypercalcaemia due to malignancy. *Lancet* 1990; **335**, 170–1.

25. Alexanian R, Haut A, Khan AU, *et al.* Treatment for multiple myeloma. Combination chemotherapy with different melphalan dose regimens. *JAMA* 1969; **208**, 1680–5.

26. Gregory WM, Richards MA, Malpas JS. Combination chemotherapy versus melphalan and prednisolone in the treatment of multiple myeloma: an overview of published trials. *J Clin Oncol* 1992; **10**, 334–42.

27. Bergsagel DE. Melphalan–prednisone versus drug combinations for plasma cell myeloma. *Eur J Haematol* 1989; **43**, 117–23.

28. Belch A, Shelley W, Bergsagel D, *et al.* A randomized trial of maintenance versus no maintenance melphalan and prednisone in responding multiple myeloma patients. *Br J Cancer* 1988; **57**, 94–9.

29. Fernberg JO, Johansson BO, Lewensohn R, *et al.* Oral dosage of melphalan and response to treatment in multiple myeloma. *Eur J Cancer* 1990; **26**, 393–6.

30. Chronic Leukaemia–Myeloma Task Force: Guidelines for protocol studies. *Cancer Chemother Rep* 1973; **4**, 145.

31. Gore ME, Selby PJ, Viner C, *et al.* Intensive treatment of multiple myeloma and criteria for complete remission. *Lancet* 1989; **2**, 879–82.

32. Alexanian R, Salmon S, Gutterman J, *et al.* Chemoimmunotherapy for multiple myeloma. *Cancer* 1981; **47**, 1923–9.

33. Garewal H, Durie BG, Kyle RA, *et al.* Serum beta 2 microglobulin in the initial staging and subsequent monitoring of monoclonal plasma cell disorders. *J Clin Oncol* 1984; **2**, 51–7.

34. Alexanian R, Dimopoulos M. The treatment of multiple myeloma. *N Engl J Med* 1994; **330**, 484–9.

35. Riccardi A, Gobbi PG, Ucci G, *et al.* Changing clinical presentation of multiple myeloma. *Eur J Cancer* 1991; **27**, 1401–5.

36. Alexanian R, Salmon S, Bonnet J, *et al.* Combination therapy for multiple myeloma. *Cancer* 1977; **40**, 2765–71.

37. Goldie JH, Coldman AJ, Gudauskas GA. Rationale for the use of alternating non-cross-resistant chemotherapy. *Cancer Treat Rep* 1982; **66**, 439–49.

38. Boccadoro M, Marmont F, Tribalto M, *et al.* Multiple myeloma: VMCP/VBAP alternating combination chemotherapy is not superior to mel-

phalan and prednisone even in high-risk patients. *J Clin Oncol* 1991; **9**, 444–8.
39. Hjorth M, Hellquist L, Holmberg E, *et al*. Initial treatment in multiple myeloma: no advantage of multidrug chemotherapy over melphalan–prednisone. The Myeloma Group of Western Sweden. *Br J Haematol* 1990; **74**, 185–91.
40. MacLennan ICM, Cuzick J. Objective evaluation of the role of vincristine in induction and maintenance therapy for myelomatosis. Medical Research Council working party on leukaemia in adults. *Br J Cancer* 1985; **52**, 153–8.
41. Osterborg A, Ahre A, Bjorkholm M, *et al*. Alternating combination chemotherapy (VMCP/VBAP) is not superior to melphalan/prednisone in the treatment of multiple myeloma patients stage III — a randomized study from MGCS. *Eur J Haematol* 1989; **43**, 54–62.
42. Pavlovsky S, Corrado C, Santarelli MT, *et al*. An update of two randomized trials in previously untreated multiple myeloma comparing melphalan and prednisone versus three- and five-drug combinations: an Argentine Group for the Treatment of Acute Leukemia study. *J Clin Oncol* 1988; **6**, 769–75.
43. Peest D, Deicher H, Coldewey R, *et al*. Induction and maintenance therapy in multiple myeloma: a multicenter trial of MP versus VCMP. *Eur J Cancer Clin Oncol* 1988; **24**, 1061–7.
44. Tribalto M, Amadori S, Cantonetti M, *et al*. Treatment of multiple myeloma: a randomized study of three different regimens. *Leukaemia Res* 1985; **9**, 1043–9.
45. Durie BG, Dixon DO, Carter S, *et al*. Improved survival duration with combination chemotherapy induction for multiple myeloma: a Southwest Oncology Group study. *J Clin Oncol* 1986; **4**, 1227–37.
46. Maclennan ICM, Chapman C, Dunn J, *et al*. Combined chemotherapy with ABCM versus melphalan for treatment of myelomatosis. *Lancet* 1992; **339**, 200–5.
47. Samson D, Gaminara E, Newland AC. Infusion of vincristine and doxorubicin with oral dexamethasone as first-line therapy for myeloma. *Lancet* 1989; **2**, 882–5.
48. Forgeson G, Selby P, Lakhani S. Infused vincristine and Adriamycin with high-dose methylprednisolone (VAMP) in advanced previously treated myeloma patients. *Br J Cancer* 1988; **58**, 469–73.
49. Fitzpatrick PJ, Rider WD. Half body radiotherapy. *Int J Radiat Oncol Biol Phys* 1976; **1**, 197–207.
50. Giles FJ, De Lord C, Gaminara EJ, *et al*. Systemic irradiation therapy of myelomatosis — the therapeutic implications of the technique. *Leukaemia and Lymphoma* 1990; **1**, 227–33.
51. Salmon SE, Tesh D, Crowley J, *et al*. Chemotherapy is superior to sequential hemibody irradiation for remission consolidation in multiple myeloma: a Southwest Oncology Group study. *J Clin Oncol* 1990; **8**, 1575–84.
52. Singer CR, Tobias JS, Giles F, *et al*. Hemibody irradiation. An effective second-line therapy in drug-resistant multiple myeloma. *Cancer* 1989; **63**, 2446–51.
53. McSweeney EN, Tobias JS, Blackman G, *et al*. Double hemibody irradiation (DHBI) in the management of relapsed and primary chemoresistant multiple myeloma. *Clin Oncol* 1993; **5**, 378–83.
54. Prato FS, Kurdyak R, Saibil EA, *et al*. The incidence of radiation pneumonitis as a result of single fraction upper body irradiation. *Cancer* 1977; **39**, 71–8.
55. Van Dyk J, Keane TJ, Kan S, *et al*. Radiation pneumonitis following large single dose irradiation: a re-evaluation based on absolute dose to lung. *Int J Radiat Oncol Biol Phys* 1981; 7, 461–7.
56. Hoskin PJ, Ford HT, Harmer CL. Hemibody irradiation (HBI) for metastatic bone pain in two histologically distinct groups of patients. *Clin Oncol*

1989; **1**, 67–9.

57. Coleman M, Saletan S, Wolf D, *et al.* Whole bone marrow irradiation for the treatment of multiple myeloma. *Cancer* 1982; **49**, 1328–33.

58. Tobias JS, Richards JD, Blackman GM, *et al.* Hemibody irradiation in multiple myeloma. *Radiother Oncol* 1985; **3**, 11–16.

59. Thomas PJ, Daban A, Bontoux D. Double hemibody irradiation in chemotherapy-resistant multiple myeloma. *Cancer Treat Rep* 1984; **68**, 1173–5.

60. MacKenzie MR, Wold H, George C, *et al.* Consolidation hemibody radiotherapy following induction combination chemotherapy in high-tumor-burden multiple myeloma. *J Clin Oncol* 1992; **10**, 1769–74.

61. Giles FJ, McSweeney EN, Richards JD, *et al.* Prospective randomised study of double hemi-body irradiation with and without subsequent maintenance recombinant alpha 2b interferon on survival in patients with relapsed multiple myeloma. *Eur J Cancer* 1992; **28A**, 1392–5.

62. Collins VP, Loeffler RK. The therapeutic use of single doses of total body irradiation. *Am J Roentgenol* 1956; **75**, 542–7.

63. Barlogie B, Alexanian R, Dicke KA, *et al.* High-dose chemoradiotherapy and autologous bone marrow transplantation for resistant multiple myeloma. *Blood* 1987; **70**, 869–72.

64. Barlogie B, Epstein J, Selvanayagam P, *et al.* Plasma cell myeloma — new biological insights and advances in therapy. *Blood* 1989; **73**, 865–79.

65. Attal M, Harousseau JL, Stoppa AM, *et al.* High dose therapy in multiple myeloma; a prospective randomised study of the Intergroupe Français du Myeloma. *Blood* 1993; **82** (Suppl 1), 776.

66. Latini P, Aristei C, Aversa F, *et al.* Lung damage following bone marrow transplantation after hyperfractionated total body irradiation. *Radiother Oncol* 1991; **22**, 127–32.

67. Gahrton G, Tura S, Ljungman P, *et al.* Allogeneic bone marrow transplantation in multiple myeloma. European Group for Bone Marrow Transplantation. *N Engl J Med* 1991; **325**, 1267–73.

68. Tura S, Cavo M, Rosti G, *et al.* Allogeneic bone marrow transplantation for multiple myeloma. *Bone Marrow Transplantation* 1989; **4** (Suppl 4), 106–8.

69. Bensinger WI, Buckner CD, Clift RA, *et al.* Phase I study of busulfan and cyclophosphamide in preparation for allogeneic marrow transplant for patients with multiple myeloma. *J Clin Oncol* 1992; **10**, 1492–7.

70. Samson D. The current position of allogeneic and autologous BMT in multiple myeloma. *Leukaemia and Lymphoma* 1992; **7** (Suppl 1), 33–8.

71. McElwain TJ, Powles RL. High dose intravenous melphalan for plasma cell leukaemia and myeloma. *Lancet* 1983; **2**, 322–4.

72. Selby PJ, McElwain TJ, Nandi AC, *et al.* Multiple myeloma treated with high dose intravenous melphalan. *Br J Haematol* 1987; **66**, 55–62.

73. Cunningham D, Paz-Ares L, Gore ME, *et al.* High-dose melphalan for multiple myeloma: long-term follow-up data. *J Clin Oncol* 1994; **12**, 764–8.

74. Barlogie B, Hall R, Zander A, *et al.* High dose melphalan with autologous bone marrow transplantation for multiple myeloma. *Blood* 1986; **67**, 1298–301.

75. Attal M, Huguet F, Schlaifer D, *et al.* Intensive combined therapy for previously untreated aggressive myeloma. *Blood* 1992; **79**, 1130–6.

76. Williams CD, McSweeney EN, Mills W, *et al.* Autologous bone marrow transplantation in multiple myeloma: a single centre experience of 23 patients. *Leukaemia and Lymphoma* 1994; **15**, 273–9.

77. Cunningham D, Paz-Ares L, Milan S, *et al.* High-dose melphalan and autologous bone marrow transplantation as consolidation in previously untreated myeloma. *J Clin Oncol* 1994; **12**, 759–63.

78. Alexanian R, Dimopoulos M, Smith T, *et al.* Limited value of myeloablative therapy for late multiple myeloma. *Blood* 1994; **83**, 512–16.

79. Jagannath S, Barlogie B, Dicke K, *et al.* Autologous bone marrow transplantation in multiple myeloma: identification of prognostic factors. *Blood* 1990; **76**, 1860–6.
80. Anderson KC, Barut BA, Ritz J, *et al.* Monoclonal antibody-purged autologous bone marrow transplantation therapy for multiple myeloma. *Blood* 1991; **77**, 712–20.
81. Anderson KC, Andersen J, Soiffer R, *et al.* Monoclonal antibody-purged bone marrow transplantation therapy for multiple myeloma. *Blood* 1993; **77**, 712–20.
82. Chiu EKW, Ganeshaguru K, Hoffbrand AV, *et al.* Circulating monoclonal B lymphocytes in multiple myeloma. *Br J Haematol* 1989; **72**, 28–31.
83. Dreyfus F, Melle J, Quarre MC, *et al.* Contamination of peripheral blood by monoclonal B cells following treatment of multiple myeloma by high-dose chemotherapy. *Br J Haematol* 1993; **85**, 411–12.
84. Jagannath S, Vesole DH, Glenn L, *et al.* Low-risk intensive therapy for multiple myeloma with combined autologous bone marrow and blood stem cell support. *Blood* 1992; **80**, 1666–72.
85. Fermand JP, Chevret S, Ravaud P, *et al.* High-dose chemoradiotherapy and autologous blood stem cell transplantation in multiple myeloma: results of a phase II trial involving 63 patients. *Blood* 1993; **82**, 2005–9.
86. Schiller G, Vescio R, Lee M, *et al.* Transplantation of autologous CD34-positive peripheral blood stem cells as treatment for multiple myeloma. *Blood* 1993; **82** (Supp 1), 778.
87. Einhorn S, Fernberg JO, Grandér D, *et al.* Interferon exerts a cytotoxic effect on primary human myeloma cells. *Eur J Cancer Clin Oncol* 1988; **24**, 1505–10.
88. Grandér D, von Stedingk LV, von Stedingk M, *et al.* Influence of interferon on antibody production and viability of malignant cells from patients with multiple myeloma. *Eur J Haematol* 1991; **46**, 17–25.
89. Klein B, Zhang X-G, Jourdan M, *et al.* Interleukin-6 is the central tumor growth factor in vitro and in vivo in multiple myeloma. *Eur Cytokine Network* 1990; **1**, 193–201.
90. Ludwig H, Cortelezzi A, Scheithauer W, *et al.* Recombinant interferon alpha-2C versus polychemotherapy (VMCP) for treatment of multiple myeloma: a prospective randomised trial. *Eur J Cancer Clin Oncol* 1986; **22**, 1111–16.
91. Quesada JR, Alexanian R, Hawkins M, *et al.* Treatment of multiple myeloma with recombinant alpha-interferon. *Blood* 1986; **67**, 275–8.
92. Ähre A, Björkholm M, Österborg A, *et al.* High doses of natural alpha-interferon (alpha-IFN) in the treatment of multiple myeloma — a pilot study from the Myeloma Group of Central Sweden (MGCS). *Eur J Haematol* 1988; **41**, 123–30.
93. Ohno R, Kimura K. Treatment of multiple myeloma with recombinant interferon alpha-2a. *Cancer* 1986; **57**, 1685–8.
94. Österborg A, Björkholm M, Bjoreman M, *et al.* Natural interferon-alpha in combination with melphalan/prednisone versus melphalan/prednisone in the treatment of multiple myeloma stages II and III: a randomised study from the Myeloma Group of Central Sweden. *Blood* 1993; **81**, 1428–34.
95. Cooper MR, Dear K, McIntyre OR, *et al.* A randomised clinical trial comparing melphalan/prednisone with or without interferon alpha-2b in newly diagnosed patients with multiple myeloma: a Cancer and Leukemia Group B study. *J Clin Oncol* 1993; **11**, 155–60.
96. Aitchison R, Williams A, Schey S, *et al.* A randomised trial of cyclophosphamide with and without low dose alpha-interferon in the treatment of newly diagnosed myeloma. *Leukaemia and Lymphoma* 1993; **9**, 243–6.
97. Westin J. Interferon therapy during the plateau phase of multiple myeloma: an update of a Swedish multicentre study. *Semin Oncol* 1991; **27** (Suppl 4), 45–8.
98. Peest D, Deicher H, Coldewey R, *et al.* Melphalan and prednisone (MP)

versus vincristine, BCNU, Adriamycin, melphalan and dexamethasone (VBAMDex) induction therapy and interferon maintenance treatment in multiple myeloma. *Onkologie* 1990; **13**, 43–4.

99. Österborg A, Mellstadt H. The mechanisms of action and the role of alpha interferon in the therapy of myeloma. In: D Crowther, ed, U Veronesi, Series ed, *Interferons: Mechanisms of Action and Role in Cancer Therapy*, Monographs: European School of Oncology. Berlin, Heidelberg: Springer Verlag, 1991; 25–31.

100. Salmon SE, Crowley J. Impact of glucocorticoids and interferon on outcome in multiple myeloma. *Proc ASCO* 1992; **11**, 316.

101. Attal M, Huguet F, Schlaifer D, *et al.* Maintenance and treatment with recombinant alpha interferon after autologous bone marrow transplantation for aggressive myeloma in first remission after conventional induction therapy. *Bone Marrow Transplant* 1991; **8**, 125–8.

102. Neri A, Baldini L, Trecca D, *et al.* P53 gene mutations in multiple myeloma are associated with advanced forms of malignancy. *Blood* 1993; **81**, 128–35.

103. Gahrton G, Tura S, Ljungman P, *et al.* Prognostic factors in allogeneic bone marrow transplantation for multiple myeloma. *J Clin Oncol* 1995; **13**, 1312–22.

104. Attal M, Harousseau JL, Stoppa AM, *et al.* High dose therapy in multiple myeloma: a prospective randomised study of the 'Intergroup Français du Myelome' (IFM). *Blood* 1993; **82** (Suppl 1), 198a (776).

# 14 Total body irradiation in bone marrow transplantation and advanced lymphomas: a comprehensive overview

*Craig L Silverman and Stuart L Goldberg*

## Introduction

The use of total body irradiation (TBI) either by itself for low-grade lymphomas, or in conjunction with bone marrow transplantation (BMT) for leukaemias, lymphomas and solid tumours, arose as a by-product of observations of the haematological effects in the nuclear explosion victims at both Hiroshima and Nagasaki. The exposure of the entire body to a high dose of irradiation is a relatively simple concept; however, the radiobiological origins, physical and technical considerations, and concerns about the acute and long-term side-effects make it complicated.

## Total body irradiation for bone marrow transplantation

### Goals

Any conditioning TBI regimen used to prepare patients for BMT must perform three essential functions, namely:

1. sufficient immunosuppression to allow engraftment of foreign donor marrow for allogeneic transplants;
2. eradication or reduction of the systemic disease; and
3. provision of sufficient marrow space for the donor marrow.

It is now felt that while TBI should be a benefit in accomplishing all three objectives, the major role, especially in conjunction with allogeneic BMT, is its immunosuppressive effects.[1,2] Gale *et al*. believe that the major role is to allow engraftment of donor immune cells to establish a graft vs leukaemic cell (GvL) reaction. Any reduction in leukaemic cell burden accomplished by direct effects is caused by promoting the GvL reaction.[2]

## Radiobiological considerations

For humans exposed to whole body irradiation, the critical organ is the bone marrow. The tolerance of bone marrow is approximately 4 Gy, which will kill approximately 50% of patients exposed without subsequent rescue ($LD_{50}$). With exposure to single doses above 10 Gy, fatal gastrointestinal syndrome is virtually inevitable. Following doses of 3–8 Gy, fatal haemopoietic syndrome results.[1,3,4] It was from these observations that the concept of an acceptable single-fraction total body irradiation dose was initially developed.

Laboratory studies have determined that the $LD_{50}$ of lymphocytes is approximately 0.9–1.2 Gy.[5] Caldwell and Lammerton determined that leukaemic cells, in particular, are very sensitive to even small doses of fractionated irradiation due to intrinsic repair mechanisms.[6] Peters et al.,[7] and later Shank et al.,[8] then postulated that hyperfractionated protocols could be developed that should be equally lethal for leukaemic cells and host bone marrow cells as a single-fraction treatment, while improving normal-tissue tolerance in especially sensitive organs, such as the lung, by allowing repair of sublethal radiation damage to occur between fractions. Storb et al. have recently shown this equivalency by demonstrating that single-dose total body irradiation and fractionated total body irradiation at a dose rate of 0.1 Gy/min have comparative marrow effects in dogs.[9]

These studies, coupled with the work of Deeg[10] in assessing both acute and delayed toxicities of single-fraction TBI, have spurred the development of the present multiple-fractionated TBI protocols. Other important radiobiological principles to consider include dose rate, fractionation, and total dose.[11]

Dose-rate considerations are of extreme interest. Since all treatments are performed at extended distance, dose rates between 0.03 and 1.0 Gy/min are possible. Too low a dose rate may allow repair of sublethal damage to occur, which impairs the effectiveness of the irradiation in eradicating host immune cells or tumour cells. Extremely high dose rates may cause irreversible long-term damage in vital organ systems. Initial treatment protocols were often extremely long in overall treatment time, frequently requiring 3–4 hrs and even as long as 7–8 hrs to deliver the treatment. Fryer et al. determined that, for single-fraction treatment of 10 Gy, dose rates less than or equal to 0.5 Gy/min led to significantly decreased incidence of interstitial pneumonia without compromising engraftment or relapse rate.[12] Ozsahin et al. prospectively evaluated two different dose-rate schedules for a single fraction of 10 Gy delivered to fifty-seven patients.[13] They evaluated 0.15 Gy/min vs 0.06 Gy/min treatments. Overall survival, relapse-free survival and engraftment were identical but they did note that interstitial pneumonitis was higher in the 0.15 Gy/min patient arm. Kim et al., using only 7.5 Gy at doses up to 0.26 Gy/min reported a similar result (see Table 14.1).[14]

For multiple-fractionated TBI, dose rate may not matter. Ozsahin et al.

**Table 14.1** Summation of dose–dose rate–fractionation effects

| | Decreased relapse rate | | Decreased complication rate | |
|---|---|---|---|---|
| | Yes | No | Yes | No |
| Dose rate (single fraction) | — | — | Fryer et al.[12]<br>Kim et al.[14]<br>Ozsahin et al.[13] | —<br>—<br>— |
| Dose rate (multiple fractions) | Scarpati et al.[15] | Kim et al.[14]<br>Ozsahin et al.[13] | —<br>— | —<br>— |
| Total dose | Buckner et al.[26] | Cossett et al.[25]<br>Kim et al.[14]<br>Messner et al.[23]<br>Socie et al.[21]<br>Thomas et al.[19] | —<br>—<br>—<br>— | —<br>—<br>—<br>—<br>— |
| Multiple fractions | Dinsmore et al.[20]<br>Kim et al.[14] | Ozsahin et al.[13]<br>Socie et al.[21]<br>Thomas et al.[19] | Thomas et al.[19] | Kim et al.[14]<br>Ozsahin et al.[13]<br>Weiner et al.[38] |

also evaluated multiple-fractionated treatments of 12 Gy in six fractions at either 0.06 Gy/min or 0.03 Gy/min. No significant differences in survival, relapse-free survival or lung complications were noted.[13] Scarpati *et al.*, however, using 9.9 Gy in three fractions over 3 days did feel that higher dose rates were correlated with decreased relapse in their leukaemic patients.[15] Based on Vriesendorp's radiobiological model, higher dose rates of 0.25–0.30 Gy/min may be better in accomplishing immunosuppression as well as decreasing the predominant lung toxicity when combined with multiple fractions, moderate fraction size (3–4 Gy), and a short overall treatment time of less than 4 days.[16]

## Single vs multiple fractions

Radiobiological modelling has demonstrated that fractionated TBI should have several advantages over single-fraction TBI. These include increased sparing of normal tissue due to repair of sublethal damage and increased leukaemic cell kill rate, possibly due to cell cycle effects.[7,8,12,16] Deeg *et al.* showed these concepts to be valid in dogs.[17] Storb *et al.* have also demonstrated the equivalent biological effect in canines between single- and multiple-dose treatments,[9] while Tarbell *et al.* have used a murine model.[18] In a randomized human trial, Thomas *et al.* demonstrated the superiority of multiple fractions to a single fraction in patients with leukaemia. Though a larger total dose was needed, a similar immunosuppressive effect was obtained, and engraftment and relapse rates were similar. Survival was significantly improved due to a decrease in acute complications.[19]

Dinsmore *et al.* also demonstrated a decrease in leukaemic relapse using multiple fractions,[20] while Kim *et al.*[14] demonstrated a similar trend toward decreased relapse rate and improved survival when comparing patients treated with single-fraction TBI to hyperfractionated TBI. Socie *et al.*[21] could not demonstrate a survival benefit of single vs multiple treatments. It appears that the true superiority of multiple-fractionated protocols may be in decreasing the incidence of such fatal complications as radiation pneumonitis,[13–15,17,19] as well as veno-occlusive disease.[13,19]

## Total dose

Initially, 10 Gy was selected, based on observations that 8 Gy gave insufficient immunosuppression.[22] Messner *et al.*, however, with a more aggressive chemoablative regimen have achieved similar long-term survivorship for patients with acute myeloblastic leukaemia, acute lymphoblastic leukaemia, and chronic myeloblastic leukaemia, using only 5-Gy single-fraction treatment.[23] Kim *et al.* used only 7.5 Gy with similar results.[14] For multiple-fractionated TBI protocols, dose equivalency to single-fraction treatment was theoretically calculated based on cell survival curve parameters, the assumption of complete repair between fractions and insignificant repopulation between fractions.[24] Ozsahin *et al.*, in a randomized protocol, demonstrated similar engraftment in patients receiving either a 10-Gy single fraction or 12 Gy in six fractions over 3 days.[13] Retrospective studies essentially showing equivalency of regimens are common.[14,19,21,25] One randomized study comparing 12 Gy vs 15.75 Gy did show a significant decrease in relapse rate but the relapse rate was abnormally high in the 12-Gy arm compared with most studies.[26,83] Gale *et al.*[2] felt that the total dose might need to be decreased based on lack of definitive proof of improvement of engraftment with present dose regimens and present level of complications. On the other hand, total dose may need to be altered upward as the goals of TBI change, especially in peripheral stem cell transplants, and autologous BMT, where its role may be more cytotoxic effects.

## Physical considerations

There are significant physical considerations that must be dealt with during the treatment of any patient with TBI. These include the position of the patient, energy of the beam, treatment distance, homogeneity of the dose, dose rate, number of fractions, as well as protection of the lung, liver and other critical structures. Dosimetric problems of TBI are considerable, as demonstrated by a lengthy American Association of Physicists in Medicine report.[27] The contour of the various body tissues, homogeneities within the body, and off-axis dose considerations can lead to considerable differences in dose within any single patient, between patients and between institutions.

## Patient positioning

There may be as many patient positioning techniques as there are institutions presently doing TBI. The technique is variable since no present equipment is truly dedicated to doing TBI alone, and therefore the technique is usually adapted to accommodate the specific machine and perhaps, more importantly, the physical dimensions of the treatment room itself. There are multiple techniques presently in use (Fig. 14.1).[28] The two major techniques remain either anterior/posterior (AP) or lateral. Homogeneity of dose distribution and lung protection are the major considerations of any set-up. An AP technique as described by Shank *et al.* alternates treating anteriorly and posteriorly with the patient standing, strapped to a vertical stand or in a semiseated position. Individually designed half value lung blocks are used with electron beam boosts to the blocked areas of the ribs and soft tissues.[24] Homogeneity of dose is quite excellent. As a general rule, AP diameters of the major areas of the body — head, thorax, abdomen, pelvis, etc. — are less variable than lateral diameters. To treat patients anteroposterior/posteroanterior (AP/PA), however, requires large treatment distances of 4 m or more.

A lateral set-up is usually easier for the patients to maintain, and more reproducible, but protection of the lungs is more problematic. It is usually accomplished by the use of the upper arms themselves to help absorb the dose. This technique is better suited to facilities that have shorter treatment distances available to them since the patient must be placed in a semifoetal position to fit within the beam. At our institution only a 3.26-m distance is required to treat patients in the lateral position but 4.25–4.5 m would be required for an AP/PA set-up. In order to irradiate adequately the superficial tissues of the skin, a beam-scattering lucite screen is used to generate secondary electrons.

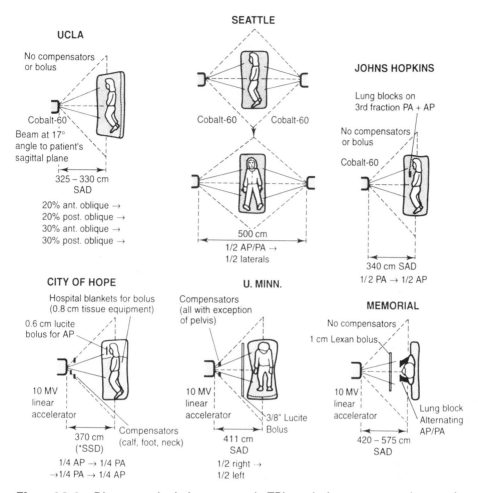

**Fig. 14.1** Diagram depicting several TBI techniques presently used. (Reprinted from Shank, *Int J Radiat Oncol Biol Phys* 1983; **9**, 1925–31.[28])

## Dose specification

The dose is usually calculated at the mid-plane of the abdomen, specifically the umbilicus.[29] Dose inhomogeneity occurs because of off-axis beam dosimetry, as well as the differing diameters of the head, thorax, abdomen, pelvis, etc. This is of more concern when treating in the lateral position. Some of that inhomogeneity can be eliminated by the construction of a compensating filter, usually of aluminium, to compensate for the difference in diameters. The head, in particular, is of concern due to its smaller lateral diameter compared with the diameter of the umbilicus, as well as its relative position away from the beam-scattering lucite shield.

To assess the quality assurance, at our institution both diode readings as well as thermoluminescent dosimetry (TLD) measurements are obtained on both sides of the head and neck, shoulders, mid-mediastinum, umbilicus, pelvis, thighs, knees and ankles. We have consistently demonstrated excellent homogeneity using compensating filters as well as an additional head bolus (Table 14.2). All patients have received ±10% of the prescribed dose to all tissues, fraction-to-fraction, as well as from patient to patient. It is this attention to detail that we believe has helped to demonstrate that the lateral technique can yield similar dosimetry and homogeneity as the AP/PA technique.

**Table 14.2**  Typical patient TLD/diode readings — lateral technique

|  | Diameter (cm) | Diodes (Gy) | TLD (Gy) |
| --- | --- | --- | --- |
| Head | 17 | 2.08/2.18 | 1.84/1.83 |
| Neck/shoulders | 49.5 | 2.45/2.40 | 1.94/2.06 |
| Mid-mediastinum | 36.5 | 2.06/2.02 | 1.90/1.98 |
| Umbilicus | 39.5 | 2.08/2.03 | 2.17/2.18 |
| Pelvis | 41 | 2.14/2.25 | 2.13/2.21 |
| Mid-thigh | 40 | 2.11/2.16 | 2.19 |
| Knees | 25.5 | 2.26/2.08 | 2.34 |
| Ankles | 13.5 | 1.95/1.90 | 2.00 |

TLD: thermoluminescent diode.

## Energy

The original TBI treatments were usually given with the cobalt-60 machine. Newer technology with sophisticated linear accelerators can create treatment beams of 10 MeV or higher. This does lead to better homogeneity, especially with larger treatment diameters in the lateral treatment position. However, a beam spoiler, usually a lucite screen, needs to be employed to generate secondary electrons to irradiate the more superficial tissues. Even a beam spoiler, however, may preferentially underdose the head due to its increased distance from the beam spoiler. Additional tissue equivalent bolus material is needed to homogenize further the dose to the head with energies of 10 MeV or higher.

## Acute toxicities

TBI-induced acute toxicity is a relatively minor consideration for patients undergoing bone marrow transplantations for most diseases. It is often difficult to separate TBI-induced toxicity from chemotherapy-induced toxicities. Most patients receive chemotherapy either immediately before or simultaneously with TBI administration. Spitzer *et al.* noted that nausea and vomiting was much less present in hyperfractionated protocols and actually decreased with each successive fraction.[30] Our experience is similar. Most patients are likely to be acutely nauseated during the first 48 hrs of the TBI treatment but few have prolonged nausea and vomiting, especially with aggressive antiemetic therapy. Syncope has been noted in some patients, especially those treated standing with an AP/PA technique;[24] mild skin erythema has also been noted. At 5–7 days after irradiation, patients can develop oral mucositis. Acute parotitis has also been noted on the first day, as well as a decrease in saliva and tear production in the occasional patient;[31] reversible alopecia also occurs. Most patients also develop a fever which may be related to the release of pyrogenic factors from tumour death.

## Delayed toxicity — lung

It became clear very early in the initially reported series from Seattle and Toronto that the most sensitive tissue was the lung.[32,33] Thomas *et al.*,[32] and later Keane *et al.*,[34] described a syndrome of interstitial pneumonitis that occurred in over 50% of their patients and was fatal in one-third. This syndrome occurred between 10 and 120 days postirradiation, peaking at about Day 50. It appears similar to radiation pneumonitis seen after conventional thoracic irradiation.[34,35] The pathogenesis of interstitial pneumonitis is often associated with infectious agents – cytomegalovirus (CMV) in particular,[36] graft vs host disease (GvHD),[37,38] chemotherapeutic agents such as busulphan and cyclophosphamide,[39] and immunosuppression, as well as intrinsic pulmonary conditions.[40] Penney *et al.* documented the pathological effects of single and fractionated irradiation in mice and showed the relative improvement in the pathological picture with fractionated treatment compared to single-dose treatment.[41]

## Dose-fractionation factors

For single-fraction total body irradiation, the actuarial incidence of acute radiation pneumonitis was found to increase from 29% to 84% for uncorrected doses of 8–10 Gy, with a threshold of approximately 7.5 Gy.[12,33–35] In Van Dyk *et al.*'s analysis, a sigmoid dose–response curve was found, rising very steeply at 9.3–10.6 Gy.[35] Tait *et al.* compared subclinical changes in diffusing capacity (DLCO), transfer coefficient (KCO) and total lung capacity in patients receiving 8-Gy single-fraction TBI vs 12-Gy fractionated TBI. Single-fraction TBI induced more severe gas transfer impairment with slower and more incomplete recovery. $FEV_1/FVC$ was stable in patients not developing concomitant GvHD.[42]

Many investigators have evaluated the possible benefits of multiple fractionation and the development of interstitial pneumonitis (Table 14.3). In

**Table 14.3** Interstitial pneumonitis: does multiple fractionation reduce incidence?

| Yes | No |
| --- | --- |
| Bamberg *et al.*[43,a] | Kim *et al.*[14,a] |
| Cossett *et al.*[25,a] | Ozsahin *et al.*[13,b] |
| Inoue *et al.*[45,a] | Thomas *et al.*[19,a] |
| Keane *et al.*[34,a] | Weiner *et al.*[38,b] |
| Pino y Torres *et al.*[44,a] | |
| Shank *et al.*[24,a] | |
| Socie *et al.*[21,a] | |
| Tait *et al.*[42,a] | |

[a]Single institution retrospective comparison.
[b]Prospective randomized trial.

an early review of the Seattle experience, Thomas *et al.* evaluated a 10-Gy single fraction vs 12 Gy in six fractions. They found no significant decrease in the incidence of interstitial pneumonitis.[19] Kim *et al.* also found no difference when they compared their non-randomized series of 7.5-Gy single-fraction TBI vs 13.2 Gy at 1.65 Gy twice-a-day for 4 days.[14] In a randomized series, Ozsahin *et al.* analysed their patients and found no significant difference in the development of interstitial pneumonitis between single- and multiple-fractionated patients.[13] Weiner *et al.* reviewed the International Bone Marrow Transplant Registry data and failed to demonstrate any evidence of lung sparing with fractionated TBI.[38] Socie *et al.*, however, did find a statistically significant difference, with 37.5% for single-fraction treatment and 17.7% for multiple-dose TBI in their series of patients.[21]

There are numerous single institutional series comparing older single-fraction results that do support the belief that fractionated TBI does indeed significantly decrease the incidence of interstitial pneumonitis from the 45–50% range down to 15–30%.[24,25,34,43–45]

Dose rate may play as important a role as fractionation. Ozsahin *et al.* did show that single-fraction TBI at 0.15 Gy/min caused more interstitial pneumonitis than at 0.06 Gy/min. No such difference was found in the multiple-fractionated patients, though the dose rates compared were quite close (0.06 Gy/min vs 0.03 Gy/min).[13] This observation of the protective pulmonary effects of low dose rate has been found by others as well[24,37,46,47] in a review of their single institution results.

## Other late complications

Veno-occlusive disease (VOD) is a poorly understood phenomenon that may account for 5–10% of BMT-related deaths.[48] The true diagnosis must be made on both biopsy and clinical means but often the clinical picture of icterus, hepatalgia, hepatomegaly, weight gain, and ascites is sufficient.[49] VOD may be due to microangiopathic damage exacerbated by a synergistic effect between the TBI and chemotherapy. In single institutional studies,[10,19,25,50] the incidence significantly dropped with the change in TBI fractionation from single fraction to multiple fraction. However, McDonald *et al.* could find no decrease with fractionation in their series.[49] Ozsahin *et al.* reported an incidence of 6% in their series and could find no difference between either high-dose-rate or low-dose-rate treatment or in the single-fraction vs multiple-fractionated patients.[13]

## Cataract

Because the orbit and globe must be encompassed in the TBI field, especially in leukaemic patients, the incidence of cataracts can be significant. The elderly appear at highest risk. In Deeg *et al.*'s review of the Seattle experience, there was an incidence of up to 80% at 6 years in their 10-Gy single-fraction patients.[51] At the Hôpital Tenon in Paris, the incidence in single-fraction patients was reported at 20%, though the mean follow-up was relatively short.[13,52] After the switch to multiple-fractionated protocols, there was a dramatic decrease in the incidence of cataract formation to only 6%. In the Seattle experience, it decreased from 80% at 6 years to only

19% at 5 years.[51] Kim *et al.* and Ozsahin *et al.* noted a similar decrease with multiple fractions.[13,14,52] There also seems to be a dose-rate effect, with patients exposed to low dose rates developing cataracts only one-third as commonly as those exposed to dose rates of 0.15 Gy/min.[52]

## Renal dysfunction

Renal dysfunction has been well documented in animal systems, developing 3–7 months following bone marrow transplantation and total body irradiation.[53] Tarbell *et al.* have reported on patients treated for either neuroblastoma or acute lymphoblastic leukaemia (ALL) developing similar renal dysfunction. The incidence can be quite high with five out of seven patients with neuroblastoma and six out of seventeen with ALL developing significant renal dysfunction.[54] Haemolytic-uraemic syndrome (HUS) can also occur.[55]

## Liver

Moulder *et al.* have evaluated the late effects of TBI on liver function in animal systems. They evaluated numerous chemotherapeutic agents known to be primarily metabolized by the liver and found that the pharmacokinetics of all of the agents were affected. The pathology of the liver at autopsy demonstrated effects more consistent with late radiation damage, than with VOD.[56]

## Hormone effects

Thyroid dysfunction, primarily hypothyroidism, has been noted in several series. Sklar *et al.* at the University of Minnesota demonstrated that ten out of twenty-three patients developed either clinical or biochemical evidence of hypothyroidism following TBI and BMT.[57] Unpublished data from the Children's Hospital of Philadelphia demonstrated that only two out of forty-four patients developed hypothyroidism after multiple-fractionated TBI at low dose rate (August, personal communication). Growth hormone has been extensively investigated as well. Deeg felt that there was a significant disturbance in the growth of paediatric patients following TBI and BMT.[10] However, Serota *et al.* studied the linear growth of twenty children treated with cytoxan and no more than 8 Gy TBI at 0.05–0.10 Gy/min. Unlike the Seattle experience, Serota's group found no significant change in height percentiles in the absence of GvHD, interstitial pneumonia, or tumour relapse.[58] Gonadal function has been studied in long-term survivors. In males, although Leydig cell function was not compromised, germinal epithelium and spermatogenesis were damaged; in prepubescent females, follicle-stimulating hormone (FSH) and luteinizing hormone (LH) levels remained normal.[59]

## Secondary malignancies

The incidence of secondary malignancies is reportedly low in numerous series,[10,58–60] although the follow-up is relatively short. Further longitudinal evaluation is needed to determine the true risk to patients.

## The role of total body irradiation in the treatment of advanced low-grade lymphomas

Low dose TBI for favourable but advanced lymphomas has been used extensively for the last 20–25 years, often competing with multiagent chemotherapy regimens. A number of randomized studies have been performed comparing the effectiveness of TBI to either single- or multiagent chemotherapy. Johnson *et al.* reported the National Cancer Institute (NCI) trial evaluating multiple-agent chemotherapy of cyclophosphamide, vincristine, and prednisone (CVP) vs TBI for Stage III–IV poorly differentiated lymphocytic lymphoma. Overall response rate and survival were essentially identical between modalities, though late relapses were more common in the TBI arm and several cases of acute leukaemia developed.[61,62] The addition of TBI to CVP added nothing. Rubin *et al.* reported the Eastern Cooperative Oncology Group (ECOG) study evaluating TBI vs chlorambucil plus prednisone in active-phase chronic lymphocytic leukaemia. No difference was seen in any major parameter evaluated.[63] Hoppe *et al.* reported a three-arm prospectively randomized Stanford University trial comparing TBI to either single-agent chemotherapy or to combination chemotherapy. No difference was seen in either survival or relapse-free survival. Overall duration of therapy as well as acute side-effects was worse in either chemotherapy arm compared with the TBI arm.[64] Meerwaldt *et al.* evaluated the European study comparing low dose TBI with combination chemotherapy for advanced follicular lymphomas.[65] The patients were treated with either 0.10 Gy three times a week to a total of 25 Gy if haematologically stable, or the most aggressive out-patient multiagent chemotherapy regimen possible — cyclophosphamide, Adriamycin, teneposide (VM-26) and prednisone plus consolidated radiotherapy to areas of bulk disease. They found no significant differences in either complete response or freedom from disease progression. Patients treated with TBI did have more Grade III/IV haematological toxicities but no long-term effects, confirming an earlier study.[66] Mendenhall *et al.* reported on a 10-year follow-up study evaluating the role of TBI for Stage II–IV non-Hodgkin's lymphoma. Patients were treated with either 0.10 Gy per fraction, five days a week to doses of 2–3 Gy with a split, if necessary, or 0.15 Gy twice a week to a total of 1.5 Gy. Dose rates were between 0.03 Gy/min and 0.07 Gy/min. They reported a 77% complete response rate with a median duration response of 3.8 years for the favourable histologies, compared with only 35% with a shorter duration in the unfavourable histologies. They also found that previously untreated patients fared much better than patients who had previously been treated with extensive chemotherapy.[67]

The trend is to either observe or treat these favourable, follicular tumours with single- or multiagent chemotherapy. The true measure of effectiveness is to evaluate not only complete response rates, duration of long-term response, and survival, but also patient convenience, as well as acute and delayed morbidity. TBI seems to be a reasonable alternative to prolonged courses of multiagent chemotherapy and appears to offer less acute and long-term morbidity with similar complete response rates, as well as median duration of responses.[61–65,67]

# Clinical applications of TBI in bone marrow transplantation

## Aplastic anaemia

Aplastic anaemia is a disease of bone marrow failure characterized by severe pancytopenia and a hypoplastic marrow. Patients with granulocyte counts of less than $0.5 \times 10^9/l$, platelet counts of less than $20 \times 10^9/l$, and reticulocyte counts of less than 1% have an extremely poor prognosis, with mortality rates of 80–90% within the first 6 months following diagnosis. The disease has been associated with a variety of medications (including chloramphenicol, gold, and antithyroid medications), hepatitis, paroxysmal nocturnal haemoglobinuria, and other environmental/occupational factors.

Marrow replacement through allogeneic BMT is the preferred treatment for patients under the age of 55, leading to cures in upwards of 80% of patients.[68] The main impediments to successful transplantation are graft rejection and treatment-related toxicity including GvHD. The major goal of the conditioning regimen is to provide sufficient immunosuppression to allow donor marrow engraftment. Unless there is a coexisting clonal abnormality (such as myelodysplasia), there is no need for the preparative regimen to eliminate residual recipient marrow cells.

In patients felt to be at low risk for graft rejection (few prior transfusions/allosensitizations, full HLA-matched sibling transplants), cyclophosphamide alone, without irradiation, may provide sufficient immunosuppression. This conditioning regimen avoids the potential long-term toxicities of radiotherapy. However, in patients felt to be at high risk for graft rejection (multiple prior blood exposures, HLA-mismatched transplants, unrelated transplants), more aggressive immunosuppression is required. In these situations, combinations of cyclophosphamide and antithymocyte globulin (ATG),[69] the addition of buffy coat marrow,[70] or the inclusion of radiation into the conditioning regimen have been used successfully.[71,72] Patients who experience graft rejection may occasionally be salvaged with immediate second transplants using either radiation-based regimens or the cyclophosphamide/ATG regimen.

A recent retrospective analysis of 595 transplants, by the International Bone Marrow Transplant Register (IBMTR), noted a 5-year actuarial survival of 63% among patients transplanted worldwide for severe aplastic anaemia. The incidences of acute and chronic GvHD were 40% and 45%, respectively. Graft rejection occurred in 10%. No differences in long-term survival between varying conditioning regimens (cyclophosphamide alone, cyclophosphamide plus limited-field radiotherapy, or cyclophosphamide plus TBI) could be recognized, although the reasons for the choice of regimen were not adequately addressed. This review noted that the inclusion of radiotherapy decreased the incidence of graft rejection. However, this was accomplished at the expense of greater toxicity and GvHD.[73]

Currently the role of radiotherapy in the treatment of severe aplastic anaemia is unclear. Although TBI and total lymphoid irradiation produce sufficient immunosuppression to allow engraftment of donor marrow in high-risk cases (including highly transfused patients, mismatched grafts, and previously rejected grafts), concerns regarding long-term toxicity have fuelled the search for better conditioning regimens. The success of the cyclophosphamide/ATG regimen has further diminished enthusiasm for radiotherapy-based regimens.

## Chronic myelogenous leukaemia (CML)

CML is a haematological malignancy characterized by a translocation of the *abl* oncogene (located on chromosome 9) to the *bcr* region (on chromosome 22). Clinically, the disease can be divided into three phases. In the 'chronic phase', the disease consists of leukocytosis, thrombocytosis, splenomegaly and minimal systemic symptoms. After a variable period (2–5 years on average), the disease enters an 'accelerated phase' during which additional cytogenetic abnormalities arise and symptoms progress. Finally, the disease terminates in a 'blastic phase' which resembles acute leukaemia but unfortunately usually fails to respond to therapy. Conventional dose chemotherapy has been unsuccessful in altering this progressive course. Interferon may prolong the chronic phase and yield occasional cytogenetic remissions but most patients still progress to a blast crisis.[74]

Allogeneic BMT is a curative treatment and represents a major advance in the therapy of CML. Data from the IBMTR, which now includes more than 2000 CML patients, indicate that patients transplanted in the chronic phase have a 50–60% probability of long-term disease-free survival.[75] Single institution studies of optimally selected patients (i.e. transplanted within the first year of diagnosis) have achieved survival rates exceeding 80% at 2 years.[76] For patients lacking an HLA-matched sibling donor, results from unrelated volunteer donors (2-year disease-free survival rates of 45%) have been encouraging.[77] Autologous marrow grafting represents a new approach with promising preliminary responses.

The conditioning regimen for allogeneic CML transplants must both eradicate the clonal disorder and provide sufficient immunosuppression for donor engraftment. The most widely used regimens are combinations of cyclophosphamide and TBI, pioneered at the Fred Hutchinson Cancer Research Center,[78] and chemotherapy regimens of busulphan and cyclophosphamide, pioneered at Johns Hopkins University[79] and subsequently modified.[80] A recent Phase III trial comparing these two approaches found both to be effective and did not reveal any differences in major treatment or result parameters (Fig. 14.2).[81] One hundred and forty-two patients with chronic-phase CML under the age of 55, undergoing HLA-identical sibling transplants, were randomized to receive cyclophosphamide (120 mg/kg) with either TBI (12 Gy in six fractions) or busulphan (16 mg/kg). After a median follow-up of 3 years, there were no statistically significant differences in long-term control of disease with either regimen. Approximately 80% of patients in both arms remain alive and the relapse rate is approximately 10%.

An alternative radiation-based regimen, pioneered at Stanford University and the City of Hope Hospital, using hyperfractionated TBI (13.2 Gy in eleven fractions over 4 days) and etoposide (60 mg/kg) has yielded similar excellent results. With a median follow-up of 30 months, 79% of patients receiving this regimen remain in complete remission.[82]

Attempts to decrease relapse by increasing the radiation dose have met

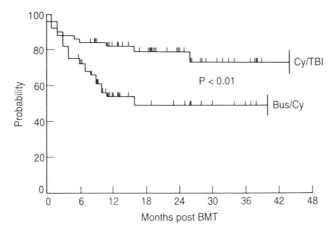

**Fig. 14.2** Comparison of cyclophosphamide/TBI vs busulphan/cyclophosphamide. Actuarial probability of disease-free survival. Tick marks represent living patients who did not relapse. (Reprinted from Clift *et al.*, *Blood* 1994; **84**, 2036–43.[81])

with mixed results. Although a fractionated schedule of 15.75 Gy yielded fewer relapses than 12 Gy, an increase in treatment-related mortality resulted in a decrease in overall survival for the high dose group.[26,83]

Presently the role of TBI in the treatment of CML appears well established. The expanding use of alternative donors in this disease (i.e. unrelated transplants) suggests that TBI will continue to play an important role.

## Acute myelogenous leukaemia (AML)

Although tremendous improvements in the treatment of AML have occurred over the past two decades, only 25–35% of patients are cured of their disease.[84] Conventional standard treatment typically consists of induction chemotherapy followed by some form of postremission therapy. A variety of induction regimens (including 3 days of cytarabine and 7 days of daunorubicin) achieve initial remission rates of 60–85%. Postremission therapy to suppress residual leukaemic clones may include consolidation therapy (abbreviated courses of the same regimen utilized to achieve remission) and/or intensification regimens (different agents given with the intensity to produce substantial marrow aplasia).

Ultrahigh dose therapy, such as allogeneic and autologous BMT, has been used as a form of intensification treatment for patients in initial remission or as a salvage treatment for patients with primary refractory or recurrent disease. The optimal timing of transplantation as part of the overall treatment approach is currently an area of intense investigation. In a recent European Oncology Research and Treatment Centre – (EORTC–GIEMA) randomized comparative trial of transplantation versus intensive conventional dose chemotherapy for patients in first remission, an improvement was noted in disease-free survival at 4 years in favour of allogeneic (54%)

and autologous BMT (49%) compared with conventional consolidation treatment (30%). However, the overall survival for remitters in the three arms was similar as patients who relapsed following traditional chemotherapy could occasionally be salvaged with delayed transplants.[85] An intergroup trial (ECOG3489/SWOG9034/CALGB9120) comparing transplantation with intensification conventional dose chemotherapy is nearing completion and will hopefully further clarify the optimal treatment strategy. For patients in second or later remission, standard dose chemotherapy rarely leads to durable remissions. BMT is the treatment of choice in these advanced cases.

Most patients undergoing allogeneic or autologous transplantation for AML have received either the cyclophosphamide/TBI or busulphan/cyclophosphamide regimen.[86] Both intensive preparative regimens are effective in eradicating the leukaemic clone(s) and provide sufficient immunosuppression of the recipient to allow permanent and functional allogeneic marrow engraftment. As in CML transplants, attempts to increase the radiation dose (from 12 to 15.75 Gy by fractionated schedules) have yielded decreased relapse rates but at the expense of increased toxicity, resulting in no difference in overall relapse-free survival.[87] Novel regimens including the substitution of etoposide or melphalan for cyclophosphamide in combination with TBI, or the addition of other chemotherapeutic agents to the combination (most notably cytarabine), also retain significant antileukaemic activity.

Three studies have attempted to define the value of radiotherapy as part of the allogeneic transplant preparative regimen for acute leukaemia. A French collaborative trial suggested that TBI-containing regimens might be superior to the combination of busulphan/cyclophosphamide in early disease.[88] One hundred and one patients with AML in first complete remission were randomized to receive either cyclophosphamide (120 mg/kg) with TBI (10-Gy single dose — seven patients; fractionated 12 Gy — forty-three patients) or busulphan (16 mg/kg) with cyclophosphamide (120 mg/kg — fifty-one patients). Patients were matched for age, sex, FAB classification, white blood cell count at the time of diagnosis, and the duration between the diagnosis and BMT. The outcome for the cyclophosphamide/TBI regimen at 2 years was better for probability of disease-free survival (72% vs 47%), overall survival (75% vs 51%), relapse (14% vs 34%) and transplant-related mortality (8% vs 27%) (Fig. 14.3). Although the relapse rate in the busulphan/cyclophosphamide group was higher than that noted in other reports, the authors suggested that this was due to the short interval between diagnosis and transplantation, allowing more patients to undergo transplantation in both arms while still at risk. In addition, the decreased toxicity of radiotherapy in this study, compared with other trials, was attributed to the adoption of lung-shielding techniques (to a median lung dose of 8.8 Gy).

Similar support for radiation-based transplant regimens in the treatment of leukaemia has been provided by a recent report from the Nordic Bone Marrow Transplant Group.[89] However, this study indicated that the benefit of radiotherapy might be largely a result of decreased toxicity. In the randomized trial of 167 patients, the busulphan/cyclophosphamide regimen was associated with increased treatment-related toxicities, including GvHD, VOD, and haemorrhagic cystitis, compared with cyclophosphamide/TBI.

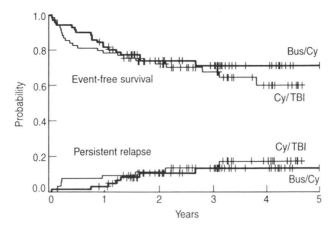

**Fig. 14.3** The probabilities of event-free survival and of developing cytogenic relapse for patients transplanted after the cyclophosphamide/TBI or busulphan/cyclophosphamide regimens. (Reprinted from Blaise *et al., Blood* 1992; **79**, 2578–82.[88])

This resulted in an increase in therapy-related mortality (busulphan 28% vs TBI 9%; $P = 0.006$) that was striking in patients with advanced-stage disease (beyond first remission or chronic phase). These differences in toxicity translated into improved 3-year actuarial survival for the TBI regimen (TBI 76% vs busulphan 62%; $P < 0.03$). However, in contrast to the French study, no statistical differences in relapse-free survival could be documented between the regimens. Relapse rates were similar with both conditioning regimens. Thus, the benefits of TBI in this study were restricted to a reduction in toxicity rather than an increase in disease control. The authors were unable to explain the differences in disease-free survival between AML first remission patients in their study and the French study (busulphan: 47% French vs 83% Nordic; TBI: 73% French vs 58% Nordic).

In contrast, a Southwest Oncology Group (SWOG) trial comparing busulphan/cyclophosphamide with a regimen of TBI and etoposide among patients with advanced leukaemias (beyond first remission) noted similar toxicity and survival rates.[90] One hundred and twenty-two patients were randomized to the two regimens. The 2-year disease-free survival for good-risk patients (second remission or accelerated phase CML) was 55% with TBI/etoposide compared with 34% with busulphan/cyclophosphamide ($P = 0.30$). Poor-risk patients had 2-year survivals of 17% vs 24% ($P = 0.81$). No differences between treatment-related toxicities or GvHD were reported. These studies point to the need for further comparisons to define the role of radiotherapy in the treatment of AML, and the need to develop more effective antileukaemic regimens that have tolerable safety profiles.

## Acute lymphoblastic leukaemia (ALL)

ALL represents a heterogeneous family of diseases. With current intensive chemotherapy regimens, most children enter prolonged remissions and over

60% are cured. However, the outlook for adults with ALL is not optimistic with only 20–30% obtaining long-term survival. Poor prognostic factors include an initial white cell count of over 50 000/μl, age less than 2 or older than 10 years, abnormal chromosomal karyotypes including t(8;14), t(4;11) and t(9;22), B-cell phenotype, and inability to achieve remission by 14 days following induction therapy.[91]

As in AML, the optimal timing of transplantation in ALL is currently under investigation.[92] In children, intensive chemotherapy without transplantation may salvage relapses. In adults, allogeneic transplantation at time of second remission has become standard therapy. Autologous transplants following relapse have been plagued by high relapse rates and may not be effective in some subtypes such as Philadelphia chromosome-positive ALL. The use of transplantation in high-risk cases at the time of first remission is an active area of research.

Most patients undergoing transplantation for ALL have received radiotherapy-based transplant regimens. Results from the IBMTR show a 44% and 62% relapse-free survival for adults and children, respectively, undergoing allogeneic transplantation in first remission.[26] In advanced disease, the disease-free survivals are 24% and 40%, respectively. Because relapse remains the major cause of death in ALL, new preparative regimens are being explored.[93,94]

ALL frequently involves the central nervous system (CNS), either at the time of diagnosis or at relapse. Consequently, most patients receive some form of CNS prophylaxis. Prior intrathecal therapy or CNS irradiation does not necessarily preclude the use of TBI in these patients. However, caution needs to be exercised in patients who will be undergoing transplantation after suffering a CNS relapse. These patients should not receive reirradiation in an attempt to eradicate CNS disease prior to transplant because this approach may lead to excessive toxicity. Such patients can be managed with intrathecal ARA-C or methotrexate until the time of transplant. For those individuals with no prior history of central nervous system disease, post-transplantation intrathecal chemotherapy should be administered, as TBI alone does not provide sufficient prophylaxis.

## Myelodysplastic and myeloproliferative syndromes

Myelodysplastic and myeloproliferative disorders represent clonal haematological diseases that are amenable to aggressive treatment with transplantation. In the preleukaemic syndromes, the goal of the transplant preparatory regimen is to eradicate the malignant clone. Cyclophosphamide with TBI (12 Gy) has yielded a 54% 4-year actuarial survival among patients with refractory anaemia and refractory anaemia with ringed sideroblasts.[95] However, in the more aggressive myelodysplastic syndromes (refractory anaemia with excess blasts and refractory anaemia with excess blasts in transition), relapse of disease remains common, suggesting that even more aggressive preparatory regimens are needed. Non-irradiation-based regimens, such as busulphan/cyclophosphamide, have been used sparingly and as yet there are no comparative trials.

Few transplants have been performed for the myeloproliferative disorders (polycythaemia vera, essential thrombocytosis, myeloid metaplasia with myelofibrosis, juvenile chronic myeloid leukaemia) other than CML. The value of radiotherapy in the conditioning regimens for these disorders is unknown.

## Multiple myeloma

Multiple myeloma is a progressive neoplastic disorder of plasma cells with a median postdiagnosis survival of only 3 years. Conventional chemotherapy typically results in initial responses but eventually the disease becomes refractory. Most patients with myeloma are elderly and are unable to tolerate transplant protocols. However, early results suggest that aggressive transplant schemata may be beneficial for younger patients. In addition, as improvements in supportive care continue, high dose therapy may eventually become an attractive option for selected elderly individuals.

It has long been recognized that multiple myeloma is a disease highly sensitive to the effects of irradiation. Allogeneic BMT is a potentially curative approach for young patients able to tolerate very aggressive therapy. Two large series have demonstrated long-term actuarial survivals of approximately 40% using either variations of the cyclophosphamide/TBI regimen or the busulphan/cyclophosphamide regimen.[96,97]

Autologous transplants, with their safer toxicity profile, are more commonly used in this disease, given the age of the diseased population.[98] A variety of either radiation-containing or all-chemotherapy preparative regimens have been attempted. Melphalan alone, at maximally tolerated doses (200 mg/m$^2$), or combinations of melphalan with TBI produce high complete remission rates in the 40–50% range when applied in patients with chemosensitive disease.[99] To date, there have been no direct comparative trials of radiation with chemotherapy in this disease although survival rates have been similar in uncontrolled series. A recently inaugurated intergroup trial is exploring the relative values of allogeneic transplantation, autologous transplantation using melphalan/TBI regimens vs conventional dose therapy.

## Non-Hodgkin's lymphoma

The non-Hodgkin's lymphomas are composed of a spectrum of lymphoproliferative disorders with varying histologies and natural histories.[100] The Working Formulation schema has attempted to classify these diseases according to their response to therapy by subdividing them into low-, intermediate-, and high-grade histologies.[101] In general, low-grade histologies follow a relatively benign course over several years, but are rarely cured with conventional therapy. In contrast, intermediate- and high-grade histologies follow a much more aggressive course, but may be cured with conventional chemotherapy in 40–50% of cases. Although several aggressive chemotherapy regimens have been developed over the past two decades, the CHOP regimen (cyclophosphamide, doxorubicin, vincristine, prednisone) yields comparable survival results with less toxicity, and currently remains the best initial treatment.[102] A predictive model to identify patients, at diagnosis, with a low chance for cure based on patient age, disease stage, performance status, serum LDH, and presence of extranodal disease, may prove useful in directing appropriate patients into clinical studies of high dose therapy.[103]

High dose therapy with stem cell rescue has become the treatment of choice for patients suffering relapse of intermediate- or high-grade histology non-Hodgkin's lymphoma. Aggressive treatment may salvage 30–40% of those with chemosensitive relapse and a small but significant proportion of patients with primary refractory or chemoresistant relapse.[104] Recently, the use of high dose regimens as initial treatment in patients with high-risk disease and in patients with low-grade histologies has entered clinical investigation. The majority of these transplants have used autologous marrow or peripheral blood stem cells as the source of haemopoietic rescue. Although allogeneic marrow may provide a graft versus lymphoma effect, the higher toxicity of this therapy has discouraged its widespread use.

In the autologous setting, the goal of the preparative regimen is to provide maximal antitumour effect rather than additional immunosuppression. Therefore, most autologous transplants for intermediate- and high-grade lymphomas have used chemotherapy-based regimens rather than TBI.[105] Exceptions to this trend have been in the low-grade lymphomas and lymphoblastic lymphomas. Comparative trials of varying regimens have not yet been performed.

At present, the role of radiotherapy in autologous bone marrow transplants (ABMT) for treatment of non-Hodgkin's lymphoma remains unclear. Rather than using TBI, many investigators have advocated localized radiotherapy to sites of bulk disease, either before transplant or as 'consolidation' following transplantation as we have been doing at our institution. Although it has been difficult to show survival advantages with either approach among complete responders, radiotherapy has been effective consolidation for patients who have achieved only a partial remission following BMT.[106]

## Hodgkin's disease

Hodgkin's disease is curable in approximately 75% of all patients.[107] Autologous transplantation using chemotherapy-based regimens is effective in salvaging 20–40% of patients who fail to achieve an initial complete remission or who relapse within 1 year of completing initial therapy.[108,109] Patients experiencing late relapse frequently benefit from either repeating the initial chemotherapy regimen or salvage radiotherapy rather than proceeding to a potentially toxic high dose treatment.

TBI is rarely used in patients undergoing transplantation for Hodgkin's disease. Since most patients have received some thoracic radiotherapy as part of their initial treatment, as well as pulmonary toxic chemotherapy, TBI carries an excessively high risk of pulmonary toxicity and is generally avoided.[110] In those patients who have not received prior mediastinal radiotherapy, total body irradiation preparative regimens may be efficacious, though at present we have adopted a regimen of high dose chemotherapy with aggressive local radiotherapy to bulky disease sites with good initial results.

## Solid tumours

The success of high dose chemotherapy in haematological malignancies has spurred the development of dose-intensive treatment of solid tumours. Over the past 5 years, the number of autologous transplants performed in the United States, as reported to the North American Autologous Bone Marrow Transplant Registry, has increased at a rate of over 20% per year and the yearly total now exceeds allogeneic transplantation. Breast cancer and lymphoma are the most common indications, but over 200 autologous transplants per year are performed for other solid tumours.[111] The indications for transplantation in chemosensitive solid tumours and the role of TBI or local irradiation remain areas of investigation.

### Breast cancer, germ cell tumours and ovarian carcinoma

TBI has not played a major role in the preparative regimens of these chemosensitive tumours. Most autologous transplant regimens have contained combinations of alkylating chemotherapeutic agents. The use of consolidative radiotherapy to sites of bulk disease, such as to the breast and axilla, has been advocated by some investigators.

### Neuroblastoma

Neuroblastoma is the most common solid malignancy of early childhood occurring outside the central nervous system. The tumour is chemoresponsive and radioresponsive. However, only 10–15% of children over 1 year old with Stage IV disease survive for more than 2 years with conventional therapy. Because of the low cure rate, the responsiveness of the tumour to initial therapy, a documented dose–response relationship between neuroblastoma and active agents, and the frequent achievement of a minimal disease state with induction therapy, neuroblastoma has been considered a candidate solid tumour for high dose trials.

Preparative transplantation regimens for neuroblastoma frequently include combinations of melphalan and TBI. In nine studies, involving over 400 advanced-disease patients transplanted in first remission, approximately a third of the children are disease free 3–4 years after autografting.[112] Similar results have been reported in 489 Stage IV patients with 2- and 5-year actuarial survival rates of 43% and 26%, respectively.[113] Favourable prognostic factors in this series included age less than 12 months at diagnosis, primary tumour size less than 10 cm, transplantation after 1987, and healed bone metastasis prior to BMT. The European Neuroblastoma Study Group (ENSG) conducted a randomized unpurged ABMT trial and noted improvement in survival and disease-free survival in those children receiving high dose therapy, although late relapses continued to occur, leading to only marginal improvement in overall survival.[114]

Among those patients with high-risk disease at presentation, in whom the need for BMT is anticipated, the dose of local irradiation given to vital structures during the induction phase must be limited. Delay in irradiation to the pelvis until the marrow is harvested should also be considered.

The high relapse rate following ABMT in neuroblastoma has raised concerns that contaminated marrow may be a source of disease reseeding.

Gene-marking studies have confirmed that infused tumour cells can be identified in relapse tissue.[115] Thus far, attempts to purge the marrow of disease have not had a notable impact on relapses. Improvements in purging techniques and/or alternative sources of haemopoietic stem cells, such as autologous peripheral blood stem cells (PBSC) or allogeneic marrow, may play an important role in this disease. Unfortunately, PBSC collections may not be tumour free. Circulating neoplastic neuroblastoma cells could be detected in 75% of peripheral blood specimens analysed at diagnosis, in 36% during therapy, and in 14% of PBSC harvests. Six of thirteen patients with minimal or no bone marrow disease had positive blood specimens.[116]

### Small cell lung cancer (SCLC)

Early results of high dose therapy in small cell lung cancer, which have frequently employed TBI, have been disappointing. Four consecutive studies by Souhami et al.[117] involving single-agent ABMT, double ABMT, induction chemotherapy followed by ABMT, and multiagent ABMT failed to result in improvements of survival over standard dose chemotherapy in limited-stage small cell lung cancer. The implications of these studies are that although there is a chemosensitive component of the tumour that can be reduced (yielding high initial response rates), a chemotherapy-resistant clone regenerates that cannot be eradicated, even with high dose therapy. Thus, it is not surprising that a randomized trial of ABMT as consolidation in responding SCLC patients revealed improvement in the relapse-free survival,[118] but similar overall survival rates. Recently, the addition of local radiotherapy to gain local control in sites of prior bulk disease following a chemotherapy-based transplant regimen has yielded encouraging results. Investigators at the Dana-Farber Cancer Institute have reported a disease-free survival of 52% at a median follow-up of 3 years in twenty-five patients with limited disease who were transplanted in complete remission (CR) or near CR.[119]

### Sarcoma

Although highly sensitive to chemotherapy and radiotherapy, metastatic Ewing's sarcoma is curable in less than 30% of children. High dose bone marrow consolidation trials performed in first remission have resulted in a 30–63% disease-free survival at 3–4 years.[120] In contrast, patients treated in relapse typically progress early, confirming a trend noted in most solid tumours that the greatest benefit of BMT occurs in chemotherapy-responsive patients treated early in their disease course. Several small series have used TBI as part of the conditioning regimen.[121]

### Thalassaemia and other genetic disorders

Allogeneic bone marrow transplantation has been applied in the treatment of a variety of genetic disorders including thalassaemia major, Fanconi's anaemia, severe combined immunodeficiency, Wiskott–Aldrich syndrome, sickle cell anaemia, and the lysosomal storage diseases.[122–125] Concerns regarding late toxicities in the paediatric setting, especially growth and developmental retardation and potential carcinogenesis, have limited the use of TBI-containing regimens in these non-neoplastic disorders.

## Transplantation involving alternative donors

A major limitation to widespread application of bone marrow transplantation for many patients is the inability to locate an HLA-matched sibling donor. In these individuals, transplants from HLA-partially-matched related donors or unrelated donors may be attempted. Preliminary results of the first 464 transplants facilitated by the National Marrow Donor Program have been encouraging.[126] The rates of disease-free survival at 2 years among patients with good-risk and poor-risk leukaemia are 40% and 19%, respectively. Among patients with congenital disorders, the survival has been 52%, and among patients with aplastic anaemia it has been 29%. Unfortunately, these transplants are complicated by a high degree of GvHD and an increased incidence of graft rejection. Therefore, the conditioning regimen must be aggressive in providing immunosuppression.

TBI is commonly included in the preparative regimen because of its excellent immunosuppressive qualities, the importance of which was underscored by a study from the Seattle transplant group. Using genotypically matched HLA-identical sibling donors, less than 2% of 930 transplants for haematological malignancies were complicated by graft failure. This contrasted with a 12% rate in 276 patients transplanted from HLA-haploidentical partially matched donors. The rate of graft failure in the haploidentical group varied with the degree of immunosuppression provided by the radiotherapy. Seventeen per cent of patients conditioned with 12 Gy, six fractions, 6 days TBI; 12% of patients conditioned with 15.75 Gy; 9% of patients conditioned with 13.2–14.4 Gy at 1.2 Gy, three times a day for eleven to twelve fractions; and 5% of patients given 10 Gy in a single dose experienced graft failure.[127] These findings have led to the inclusion of TBI in most unrelated and haploidentical transplants.

# The future role of TBI

BMT has emerged as an effective treatment for a variety of haematological malignancies, genetic disorders and solid tumours. TBI, with its broad antineoplastic activity and excellent immunosuppressive qualities, is an important part of many current conditioning regimens.

However, the future role of TBI in transplantation is unclear. Among those diseases with a high degree of chemoresistance, such as advanced leukaemias and refractory lymphomas, radiotherapy-based transplantation is likely to continue. New methods to target radiotherapy directly to sites of disease, which are under development, would further this use.[128] Additionally, radiotherapy-based regimens, because of their superior immunosuppression, will remain important for unrelated-donor transplants. Nevertheless, the increasing role of autologous transplantation (especially in solid tumours and as part of gene therapy), which does not rely on immunosuppressive qualities, may lead to a gradual reduction in the overall use of TBI. Current investigations on post-transplant immunotherapy, designed to simulate the immunological effects of graft versus tumour without the undesirable GvHD, will further expand the use of autologous transplantation among haematological malignancies and may lead to a subsequent reduction in the role of TBI.

# Conclusions

As the indications for transplantation change, so must the role of TBI change — more antitumour effect when chemoresistant tumour eradication is the goal; better immunosuppression when GvHD occurs, especially when dealing with partially matched transplants. The challenge is two-fold — to develop less-toxic TBI regimens while improving antitumour effects. We agree with the viewpoint expressed by Dr Gale and his associates that TBI remains an important factor, especially in T-cell-depleted transplants, but continued careful re-examination of techniques and results is mandatory.[2] Dr Thomas has expressed concerns that perhaps the limits of TBI have been established and that new directions must be explored, such as monoclonal antibodies and bone-seeking radioisotopes.[78] We agree that research along these lines must continue, as well as continuing to develop innovative integration of chemotherapy and irradiation of biological modifiers such as radioprotectors or sensitizers. Understanding more about the dose-rate effects and more effective shielding of vital dose-limiting structures are required, as well as improvement in the management of interstitial pneumonitis, VOD, and other acute and long-term effects that have been associated with the present regimens.

# References

1. Vriesendorp HM. Radiobiological speculations on therapeutic total body irradiation. Critical Review. *Hematol Oncol* 1990; **10**, 211–21.
2. Gale RP, Buttarini A, Bortin MM. What does total body irradiation do in bone marrow transplants for leukemia? *Int J Radiat Oncol Biol Phys* 1991; **20**, 631–4.
3. Jammett H, Mathé G, Pendic M. *et al.* Etude de six cas d'irradiation totalle aigue accedetelle. Review Franc Etudes. *Clin Biol* 1959; **4**, 210–25.
4. Hall EJ (ed). *Radiobiology for the Radiologist.* Philadelphia, PA: JB Lippincott and Co, 1988; 366–76.
5. Dutreix J, Wambersie A, Loierette M, *et al.* Time factors in total body irradiation. *Pathol Biol* 1979; **27**, 365–71.
6. Caldwell WL, Lammerton LF. Increased sensitivity of *in vitro* murine leukemic cells to fractionated x-rays. *Nature* 1965; **208**, 168–70.
7. Peters LJ, Withers HR, Cundiff JH. Radiological considerations in the use of total body irradiation for bone marrow transplantation. *Radiology* 1979; **131**, 243–7.
8. Shank B, Andreef M, Li D. Cell survival kinetics in peripheral blood in bone marrow during total body irradiation for marrow transplantation. *Int J Radiat Oncol Biol Phys* 1983; **9**, 1613–23.
9. Storb R, Raff RF, Graham T, *et al.* Marrow toxicity of fractionated vs single

dose total body irradiation is identical in a canine mode. *Int J Radiat Oncol Biol Phys* 1993; **26**, 275–83.

10. Deeg HJ. Acute and delayed toxicities of total body irradiation. *Int J Radiat Oncol Biol Phys* 1983; **9**, 1933–9.

11. Evans RG. Radiobiological considerations in magna-field irradiation. *Int J Radiat Oncol Biol Phys* 1983; **9**, 1907–11.

12. Fryer C, Fitzpatrick P, Ryder W. Radiation pneumonitis. *Int J Radiat Oncol Biol Phys* 1978; **4**, 931–7.

13. Ozsahin M, Pene F, Touboul E, et al. Total body irradiation before bone marrow transplantation. *Cancer* 1992; **69**, 2853–65.

14. Kim TH, McGlane PB, Ramsay N. Comparison of two total body irradiation regimens in allogeneic bone marrow transplantation for acute non-lymphoblastic leukemia in first remission. *Int J Radiat Oncol Biol Phys* 1990; **19**, 889–97.

15. Scarpati D, Frassoni MD, Vitale V. Total body irradiation in acute myeloid leukemia and chronic myeloid leukemia: influence of dose and dose rate on leukemic relapse. *Int J Radiat Oncol Biol Phys* 1989; **17**, 5478–552.

16. Vriesendorp HM. Prediction of effects of therapeutic total body irradiation in man. *Radiother Oncol* 1990; **18**, 37–52.

17. Deeg HJ, Storb R, Longton G, et al. Single dose or fractionated total body irradiation and autologous marrow transplant in dogs: effects of exposure rate, fraction size, and fractionation interval on acute and delayed toxicity. *Int J Radiat Oncol Biol Phys* 1988; **15**, 647–53.

18. Tarbell NJ, Amato DA, Down JD, et al. Fractionation and dose rate effects in mice. *Int J Radiat Oncol Biol Phys* 1987; **13**, 1065–9.

19. Thomas ED, Clift RA, Herman J, et al. Marrow transplantation for acute non-lymphoblastic leukemia and first remission using fractionated or single-dose irradiation. *Int J Radiat Oncol Biol Phys* 1982; **8**, 817–21.

20. Dinsmore R, Kirkpatrick D, Flomenberg N. Allogeneic bone marrow transplantation for patients with acute lymphoblastic leukemia. *Blood* 1983; **62**, 381–8.

21. Socie G, Devergie A, Gerinsky T, et al. Influence of fractionation of total body irradiation on complications and relapse rate for chronic myelogenous leukemia. *Int J Radiat Oncol Biol Phys* 1991; **20**, 397–404.

22. Thomas ED, Ashley CA, Lochte HE. Homografts of bone marrow in dogs after lethal total body irradiation. *Blood* 1959; **14**, 720–36.

23. Messner HA, Fyles G, Meharchment J. Long term survival of bone marrow transplantation recipients with AML, ALL, and CML after preparation with chemotherapy and total body irradiation of 500 cGy. *J Cell Biochem* 1988, Suppl 12C, 92.

24. Shank B, Hopfan S, Kim JH, et al. Hyperfractionated total body irradiation for bone marrow transplantation. *Int J Radiat Oncol Biol Phys* 1981; **7**, 1109–15.

25. Cossett JM, Baume D, Pico JL, et al. Single dose versus hyperfractionated total body irradiation before allogenic bone marrow transplant. *Radiother Oncol* 1989; **15**, 151–60.

26. Buckner CD, Clift RA, Appelbaum FR. A randomized trial of 12.0 or 15.75 Gy of total body irradiation in patients with acute non-lymphoblastic leukemia and chronic myelogenous leukemia followed by marrow transplantation. *Exper Hematol* 1989; **17**, 522–9.

27. Van Dyke, Galvin JM, Glasco GP, et al. The physical aspects of total and hemibody photon irradiation. A report of Task Group 29 Radiation Therapy Committee: *AAPM Report No 17*. New York: American Association of Physicists in Medicine, June 1986.

28. Shank B. Techniques of magna field irradiation. *Int J Radiat Oncol Biol Phys*

1983; **9**, 1925–31.

29. Galvin JM. Calculation and prescription of dose for total body irradiation. *Int J Radiat Oncol Biol Phys* 1983; **9**, 1919–24.

30. Yahalom J, Fuks ZY. Strategies for the use of total body irradiation as systemic therapy in leukemias and lymphomas. In: JO Armitage, KH Antman, eds, *High-Dose Cancer Therapy*. Baltimore, MD: Williams & Wilkins, 1992; 156–8.

31. Gluckman E, Devergie A, Dutreix A, *et al*. Total body irradiation in bone marrow transplantation. Hôspital Saint Louis results. *Path Biol* 1979; **27**, 349–52.

32. Thomas ED, Buckner CD, Banaji M, *et al*. One hundred patients with acute leukemia with chemotherapy, total body irradiation and allogenic marrow transplantation. *Blood* 1977; **49**, 511–33.

33. Fitzpatrick PJ, Rider WD. Half-body radiotherapy. *Int J Radiat Oncol Biol Phys* 1976; **1**, 197–207.

34. Keane TJ, Van Dyk KW, Ryder WD. Interstitial pneumonitis following total body irradiation. *Int J Radiat Oncol Biol Phys* 1981; **7**, 1365–70.

35. Van Dyk J, Keane TJ, Kan S. Radiation pneumonitis following a large single dose of irradiation. A re-evaluation based on absolute dose to lung. *Int J Radiat Oncol Biol Phys* 1981; **7**, 461–7.

36. Neiman PE, Reeves W, Ray G, *et al*. A prospective analysis of interstitial pneumonia and opportunistic viral infections among recipients of allogenic bone marrow grafts. *J Infect Dis* 1977; **136**, 754–67.

37. Barrett A, Depledge MH, Powles RL. Interstitial pneumonitis following bone marrow transplantation after low dose rate TBI. *Int J Radiat Oncol Biol Phys* 1983; **9**, 1029–33.

38. Weiner RS, Bortin MM, Gale RP, *et al*. Interstitial pneumonitis after bone marrow transplantation. *Ann Intern Med* 1986; **104**, 168–75.

39. Ginsberg SJ, Comis RL. The pulmonary toxicity of antineoplastic agents. *Semin Oncol* 1982; **9**, 34–51.

40. Depledge MH, Barrett A, Powles RL. Lung function after bone marrow grafting. *Int J Radiat Oncol Biol Phys* 1983; **9**, 145–51.

41. Penney DP, Seimann DW, Rubin P, *et al*. Morphological correlates of fractionated radiation of the mouse lung: early and late effects. *Int J Radiat Oncol Biol Phys* 1994; **29**, 789–804.

42. Tait RC, Burnett AK, Robertson AG, *et al*. Subclinical pulmonary function defects following autologous and allogenic bone marrow transplantation relationship to total bone irradiation and graft vs host disease. *Int J Radiat Oncol Biol Phys* 1991; **20**, 1219–27.

43. Bamberg M, Beelen DW, Mahmoud HK, *et al*. The incidence of interstitial pneumonitis. Comparison of total body irradiation schedules for allogeneic bone marrow transplantation. *Strahlenther Onkol* 1986; **162**, 218–22.

44. Pino y Torres JL, Bross DS, Lam W, *et al*. Risk factors and interstitial pneumonitis following allogeneic bone marrow transplantation. *Int J Radiat Oncol Biol Phys* 1982; **8**, 1301–7.

45. Inoue T, Masaoka T, Shibata H. Interstitial pneumonias following allogenic bone marrow transplantation in the treatment of leukemia. *Strahlenther Onkol* 1988; **164**, 729–33.

46. Rindgen O, Baryd I, Johannson B. Increased mortality by septicemia, interstitial pneumonitis, and pulmonary fibrosis among bone marrow transplant recipients receiving an increased mean dose rate of total body irradiation. *Acta Radiol Oncol* 1983; **22**, 423–8.

47. Cordonnier C, Bernaudin JF, Bierling P, *et al*. Pulmonary complications occurring after allogenic bone marrow transplantation. *Cancer* 1986; **58**, 1047–54.

48. Ganem G, Girardin MFSM, Kuentz M, *et al*. Veno-occlusive disease of the

liver after allogenic bone marrow transplantation in man. *Int J Radiat Oncol Biol Phys* 1988; **14**, 879–84.

49. McDonald GB, Sharma T, Matthews DE, *et al.* Veno-occlusive disease of the liver after bone marrow transplantation. *Hepatology* 1984; **4**, 116–22.

50. Baume D, Cossett JM, Pico JL. Maladie veino-occlusive de foie apres graft de moelle osseuse. *Presse Medicine* 1987; **16**, 1559–63.

51. Deeg HJ, Flournoy N, Sullivan K, *et al.* Cataracts after total body irradiation and marrow transplantation — effect of dose fractionation. *Int J Radiat Oncol Biol Phys* 1984; **10**, 957–64.

52. Ozsahin M, Belkacemi Y, Pene F, *et al.* Total body irradiation cataract incidence. A randomized comparison of two instantaneous dose rates. *Int J Radiat Oncol Biol Phys* **28**, 343–7.

53. Bergstein J, Andreoli SP, Probizer AJ, *et al.* Radiation nephritis following total body irradiation and cyclophosphamide in preparation for bone marrow transplantation. *Transplantation* 1986; **41**, 63–6.

54. Tabell NJ, Guinan EC, Neimeyer C, *et al.* Late onset of renal dysfunction in survivors of bone marrow transplantation. *Int J Radiat Oncol Biol Phys* 1988; **15**, 99–104.

55. Rabinowe RN, Soiffer RJ, Tarbell NJ, *et al.* Hemolytic uremic syndrome following bone marrow transplantation in adults with hematological malignancies. *Blood* 1991; **77**, 1837–44.

56. Moulder JE, Fish BL, Holcenberg JS, *et al.* Hepatic function and drug pharmacokinetics after total body irradiation plus bone marrow transplantation. *Int J Radiat Oncol Biol Phys* 1990; **19**, 1389–96.

57. Sklar C, Kim T, Ramsay N. Thyroid dysfunction among long term survivors of bone marrow transplantation. *AACR/ASCO Proc* 1982; **23**, 157.

58. Serota FT, Burkey PA, August CS, *et al.* Total body irradiation as preparation for bone marrow transplantation in the treatment of acute leukemia in aplastic anemia. *Int J Radiat Oncol Biol Phys* 1983; **9**, 1941–9.

59. Stewart PS, Buckner CD, Clift RA *et al.* Allogenic marrow grafting for acute leukemias: a follow-up of long-term survivors. *Exper Hematol* 1982; **7**, 509–18.

60. Witherspoon RP, Fischer LD, Schoch G, *et al.* Secondary cancers after bone marrow transplantation for leukemia or aplastic anemia. *N Engl J Med* 1989; **321**, 784–7.

61. Johnson RE, Canellos GP, Young RC, *et al.* Chemotherapy vs total body irradiation for Stage III–IV poorly differentiated lymphocytic lymphoma. *Cancer Treat Rep* 1978; **62**, 321–5.

62. Young RC, Johnson RE, Canellos GP, *et al.* Randomized comparisons of chemotherapy and radiotherapy alone or in combination. *Cancer Treat Rep* 1977; **61**, 1153–9.

63. Rubin P, Bennett JM, Begg C, *et al.* The comparison of total body irradiation vs chlorambucil plus prednisone for remission induction of active chronic lymphocytic leukemia: an ECOG study. *Int J Radiat Oncol Biol Phys* 1981; **7**, 1623–32.

64. Hoppe RT, Kushlan P, Kaplan HS, *et al.* The treatment of advanced stage favorable histology non-Hodgkin's lymphoma. A preliminary report of a randomized trial comparing single agent chemotherapy, combination chemotherapy and whole body irradiation. *Blood* 1981; **58**, 592–8.

65. Meerwaldt JH, Carde P, Burgers JM, *et al.* Low dose total body irradiation vs combination chemotherapy for lymphomas with follicular growth patterns. *Int J Radiat Oncol Biol Phys* 1991; **21**, 1167–72.

66. Lybeert MLM, Meerwaldt JH, Denebe W, *et al.* Long term results of low dose total body irradiation for advanced non-Hodgkin's lymphoma. *Int J Radiat Oncol Biol Phys* 1987; **13**, 1167–72.

67. Mendenhall NP, Noyse WD, Million RR. Total body irradiation for Stage

II–IV non-Hodgkin's lymphoma: 10 year follow-up. *J Clin Oncol* 1989; **7**, 67–74.

68. Storb R, Longton G, Anasetti C, *et al*. Changing trends in marrow transplantation for aplastic anemia. *Bone Marrow Transplant* 1992; **10** (Suppl 1), 45–52.

69. Storb R, Etzioni R, Anasetti C, *et al*. Cyclophosphamide combined with antithymocyte globulin in preparation for allogeneic marrow transplants in patients with aplastic anemia. *Blood* 1994; **84**, 941–9.

70. Storb R, Doney KC, Thomas ED, *et al*. Marrow transplantation with or without donor buffy coat cells for 56 transfused aplastic anemia patients. *Blood* 1994; **59**, 236–46.

71. McGlave PB, Haake R, Miller W, *et al*. Therapy of severe aplastic anemia in young adults and children with allogeneic bone marrow transplantation. *Blood* 1987; **70**, 1325–30.

72. Gluckman E, Socie G, Devergie A, *et al*. Bone marrow transplantation in 107 patients with severe aplastic anemia using cyclophosphamide and thoraco-abdominal irradiation: long-term follow-up. *Blood* 1991; **78**, 2451–5.

73. Gluckman E, Horowitz MM, Champlin RE, *et al*. Bone marrow transplantation for severe aplastic anemia: influence of conditioning and graft-versus-host disease prophylaxis regimens on outcome. *Blood* 1992; **79**, 269–75.

74. Kantarjian HM, Deisseroth A, Kurzrock R, *et al*. Chronic myelogenous leukemia: a concise update. *Blood* 1993; **82**, 691–703.

75. Champlin R, McGlave P. Allogeneic bone marrow transplantation for chronic myeloid leukemia. In: SJ Forman, KG Blume, ED Thomas, eds, *Bone Marrow Transplantation*. Cambridge, MA: Blackwell Scientific Publications, 1994; 595–606.

76. Thomas ED, Clift RA, Fefer A, *et al*. Marrow transplantation for the treatment of chronic myelogenous leukemia. *Ann Intern Med* 1986; **104**, 155–63.

77. McGlave P, Bartsch G, Anasetti C, *et al*. Unrelated donor marrow transplantation therapy for chronic myelogenous leukemia: initial experience of the National Marrow Donor Program. *Blood* 1993; **81**, 543–50.

78. Thomas ED. Total body irradiation regimens for marrow grafting. *Int J Radiat Oncol Biol Phys* 1990; **19**, 1285–8.

79. Santos GW, Tutschka PJ, Brookmeyer R, *et al*. Marrow transplantation for acute nonlymphocytic leukemia after treatment with busulfan and cyclophosphamide. *N Engl J Med* 1983; **309**, 1347–53.

80. Tutschka PJ, Copelan EA, Klein JP. Bone marrow transplantation for leukemia following a new busulfan and cyclophosphamide regimen. *Blood* 1987; **70**, 1382–8.

81. Clift RA, Buckner CD, Thomas ED, *et al*. Marrow transplantation for CML: a randomized study comparing cyclophosphamide and TBI with busulfan and cyclophosphamide. *Blood* 1994; **84**, 2036–43.

82. Blume K, Forman S. High dose etoposide (VP-16)-containing preparatory regimens in allogeneic and autologous bone marrow transplantation for hematologic malignancies. *Semin Oncol* 1992; **19** (Suppl 13), 63–6.

83. Clift RA, Buckner CD, Appelbaum FR, *et al*. Allogeneic marrow transplantation in patients with chronic myelogenous leukemia in the chronic phase: a randomized trial of two irradiation regimens. *Blood* 1991; 77, 1660–5.

84. Stone RM, Mayer RJ. Treatment of the newly diagnosed adult with de novo acute myeloid leukemia. *Hematol Oncol Clin North Am* 1993; 7, 47–64.

85. Zittoun R, Mandelli F, Willhelmz R, *et al*. Prospective phase III study of autologous bone marrow transplantation (ABMT) v short intensive chemotherapy (IC) v allogeneic bone marrow transplantation (allo-BMT) during first complete remission (CR) of acute myelogenous leukemia (AML). Results of the EORTC–GIEMA AML 8A trial. *Blood* 1993; **82** (Suppl 1), 85a.

86. Gorin NC. High-dose therapy for acute myelogenous leukemia. In: JO Armitage, KH Antman, eds, *High-Dose Cancer Therapy*. Baltimore, MD: Williams & Wilkins, 1992; 569–606.
87. Clift RA, Buckner CD, Appelbaum FR, *et al.* Allogeneic marrow transplantation in patients with acute myeloid leukemia in first remission: a randomized trial of two irradiation regimens. *Blood* 1990; **76**, 1867–71.
88. Blaise D, Maraninchi D, Archimbaud E, *et al.* Allogeneic bone marrow transplantation for acute myeloid leukemia in first remission: a randomized trial of a busulfan/cytoxan vs cytoxan/total body irradiation as preparative regimen: a report from the Groupe d'Etudes de la Greffe de Moelle Osseuse. *Blood* 1992; **79**, 2578–82.
89. Ringden O, Ruutu T, Remberger M, *et al.* A randomized trial comparing busulfan with total body irradiation as conditioning in allogeneic marrow transplant recipients with leukemia: a report from the Nordic Bone Marrow Transplantation Group. *Blood* 1994; **83**, 2723–30.
90. Blume KG, Kopecky KJ, Henslee-Downey JP, *et al.* A prospective randomized comparison of total body irradiation–etoposide versus busulfan-cyclophosphamide as preparatory regimens for bone marrow transplantation in patients with leukemia who were not in first remission: a Southwest Oncology Group Study. *Blood* 1993; **81**, 2187–93.
91. Poplack DG. Clinical manifestations of acute lymphoblastic leukemia. In: R Hoffman, EJ Benz Jr, SJ Shattil, *et al.*, eds, *Hematology: Basic Principles and Practice*. New York: Churchill–Livingstone, 1991; 776–84.
92. Ramsay NKC, Kersey JH. Indications for marrow transplantation in acute lymphoblastic leukemia. *Blood* 1990; **75**, 815–18.
93. Bortin MM, Barrett AJ, Horowitz MM, *et al.* Progress in allogeneic bone marrow transplantation for acute lymphoblastic leukemia in the 1980s: a report from the IBMTR. *Leukemia* 1992; **6** (Suppl 2), 196–7.
94. Barrett AJ. Allogeneic bone marrow transplantation for acute lymphoblastic leukemia. *Leukemia* 1992; **6** (Suppl 2), 139–43.
95. Anderson JE, Appelbaum FR, Fisher LD, *et al.* Allogeneic bone marrow transplantation for 93 patients with myelodysplastic syndrome. *Blood* 1993; **82**, 677–81.
96. Gahrton G, Tura S, Ljungman P, *et al.* Allogeneic bone marrow transplantation in multiple myeloma. *N Engl J Med* 1993; **325**, 1267–73.
97. Bensinger WI, Buckner CD, Clift RA, *et al.* A phase I study of busulfan and cyclophosphamide in preparation for allogeneic marrow transplant for patients with multiple myeloma. *J Clin Oncol* 1992; **10**, 1492–7.
98. Barlogie B, Gahrton G. Bone marrow transplantation in multiple myeloma — a review. *Bone Marrow Transplant* 1991; **7**, 71–9.
99. Barlogie B, Jagannath S. Autologous bone marrow transplantation for multiple myeloma. In: SJ Forman, KG Blume, ED Thomas, eds, *Bone Marrow Transplantation*. Cambridge, MA: Blackwell Scientific Publications, 1994; 754–66.
100. Armitage JO. Treatment of non-Hodgkin's lymphoma. *N Engl J Med* 1993; **328**, 1023–30.
101. The Non-Hodgkin's Lymphoma Pathologic Classification Project. National Cancer Institute sponsored study of classifications of non-Hodgkin's lymphomas: summary and description of a working formulation for clinical usage. *Cancer* 1982; **49**, 2112–35.
102. Fisher RI, Gaynor ER, Dahlberg S, *et al.* Comparison of a standard regimen (CHOP) with three intensive chemotherapy regimens for advanced non-Hodgkin's lymphoma. *N Engl J Med* 1993; **328**, 1002–6.
103. The International Non-Hodgkin's Lymphoma Prognostic Factors Project. A predictive model for aggressive non-Hodgkin's lymphoma. *N Engl J Med* 1993;

329, 987–94.

104. Philip T, Armitage JO, Spitzer G, et al. High dose therapy and autologous bone marrow transplantation after failure of conventional chemotherapy in adults with intermediate grade or high grade non-Hodgkin's lymphoma. *N Engl J Med* 1987; **316**, 1493–8.

105. Bierman PJ, Armitage JO. Autologous bone marrow transplantation for non-Hodgkin's lymphoma. In: SJ Forman, KG Blume, ED Thomas, eds, *Bone Marrow Transplantation.* Cambridge, MA: Blackwell Scientific Publications, 1994; 683–95.

106. Goldstone AH, Singer CRJ, Gribben JG, et al. Fifth report of EBMTG experience of ABMT in malignant lymphoma. *Bone Marrow Transplant* 1988; **3** (Suppl 1), 33–6.

107. Urba WJ, Longo DL. Hodgkin's disease. *N Engl J Med* 1992; **326**, 678–87.

108. Philips GL. Transplantation for Hodgkin's disease. In: SJ Forman, KG Blume, ED Thomas, eds, *Bone Marrow Transplantation.* Cambridge, MA: Blackwell Scientific Publications, 1994; 696–708.

109. Bierman PJ, Armitage JO. Role of autotransplantation in Hodgkin's disease. *Hematol Oncol Clin North Am* 1993; **7**, 591–611.

110. Pecego R, Hill R, Appelbaum FR, et al. Interstitial pneumonitis following autologous bone marrow transplantation. *Transplantation* 1986; **42**, 515–17.

111. Armitage JO, Horowitz MM. Increasing use of autotransplants to treat malignancy. *Blood* 1993; **82** (Suppl 1), 673a.

112. Graham-Pole JR. Myeloablative treatment supported by marrow infusions for children with neuroblastoma. In: JO Armitage, KH Antman, eds, *High-Dose Cancer Therapy.* Baltimore, MD: Williams & Wilkins, 1992; 735–49.

113. Ladenstein R, Lasset C, Hartmann O, et al. The Lyon and the EBMT data on megatherapy (MGT) in neuroblastoma followed by bone marrow rescue. *Bone Marrow Transplant* 1992; **10** (Suppl 2), 14.

114. Pinkerton CR. ENSG-1 randomized study of high-dose melphalan in neuroblastoma. *Bone Marrow Transplant* 1991; **7** (Suppl 3), 112–13.

115. Brenner MK, Rill DR, Holladay M, et al. Gene transfer in autologous bone marrow transplantation. Paper presented at Fourth International Symposium on Bone Marrow Purging and Processing, Orlando, FL, 16–17 September 1993.

116. Moss TJ, Sander DG, Lasky LC, et al. Contamination of peripheral blood stem cell harvests by circulating neuroblastoma cells. *Blood* 1990; **76**, 1879–83.

117. Souhami RL, Hajichristou HT, Miles DW, et al. Intensive chemotherapy with autologous bone marrow transplantation for small-cell lung cancer. *Cancer Chemother Pharmacol* 1989; **24**, 321–5.

118. Humblet Y, Symann M, Bosly A, et al. Late intensification chemotherapy with autologous bone marrow transplantation in selected small-cell carcinoma of the lung: a randomized study. *J Clin Oncol* 1987; **5**, 1864–73.

119. Elias AD, Ayash L, Wheeler C, et al. High dose combined alkylating agents supported by autologous bone marrow with chest radiotherapy for responding limited stage small cell lung cancer. *Proc ASCO* 1992; **11**, 296a.

120. Antman KH, Elias A, Fine HA. Dose-intensive therapy with autologous bone marrow transplantation in solid tumors. In: SJ Forman, KG Blume, ED Thomas, eds, *Bone Marrow Transplantation.* Cambridge, MA: Blackwell Scientific Publications, 1994; 767–88.

121. Burdach S, Juergens H, Peters C, et al. Myeloablative radiochemotherapy and hematopoietic stem-cell rescue in poor-prognosis Ewing's sarcoma. *J Clin Oncol* 1993; **11**, 1482–8.

122. Brochstein JA. Bone marrow transplantation for genetic disorders. *Oncology* 1992; **6**, 51–6.

123. Lucarelli G, Galimberti M, Polchi P, et al. Bone marrow transplantation for

patients with thalassemia. *N Engl J Med* 1990; **322**, 417–21.

124. Hows JM, Chapple M, Marsh JCW, *et al*. Bone marrow transplantation for Fanconi's anemia: the Hammersmith experience 1977–89. *Bone Marrow Transplant* 1989; **4**, 629–34.
125. Lenarsky C, Parkman R. Bone marrow transplantation for the treatment of immune deficiency states. *Bone Marrow Transplant* 1990; **6**, 361–9.
126. Kernan NA, Bartsch G, Ash RC *et al*. Analysis of 462 transplantations from unrelated donors facilitated by the National Marrow Donor Program. *N Engl J Med* 1993; **328**, 593–602.
127. Anasetti C, Amos D, Beatty PG, *et al*. Effect of HLA compatibility on engraftment of bone marrow transplants in patients wtih leukemia or lymphoma. *N Engl J Med* 1989; **320**, 197–204.
128. Vriesendorp HM, Quadri SM, Williams JR. Radioimmunoglobulin therapy. In: JO Armitage, KH Antman, eds, *High-Dose Cancer Therapy*. Baltimore, MD: Williams & Wilkins, 1992; 84–123.

# 15 The role of radiation therapy in endometrial carcinoma

*Nina Einhorn*

## Historical review

Surgery as a treatment for endometrial carcinoma developed during the nineteenth century, but at that time the primary mortality was high; Schottlaender and Kermauner reported 18% in 1912.[1] This substantial mortality was the primary reason for radiotherapy already being introduced in 1908 in Paris.[2] Forsell reported on three cases of carcinoma of the endometrium treated by radiotherapy in 1914.[3] He emphasized the value of radiotherapy where no other type of treatment could be effective, but Heyman extended this treatment to clinically operable cases[4] and in 1930 he introduced so called 'packing methods'.[5-7] The results with radiotherapy alone were encouraging in the years 1914–30, when only 41% survived in more selected patients who underwent surgery, compared with 33% of all patients treated with radiotherapy alone. During the 1930s, surgery and radiotherapy began to be used in combination, and the survival rate increased to 60%. Advances in anaesthesia, antibiotics and surgical techniques considerably improved the survival rate in operable endometrial carcinoma, but also moved the treatment modalities towards primary surgery, especially in patients with good prognostic factors.

## Epidemiology

Adenocarcinoma of the endometrium is the fourth commonest cancer in women.[8] There was a significant increase in incidence of carcinoma of the endometrium during the 1970s, especially in the western world. It is not entirely certain whether this apparent increase is related to:

1. an increased elderly population;
2. unopposed oestrogen administration, which was frequently given during the 1960s;
3. better nutrition;
4. better diagnostic tools.

There are still extensive geographical differences in the incidence of carcinoma of the endometrium. In the United States, the peak incidence is found in the San Francisco area, with 25.7 cases per 10 000 women, which can be compared with Sweden, 13.2, and Nagpur, India, 1.2 women per 100 000.[9,10]

Endometrial carcinoma is predominantly a disease of older women. The highest incidence is found among women of 65–69 years of age. Only 0.5% of the cases occur in women under 40 years of age (Table 15.1).

**Table 15.1**   Number of new cases of endometrial carcinoma by age at diagnosis in Sweden, 1990

| Age at diagnosis | New cases | Incidence per 100 000 |
|---|---|---|
| 25–29 | 1 | 0.3 |
| 30–34 | 0 | — |
| 35–39 | 4 | 1.4 |
| 40–44 | 12 | 3.7 |
| 45–49 | 47 | 16.2 |
| 50–54 | 81 | 35.4 |
| 55–59 | 120 | 56.7 |
| 60–64 | 156 | 70.5 |
| 64–69 | 186 | 77.8 |
| 70–74 | 141 | 67.1 |
| 75–79 | 122 | 65.8 |
| 80–84 | 89 | 66.3 |
| 85 + | 55 | 59.0 |

Source: the Cancer Registry, *Incidence in Sweden* 1990. Stockholm: National Board of Health and Welfare, 1993.[8]

# Aetiology

The aetiological factors are well established and it is generally accepted that endometrial cancer is an oestrogen-dependent neoplasm. Obesity, nulliparity and late menopause have been classically associated with endometrial carcinoma. The unopposed use of oestrogens was documented during the 1970s as the cause of a 1.5-fold increase in the number of patients with endometrial carcinoma in the United States.[11] There are other conditions where endogenous oestrogens may contribute to the development of endometrial carcinoma. An increased incidence of endometrial carcinoma has been found in patients with granulosa theca cell tumours,[12] as well as in polycystic ovary syndrome and ovarian dysgenesis.[13,14]

Diagnosis is usually made as a result of bleeding in postmenopausal

**Table 15.2** Distribution according to stages

| Stage | Distribution | % |
|-------|-------------|---|
| I | 12 822 | 72 |
| II | 2 674 | 15 |
| III | 1 636 | 9 |
| IV | 591 | 3 |

Source: Pettersson (ed), *Annual Report on the Results of Treatment of Gynecological Cancer*, Vol 21. Stockholm: Elsevier, 1991.[16]

women. Because this is usually an early symptom, the majority of patients with endometrial carcinoma will be diagnosed in the early stages (Table 15.2).

# Staging

Until 1981, the staging of endometrial carcinoma was entirely clinical, i.e. based on careful physical examination and preoperative investigation. At the time of laparotomy the disease might be more or less advanced than the clinical staging indicated, but it did not allow the investigator to change the clinical stage on the basis of the operative findings (Table 15.3).

Clinical staging had its positive side, as it could be used for all patients — those who because of their general condition were not suitable for surgery, as well as those to whom preoperative treatment was offered, and also those who were operated upon primarily. Criticism of clinical staging focused mainly on the differences in preoperative and peroperative findings. It should still be recognized that clinical staging supports the basic aims of the staging system, such as simplicity, practicality, credibility and usefulness to all clinicians dealing with the disease. The staging system was never

**Table 15.3** FIGO clinical staging of carcinoma of the corpus uteri

| | |
|---|---|
| Stage 0 | Atypical endometrial hyperplasia, carcinoma *in situ* Histological findings are suspicious of malignancy |
| Stage I | The carcinoma is confined to the corpus |
|     Stage Ia | The length of the uterine cavity is 8 cm or less |
|     Stage Ib | The length of the uterine cavity is more than 8 cm |
| Stage II | The carcinoma has involved the corpus and the cervix, but has not extended outside the uterus |
| Stage III | The carcinoma has extended outside the uterus, but not outside the true pelvis |
| Stage IV | The carcinoma has extended outside the true pelvis or has obviously involved the mucosa of the bladder or rectum. A bullous oedema, as such, does not permit a case to be allotted to Stage IV |
|     Stage IVa | Spread of the growth to adjacent organs such as urinary bladder, rectum, sigmoid, or small bowel |
|     Stage IVb | Spread to distant organs |

meant to be a guideline for treatment, but rather a tool to be used by all physicians dealing with endometrial carcinoma.

In 1988, the International Federation of Gynaecology and Obstetrics (FIGO) Cancer Committee decided to change the clinical staging of carcinoma of the endometrium to a surgical staging system (Table 15.4) to facilitate the tailoring of adjuvant therapy to surgical findings. By introducing surgical staging, the pressure towards primary surgery in endometrial carcinoma increased in the gynaecological oncology community. The decision created controversy and an intensive debate which still continues. Nevertheless, the decision on surgical staging did change the attitude towards primary surgical treatment of patients with endometrial carcinoma. Another contributory factor of this change in attitude is the development of anaesthesiology and general care of surgically treated patients, which allows surgery to be performed even at advanced ages.

Surprisingly enough, very few randomized studies have been performed in carcinoma of the endometrium. The decision on surgical staging and, consequently, in favour of primary surgery, was made on the basis of the prognostic factors found during the Gynecologic Oncology Group (GOG) study of endometrial carcinoma[15] rather than through comparative studies on treatment methods. There are still important questions concerning preoperative radiotherapy which cannot be answered unanimously today.

**Table 15.4**   FIGO surgical staging of carcinoma of the corpus uteri

| | | |
|---|---|---|
| Stage Ia | Grade 1, 2, 3 | Tumour limited to endometrium |
| Stage Ib | Grade 1, 2, 3 | Invasion to < 1/2 myometrium |
| Stage Ic | Grade 1, 2, 3 | Invasion ≥ 1/1 myometrium |
| Stage IIa | Grade 1, 2, 3 | Endocervical glandular involvement only |
| Stage IIb | Grade 1, 2, 3 | Cervical stromal invasion |
| Stage IIIa | Grade 1, 2, 3 | Tumour invades serosa and/or adnexae and/or positive peritoneal cytology |
| Stage IIIb | Grade 1, 2, 3 | Vaginal metastases |
| Stage IIIc | Grade 1, 2, 3 | Metastases to pelvic and/or para-aortic lymph nodes |
| Stage IVa | Grade 1, 2, 3 | Tumour invasion of bladder and/or bowel mucosa |
| Stage IVb | Grade 1, 2, 3 | Distant metastases including intra-abdominal and/or inguinal lymph nodes. |

# Prognostic factors

Several prognostic factors have been shown to correlate with the outcome in patients with carcinoma of the endometrium. The most important prognostic variable is the *stage* of the disease.[16] *Age* is another important prognostic factor, older patients having a worse prognosis than younger ones.[17-19] It is recognized that there are *histopathological types* of carcinoma of the endometrium where the prognosis is relatively poor. These include adenosquamous carcinoma, papillary serous carcinoma and clear cell carcinoma.[20-25] A very strong correlation exists between *histological grade, myometrial invasion* and prognosis. The GOG study provides the most relevant information on these factors.[15,26] *Vascular space invasion* is also recognized as an important risk factor in carcinoma of the endometrium.[27]

The significance of positive *peritoneal cytology* is controversial. It seems that positive peritoneal cytology is not an independent prognostic factor but integrated with grade and depth of myometrial invasion.[28] Some of the publications reflect extremely different beliefs in the significance of the peritoneal cytology.[29,30] This discrepancy in the reported results may reflect the difficulty of cytological interpretation, especially of peritoneal washings.

*Lymph node metastasis* — pelvic and para-aortic — is of very great prognostic value. The incidence of lymph node metastasis increases with histological grade and myometrial invasion. For Grade 1, positive pelvic nodes will be found in 3.1% and para-aortic nodes in 1.9%; for Grade 2, in 11.3% and 7.5%, respectively; and for Grade 3 in 24.7% and 16.0%, respectively. In patients with no myometrial invasion, 2.0% of positive pelvic nodes and 1.1% of positive para-aortic nodes were found, compared with 5.2% and 3.0%, respectively, in patients with inner-third myometrial invasion; for middle-third myometrial invasion, 13.2% pelvic and 7.1% positive para-aortic nodes; and for outer-third myometrial invasion, 31.8% and 21.8%, respectively.[15,31]

During recent years the *DNA ploidy and S-phase fraction* have been shown to be of prognostic value; but the problem of methodology remains unsolved. Some investigators believe in flow cytometry,[32] others in photographic methods.[33]

# Diagnosis

The main controversy nowadays centres around the question of whether the prognostic variables should be established preoperatively, thus opening the possibility of giving preoperative irradiation to patients with poor prognostic factors; or whether the primary surgery should establish the prognostic variables and tailor the adjuvant therapy postoperatively.

By using modern techniques, all the important prognostic factors can be established preoperatively. Careful palpation in anaesthesia, as well as fractionated curettage, will supply information about the probable stage, histology, grade, and DNA content. The depth of myometrial infiltration can be established preoperatively either by ultrasound or by magnetic resonance imaging (MRI). The possibility of lymph node metastasis cannot be excluded without total pelvic and para-aortic lymph node dissection. This special diagnostic tool, which seems to be necessary for performing a full staging procedure according to the new FIGO classification, is again subject to debate. Many patients with endometrial carcinoma are unsuitable for extensive surgery with full lymph node dissection. In addition, extensive dissection of lymph nodes, when combined with irradiation, can cause excessive morbidity. Moreover, many endometrial cancer patients are operated upon in small community hospitals where few or none of the physicians are trained in performing radical surgery with lymph node dissection. In view of all these difficulties, sampling of the lymph nodes has been suggested as a compromise. What sampling of the lymph nodes really means is not well defined. The purpose of the procedure is to dissect the lymph nodes which are clearly enlarged — a method with low sensitivity and specificity.

Another diagnostic procedure which has been incorporated into the new FIGO staging is peritoneal washing. Even this procedure has created debate, as not all cytologists will agree on the interpretation of the findings.

As a consequence of the problems mentioned, even if the 1988 FIGO staging has moved the trend towards primary surgery, such surgery at many centres is not performed according to the full staging requirement.

# Radiotherapy as a treatment method in endometrial cancer — Stage I and II

Radiotherapy can be applied both as intracavitary treatment or externally. As mentioned before, intracavitary treatment was introduced very early in this century. During the 1930s, the packing method was developed by Heyman[4] and became widely used. The survival rate achieved by radiotherapy alone proves that carcinoma of the endometrium is a very radiosensitive tumour, and high curability can be achieved. During the 1940s and 1950s radiotherapy was used on its own, even in cases suitable for surgery, but with the development of better anaesthesiology and postoperative care, a combination therapy began to be used and has shown about 15–20% better results in long-term survival than radiotherapy alone.[34,35]

Current controversies includes:

1. the correct sequence of irradiation and surgery;
2. the technique of irradiation.

Preoperative irradiation has previously been widely used, its rationale being as follows:

1. The irradiated cancer cells are less clonogenic and less amenable to implantation by surgical manipulation.
2. Tumour shrinkage promotes a better surgical procedure, and sterilization of peripheral tumour extension renders non-resectable tumours resectable.
3. The dose distribution given by intracavitary treatment influences nodal metastases.
4. The amount of residual tumour will be greater in the non-preoperatively treated group, and a larger number of patients would need postoperative irradiation, with greater morbidity and complication rates.

Is there any evidence for these postulates? Macasaet et al.[36] reported a 5-year survival rate of 77% for patients with viable residual tumour and 94% for patients without residual tumour, following preoperative intracavitary radiotherapy. McCabe and Sagerman[37] observed 14% failures when residual disease was present and only 3% when there was none. Macasaet, as well as Komaki, Toonkel and their coworkers,[36,38,39] found decreased survival rate associated with residual deep endometrial penetration when compared with lesser extent of residual tumour. In the Macasaet material, two treatment methods were identified — radiotherapy followed by surgery, and surgery followed by radiotherapy. Patients without residual tumour, when recurred, had only distant metastases and no evidence of pelvic recurrence.

In Komaki *et al.*'s analysis, patients with no residual tumour had a 96% 5-year survival rate, against 65% for those who had residual disease. Some of the studies analysed the value of preoperative irradiation in moderately and poorly differentiated tumours. In moderately differentiated tumours, two studies[40,41] showed a better 5-year survival for patients preoperatively treated with irradiation compared with primary surgery. The first study presents a 4% recurrence rate in patients of the preoperatively treated group compared with 18% in patients who were primarily operated upon. In the second study, which represents a large Canadian group of 2719 patients, comparing preoperative and postoperative irradiation, the 5-year survival rates were 86% and 82%, respectively, but the complication rate was 4% for the first group and 12% for the second. The conclusion was that it was safer to give preoperative rather than postoperative treatment. The same conclusion was reached by Surwit *et al.*[42] who compared an unselected patient population treated in two different ways in the Stockholm region. One group was operated upon primarily and the other was treated with preoperative irradiation. For the Grade 2 group, the survival rate was similar: 89% for preoperatively treated patients and 91% for postoperatively treated patients; but there was a difference for Grade 3 patients: 90% survival for the preoperatively treated patients and 75% for those postoperatively treated. What was important in this study was that the number of patients with deep myometrial invasion was considerably larger in the primarily operated patient group, who consequently had to be subject to postoperative external irradiation.   Another study, by Bedwinek *et al.*,[43] of patients with poorly differentiated tumours showed that residual tumour had a high influence on the survival rate, resulting in a highly significant difference in the survival rate for patients with no residual tumour and those with residual tumour: 93% and 67% 5-year survival rate, respectively. The author also observed a highly significant difference in survival for different mg/hr (MGH) applications in the uterus. Thirty-eight per cent of the patients with less than 2500 MGH had pelvic failures compared with 8% for patients for whom 2500–3500 MGH were delivered, and 0% for patients for whom more than 3500 MGH was delivered. The conclusion was that intrauterine irradiation would appear to be a very important surgical adjunct, at least for Grade 3 lesions. In another retrospective analysis made by Jazy *et al.*,[44] the preoperative radiotherapy group had only 4% incidence of deep myometrial invasion vs 31% in patients treated postoperatively. Of interest in this study was that in the preoperative group, the depth of infiltration was not correlated with the differentiation grade. The patients treated with preoperative irradiation had an increased survival rate both for 5- and 10-year observation periods. Some authors point out that preoperative irradiation also influences the incidence of positive pelvic nodes found later in surgery.[45] The rationale behind this postulate is that the low dose of irradiation delivered to the pelvic wall has some influence on the nodal metastases and survival rate.

Several other authors claim, on the basis of analysis of a large number of retrospective studies, that patients with bad prognostic factors should be treated preoperatively with irradiation.[46–53]

Through the decision on surgical staging, primary preoperative irradiation became discredited among leading gynaecological oncologists. There are several reasons why primary surgery became more and more attractive in the treatment of endometrial carcinoma, and there is no doubt that in patients with good prognostic factors this approach is justified, although unfortunately no real scientific proof has been offered to justify primary surgery in patients with poor prognostic factors.

## Postoperative external irradiation

Several studies have reported that external irradiation is indicated as adjuvant postoperative treatment in patients with poor prognostic factors found during surgery, such as myometrial invasion, poor differentiation and advanced stages of endometrial cancer, as well as in patients with lymph node involvement.[54–57] A randomized study performed in Norway focused on postoperative irradiation in Stage I disease, where all patients, after surgery, primarily received intravaginal irradiation and were then randomized between external irradiation and observation. A better survival with external irradiation was observed only in patients with poor differentiation and deep myometrial invasion.[11]

## Intravaginal irradiation

It has been a general belief, based on several studies, that in patients treated by hysterectomy alone vaginal recurrence will occur in up to 18% of Stage I and II tumours. With intravaginal irradiation, the incidence of vaginal metastases is reduced to about 1%.[58–64] In tumours with poor prognostic factors, such as Grade 3 and deep myometrial invasion, the vaginal recurrence is even more frequent.[65–67] In the latest Annual Report,[9] data collected from 113 institutions were analysed. Comparison between treatment results in Stage I of primary surgery versus primary surgery plus vaginal irradiation for Grade 1, 2 and 3, respectively, was based on 4865 patients (Table 15.5).

Recently, two studies regarding the influence of vaginal irradiation in low- and high-risk patients have been presented. The first, by Elliott *et al.*, analysed results of treatment of 927 patients in FIGO Stage I and II

**Table 15.5** Results of treatment with and without postoperative vaginal irradiation

| Treatment | Grade 1 | | Grade 2 | | Grade 3 | |
|---|---|---|---|---|---|---|
| | No. | Survival (%) | No. | Survival (%) | No. | Survival (%) |
| Primary surgery | 1688 | 91 | 661 | 80 | 193 | 68 |
| Primary surgery + vaginal radiotherapy | 1381 | 98 | 676 | 90 | 97 | 75 |

endometrial cancer.[68] The patients were divided into low-risk Stage I (Grades 1 or 2 — lesions confined to the inner third of the myometrium), high-risk Stage I (Grade 3 and/or invasion of the middle third of the myometrium or beyond), and FIGO Stage II tumours, which in the analysis are incorporated with other high-risk tumours. In 492 patients, surgery was the only treatment, in 145 patients the vaginal vault was irradiated, and in 290 patients the whole vagina was irradiated. Of high-risk patients treated with surgery alone, 12% developed vaginal recurrence, and of patients treated with surgery and irradiation of the vault, 4.7% developed vaginal recurrence. In the same category of patients, when the whole vagina was irradiated, 1.1% developed vaginal metastasis. For the low-risk group there was, for patients treated with surgery alone, a 3.2% vaginal recurrence rate and for surgery plus vault irradiation, a 5% recurrence rate. Low-risk patients treated with whole-vagina irradiation had no recurrences at all. Of patients developing isolated vaginal recurrence, 43% were dead within 1 year, and 77% within 5 years; only 10% survived the vaginal recurrence for 10 years.

In the recently presented study of the Danish Endometrial Cancer Group (DEMCA), patients are basically divided into low- and high-risk groups: low — Grade 1 and 2, less than 50% myometrial invasion; high — Grade 1 and 2, more than 50% myometrial invasion, and all patients in Grade 3 and also all operable patients in Stage II and III. All patients were primarily operated upon. Low-risk patients received no postoperative treatment and high-risk patients received external irradiation (45 Gy in twenty-two fractions). During follow-up of 56–80 months, there was 7% recurrence in the low-risk group and 22% in the high-risk group. Of 580 low-risk-group patients, forty developed recurrence, sixteen in the vagina, thirteen of whom were salvaged by irradiation.[69]

The conclusions of these recent studies are contradictory in respect of the possibility of cure from vaginal recurrence. The Danish study had a shorter observation time, but in the Australian study nearly half of the patients with vaginal recurrence died from cancer within 1 year, while thirteen of sixteen vaginal recurrences in the low-risk group in the Danish study are without evidence of disease. The conclusion is that risk of vaginal recurrence in low-risk groups is small — only a few per cent. In the Australian and Danish studies, in low-risk patients vaginal recurrence did not occur in more than 3.2% and 2.7%, respectively. The question remains whether it is justifiable to treat *all* patients with total vaginal irradiation to reduce the recurrence rate to virtually zero.

## Inoperable patients — clinical Stages I–II

Irradiation therapy is used as the only treatment method for patients who, because of age or poor general condition, are considered to be inoperable.[70–76] Five-year survival rate for this type of patient varies between 70% and 80% for Stage I and 50% and 60% for Stage II.[35,77,78]

# Advanced stages

Intracavitary radiotherapy in combination with external radiotherapy is the dominant method used for non-operable advanced endometrial carcinoma in Stages III and IV. The disease-specific survival in a review of recent series of endometrial carcinoma treated with irradiation alone in Stages III and IV varies between 10% and 49%.[70-78]

# Curative and palliative treatment of recurrent disease

There are several publications indicating that radiation therapy plays an important role in treating local recurrence. Intracavitary treatment may have a curative effect on vaginal metastases. For other localizations, external irradiation therapy may provide exceptionally good palliative treatment, and in individual cases it may even have a curative effect.[79-83]

# Techniques

### Intrauterine brachytherapy

Brachytherapy may be applied by the use of Heyman–Simon capsules or Fletcher–Suit applicators for low dose treatment. Both Heyman–Simon capsules and Fletcher–Suit applicators are afterloading devices, which can also be used in a remote closed system preventing occupational irradiation exposure. To apply a high dose rate, the so-called bulb technique with a single intrauterine applicator has been developed.[5,84] A tumoricidal dose of 60–100 Gy will be given with two Heyman or Heyman–Simon applicators, resulting in 30 Gy being given 1.5 cm from the applicator. With a Fletcher–Suit applicator, a higher dose of 60 Gy is usually given 1.5 cm from the surface of the endometrial cavity (Figs 15.1–15.3).

### Intracavitary vaginal treatment

Using Manchester or Stockholm techniques, both low dose and high dose are in use — nowadays, mostly with an afterloading system. The aim is to give 60 Gy to the vaginal epithelium (Figs 15.4 and 15.5).[84,85]

### External irradiation

External irradiation has been used as either a preoperative or a postoperative treatment in patients with poor prognostic factors. The dosage varies between 40 and 50 Gy to the pelvis including the obturator foramina and the upper border between L4 and L5, with a lateral border 1 cm outside the pelvic cavity. Usually a two-field technique is used but, occasionally, also a four-field technique. In some departments, a four-field plan is used routinely.

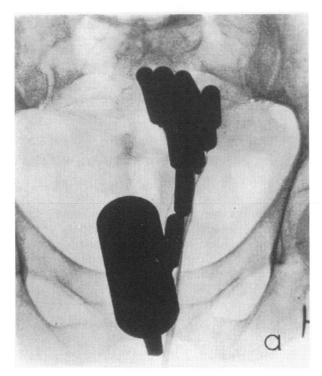

**Fig. 15.1**   Radiograph of Heyman's packing and vaginal cylinder.

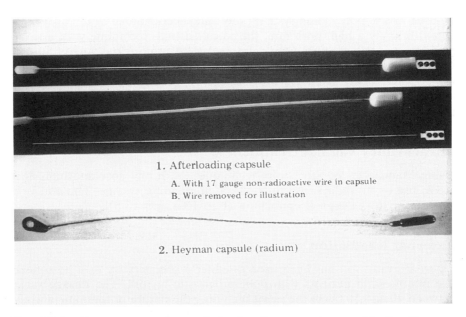

**Fig. 15.2**   Heyman capsules and afterloading capsules used in the Norman Simon system.

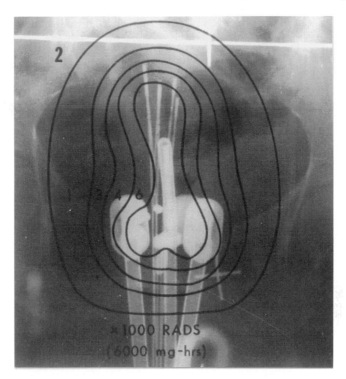

**Fig. 15.3** Radiography of Simon–Heyman system and vaginal colpostats according to Fletcher–Suit system. (Reprinted, with permission, from Perez CA, Brady LW, eds, *Principles and Practice of Radiation Oncology*. Philadelphia: JB Lippincott, 1987; 977.)

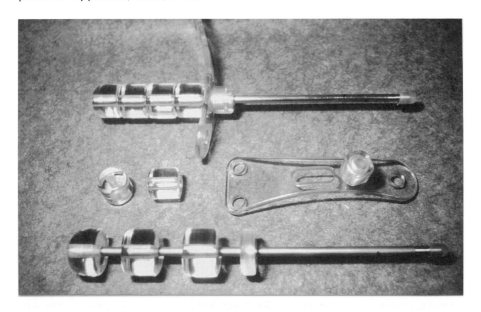

**Fig. 15.4** Afterloading vaginal cylinder used in the Stockholm technique.

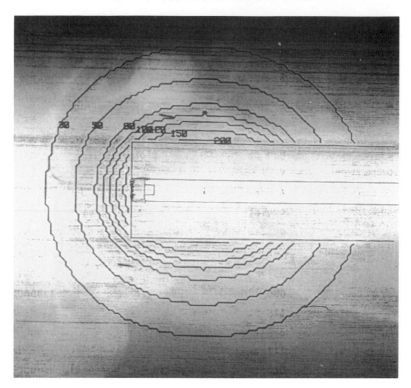

**Fig. 15.5** Isodose curves from afterloading vaginal cylinder in treatment according to the Stockholm technique.

## Extended-field irradiation

In about 17% of the endometrial cancer cases, para-aortic lymph node engagement can be demonstrated. Previously it was believed that para-aortic engagement gave no chance of a curative result. Recent reports have shown that irradiation may have a successful impact on survival, and survival rates of 25–55% have been presented in several reports.[86-89]

# Conclusions

In the past, radiotherapy had a more clearly defined role in the treatment of endometrial carcinoma. Taking into consideration all the important prognostic factors we recognize today, we are justified in claiming that patients with good prognostic factors — highly differentiated tumours, less than 50% invasion of the myometrium — may not need any adjuvant therapy. Some of the newer prognostic factors, such as DNA content and S-phase, as well as further developments in the field of molecular biology, may provide better opportunities in the future to select patients with good prognosis. It will then be necessary to make treatment decisions for patients with poor prognostic factors, and even if the recently revised staging method pushes towards primary surgery there is probably a group of patients in whom preoperative irradiation would be of benefit in Stages I and II. Postoperative irradiation should certainly be given to patients with poor prognostic factors. It is important to point out that adenocarcinoma of the endometrium is a highly radiosensitive tumour, and that radiotherapy alone plays a curative role in the treatment of patients unfit for surgery because of advanced-stage disease or bad general condition. However, it has to be remembered that high-quality precision radiotherapy is essential if the best results are to be obtained.

# References

1. Schottlaender J, Kermauner F. *Zur Kenntnis der Uteruskarzinoms*. Berlin: S Karger Verlag, 1912.
2. Laborde S. *La Curie Therapie des Cancer*. Paris: Masson, 1925; 234–5.
3. Forsell G. Erfarenheter om radiumbehandling av underlivskräfta vid Radiumhemmet i Stockholm 1910–1913. *Hygiea* 1914; **76**, 1170.
4. Heyman J. Our experience at Radiumhemmet with radiological treatment of cancer of the corpus uteri. *Acta Radiol* 1926; **6**, 566.
5. Heyman J. The so-called Stockholm method and the results of treatment of uterine cancer at the Radiumhemmet. *Acta Radiol* 1935; **16**, 129.
6. Heyman J. The Radiumhemmet method of treatment and results in cancer of the corpus of the uterus. *J Obstet Gynaecol Br Emp* 1936; **43**, 655.
7. Heyman J, Reuterwall O, Benner S. The Radiumhemmet experience with radiotherapy in cancer of the corpus of the uteri. *Acta Radiol* 1941; **22**, 14.
8. Cancer Registry. *Incidence in Sweden 1990*. Stockholm: National Board of Health and Welfare, 1993.
9. Devesa SS, Silverman DT, Young JL Jr, *et al*. Cancer incidence and mortality trends among whites in the Unites States. *JNCI* 1987; **79**, 701–7.
10. Whelan SL, Parkin DM, Masuyer E. Patterns of cancer in five continents. *IARC Scientific Publications, No 102*. Lyon: IARC, 1990.
11. Smith DC, Prentice R, Thompson DJ, *et al*. Association of exogenous estrogen and endometrial carcinoma. *N Engl J Med* 1975; **293**, 1164.
12. Norris HJ, Taylor HG. Prognosis of granulosa thecal tumor of the ovary. *Cancer* 1968; **21**, 255.
13. Fechner RE, Kaufman RH. Endometrial adenocarcinoma in Stein–Leventhal syndrome. *Cancer* 1974; **34**, 444–52.
14. Coulam CB, Annegers JF, Krantz JS. Chronic anovulation syndrome and associated neoplasia. *Obstet Gynecol* 1983; **61**, 403–7.
15. Boronow RC, Morrow CP, Creasman WT, *et al*. Surgical staging in endometrial cancer: clinicopathologic findings of a prospective study. *Obstet Gynecol* 1984; **63**, 825.
16. Pettersson F (ed). *Annual Report on the Results of Treatment of Gynecological Cancer*, Vol 21. Stockholm: Elsevier, 1991.
17. Malkasian GD, Annegers JF, Fountain KS. Carcinoma of the endometrium: stage I. *Am J Obstet Gynecol* 1980; **136**, 872.
18. Aalders J, Abeler V, Kolstad P, *et al*. Postoperative external irradiation and prognostic parameters in stage I endometrial carcinoma. *Obstet Gynecol* 1980; **56**, 419.
19. Quinn MA, Kneale BJ, Fortune DW. Endometrial carcinoma in premenopausal women: a clinicopathological study. *Gynecol Oncol* 1985; **20**, 298.
20. Silverberg SG, Bolin MG, De Giorgi LS. Adenoacanthoma and mixed adenosquamous carcinoma of the endometrium: a clinicopathologic study.

*Cancer* 1972; **30**, 1307.

21. Julian CG, Daikolu NH, Gillespie A. Adenoepidermoid and adenosquamous carcinoma of the uterus: a clinicopathologic study of 118 cases. *Am J Obstet Gynecol* 1977; **128**, 106.

22. Ng ABP, Reagan JW, Storassli JP, *et al.* Mixed adenosquamous carcinoma of the endometrium. *Am J Clin Pathol* 1973; **59**, 765.

23. Lauchlan SC. Tubal (serous) carcinoma of the endometrium. *Arch Pathol Lab Med* 1981; **15**, 615.

24. Jeffrey JF, Krepart GV, Lotocki RJ. Papillary serous adenocarcinoma of the endometrium. *Obstet Gynecol* 1986; **67**, 670.

25. Webb GA, Lagios MD. Clear cell carcinoma of the endometrium. *Am J Obstet Gynecol* 1987; **156**, 1486–91.

26. Morrow CP, Bundy BN, Kurman RJ, *et al.* Relationship between surgical–pathological risk factors and outcome in clinical stage I and II carcinoma of the endometrium: a Gynecologic Oncology Group study. *Gynecol Oncol* 1991; **40**, 55–65.

27. Hansson MB, Van Nagell JR, Powell DE, *et al.* The prognostic significance of lymph–vascular space invasion in stage I endometrial cancer. *Cancer* 1985; **55**, 1753.

28. Grimshaw RN, Tupper WC, Frazer RC, *et al.* Prognostic value of peritoneal cytology in endometrial carcinoma. *Gynecol Oncol* 1990; **36**, 97–100.

29. Creasman WT, DiSaia PJ, Blessing J, *et al.* Prognostic significance of peritoneal cytology in patients with endometrial cancer and preliminary data concerning therapy with intraperitoneal radiopharmaceuticals. *Am J Obstet Gynecol* 1981; **141**, 921,

30. Yazigi R, Piver S, Blumenson L. Malignant peritoneal cytology as a prognostic index in stage I endometrial cancer. *Obstet Gynecol* 1983; **62**, 359.

31. Morrow CP, Smart G, eds. *Gynaecological Oncology — Proceedings of the Second International Conference on Gynaecological Cancer, Edinburgh.* New York: Springer-Verlag, 1984.

32. Lindahl B, Alm P, Killander D, *et al.* Flow cytometric DNA analysis of normal and cancerous human endometrium and cytological–histopathological correlations. *Anticancer Res* 1987; 7, 781–9.

33. Moberger B. DNA content and prognosis in endometrial carcinoma: a clinical and methodological study. *Diss Abstr Int (C)* 1989; **51**, 72.

34. Karlstedt K. Carcinoma of the uterine corpus. Dissertation. *Acta Radiol* 1968; Suppl 282.

35. Joelsson I, Sandri A, Kottmeier H-L. Carcinoma of the uterine corpus. *Acta Radiol* 1973; Suppl 334.

36. Macasaet M, Brigati D, Boyce J, *et al.* The significance of residual disease after radiotherapy in endometrial carcinoma: clinicopathologic correlation. *Am J Obstet Gynecol* 1980; **138**, 557–63.

37. McCabe J, Sagerman RH. Treatment of endometrial cancer in a regional radiation therapy center. *Cancer* 1979; **43**, 1052–7.

38. Komaki R, Cox JD, Hartz A, *et al.* Influence of preoperative irradiation on failures of endometrial carcinoma with high risk of lymph node metastasis. *Am J Clin Oncol* 1984; 7, 661–8.

39. Toonkel LM, Fix I, Jacobson LH, *et al.* Myometrial penetration of endometrial carcinoma as a prognostic factor for patients receiving pre- or postoperative radiation therapy. *Am J Clin Oncol* 1984; 7, 669–73.

40. Wharam MD, Phillips TL, Bagshaw MA. The role of radiation therapy in clinical stage I carcinoma of the endometrium. *J Radiat Oncol Biol Phys* 1976; **1**, 1081–9.

41. Starreveld AA, Shankowsky HA, Koch M. Canadian Association of Radiologists: treatment results in 2719 patients with carcinoma of the

endometrium 1973–1977. *J Can Assoc Radiol* 1987; **38**, 96–105.

42. Surwit EA, Joelsson I, Einhorn N. Adjunctive radiation therapy in the management of stage I cancer of the endometrium. *Obstet Gynecol* 1981; **58**, 590–5.

43. Bedwinek J, Galakatos A, Camel M, *et al*. Stage I, grade III adenocarcinoma of the endometrium treated with surgery and irradiation. *Cancer* 1984; **54**, 40–7.

44. Jazy FK, Shehata WM, Dobrogorski OJ, *et al*. Pre-operative versus postoperative irradiation in stage I carcinoma of the endometrium. *Clin Oncol* 1983; **9**, 281–8.

45. Landgren RD, Fletcher GH, Galager HS, *et al*. Treatment failure sites according to irradiation technique and histology in patients with endometrial cancer. *Cancer* 1977; **40**, 131–5.

46. Grigsby PW, Perez CA, Kuten A, *et al*. Clinical stage I endometrial cancer: results of adjuvant irradiation and patterns of failure. *Int J Radiat Oncol Biol Phys* 1991; **21**, 379–85.

47. Jazy FK, Shehata WM, Dobrogorski OJ, *et al*. Pre-operative versus postoperative irradiation in stage I carcinoma of the endometrium. *Clin Oncol* 1983; **9**, 281–8.

48. Vaeth JM, Fontanesi J, Tralins AH, *et al*. External radiation therapy of stage I cancer of the endometrium: a need for reappraisal of this adjunctive modality. *Int J Radiat Oncol Biol Phys* 1988; **15**, 1291–7.

49. Sause WT, Fuller DB, Smith WG, *et al*. Analysis of preoperative intracavitary cesium application versus beam radiation in stage I endometrial carcinoma. *Int J Radiat Oncol Biol* 1990; **18**, 1011–17.

50. Stokes S, Bedwinek J, Kao M-S, *et al*. Treatment of stage I adenocarcinoma of the endometrium by hysterectomy and adjuvant irradiation: a retrospective analysis of 304 patients. *Int J Radiat Oncol Biol Phys* 1986; **12**, 339–44.

51. Calitchi E, Lobo PA, Martin M, *et al*. The role of radiation therapy in the treatment of adenocarcinoma of the corpus uteri stage I. A ten year experience. *Acta Radiol Oncol* 1984; **23**(6), 461–4.

52. Reisinger SA, Staros EB, Feld R, *et al*. Preoperative radiation therapy in clinical stage II endometrial carcinoma. *Gynecol Oncol* 1992; **45**, 174–8.

53. Kinsella TJ, Bloomer WD, Lavin PT, *et al*. Stage II endometrial carcinoma: 10-year follow-up of combined radiation and surgical treatment. *Gynecol Oncol* 1980; **10**, 290–7.

54. Gagon JD, Moss WT, Gabourel LS, *et al*. External irradiation in the management of stage II endometrial carcinoma. A logical approach. *Cancer* 1979; **44**, 1247–51.

55. Cox JD, Komaki R, Wilson JF, *et al*. Locally advanced adenocarcinoma of the endometrium: results of irradiation with and without subsequent hysterectomy. *Cancer* 1980; **45**, 715–19.

56. Potish RA. Abdominal radiotherapy for cancer of the uterine cervix and endometrium. *Int J Radiat Oncol Biol Phys* 1989; **16**, 1453–8.

57. Torrisi JR, Barnes WA, Poposcu G, *et al*. Postoperative adjuvant external-beam radiotherapy in surgical stage I endometrial carcinoma. *Cancer* 1989; **64**, 1414–17.

58. Nguyen TD, Froissart D, Panis X. Systemic irradiation of the vaginal vault in stage I endometrial carcinoma. *Radiother Oncol* 1988; **12**, 171–6.

59. Joslin CA, Vaishampayan GV, Mallik A. The treatment of early cancer of the corpus uteri. *Br J Radiol* 1977; **50**, 38–45.

60. Piver MS, Yazigi R, Blumenson L, *et al*. A prospective trial comparing hysterectomy, hysterectomy plus vaginal radium, and uterine radium plus hysterectomy in stage I endometrial carcinoma. *Cancer* 1990; **15**, 1133.

61. Salazar OM, Feldstein ML, Depapp EW, *et al*. Endometrial carcinoma: analysis of failures with special emphasis on the use of initial preoperative external pelvic radiation. *Int J Radiat Oncol Biol Phys* 1977; **2**, 1101–7.

62. Bliss P, Cowie VJ. Endometrial carcinoma: does the addition of intracavitary vault caesium to external beam therapy postoperatively result in improved control or increased morbidity? *Clin Oncol* 1992; **4**, 373–6.

63. Frick HC, Munnell EW, Richart RM, *et al.* Carcinoma of the endometrium. *Am J Obstet Gynecol* 1983; **115**, 663–76.

64. Sorbe BG, Smeds A. Post operative vaginal radiation with high dose rate afterloading technique in endometrial carcinoma stage I. *Int J Radiat Oncol Biol Phys* 1990; **18**, 305–14.

65. Aalders JG, Abeler V, Kolstad P. Recurrent adenocarcinoma of the endometrium: a clinical and histopathological study of 379 patients. *Gynecol Oncol* 1984; **17**, 85–103.

66. Curran WJ, Whittington R, Peters AJ, *et al.* Vaginal recurrences of endometrial carcinoma: the prognostic value of staging by a primary vaginal carcinoma system. *Int J Radiat Oncol Biol Phys* 1988; **15**, 803–8.

67. Mandell L, Daffatreyudu N, Anderson L, *et al.* Postoperative vaginal radiation of endometrial cancer using a remote overloading technique. *Int J Radiat Oncol Biol Phys* 1985; **11**, 473–8.

68. Elliott P, Green D, Coates A, *et al.* The efficacy of postoperative vaginal irradiation in preventing vaginal recurrence in endometrial cancer. *Int J Gynecol Cancer* 1994; **4**, 84–93.

69. Kvist Poulsen H, and Danish Endometrial Cancer Group (DEMCA). Uniform guidelines for treatment of endometrial cancer in the total Danish population: five-year follow-up. Abstract presented at the *4th Biennial Meeting of the International Gynecologic Cancer Society*, Stockholm, 1993.

70. Kupelian PA, Eifel PJ, Tornos C, *et al.* Treatment of endometrial carcinoma with radiation therapy alone. *Int J Radiat Oncol Biol Phys* 1993; **27**, 817–24.

71. Lehoczky O, Bosze P, Unger L, *et al.* Stage I endometrial carcinoma: treatment of nonoperable patients with intracavitary radiation therapy alone. *Gynecol Oncol* 1991; **43**, 211–16.

72. Landgren RC, Fletcher GH, Delclos L, *et al.* Irradiation of endometrial cancer in patients with medical contraindication to surgery or with unresectable lesions. *Am J Roentgenol* 1976; **126**, 148–54.

73. Abayomi O, Tak W, Emami B, *et al.* Treatment of endometrial carcinoma with radiation therapy alone. *Cancer* 1982; **49**, 2466–9.

74. Rustowski J, Kupse W. Factors influencing the results of radiotherapy in cases of inoperable endometrial cancer. *Gynecol Oncol* 1982; **14**, 185–93.

75. Varia M, Rosenman J, Halle J, *et al.* Primary radiation therapy for medically inoperable patients with endometrial carcinoma — stage I–II. *Int J Radiat Oncol Biol Phys* 1987; **13**, 11–15.

76. Wang ML, Hussey DH, Vigliotti APG, *et al.* Inoperable adenocarcinoma of endometrium: radiation therapy. *Radiology* 1987; **165**, 561–5.

77. Taghian A, Pernot M, Hofstetter S, *et al.* Radiation therapy alone for medically inoperable patients with adenocarcinoma of the endometrium. *Int J Radiat Oncol Biol Phys* 1988; **15**, 1135–40.

78. Rouanet P, Dubois JB, Gely S, *et al.* Exclusive radiation therapy in endometrial carcinoma. *Int J Radiat Oncol Biol Phys* 1993; **26**, 223–8.

79. Poulsen MG, Roberts SJ. The salvage of recurrent endometrial carcinoma in the vagina and pelvis. *Int J Radiat Oncol Biol Phys* 1988; **15**, 809–13.

80. Greven K, Olds W. Isolated vaginal recurrences of endometrial adenocarcinoma and their management. *Cancer* 1987; **60**, 419–21.

81. Lederman GS, Niloff JM, Redline R, *et al.* Late recurrence in endometrial carcinoma. *Cancer* 1987; **59**, 825–8.

82. Halle JS, Rosenman JG, Varia MA, *et al.* 1000 cGy single dose palliation for advanced carcinoma of the cervix or endometrium. *Int J Radiat Oncol Biol Phys* 1986; **12**, 1947–50.

83. Pirtoli L, Ciatto S, Cionini L, *et al.* Salvage with radiotherapy of postsurgical relapses of endometrial cancer. *Tumori* 1980; **66**(4), 475–80.

84. Björnsson M, Sorbe B. Intracavitary irradiation of endometrial carcinomas of the uterus in stage I using a 'bulb technique': physical basis. *Br J Radiol* 1982; **55**, 56–9.

85. Einhorn N. The role of preoperative radiotherapy in the treatment of carcinoma of the endometrium. In: E. Survit, and D. Alberts, eds, *Endometrial Cancer.* Boston: Kluwer Academic Publishers, 1989; 53–61.

86. Potish RA, Twiggs LB, Adcock LL, *et al.* Para-aortic lymph node radiotherapy in cancer of the uterine corpus. *Obstet Gynecol* 1985; **65**, 251–6.

87. Rose PG, Cha SD, Tak WK, *et al.* Radiation therapy for surgically proven para-aortic node metastasis in endometrial carcinoma. *Int J Radiat Oncol Biol Phys* 1992; **24**, 229–33.

88. Corn BW, Lanciano RM, Greven KM, *et al.* Endometrial cancer with para-aortic adenopathy: patterns of failure and opportunities for cure. *Gynecol Oncol* 1992; **45**, 174–8.

89. Hicks ML, Piver MS, Puretz JL, *et al.* Survival in patients with para-aortic lymph node metastases from endometrial adenocarcinoma clinically limited to the uterus. *Int J Radiat Oncol Biol Phys* 1993; **26**, 607–11.

# 16 Radiation therapy for ovarian cancer: an underutilized modality?

*Gerard Morton and Gillian M Thomas*

## Introduction

Cancer of the ovary accounts for 4% of all female incident cancers and is the fourth leading cause of cancer death.[1] It is frequently advanced at presentation, being localized in only 23% of cases. The 5-year survival in the United States is approximately 40%, a moderate improvement on the 32% survival of patients treated 30 years ago.[1] Factors which may have contributed to improvement in outcome include better understanding of the disease, advances in surgery, the introduction of megavoltage radiotherapy and the use of chemotherapy. Some evidence suggests that cisplatin may have improved 5-year survival by 10%,[2] although other factors, including a selection bias in patients treated, are also contributory. Unfortunately, the long-term survival for patients with advanced disease is still only 4–8%.[3,4]

Unlike most solid tumours, haematogenous spread beyond the cavity of origin is unusual, even at time of relapse. Gross or occult spread to the upper abdomen is common at presentation. Without careful surgical exploration, occult transperitoneal metastases can easily be overlooked. Staging peritoneoscopy performed on patients considered to have disease limited to the pelvis at the time of initial surgery, but without careful exploration, has revealed over 20% to have previously unsuspected diaphragmatic metastases.[5,6] The high rate of transcoelomic spread at presentation is reflected in the predominant intra-abdominal pattern of relapse. Patients dying from ovarian cancer generally have diffuse intraperitoneal carcinomatosis and bowel obstruction. Eighty-five per cent of relapses occur within the abdomen, even after apparent initial surgical clearance of disease. Because of the high recurrence rate after surgery alone, postoperative adjuvant treatment is mandatory in almost all patients. Ovarian carcinoma is sensitive to both chemotherapy and radiotherapy. Postoperatively, a low dose of radiotherapy directed to the whole abdomen is capable of decreasing the risk of intra-abdominal recurrence and improving survival in selected patients with a small or microscopic tumour burden.

Surgery is the standard initial management. This has the dual purpose of removing gross disease (debulking) and assessing the peritoneal cavity for evidence of spread. The volume of disease remaining after initial surgery has emerged as an important prognostic factor.[7,8] Griffiths[9] first documented a strong relationship between the maximum diameter of residual disease and median survival in a group of patients treated postoperatively with melphalan. Several reports using cisplatin-based combination chemotherapy also document a greater survival among patients 'optimally cytoreduced' compared with patients whose largest residuum measures > 1 cm or 2 cm.[10-14] Cytoreductive surgery has a number of potential benefits to the patient: several logs of tumour may be readily removed, thus increasing the chances of eradicating residual disease with adjuvant chemotherapy or radiotherapy; the mechanical effect of removing gross disease can improve the patient's quality of life[15] and relieve or delay obstructive symptoms; access of chemotherapy to the tumour may be improved. Although it is not certain that the process of debulking itself, rather than the favourable biology of debulkable tumours, is responsible for the beneficial effects of surgery,[16] a standard recommended surgical procedure includes maximal cytoreduction if 'optimal' postoperative residuum can be achieved without excessive morbidity. Meticulous intraoperative staging is required in patients with apparently early-stage disease to determine the extent of spread and the most appropriate type of adjuvant treatment. At laparotomy, the presence and volume of ascites is noted and checked for malignant cells. Peritoneal washings with saline are performed in the absence of ascites. Local invasion and dense adherence by the primary tumour is recorded. The entire peritoneal surface should be inspected and palpated. Any suspicious nodules or plaques should be excised and areas of adhesion biopsied. In the absence of any macrosopic intra-abdominal disease, blind biopsies of the peritoneal surface are performed followed by an infracolic omentectomy. Biopsies are taken from the pelvic peritoneum, the paracolic gutters, and the surface of the diaphragm. Para-aortic lymph node spread occurs in 4% of patients with Stage I and 19.5% with Stage II,[17] with a good correlation between clinical and pathological findings. Pelvic and para-aortic nodes should be carefully palpated with biopsy if they are clinically suspicious or if the lesion is of higher grade. The need for routine lymphadenectomy is uncertain.[18]

Because of the high relapse risk following surgery alone, further therapy is required in all but a small proportion of patients (Stage I, Grade 1).[19] Curative radiotherapy is directed to the whole abdomen and pelvis in selected patients whose bulk of residual disease is such that it can be cured with a tolerable dose of radiation. Patients suitable for treatment with primary radiotherapy have no macroscopic disease in the abdomen and, at most, small-volume disease in the pelvis. The dose of radiotherapy required to acheive control of this burden of disease is within normal-tissue tolerance. With a greater volume of residual disease (macroscopic disease in the abdomen or 'bulky' disease in the pelvis), radiotherapy is no longer a curative treatment as the dose of radiation required would be excessive. In patients with bulky postoperative residuum or inoperable disease, cisplatin-based chemotherapy can produce a high response rate with the possibility of an improvement in median survival time. Unfortunately, there remains a high relapse rate within the abdomen, even in patients who have obtained a complete response. Although ineffective as primary treatment, radiotherapy may have a role as 'consolidative' treatment to decrease intra-abdominal recurrence risk in patients who have obtained a favourable response to chemotherapy. Finally, local radiotherapy is a very effective palliative treatment in patients with symptomatic recurrent disease, even in patients who are resistant to further chemotherapy.

# Radiobiological considerations

The dose of radiation required to eradicate a tumour varies with tumour size, which reflects the number of clonogenic malignant cells present. From clinical data, Fletcher related tumour control probability to tumour size and radiation dose.[20] A dose of 50 Gy had a 50% probability of controlling metastatic squamous carcinoma in cervical lymph nodes measuring 2–3 cm in diameter. A dose of 70 Gy increased tumour control to 80%. Larger nodes required a higher dose and smaller nodes a lower dose to achieve the same tumour control probability (TCP). Subclinical disease in lymph nodes from either breast or head and neck primaries had a TCP of 60–70% with 30–35 Gy, 80–90% with 40 Gy, and over 90% with a dose of 50 Gy. It is likely that a similar relationship between TCP, dose, and volume of disease exists for carcinoma of the ovary. Assuming that tumour cure requires the eradication of the last remaining clonogenic cell, the probability of cure ($P_{cure}$) is an exponential function of the average number of remaining clonogens, $x$, which, in turn, is the product of the initial number of clonogens, $M$, and the surviving fraction, SF.

$$P_{cure} = e^{-x} = e^{-M \cdot SF} \tag{16.1}$$

As the average number of surviving clonogens decreases from 1 to 0.1, the probability of cure would increase from 37% to 90%. If a given dose of radiotherapy produced a 90% cure rate, increasing the number of initial clonogens by a factor of ten would reduce the cure rate to 37%, assuming that the surviving fraction remains unchanged. The number of clonogens is generally proportional to the volume of the tumour. The volume of a spherical tumour is proportional to the cube of the diameter. Doubling a diameter would increase the number of cells by a factor of eight, and for a given dose of radiation reduce control probability from, say, 90% to 45%. The effect of an increase in clonogen number is even more marked if the tumour is 'just curable' with the dose of radiation used. If a tumour has only a 50% probability of cure, a four-fold or eight-fold increase in average number of surviving clonogens would reduce control probability to 6% and < 1%, respectively.

These considerations underline the importance of the amount of postoperative residual disease in patients considered for radiotherapy. The maximum diameter of tumour residuum is a good indicator of the number of clonogenic cells present and the subsequent probability of cure with post-operative radiotherapy. The location of the residual disease is critical. The maximum dose of radiation which can be delivered is limited by the toler-ance of normal tissues within the target volume. In the upper abdomen, the liver has a $TD_{5/5}$ (dose which results in a 5% complication rate at 5 years) of 30 Gy, with renal tolerance around 23 Gy.[21] Although the renal dose can easily be limited with the use of appropriate shielding, it is not possible to limit the hepatic dose without also limiting the dose to the infe-rior surface of the diaphragm, which reduces the dose to a critical part of the target volume. The dose to the upper abdomen is therefore usually lim-ited to below about 27.5 Gy. This dose of radiation has a moderate prob-ability (perhaps 50%) of eradicating microscopic disease, with a low risk of complications. Patients with any macroscopic disease in the upper abdomen have a much greater number of clonogenic cells with an exponential decrease in cure probability with achievable radiation dose, and are there-fore not suitable for primary postoperative radiotherapy. Similarly, volume of residual disease in the pelvis determines the probability of tumour con-trol with radiotherapy,[22] although the pelvis can tolerate a much larger dose. With postoperative radiotherapy, the 5-year survival is only 8% in patients with bulky residuum (for which an incomplete bilateral salpingo-oophorec-tomy and hysterectomy (BSOH) served as a surrogate), compared with 42–79% among patients with a completed pelvic operation.[23] Patients most likely to have a curative benefit from postoperative radiotherapy to the abdomen and pelvis should therefore be without macroscopic disease in the abdomen and have, at most, small-volume (< 2 cm) residuum in the pelvis.

# Primary postoperative radiotherapy

Patients are selected for primary postoperative abdominopelvic radiother-apy based on prognostic factors following initial surgery. The most impor-tant established prognostic factors are presence of residual disease, tumour stage, tumour grade, patient age and pathology subtype.[23–29] These factors were initially identified by univariate analysis from a series of 430 patients treated at the Princess Margaret Hospital (PMH), Toronto, in 1970–6.[23] Log–rank test revealed residual disease and tumour grade to be the two most important independent variables ($P < 0.001$), followed by stage ($P = 0.002$), age ($P < 0.004$), and pathology subtype ($P = 0.058$). Patients could initially be divided into 'good prognosis' and 'poor prognosis' groups. The latter comprised patients with bulky (> 2 cm) disease in the pelvis or macroscopic disease in the abdomen. Radiotherapy was ineffective as a cura-tive treatment in this group with 5-year disease control of less than 5%. These patients (about 50% of all presenting patients) should not receive primary radiotherapy and are best managed by primary chemotherapy.

The 'good prognosis' group comprised patients with Stage I–III invasive ovarian carcinoma who had had optimal surgery, i.e. no residual disease in the abdomen and, at most, small-volume residuum in the pelvis. Despite the name, this group consists of patients with widely different prognoses, from Stage I, Grade 1 disease with a 96% survival (with or without treatment)[19] to Stage III, Grade 3 disease with pelvic residuum and a recurrence-free survival of only 16%[24] despite radiotherapy. FIGO stage (Table 16.1), histological grade, and presence of residual disease have independent prognostic value within the group and enable patients to be subdivided by prognosis into low, intermediate and high risk of recurrence (Fig. 16.1). This matrix of prognostic factors was derived retrospectively from a series of 405 'good prognosis' patients treated prior to 1978 in Toronto, and then subsequently verified prospectively on a further 472 patients treated between 1979 and 1985.[30] This confirmed the ability of the prognostic matrix to predict outcome with radiotherapy. The low-risk patients account for approximately 17% and require no further treatment following surgery. The high-risk patients make up approximately 20% and have a relapse-free survival of 23–40% at 5 years, with a long-term survival of only 19%.[24,30] Most of the patients in this subgroup are therefore not cured by postoperative radiotherapy alone. The addition of chemotherapy improves duration of median survival and progression-free interval. In a comparison with historical controls treated with radiotherapy alone, six cycles of cisplatin-based chemotherapy given prior to radiotherapy increased

**Table 16.1**  International Federation of Gynaecology and Obstetrics (FIGO) staging of primary ovarian cancer

| Stage I | | Tumour limited to one or both ovaries |
|---|---|---|
| | IA | Tumour limited to one ovary; capsule intact, no tumour on ovarian surface, no malignant cells in ascites or peritoneal washings |
| | IB | Tumour limited to both ovaries; capsules intact, no tumour on ovarian surface, no malignant cells in ascites or peritoneal washings |
| | IC | Tumour limited to one or both ovaries with any of the following: capsule rupture, tumour on surface, malignant cells in ascites or peritoneal washings |
| Stage II | | Tumour involves one or both ovaries with pelvic extension |
| | IIA | Extension and/or implants on uterus and/or tubes; no malignant cells in ascites or peritoneal washings |
| | IIB | Extension to other pelvic tissues; no malignant cells in ascites or peritoneal washings |
| | IIC | Stage IIA or IIB, but with malignant cells in ascites or peritoneal washings |
| Stage III | | Tumour involves one or both ovaries with microscopically confirmed peritoneal metastasis outside the pelvis and/or regional lymph node metastasis |
| | IIIA | Microscopic peritoneal metastasis beyond the pelvis |
| | IIIB | Macroscopic peritoneal metastasis beyond the pelvis 2 cm or less in greatest dimension |
| | IIIC | Peritoneal metastasis beyond the pelvis more than 2 cm in greatest dimension and/or regional lymph node metastasis |
| Stage IV | | Distant metastasis (other than peritoneal metastasis) |

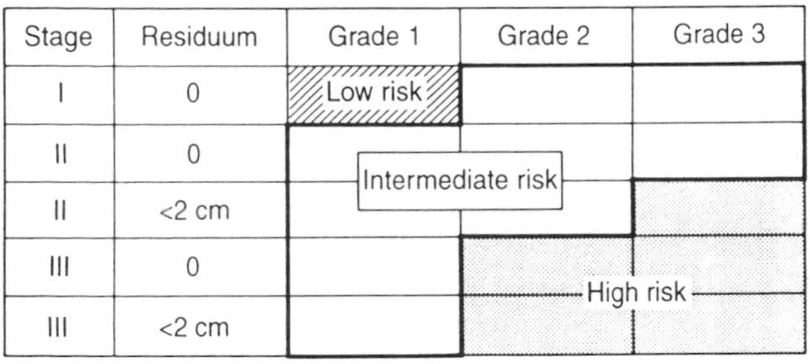

| Stage | Residuum | Grade 1 | Grade 2 | Grade 3 |
|-------|----------|---------|---------|---------|
| I | 0 | Low risk | | |
| II | 0 | Intermediate risk | | |
| II | <2 cm | | | |
| III | 0 | | High risk | |
| III | <2 cm | | | |

**Fig. 16.1** Prognostic subgroupings according to stage, residuum and grade in patients with Stages I–III, small or no tumour residuum. Abdominopelvic radiation therapy is recommended as the sole postoperative treatment in the intermediate-risk group. (Reprinted, with kind permission of Elsevier Science Ltd, from Dembo, *Int J Radiat Oncol Biol Phys* 1992; **22**, 835–45.[42])

median survival time from 2.4 to 5.7 years and 5-year relapse-free survival from 21.6% to 42.6%.[31] Although it is possible that the improvement was due to the chemotherapy alone, there is some evidence of an additive role.[32] The remaining patients (approximately two-thirds) have a relapse-free rate of 63–73% at 5 years and 57–64% at 10 years. The majority of patients within this intermediate-risk group are cured of their disease following post-operative whole abdominal radiotherapy (WAR).

Evidence for the curative potential of WAR within this group of patients emerged from early studies conducted at the PMH. In the 1970s, based on some retrospective reports, pelvic radiotherapy was generally felt to improve survival in Stage II disease.[33] WAR was restricted to patients with Stage III disease, usually with gross abdominal disease. Results were understandably quite poor. In 1971, a prospective randomized study was undertaken in Toronto which included 190 patients with Stage IB, II or asymptomatic Stage III ovarian cancer.[22] Borderline tumours were not included. Patients with Stage IB and II were randomized to pelvic radiotherapy alone, pelvic radiotherapy plus chlorambucil, or pelvic radiotherapy followed by radiotherapy to the whole abdomen. Patients with Stage III were randomized between the latter two treatments. Once again, patients with bulky residual disease (incomplete pelvic operation) fared badly, with a 21% 5-year survival irrespective of treatment received. The patients with a completed BSOH had a 5-year survival of 62% which was treatment dependent. Within this group, WAR plus pelvic boost radiotherapy gave 5- and 10-year actu-arial survivals of 78% and 64%, respectively. Pelvic radiotherapy plus chlorambucil (although not optimal by today's standards) gave lower 5- and 10-year survivals of 51% and 40%, respectively.[34] WAR was capable of con-trolling occult upper abdominal disease in approximately 30% more cases than was pelvic radiotherapy and chlorambucil within the 'good prognosis' group described above. This reduction in abdominal recurrence rate led to a similar improvement in survival.

Dembo[24] reported results of treating 415 patients with primary post-operative WAR over a 10-year period. From these data, the above prog-nostic classification was generated and an intermediate-risk group (one-third of all ovarian cancer patients) was identified with a 5-year survival in excess of 70% following WAR. Treatment was well tolerated, with serious gastro-intestinal toxicity in only 4% of patients. Several other series identified comparable groups of patients, in whom similar predictive factors were capable of defining who would do well with radiotherapy. Patients with borderline carcinoma were not included. Fuller et al.[25] reported a 71% 10-year actuarial survival in forty-two patients with Stage I–III disease, with minimal (< 0.5 cm) or no abdominal disease and < 2 cm pelvic disease. Sixty-four patients were treated with various subtotal abdominal techniques with a 10-year relapse-free survival of 40%, emphasizing the importance of adequate coverage of the whole peritoneal cavity. Surgical bowel complications occurred in 7.1%. Data from Yale[35] indicated a 77% actuarial survival at 10 years following WAR in the intermediate-risk group. Patients within the high-risk group had a survival of only 7%. Four per cent required surgery for bowel obstruction.

Several European centres had similar results. Leers and Koch[36] found a 5-year actuarial survival rate of 73% in 127 patients with Stage I–III cancer with no or minimal residual disease postoperatively. A report from the Netherlands Cancer Institute[37] indicated a 5-year recurrence-free survival of 75% in patients from the intermediate-risk group without macroscopic postoperative residual disease. Complications were related to the extent of surgery. Thirteen per cent of patients who had a staging retroperitoneal lymph node dissection developed small bowel obstruction in contrast with no bowel complications in the non-dissected patients. German data[27] revealed a 5-year survival of 75% for intermediate-risk patients and 20% for high-risk patients. Small bowel obstruction occurred in one of eighty-four patients. In 345 patients with Stage I–III carcinoma treated at Cracow,[29] the overall 5-year disease-free survival was 42%. Patients with microscopic residual disease had a 70% 5-year survival, following radiotherapy. Patients treated to the whole abdomen and pelvis had a better survival than those treated to the pelvis alone. A report from Southampton, UK,[38] of fifty-seven patients had a lower 5-year survival of 57%. As noted by the authors, however, this was not statistically different from the PMH survival of 75%.

There is, therefore, considerable evidence from several centres that, by using stage, grade and residual disease as prognostic factors, we can define a group constituting approximately 30% of all patients with invasive ovarian cancer whose survival is 75% with abdominopelvic radiotherapy. Patients with tumours of low malignant potential (borderline tumours) have a different natural history and are not included in the above series.

# Radiotherapy techniques and toxicity

The aim of treatment is to deliver an appropriate dose of radiation to all areas at risk of disease without exceeding the tolerance of normal tissues. The predominant site of relapse is within the abdomen. In the series from Salt Lake City, sixty-one of the sixty-two relapses were within the abdominal cavity.[25] Within the intermediate-risk group, the upper abdomen may contain microscopic disease only, which can be sterilized with a dose that does not exceed liver tolerance. The diaphragmatic lymphatics drain fluid from the peritoneal cavity, and the diaphragm is a frequent site of occult disease. The pelvis can fortunately tolerate a higher dose of radiotherapy and it may also contain a greater burden of disease. It is therefore taken to a higher dose than the remainder of the abdomen. There is sufficient evidence that techniques which do not include the whole abdomen in the target volume are associated with an increased risk of recurrence and decreased survival.[22, 25, 26, 29] Irradiating the upper abdomen, to include the diaphragm, decreases the risk of recurrence by 30% compared with techniques that include only the pelvis or lower abdomen. This is true for patients with Stage I and II as well as Stage III.

The target volume extends from above the domes of the diaphragm at maximal expiration to below the obturator foramina. Laterally, the fields extend beyond the skin of the flanks to include the peritoneal reflection (Fig. 16.2). Suitable beam energy is chosen to limit dose variation across

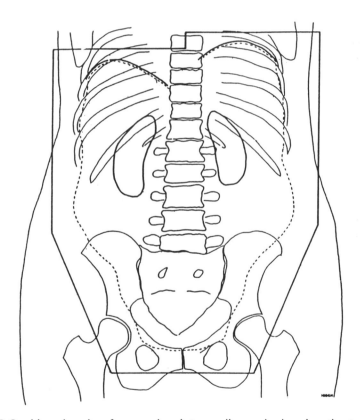

**Fig. 16.2** Line drawing from a simulator radiograph showing the treatment volume for abdominopelvic radiotherapy. A generous margin is allowed between the treatment field edges and the peritoneum, indicated by a dotted line. Note that the field extends outside the iliac crests. The kidney shielding is from the posterior to keep the renal dose between 18 and 20 Gy. The pelvic boost field is not shown. This is the posterior (prone) projection. (Reprinted, with permission, from Dembo, *Cancer* 1985; **55**, 2285–90.[24])

the target volume to within 5% of the mid-plane. The dose to the kidneys is limited to about 20 Gy by the appropriate use of shielding, such as the insertion of a posterior 5 HVL kidney shield after a mid-plane dose of 15 Gy. The remainder of the target volume may then be taken to a dose of 22.5–25 Gy in a total of twenty-two to twenty-five fractions. The pelvis may then be treated to a higher dose of 45–50 Gy. Some investigators have also given a boost dose to the para-aortic nodes and medial diaphragm, although the benefit of this is uncertain and complications may be increased.[39]

The simplest technique to treat the target volume is the open-field technique, which uses large anterior and posterior opposed fields, each field being treated daily. The dose per fraction is kept low, usually 1–1.5 Gy, to limit late toxicity. An alternative and older technique is the moving strip, in which the abdomen is treated by a 10-cm-long field which sequentially moves down the target volume in 2.5-cm steps. The prescribed dose (usually 25–28 Gy in ten to twelve fractions) is delivered completely to each point within the abdomen as the volume being irradiated gradually descends from the diaphragm to the pelvic floor. This technique is associated with a longer overall treatment time and has the potential disadvantage of allowing tumour cell reimplantation from the untreated to the already-treated volume. The dose per fraction is higher, with a theoretical greater biological efficacy, although with increased potential for late toxicity. A randomized comparison with the open-field technique reveals it to have equal efficacy with an increased incidence of late complications.[40]

Abdominopelvic radiotherapy is generally well tolerated with a low incidence of late sequelae. In an analysis of late treatment complications encountered in 598 patients treated at the PMH, 4.3% experienced small bowel obstruction, which required surgery in 2.7%.[41] Symptomatic basal pneumonitis occurred in 4%, almost exclusively in patients treated by the moving strip technique. Although transient elevation of liver enzymes was common, occurring in 44%, no patient developed late hepatic toxicity. In a review by Dembo of 1098 patients from ten reports, 5.6% of patients required surgery for bowel obstruction,[42] with deaths from bowel toxicity in 0.4%. Complications were related to the total dose, the dose per fraction, and prior surgery (especially para-aortic lymph node dissection).[36] With a dose of 22.5 Gy in twenty-two fractions to the abdomen, the risk of serious late gastrointestinal toxicity is less than 5%. Although serious toxicity is uncommon, chronic diarrhoea requiring intermittent medication occurred in 14% of the PMH series. The main acute side-effects are gastrointestinal and haematological. Transient treatment-related nausea and vomiting occurs in 61–95% of patients.[25,35,39,41] Diarrhoea occurred in 62% of the Toronto patients. In that series, treatment interruption was required in 23% of patients, with half due to myelosuppression. The myelosuppression was rarely severe and usually recovered quickly when treatment was interrupted. Ninety per cent of patients were able to complete the course of radiotherapy. Therefore, although acute toxicity is common, it is amenable to symptomatic management and settles promptly on completion of treatment. Late serious toxicity is rare with appropriate patient selection and the use of low dose per fraction.

# Chemotherapy in early disease

The relative benefit of WAR over cisplatin-based chemotherapy in early carcinoma of the ovary is unclear. Much of the chemotherapy data relates to patients with advanced disease, where it is shown to have a response rate of 70–80%. Despite the high response rates, responses may not be durable or lead to an improved long-term survival.[3,4] In contrast to response rates and negative second-look rates, the radiotherapy data tend to be older and report survival at 5, 10 and even 15 years.[22,24,29,30,35] This makes direct comparison of chemotherapy and radiotherapy data difficult. Radiotherapy has been shown to have a curative role in intermediate-risk patients with no or minimal residual disease. It is not yet established that chemotherapy can produce similar long-term survival in the same population. A randomized trial of radiotherapy and modern chemotherapy in this patient population is required to establish their relative efficacies. Unfortunately, two large cooperative groups were unable to complete randomized clinical trials comparing optimally administered WAR and cisplatin-based chemotherapy. Early study closures were due to poor patient accrual, related perhaps to strong investigator bias against one or other of the treatments and the widely divergent treatment methods.

The trial from the Italian National Institute for Cancer Research typifies the problem.[43] Seventy patients with high-risk Stage I and II ovarian cancer were randomized to either WAR or six cycles of cisplatin and cyclophosphamide. Almost a quarter (8/34) of the patients randomized to receive WAR in fact received chemotherapy instead, due either to their own or their physician's preference. This poor compliance with radiotherapy was felt to be due both to geographic lack of local radiotherapy facilities and a generalized mistrust of radiotherapy by patient and referring gynaecologist. No statistical difference in survival or recurrence-free survival was noted, although, as only 67% of patients so randomized completed the WAR, few meaningful conclusions can be drawn. A somewhat similar trial was conducted by the West Midlands Cancer Research Centre (CRC) Clinical Trials Unit.[44] Forty patients with Stage I–III carcinoma, without macroscopic disease after initial surgery, were randomized to either five cycles of cisplatin or WAR administered via a moving strip technique. In this study, only one protocol violation occurred in the radiotherapy arm. There was no difference in 5-year survival between the cisplatin and WAR arms (62% and 58%, respectively), although the power of the study was limited by the small sample size. The study was discontinued prematurely due to poor patient accrual and an unexplained bias in favour of chemotherapy. A large trial was reported from the Norwegian Radium Hospital which randomized 347 patients without residual postoperative disease to receive either six cycles of cisplatin or the intraperitoneal instillation of radioactive phosphorus.[45] Of the 169 patients randomized to receive the latter treatment, twenty-eight received WAR because of the presence of extensive intraperitoneal adhesions. It is not surprising, therefore, that there was a high rate (21%) of small bowel obstruction in the irradiated patients. The 5-year crude survival for all patients was 82%, with no difference between treatment arms. The excellent prognosis is presumably related to patient selection. Seventy-five per cent of the patients had Stage I disease, 33% had

Grade 1 and 33% had borderline histology. It is quite likely that most of the patients included in the study had a good prognosis without any post-operative treatment, and are not comparable with the intermediate-risk group in whom adjuvant WAR would be recommended. No firm conclusions can be drawn about the efficacy of chemotherapy in this group.

WAR has been compared with pelvic radiotherapy plus non-cisplatin chemotherapy in a number of clinical trials. The early PMH study of pelvic radiotherapy plus chlorambucil versus pelvic radiotherapy followed by WAR demonstrated unequivocally the superiority of WAR in patients optimally debulked.[22] In these patients, WAR reduced disease progression in the upper abdomen by 30% compared with daily chlorambucil. A study from the National Cancer Institute (NCI) of Canada randomized 257 patients with Stage I–III carcinoma between WAR, 18 months of oral melphalan and intraperitoneal radioactive phosphorus following postoperative pelvic radiotherapy.[46] The radioactive-phosphorus arm of the study was discontinued early due to toxicity, and 213 patients were randomized to the first two treatments. No difference in 5-year survival was demonstrated between WAR and pelvic radiotherapy plus melphalan (62% and 61%, respectively). Radiotherapy protocol violations were very common, however, typically leading to inadequate coverage of the target volume. In a multivariate analysis of prognostic factors, errors in radiotherapy field placement were associated with a decreased survival. In a study from Denmark, Sell *et al.* randomized 118 patients with Stage I and II ovarian cancer to either WAR or pelvic radiotherapy plus 1 year of oral cyclophosphamide.[47] Once again, there was no difference in 4-year survival between the groups (63% and 55%, respectively), although patient numbers were small.

In summary, therefore, patients at intermediate risk of tumour recurrence can have a 60–70% long-term survival when treated with WAR. One large randomized trial has demonstrated superiority of this treatment over pelvic radiotherapy plus chlorambucil. This result has not been reproduced in studies using other alkylating agents, although radiotherapy technique, different patient populations and small sample size lead to difficulty drawing firm conclusions. It is quite possible that cisplatin-based chemotherapy provides treatment results equivalent to those of WAR in intermediate-risk patients. The data, however, are not available to enable a direct comparison and the long-term survival of patients treated with chemotherapy is not yet known. Results of combined modality (cisplatin plus WAR) treatment in intermediate-risk patients are not obviously superior to results with radiotherapy alone.[48] WAR remains a well-tolerated and effective postoperative treatment for patients at intermediate risk of recurrence.

# Advanced carcinoma of the ovary

Approximately one-third of all patients presenting with carcinoma of the ovary have early disease or are rendered free of gross disease by initial surgery, and are suitably managed by primary postoperative radiotherapy. Most of the remaining patients either have bulky postoperative residua or are otherwise deemed inoperable. Current standard therapy is cisplatin-based chemotherapy, with a possible future role for Taxol as a first-line treatment. Objective response rates are typically 70–80%, with 20–30% rendered free of disease.[49] Unfortunately, responses are often not durable. The median survival of patients with advanced Stage III and IV is under 2 years, with 10-year survival of less than 10%.[2-4] Approximately half of patients clinically clear of disease following chemotherapy will be found to have residual disease at second look. Even patients who have obtained a complete pathological response have a recurrence rate of up to 63% at 10 years.[3] Neijt, *et al.* report a survival of approximately 60% at 5 years and 40% at 10 years in patients found without disease at second-look laparotomy.[2] The most important prognostic factors in patients who have obtained a complete pathological response appear to be initial tumour grade and the amount of disease present prior to the start of chemotherapy.[50,51] Rubin *et al.*[50] noted a recurrence rate of 14% in Grade 1, 36% in Grade 2, and 65% in Grade 3. Desjardins *et al.*[51] reported that both grade and extent of residual disease after initial surgery predicted risk of recurrence on multivariate analysis. The peritoneal cavity is the site of recurrence in 80–90% of cases.

Recurrent disease has a poor prognosis, with a median survival of 12 months and 5-year survival of 5% from time of relapse.[50] Patients with persistent disease after first-line chemotherapy fare very badly, with a median survival of only 6–18 months.[2] Second-line chemotherapy is usually ineffective.

Given the high intra-abdominal relapse rate, even following a very favourable response to chemotherapy, the use of WAR as a consolidative treatment following chemotherapy has been explored. The effectiveness of radiotherapy when used as primary postoperative treatment is very dependent on the amount of disease present. It has been demonstrated that macroscopic disease in the upper abdomen cannot be eradicated with any acceptable degree of probability by radiotherapy, as the dose required would exceed normal-tissue tolerance. Small volume (< 2 cm) disease in the pelvis may be amenable to curative treatment as a higher dose may be safely given. Chemotherapy, therefore, would have the effect of reducing the bulk of disease present to a volume which is amenable to cure by radiotherapy. This sequential approach also offers the potential to overcome residual drug-resistant clones by the application of radiotherapy.

The interactions between cisplatin and radiation are complex. Most experimental data indicate an enhancement of radiation effects by cisplatin, supported by some clinical data from a number of tumour sites.[52-54] This has been attributed to inhibition of repair of sublethal injury although inhibition of repair of potentially lethal damage, inhibition of tumour repopulation and other factors are also implicated.[55,56] These synergistic interactions occur when the two treatment modalities are given concurrently. Enhancement of radiation response does not occur with consolidative treatment, when many weeks elapse between completion of chemotherapy and the start of radiotherapy. In this case, the possibilities of chemotherapy-induced radiation resistance and increased normal-tissue toxicity due to stem-cell depletion warrant consideration. Tumour cell cross-resistance to cisplatin and radiotherapy has been observed, perhaps related to depletion of cellular glutathione S-transferase (GSH) levels. Early work at the National Cancer Institute (NCI) of the United States demonstrated a 1.5-fold increase in the radioresistance of ovarian cancer cell lines resistant to melphalan and cisplatin, compared with the parent cell line.[57] Similar results were reported by De Prooter *et al.* who noted that cisplatin-resistant cell lines were also resistant to radiation,[58] although interestingly the induction of radiation resistance was associated with an increase in sensitivity to cisplatin.

Another possible form of radiation resistance induced by chemotherapy is due to induction of accelerated repopulation of clonogenic cells. Accelerated repopulation would lead to a greater proportion of clonogenic cells within the tumour. The success of radiotherapy is exponentially related to the number of clonogenic cells present. Thus, the increased proportion of clonogenic cells would greatly reduce the radiocurability of a tumour deposit found prior to and after chemotherapy. Tumour cell repopulation itself leads to radioresistance unless the radiation dose is increased to compensate. A much greater dose of radiotherapy may thus be needed to eradicate the same-sized tumour found before and after chemotherapy. Finally, the response of the normal tissues needs consideration, as it is possible that prior chemotherapy may cause normal stem cell depletion with resultant difficulty in administering a sufficient dose of radiotherapy. The bone marrow is particularly sensitive to the effects of combined modality therapy, and patients heavily pretreated by chemotherapy may experience difficulty tolerating full-dose radiotherapy.

With these theoretical concerns in mind, it is possible to look at clinical experience with the use of consolidative radiotherapy. Patients have been treated with WAR with varying amounts of residual disease present and following variable numbers of prior chemotherapy regimens. There has been a tendency in most early reports to irradiate only patients with residual disease and specifically to exclude patients without disease at second-look laparotomy. It might, however, be expected that the only patient group likely to benefit would be those with no or minimal disease, and that any macroscopic residual disease would be very difficult or impossible to eradicate with achievable doses of radiotherapy. The situation is rendered more difficult as most studies have small numbers and are without a control arm.

In a review of the literature, Thomas identified twenty-eight studies where sequential multimodality therapy was applied to ovarian carcinoma.[59] Twenty-four of these were single-arm studies. Generally, patients were initially treated with one or more platinum-based chemotherapy regimens. Following this, a second-look procedure was performed, often with an attempt at secondary surgical cytoreduction. Patients with varying amounts of residual disease were included. There appeared to be a strong correlation between amount of tumour residuum prior to radiotherapy and survival. Patients with no residuum had a survival of 76% (86/113). Survival dropped to 49% (77/158) in patients with microscopic or < 5 mm residuum. Only 17% (34/202) were alive in the presence of macroscopic residuum. The data suggest that consolidative radiotherapy has no role in the face of macroscopic disease. Patients with a reasonable prognosis after consolidative radiotherapy are those with no, microscopic or minimal disease (< 5 mm) after chemotherapy. As most of the studies are single arm, it is unclear what contribution radiotherapy made to outcome. Studies which support the use of consolidative WAR in ovarian carcinoma with minimal disease are indicated in Table 16.2.

**Table 16.2** Survival results reporting benefit for sequential therapy in patients with zero or microscopic residual disease prior to radiation therapy

| Author | Number surviving/number at risk | |
| | Zero residuum | Microscopic or <5 mm |
| --- | --- | --- |
| Chiara *et al.*[60] | 6/9 | 5/11 |
| Greiner *et al.*[61] | 14/15 | 5/9[a] |
| Reddy *et al.*[62] | — | 4/5 |
| Kuten *et al.*[63] | 5/5 | 12/18 |
| Solomon *et al.*[64] | — | 4/12 |
| Kong *et al.*[65] | — | 3/5 |
| Rosen *et al.*[66] | 4/4 | 3/4 |
| Haie *et al.*[67] | 14/23 | — |
| Kersh *et al.*[68] | 1/4 | 10/15 |
| Goldhirsch *et al.*[69] | 19/24 | — |
| Menczer *et al.*[70] | 9/10[b] | — |
| Morgan *et al.*[71] | — | 8/8[a] |

[a] <1 cm residuum.
[b] Result interpreted as negative by authors.
Source: Thomas, *Gynecol Oncol* 1993; **51**, 97–103,[59] reprinted with permission.

There is a wide range of recurrence rates documented in different series of patients without residual disease prior to radiotherapy. This is related to the variable prognostic factors within different patient populations and the fact that some patients achieve their disease-free status only after secondary surgical cytoreduction. It is likely that the biology of tumours remaining after chemotherapy, but then surgically removed, is different from that of tumours which have been eradicated by first-line chemotherapy alone. Of sixty-five patients with advanced ovarian carcinoma treated by Haie *et al.*,[67] who came to second-look procedure following ciplatin-based chemotherapy, twenty-three were found without residual disease. Following WAR, 24% of patients with a negative second-look recurred at 6 years in contrast to a recurrence rate of 57% in those found to have microscopic or minimal macroscopic disease. Fuks *et al.*[72] treated twenty-five patients with WAR after chemotherapy. Fourteen had achieved a complete pathological response while a further eleven had all disease removed at second-look, so that no patient had disease detectable at the time of radiotherapy. Outcome, however, was disappointing, with an overall and disease-free survival of only 35% and 20%, respectively. Patients achieving a complete response to chemotherapy alone had a 5-year survival of 37%, which was not statistically different from the survival of 27% among patients secondarily debulked to no residuum. Tumour grade emerged as an important prognostic factor, and many patients had high-grade tumours. Interpreting the contribution of radiotherapy to outcome is compounded by various combinations of prognostic factors in different groups, small study size, frequent heavy pretreatment with both chemotherapy and surgery, and variable periods of follow-up. In the absence of a carefully conducted randomized study with groups matched for prognostic factors, it is impossible to know the value of consolidative radiotherapy.

Schray *et al.* identified tumour histological grade, volume of residual disease prior to radiotherapy, and volume of disease prior to chemotherapy as independent prognostic factors.[73] Patients with all three favourable factors (Grade 1 or 2 out of 4, microscopic rather than macroscopic disease prior to radiotherapy, and prechemotherapy residuum < 2 cm) had a disease-free survival of 67%. This decreased to 53% and 29% with two and one favourable factors, respectively. None of seventeen patients with all factors unfavourable remained disease-free. This analysis emphasizes the need to select carefully patients for consolidative treatment. Although it is not known what extra benefit came from adding radiotherapy, treating patients with high-grade carcinoma and macroscopic disease is not likely to be effective.

Many reports indicate a large proportion of patients unable to complete the planned treatment due to therapy-related toxicity. The toxicity is related to multiple factors. Patients may have received many courses of chemotherapy prior to radiotherapy — often in excess of twelve cycles of cisplatin-based chemotherapy.[73-76] This may contribute to the frequent high incidence of myelosuppression[72] with subsequent difficulty administering the planned course of radiotherapy. Several prior laparotomies is the norm, often with attempted secondary and even tertiary debulking. It is not surprising that a high rate of bowel obstruction would be recorded. The toxicity of WAR following cisplatin-based chemotherapy was analysed in a group of 105 patients with advanced ovarian carcinoma treated in Toronto.[77] Mild to moderate acute myelosuppression was common (platelet count < $100 \times 10^9$/l in 58%, < $50 \times 10^9$/l in 16%). Myelosuppression resulted in treatment delay in 9% and incomplete treatment in 12% of patients. Surprisingly, there was no relationship between the amount or type of previous chemotherapy and the degree of myelosuppression. Severe bowel obstruction occurred with an actuarial risk of 13% at 5 years. A second-look procedure and a dose of radiation to the abdomen greater than 22.5 Gy correlated with risk of bowel complications. Many reports in the literature fail to distinguish between obstruction due to recurrent tumour and that due to radiation. Review of the reports in which the cause of bowel obstruction was identified indicates a complication rate of approximately 10%.[77] Most of the toxicity associated with the use of consolidative WAR appears to stem from prior surgery rather than cisplatin chemotherapy. It is possible, though, that the use of myelosuppressive substitutes (e.g. carboplatin) may increase acute toxicity.

An unresolved issue is the relative merit of consolidative radiotherapy over consolidative chemotherapy following first-line chemotherapy. Radiotherapy offers the use of a potentially non-cross-resistant treatment modality. Prolonged chemotherapy may risk cumulative toxicity. A study from Italy randomized forty-one patients with no disease or macroscopic disease < 2 cm after cisplatin chemotherapy between consolidative WAR and three further cycles of induction chemotherapy.[78] Although there was a trend towards better outcome in the chemotherapy-treated group, the two groups were not well balanced for prognostic factors. More patients randomized to chemotherapy had achieved an initial complete response. A similar study was conducted by the North Thames Ovary Group (UK).[79] One hundred and seventeen patients with no or minimal (< 2 cm) disease after five cycles of carboplatin were randomized between consolidative WAR and a further five cycles of carboplatin. The radiotherapy was well tolerated. There was no survival difference between the two groups. However, it is unclear how many patients had macroscopic disease in the abdomen and could not have benefited from radiotherapy. When the analysis is restricted to the seventy-nine patients with no residual disease prior to radiotherapy, results were surprisingly poor, with only 25% remaining disease-free at 5 years. Consolidative radiotherapy has also been compared with 12 months of chlorambucil following initial cisplatin-based chemotherapy[80] in a randomized study. Survival was only 35% at 2 years, reflecting the fact that 50% of patients had macroscopic disease, with no difference between treatment arms.

It would appear that consolidative WAR is a reasonable option in patients who have obtained a complete response to induction chemotherapy, given the degree of efficacy and low toxicity of radiotherapy. Untreated, over 50% of these patients recur within the abdomen. Comparisons with consolidative chemotherapy are difficult to interpret because of frequent inappropriate patient selection and small numbers. Survival following radiotherapy is better for patients with lower-grade tumours and for those with optimal residual disease prior to chemotherapy. However, no consolidative therapy has been shown to improve cure rates.

## Palliative radiotherapy

Unfortunately, the majority of patients with advanced ovarian cancer die with uncontrolled intra-abdominal disease following chemotherapy. Local-field palliative radiotherapy has a major role in the relief of symptoms of pain, vaginal bleeding or discharge, and localized obstruction due to recurrent tumour. Table 16.3 summarizes the symptomatic response.

## Conclusions and future directions

Radiotherapy is an effective treatment modality for approximately one-third of all patients with carcinoma of the ovary. These include selected patients with no or minimal disease following initial surgery. Most patients with Stage II disease are suitable for treatment; Stage I patients are treated if the tumour is Grade 2 or 3; and Stage III patients are treated if the tumour is Grade 1. There must be no macroscopic disease in the abdomen. Following WAR, 60–70% of patients within this group are alive and disease-free. Significant long-term toxicity is infrequent. Data exist that show the superiority of radiotherapy over older chemotherapy regimens. Randomized comparisons with cisplatin-based chemotherapy have not been completed. Cisplatin may prove to be an effective alternative to WAR, but long-term data on efficacy are lacking.

Treatment results are disappointing in patients with advanced or recurrent disease. Although modern chemotherapy is associated with a high response rate, responses are not durable and long-term survival is poor.

**Table 16.3** Symptom response to palliative radiotherapy in advanced or recurrent carcinoma of the ovary

| Author | Pain | Obstruction | Bleeding/ discharge | Oedema | Tumour shrinkage |
|---|---|---|---|---|---|
| Hunter et al.[81] | 18/18 | 3/6 | 13/14 | | 11/13 |
| Adelson et al.[82] | 11/16 | | 15/18 | 1/5 | 25/34 |
| May et al.[83] | 12/18 | 7/11 | 4/5 | 0/2 | |
| Total | 41/52 (79%) | 10/17 (59%) | 32/37 (86%) | 1/7 (14%) | 36/47 (77%) |

Even patients who obtain a complete pathological response to chemotherapy have a high relapse rate (perhaps up to 50–60%). Radiotherapy has been explored as a means of decreasing the high intra-abdominal recurrence risk. The available data are limited. Patients with lower-grade tumours and small bulk of disease before chemotherapy are most likely to do well with WAR following a complete response. No randomized studies, however, compare consolidative radiotherapy with observation alone. WAR is therefore a reasonable treatment option in selected patients who have obtained a complete response to first-line chemotherapy. It is not an effective treatment in the face of any macroscopic disease following chemotherapy. Local-field radiotherapy is a highly effective palliative modality, with a high rate of symptom control.

Radiotherapy is frequently limited by the inability to administer a high enough dose of radiotherapy to the target volume, particularly in the upper abdomen. Gross disease cannot be controlled by standard doses of radiation. Technques to boost sites of gross tumour with intraoperative interstitial therapy have developed, which seem feasible and safe,[84] although treatment efficacy is unknown. The biologically effective radiation dose may be increased with the concurrent use of radiosensitizing agents (e.g. 5-fluorouracil, cisplatin).[55,56,85] Taxol has shown synergistic activity with radiation, although data on clinical efficacy are lacking.[86,87] It is possible that agents such as buthionine sulphoximine may have a future role in the reversal of platinum-shared radiation resistance.

The effective radiation dose may be increased with an increase in therapeutic ratio by the use of altered radiation fractionation schemes. Early reports of hyperfractionated whole abdominal radiotherapy in ovarian cancer are encouraging.[71] Hyperfractionated split-course radiotherapy may be better tolerated.[65]

# References

1. Boring CC, Squires TS, Tong T, *et al.* Cancer statistics, 1994. *CA Cancer J Clin* 1994; **44**, 7–26.
2. Neijt JP, ten Bokkel Huinink WW, van der Burg MEL, *et al.* Long-term survival in ovarian cancer. *Eur J Cancer* 1991; **27**, 1367–72.
3. Hoskins PJ, O'Reilly SE, Swenerton KD, *et al.* Ten-year outcome of patients with advanced epithelial ovarian carcinoma treated with cisplatin-based multimodality therapy. *J Clin Oncol* 1992; **10**, 1561–8.

4. Bertelsen K, Andersen JE. Long-term survival and prognostic factors in advanced epithelial ovarian cancer with special emphasis upon the effects of protocol inclusion. *Int J Gynecol Cancer* 1994; **4**, 180–7.

5. Ozols RF, Fisher RI, Anderson T, *et al.* Peritoneoscopy in the management of ovarian cancer. *Am J Obstet Gynecol* 1981; **140**, 611–19.

6. Piver MS, Barlow JJ, Lele SB. Incidence of subclinical metastasis in stage I and II ovarian carcinoma. *Obstet Gynecol* 1978; **52**, 100–4.

7. Hacker NF, Berek JS, Lagasse LD, *et al.* Primary cytoreductive surgery for epithelial ovarian cancer. *Obstet Gynecol* 1983; **61**, 413–20.

8. Delgado G, Oram DH, Petrelli EG. Stage III epithelial ovarian cancer: the role of maximal surgical reduction. *Gynecol Oncol* 1984; **18**, 293–8.

9. Griffiths CT. Surgical resection of tumour bulk in the primary treatment of ovarian cancer. *Natl Cancer Inst Monogr* 1975; **42**, 101–4.

10. Vogl SE, Pagano M, Kaplan BH, *et al.* Cisplatin-based combination chemotherapy for advanced ovarian cancer: high overall response rate with curative potential only in women with small tumor burdens. *Cancer* 1983; **51**, 2024–30.

11. Neijt JP, van der Burg MEL, Vriesendorp R, *et al.* Randomised trial comparing two combination chemotherapy regimens (Hexa-CAF vs CHAP-5) in advanced ovarian carcinoma. *Lancet* 1984; **2**, 594–600.

12. Pohl R, Dallenback-Hellweg G, Plugge T, *et al.* Prognostic parameters in patients with advanced malignant ovarian tumors. *Eur J Gynecol Oncol* 1984; **3**, 160–9.

13. Redman JR, Petroni GR, Saigo PE, *et al.* Prognostic factors in advanced ovarian cancer. *J Clin Oncol* 1986; **4**, 515–23.

14. Conte PF, Bruzzone M, Chiara S, *et al.* A randomised trial comparing cisplatin plus cyclophosphamide versus cisplatin, doxorubicin and cyclophosphamide in advanced ovarian cancer. *J Clin Oncol* 1986; **4**, 965–71.

15. Blythe JG, Wahl TP. Debulking surgery: does it increase the quality of survival? *Gynecol Oncol* 1982; **14**, 396–408.

16. Hoskins WJ, Bundy BN, Thigpen JT, *et al.* The influence of cytoreductive surgery on recurrence free interval and survival in small-volume stage III epithelial ovarian cancer: a Gynecologic Oncology Group study. *Gynecol Oncol* 1992; **47**, 159–66.

17. Buchsbaum HJ, Brady MF, Delgado G, *et al.* Surgical staging of carcinoma of the ovaries. *Surg Gynecol Obstet* 1989; **169**, 226–32.

18. Petru E, Lahousen M, Tamussino K, *et al.* Lymphadenectomy in stage I ovarian cancer. *Am J Obstet Gynecol* 1994; **170**, 656–62.

19. Dembo AJ, Davy M, Stenwig AE, *et al.* Prognostic factors in patients with stage I epithelial ovarian cancer. *Obstet Gynecol* 1990; **75**, 263–73.

20. Fletcher GH. Clinical dose–response curves of human malignant epithelial tumours. *Br J Radiol* 1973; **46**, 1–12.

21. Emami B, Lyman J, Brown A, *et al.* Tolerance of normal tissue to therapeutic radiation. *Int J Radiat Oncol Biol Phys* 1991; **21**, 109–22.

22. Bush RS, Allt WEC, Beale FA, *et al.* Treatment of epithelial carcinoma of the ovary: operation, irradiation and chemotherapy. *Am J Obstet Gynecol* 1977; **127**, 692–704.

23. Dembo AJ, Bush RS. Choice of postoperative therapy based on prognostic factors. *Int J Radiat Oncol Biol Phys* 1982; **8**, 893–7.

24. Dembo AJ. Abdominopelvic radiotherapy in ovarian cancer, a 10-year experience. *Cancer* 1985; **55**, 2285–90.

25. Fuller DB, Sause WT, Plenk HP, *et al.* Analysis of postoperative radiation therapy in stage I through III epithelial ovarian carcinoma. *J Clin Oncol* 1987; **5**, 897–905.

26. Martinez A, Schray MF, Howes AE, *et al.* Postoperative radiation therapy for epithelial ovarian cancer: the curative role based on a 24-year experience. *J Clin*

*Oncol* 1985; **3**, 901–11.

27. Lindner H, Willich H, Atzinger A. Primary adjuvant whole abdominal irradiation in ovarian cancer. *Int J Radiat Oncol Biol Phys* 1990; **19**, 1203–6.

28. Weiser EB, Burke TW, Heller PB, *et al.* Determinants of survival of patients with epithelial ovarian carcinoma following whole abdominal irradiation (WAR). *Gynecol Oncol* 1988; **30**, 201–8.

29. Reinfuss M, Kojs Z, Skolyszewski J. External beam radiotherapy in the management of ovarian carcinoma. *Radiother Oncol* 1993; **26**, 26–32.

30. Carey MS, Dembo AJ, Simm JE, *et al.* Testing the validity of a prognostic classification in patients with surgically optimal ovarian carcinoma: a 15-year review. *Int J Gynecol Cancer* 1993; **3**, 24–35.

31. Ledermann JA, Dembo AJ, Sturgeon FG, *et al.* Outcome of patients with unfavourable optimally cytoreduced ovarian cancer treated with chemotherapy and whole abdominal radiation. *Gynecol Oncol* 1991; **41**, 30–5.

32. Pickel H, Petru E, Lahousen M, *et al.* Consolidation radiotherapy following carboplatin-based chemotherapy in radically operated advanced ovarian cancer. *Am J Clin Oncol (CCT)* 1991; **14**, 184–7.

33. Bagley CM, Young RC, Canellos GP, *et al.* Treatment of ovarian carcinoma: possibilities for progress. *N Engl J Med* 1972; **287**, 856–62.

34. Dembo AJ. Radiotherapeutic management of ovarian cancer. *Semin Oncol* 1984; **11**, 238–50.

35. Goldberg N, Peschel RE. Postoperative abdominopelvic radiation therapy for ovarian cancer. *Int J Radiat Oncol Biol Phys* 1988; **14**, 425–9.

36. Leers WH, Koch HC. The evaluation of postoperative irradiation in patients with early-stage ovarian cancer. *Gynecol Oncol* 1987; **28**, 41–9.

37. van Bunningen B, Bouma J, Kooijman C, *et al.* Total abdominal irradiation in stage I and II carcinoma of the ovary. *Radiother Oncol* 1988; **11**, 305–10.

38. Macbeth FR, MacDonald H, Williams CJ. Total abdominal and pelvic radiotherapy in the management of early stage ovarian carcinoma. *Int J Radiat Oncol Biol Phys* 1988; **15**, 353–8.

39. Schray MF, Martinez A, Howes AE. Toxicity of open field whole abdominal irradiation as primary post-operative treatment in gynecological malignancy. *Int J Radiat Oncol Biol Phys* 1988; **16**, 397–403.

40. Dembo AJ, Bush RS, Beale FA, *et al.* A randomised clinical trial of moving strip versus open field whole abdominal irradiation in patients with invasive epithelial cancer of ovary. *Int J Radiat Oncol Biol Phys* 1983; **9** (Suppl 1), 97 (Abstract).

41. Fyles AW, Dembo AJ, Bush RS, *et al.* Analysis of complications in patients treated with abdomino-pelvic radiation therapy for ovarian carcinoma. *Int J Radiat Oncol Biol Phys* 1992; **22**, 847–51.

42. Dembo AJ. Epithelial ovarian cancer: the role of radiotherapy. *Int J Radiat Oncol Biol Phys* 1992; **22**, 835–45.

43. Chiara S, Conte P, Franzone P, *et al.* High-risk early-stage ovarian cancer. Randomised clinical trial comparing cisplatin plus cyclophosphamide versus whole abdominal radiotherapy. *Am J Clin Oncol (CCT)* 1994; **17**, 72–6.

44. Redman CWE, Mould J, Warwick J, *et al.* The West Midlands epithelial ovarian cancer adjuvant therapy trial. *Clin Oncol* 1993; **5**, 1–5.

45. Vergote IB, Vergote-De Vos LN, *et al.* Randomized trial comparing cisplatin with radioactive phosphorus or whole abdomen irradiation as adjuvant treatment of ovarian cancer. *Cancer* 1992; **69**, 741–9.

46. Klaassen D, Shelley W, Starreveld A, *et al.* Early stage ovarian cancer: a randomised clinical trial comparing whole abdominal radiotherapy, melphalan, and intraperitoneal chromic phosphate: a National Cancer Institute of Canada Clinical Trials Group report. *J Clin Oncol* 1988; **6**, 1254–68.

47. Sell A, Bertelsen K, Andersen JE, *et al.* Randomized study of whole-abdomen

irradiation versus pelvic irradiation plus cyclophosphamide in treatment of early ovarian cancer. *Gynecol Oncol* 1990; **37**, 367–73.

48. Hoskins PJ, Swenerton KD, Manji M, *et al.* 'Moderate risk' ovarian cancer (stage I, grade 2; stage II, grade 1 or 2) treated with cisplatin chemotherapy (single agent or combination) and pelviabdominal irradiation. *Int J Gynecol Cancer* 1994; **4**, 272–8.

49. Ozols RF, Young RC. Chemotherapy of ovarian cancer. *Semin Oncol* 1991; **18**, 222–32.

50. Rubin SC, Hoskins WJ, Hakes TB, *et al.* Recurrence after negative second-look laparotomy for ovarian cancer: analysis of risk factors. *Am J Obstet Gynecol* 1988; **159**, 1094–8.

51. Desjardins C, Pater J, Zee B, *et al.* Prognostic factors after a negative second-look laparotomy in ovarian cancer: a Canadian–Italian study. *Ann Oncol* 1992; **3** (Suppl 5), 107 (Abstract).

52. Elias A. Chemotherapy and radiotherapy for regionally advanced non-small-cell lung cancer. *Chest* 1993; **103** (Suppl 4), 362S–6S.

53. Forastiere AA. Cisplatin and radiotherapy in the management of locally advanced head and neck cancer. *Int J Radiat Oncol Biol Phys* 1993; **27**, 465–70.

54. Zietman AL, Shipley WU, Kaufman DS. The combination of cis-platin based chemotherapy and radiation in the treatment of muscle-invading transitional cell cancer of the bladder. *Int J Radiat Oncol Biol Phys* 1993; **27**, 161–70.

55. Dewit L. Combined treatment of radiation and cis-diamminedichloroplatinum (II): a review of experimental and clinical data. *Int J Radiat Oncol Biol Phys* 1987; **13**, 403–6.

56. Coughlin CT, Richmond RC. Biologic and clinical developments of cisplatin combined with radiation: concepts, utility, projections for new trials, and the emergence of carboplatin. *Semin Oncol* 1989; **16** (Suppl 6), 31–43.

57. Louie KG, Behrens BC, Kinsella TJ, *et al.* Radiation survival parameters of antineoplastic drug-sensitive and -resistant human ovarian cancer cell lines and their modification by buthionine sulfoximine. *Cancer Res* 1985; **45**, 2110–15.

58. De Pooter CM, Scalliet PG, Elst HJ, *et al.* Resistance patterns between cis-diamminedichloroplatinum (CDDP) and ionising radiation. *Cancer Res* 1991; **51**, 4523–7.

59. Thomas GM. Is there a role for consolidation or salvage radiotherapy after chemotherapy in advanced epithelial ovarian cancer? *Gynecol Oncol* 1993; **51**, 97–103.

60. Chiara S, Orsatti M, Franzone P, *et al.* Abdominopelvic radiotherapy following surgery and chemotherapy in advanced ovarian cancer. *Clin Oncol* 1991; **3**, 340–4.

61. Greiner R, Goldhirsch A, Davis BW, *et al.* Whole-abdomen radiation in patients with advanced ovarian carcinoma after surgery, chemotherapy and second-look laparotomy. *J Cancer Res Clin Oncol* 1984; **107**, 94–8.

62. Reddy S, Hartsell W, Graham J, *et al.* Whole-abdomen radiation therapy in ovarian carcinoma: its role as a salvage therapeutic modality. *Gynecol Oncol* 1989; **35**, 307–13.

63. Kuten A, Stein M, Steiner M, *et al.* Whole abdominal irradiation following chemotherapy in advanced ovarian carcinoma. *Int J Radiat Oncol Biol Phys* 1988; **14**, 273–9.

64. Solomon HJ, Atkinson KH, Coppleson JVM, *et al.* Ovarian carcinoma: abdominopelvic irradiation following reexploration. *Gynecol Oncol* 1988; **31**, 396–401.

65. Kong JS, Peters LJ, Whartin JT, *et al.* Hyperfractionated split-course whole abdominal radiotherapy for ovarian carcinoma: tolerance and toxicity. *Int J Radiat Oncol Biol Phys* 1988; **14**, 737–43.

66. Rosen EM, Goldberg ID, Rose C, *et al.* Sequential multi-agent chemotherapy

and whole abdominal irradiation for stage III ovarian carcinoma. *Radiother Oncol* 1986; 7, 223–32.

67. Haie C, Pejovic-Lenfant MH, George M, *et al.* Whole abdominal irradiation following chemotherapy in patients with minimal residual disease after second look surgery in ovarian carcinoma. *Int J Radiat Oncol Biol Phys* 1989; **17**, 15–19.

68. Kersh CR, Randall ME, Constable WC, *et al.* Whole abdominal radiotherapy following cytoreductive surgery and chemotherapy in ovarian carcinoma. *Gynecol Oncol* 1988; **31**, 113–20.

69. Goldhirsch A, Greiner R, Dreher E, *et al.* Treatment of advanced ovarian cancer with surgery, chemotherapy, and consolidation of response by whole-abdominal radiotherapy. *Cancer* 1988; **62**, 40–7.

70. Menczer J, Modan M, Brenner J, *et al.* Abdominopelvic irradiation for Stage II–IV ovarian carcinoma patients with limited or no residual disease at second-look laparotomy after completion of cisplatinum-based combination chemotherapy. *Gynecol Oncol* 1986; **24**, 149–54.

71. Morgan L, Chafe W, Mendenhall W, *et al.* Hyperfractionation of whole-abdomen radiation therapy: salvage treatment of persistent ovarian carcinoma following chemotherapy. *Gynecol Oncol* 1988; **31**, 122–34.

72. Fuks Z, Rizel S, Biran S. Chemotherapeutic and surgical induction of pathological complete remission and whole abdominal irradiation for consolidation does not enhance the cure of Stage III ovarian carcinoma. *J Clin Oncol* 1988; **6**, 509–16.

73. Schray MF, Martinez A, Howes AE, *et al.* Advanced epithelial ovarian cancer: salvage whole abdominal irradiation for patients with recurrent or persistent disease after combination chemotherapy. *J Clin Oncol* 1988; **6**, 1433–9.

74. Hoskins WJ, Lichter AS, Whittington R, *et al.* Whole abdominal and pelvic irradiation in patients with minimal disease at second-look surgical reassessment for ovarian carcinoma. *Gynecol Oncol* 1985; **20**, 271–80.

75. Hacker NF, Berek JS, Burnison CM, *et al.* Whole abdominal radiation as salvage therapy for epithelial ovarian cancer. *Obstet Gynecol* 1985; **65**, 60–6.

76. Steiner M, Rubinov R, Borovik R, *et al.* Multimodal approach (surgery, chemotherapy, and radiotherapy) in the treatment of advanced ovarian carcinoma. *Cancer* 1985; **55**, 2748–52.

77. Whelan TJ, Dembo AJ, Bush RS, *et al.* Complications of whole abdominal and pelvic radiotherapy following chemotherapy for advanced ovarian cancer. *Int J Radiat Oncol Biol Phys* 1992; **22**, 853–8.

78. Bruzzone M, Repetto L, Chiara S, *et al.* Chemotherapy versus radiotherapy in the management of ovarian cancer patients with pathological complete response or minimal residual disease at second look. *Gynecol Oncol* 1990; **38**, 392–5.

79. Lambert HE, Rustin GJS, Gregory WM, *et al.* A randomized trial comparing single-agent carboplatin with carboplatin followed by radiotherapy for advanced ovarian cancer: a North Thames Ovary Group study. *J Clin Oncol* 1993; **11**, 440–8.

80. Lawton F, Luesley D, Blackledge G, *et al.* A randomized trial comparing whole abdominal radiotherapy with chemotherapy following cisplatinum cytoreduction in epithelial ovarian cancer. West Midlands Ovarian Cancer Group trial II. *Clin Oncol* 1990; **2**, 4–9.

81. Hunter M, Lanciano R, Hogan WM. The palliation of chemotherapy failures by radiation in ovarian cancer. *Proc Ann Meet Am Soc Clin Oncol* 1993; **12**, A873 (Abstract).

82. Adelson MD, Wharton JT, Celclos L, *et al.* Palliative radiotherapy for ovarian cancer. *Int J Radiat Oncol Biol Phys* 1987; **13**, 17–21.

83. May LF, Belinson JL, Roland TA. Palliative benefit of radiation therapy in advanced ovarian cancer. *Gynecol Oncol* 1990; **37**, 408–11.

84. Porkowski M, Holloway R, Delgado G, *et al.* Radiotherapy of malignant

subdiaphragmatic implants in advanced ovarian carcinoma: a new technique. *Int J Radiat Oncol Biol Phys* 1992; **22**, 1005–8.

85. Byfield JE, Calabro-Jones P, Klisak I, *et al*. Pharmacologic requirements for obtaining sensitization of human tumour cells *in vitro* to combined 5-fluorouracil or ftorafur and x-rays. *Int J Radiat Oncol Biol Phys* 1982; **8**, 1923–33.

86. Steren A, Sevin B, Perras J, *et al*. Taxol sensitizes human ovarian cancer cells to radiation. *Gynecol Oncol* 1993; **48**, 252–8.

87. Steren A, Sevin B, Perras J, *et al*. Taxol as a radiation sensitizer: a flow cytometric study. *Gynecol Oncol* 1993; **50**, 89–93.

# 17 Results and late effects of treatment for early-stage germ cell tumours

*R Timothy D Oliver*

## Introduction

Before the advent of highly effective cisplatin-based combination chemotherapy, all cases of early-stage non-seminomatous germ cell cancer, i.e. Stage 1 and 2 patients, underwent treatment either by retroperitoneal surgery (predominantly in the USA) or by radiotherapy (in the UK).[1] From the time of the initial reports the results of these two approaches appeared equal in effectiveness (Table 17.1), though both had improved considerably during the 30-year period before the advent of cisplatin led to the first serious questioning of this status quo.

Today, retroperitoneal surgery remains the standard treatment in much

**Table 17.1** Historical overview of Stage I and Stage II malignant teratoma treatment results (for references, see Blandy *et al*.[1])

| Historical period | Orchidectomy + lymph node dissection | | Orchidectomy + para-aortic ± mediastinal radiation | |
|---|---|---|---|---|
| | *N* | Survival (%) | *N* | Survival (%) |
| Pre-1970 (5-year survival) | 568 | 51 | 421 | 60 |
| 1970–75 (3-year survival) | 185 | 68 | 184 | 72 |
| Post-1975 (2-year survival) | 117 | 94 | 71 | 90 |

of North America, with an overall cure rate (after salvage chemotherapy for the 30% who recur) in excess of 98%.[2,3] An equally high cure rate, however, is achieved for patients with Stage 1 and 2 disease in centres in the UK and elsewhere, using routine chemotherapy (including adjuvant chemotherapy for Stage 1 cases) and salvage surgery (restricted to the minority with residual masses after chemotherapy).[4-6] For the Stage 1 patients, surveillance and salvage chemotherapy for relapse appears to be equally effective.[7] For seminoma Stages 1 and 2, cure by radiation therapy is also in excess of 98%,[8] though an equally high cure rate is now achieved using chemotherapy, including single-course adjuvant carboplatin for Stage 1 cases[9] and single-agent carboplatin for Stage 2.[10]

Since there have been no randomized trials assessing long-term quality of life, the choice of which treatment modality to offer early-stage patients (for both seminoma and other germ cell tumour types) remains, at present, a matter of personal bias and judgement based on experience of the acute and late side-effects of treatment. As any trial would need more than 10 years and possibly as long as 30 years follow-up (to address the issue of late toxicity), there is an urgent need for a simple late monitoring process to generate reliable late follow-up information.

Together with a consideration of current views on histopathology of this disease and the development of chemotherapy for advanced metastatic disease, the main aim of this chapter is to review the evolution of treatment of Stage 1 and 2 disease and assess both its effectiveness and late (15–30 year) toxicities. The focus will primarily be on surgery and radiotherapy; for chemotherapy, as it is now 16 years since the first reports of its use, the question arises as to whether early indications of late toxicity make it safe for use in early-stage cases. This chapter will also consider the development of techniques to monitor for late unexpected events.

# Current views on the histogenesis and classification of germ cell cancer as it relates to treatment of early-stage disease

Cytogenetic studies in both colorectal and bladder cancer have provided the most convincing demonstration, to date, that adult solid cancers develop by a process of Darwinian-like survival of the fittest, due to a stepwise accumulation of mutations/deletions in critical DNA replication activation and suppressor genes to increase the growth efficiency of the tumour. Long before the advent of modern molecular genetics of cancer, histopathologists anticipated this concept with the introduction of tumour grading as a measure of how far the malignancy had evolved from its tissue of origin. Although the general principle has been to identify the most malignant morphological component in setting the grade, there has been some inconsistency in application, i.e. whether it is the proportion of immature cells or the degree of anaplasia which determines the intermediate or G2 stage. A new approach to this issue has recently been proposed[11] and is summarized below.

Few people today would dispute the view that all germ cell tumours except spermatocytic seminoma and mature teratoma derive from carcinoma *in situ* (CIS), which is a far cry from the situation more than 20 years ago when the view was first proposed.[12,13] In contrast to this consensus is the more uncertain situation relating to the pathological criteria for prognostication of what constitutes good-, intermediate- or poor-risk tumours, which has continued now for nearly a century since Chevassu[14] reported the first large series in 1902.

There is reasonable agreement that seminoma has a low malignant potential as is most convincingly illustrated by a personal case surviving for 20 years, untreated from the onset of primary tumour until he presented clinically with metastases. The increasing acceptance that seminoma metastases have both a radiosensitivity and a chemosensitivity closer to that of the normal spermatogonia than do non-seminoma cases would also support the concept that these are low-grade malignant tumours. Given that the morphology of individual cells within a seminoma differs little from the individual carcinoma *in situ* cell, it seems reasonable to classify such tumours as Grade 1 or well-differentiated gonocytoma using the general terminology for these tumours proposed by Grigor and Skakkebaek.[15]

It is over what constitutes an intermediate- or high-risk germ cell tumour that there is most disagreement. Analysis of clinical data and comparison with pathological subgroups is beginning to justify a new approach to classification, focusing attention on the subgroups classified as combined seminoma/malignant teratoma by Pugh[16] or mixed seminoma/non-seminoma by Mostofi.[17] This group of tumours, as well as exhibiting intermediate clinical behaviour (Table 17.2), have an intermediate cell content, with morphological similarity to what is universally accepted as the original stem cell, while the Pugh pure malignant teratoma or Mostofi non-seminoma group have none, despite more than 90% having evidence for the original stem cell, i.e. CIS in the surrounding rim of residual normal testis adjacent to the tumour. It would be reasonable to regard the former as intermediate or Grade 2 gonocytoma, while the latter could acceptably be classified as undifferentiated/anaplastic or Grade 3 gonocytoma.

Clearly, grading on its own would be inadequate to describe the multiplicity of cell types seen in the G2/G3 gonocytomas. However, it might be more appropriate to consider the non-germ-cell somatic and foetal tissues within these tumours as malignant metaplastic elements. The morphology of these components is the main basis for the multiplicity of subgroups of germ cell tumour defined by the current World Health Organization (WHO) classification[17] which treats seminoma elements equally to non-seminoma elements. If use of the term metaplastic components was accepted, this approach would then bring germ cell tumours into line with other solid cancer pathology, as is best illustrated by bladder cancer. As well as having squamous, glandular and cartilaginous malignant metaplastic variants, there is also a well documented but relatively rare choriocarcinomatous bladder cancer variant. These cases produce massive amounts of βhCG and almost universally have extensive lung metastases like the testicular variant. Their frequency in metastatic bladder cancer series is about 1–2% which is little different from the frequency of testicular choriocarcinoma. In addition, more than a third of metastatic bladder cancer patients have circulating human chorionic gonodotrophin (hCG) levels of greater than 100 iu/l.

**Table 17.2** Combined tumours as an intermediate prognosis subgroup of testicular germ cell tumours.

| | Seminoma (%) | Combined seminoma/non-seminoma (%) | Non-seminoma (%) |
|---|---|---|---|
| | $N = 248$ | $N = 116$ | $N = 241$ |
| Median age, Stage 1 | 36 yrs | 31 yrs | 29 yrs |
| Median age, metastatic patients | 42 yrs | 37 yrs | 29 yrs |
| Proportion presenting in Stage 1 | 79 | 51 | 41 |
| Relapse Stage 1, adjuvant | 1 | 6 | 0 |
| Relapse Stage 1, surveillance | 23 | 31 | 38 |
| Primary cure of all metastatic patients | 91 | 93 | 86 |
| Proportion of metastatic cases with high markers | 0 | 16 | 21 |
| Cure rate, low markers | 91 | 94 | 92 |
| Cure rate, high markers | — | 89 | 65 |

Source: Oliver *et al.*[18]

There is one subtype which does not easily fit into this proposal: how to classify mature teratoma differentiated (TD)? It is now established that the paediatric variant, like spermatocytic seminoma, lacks carcinoma *in situ* (CIS) and might therefore be classified as a non-CIS-related tumour. But more difficult still is how to explain the rare adult TD. Review of three such patients, referred over the last 15 years with this condition, demonstrated that all three had normal spermatogenesis in the rim of residual tubules abutting the tumour. One had had his tumour for more than 10 years and was diagnosed when visiting his doctor for investigation of irritable bowel syndrome; the second had had his tumour for 20 years since an episode of epididymo-orchitis; and the third was discovered in the contralateral testis of a patient who had undergone adjuvant chemotherapy. As it is known from the work of Azzopardi and Hoffbrand[19] that primary tumours can undergo rejection while metastases persist, it is possible that TD represents residual metaplastic components from gonocytomas which have undergone spontaneous regression.

It is clear that there is a need for the WHO pathological classification of testis tumours to be modified to better reflect the stem cell from which they are derived, as well as their clinical behaviour and biology. The system of grading proposed does better reflect this issue and would not cause a major disruption of the current classification which focuses primarily on the malignant metaplastic components. All that would be required would be to recognize that seminoma components within non-seminomas have a different significance from the other metaplastic elements.

# A historical perspective of the development of platinum-based chemotherapy for germ cell cancer

## Grade 2/3 germ cell cancer (non-seminoma/WHO/malignant teratoma UK)

At the time that cisplatin was first shown to have single-agent activity,[20] many groups had been assessing different combinations of the previously available drugs. Most achieved little or no benefit over the 15% complete response and 8% long-term cure achievable with single-agent actinomycin D,[21] apart from the group led by Samuels who had reported a 40% complete response, and later reported a 35% durable cure rate with high dose bleomycin and vinblastine.[22] Four major approaches with platinum-based chemotherapy for germ cell cancer have developed (Table 17.3). The first and currently dominant school (developed by Einhorn and Donohue) started by adding cisplatin to slightly reduced dosages of the Samuels bleomycin/vinblastine regimen. Initially, this group reported 64% long-term cure in their first fifty patients,[24] and in subsequent studies these results improved up to 73% cure. The first major development after bleomycin, vinblastine and platinum (BVP) from the Einhorn group was to show in a randomized trial (Table 17.4) that bleomycin, etoposide and cisplatin (BEP), though overall not significantly better than BVP, produced

**Table 17.3** Primary cisplatin-based chemotherapy regimen for metastatic Grade 2–3 germ cell cancer (for sources, see Schmoll[23])

|       | Initial report | | | Subsequent series | | |
|-------|------|---------------|---------------------|------|---------------|---------------------|
|       | Year | No. of cases | Progression free (%) | Year | No. of cases | Progression free (%) |
| BVP   | 1977 | 50 | 64 | 1981 | 171 | 73 |
| VAB   | 1981 | 45 | 49 | 1986 | 147 | 72 |
| POMB  | 1980 | 43 | 66 | 1983 | 69  | 83 |
| BOP   | 1978 | 34 | 65 | 1984 | 29  | 83 |

BVP: bleomycin, vinblastine, platinum; VAB: vinblastine, actinomycin D, bleomycin; POMB: platinum, vincristine, methotrexate, bleomycin; BOP: bleomycin, vincristine, cisplatin.

**Table 17.4** Indiana randomized trials in germ cell cancer (for sources, see Schmoll[23])

|            | All | | 'Good risk' | | 'Poor risk' | |
|------------|--------------|----------------------|--------------|----------------------|--------------|----------------------|
|            | No. of cases | Progression free (%) | No. of cases | Progression free (%) | No. of cases | Progression free (%) |
| BVP        | 121 | 66 | NA | 76 | NA | 48 |
| vs         |     |    |    |    |    |    |
| BEP        | 123 | 78 | NA | 84 | NA | 68 |
| BEP (20)   | ND | — | ND | — | 77 | 61 |
| vs         |    |   |    |   |    |    |
| BEP (40)   | ND | — | ND | — | 76 | 63 |
| BEP        | ND | — | ND | — | 125 | 42 |
| vs         |    |   |    |   |     |    |
| VIP        | ND | — | ND | — | 128 | 48 |
| BEP (× 4)  | ND | — | 96 | 92 | ND | — |
| vs         |    |   |    |    |    |   |
| BEP (× 3)  | ND | — | 88 | 92 | ND | — |

BVP: bleomycin, vinblastine, platinum; BEP: bleomycin, etoposide, cisplatin; VIP: etoposide, ifosfamide, cisplatin.
BEP (20): 20 mg/m$^2$ × 5q21; BEP (40): 40 mg/m$^2$ × 5q21.
NA: not available; ND: not done.

significantly better survival of patients with advanced bulky disease.[25] This regimen used a higher dose intensity of etoposide, i.e. 100 mg/m$^2$ for 5 days compared with 120 mg/m$^2$ for 3 days as reported in the original BEP publication by Peckham *et al.*[26] As a result, even to this day, there is a difference of opinion over dosage between the US and UK, hopefully to be resolved in the next European trial which will compare, in a 2 × 2 trial, 3 vs 5 days of cisplatin/etoposide and three vs four courses of chemotherapy. Subsequently, the Einhorn school developed a VP16-213 (etoposide), ifosfamide, cisplatin (VIP) regimen, first as a salvage regimen[27] and subsequently in a multicentre randomized trial for poor-risk patients. Despite considerably increased toxicity, the preliminary analysis has suggested only a small non-significant benefit for VIP over BEP,[28] which remains the standard over most of the world. However, in BVP and BEP the bleomycin is given by weekly intravenous bolus instead of the continuous infusion that had been used by Samuels in the original bleomycin/vinblastine studies. Lethal/bleomycin lung toxicity has been a treatment-related complication in many of the subsequent trials and many attempts have been made to avoid or discontinue the use of bleomycin (Table 17.5), although administration by prolonged infusion seems to reduce the risks and retain the therapeutic benefit.[22,29,30]

The second school of germ cell cancer chemotherapy developed at Memorial Hospital, New York, and piloted a series of vinblastine, actinomycin D and bleomycin (VAB) trials.[31,32] These were not quite as successful as the high dose vinblastine/bleomycin protocol of Samuels. In addition, by the time this group added cisplatin they had also added cyclophosphamide, failing to remember the lesson from their own institution in the 1960s when it was demonstrated that after 6-years use of the combination of methotrexate, actinomycin D and chlorambucil, overall the results were the same as with actinomycin D alone.[21] More drugs are not necessarily any better than a single drug, a point which has been learnt from study of several tumours. Because of these extra drugs in the VAB regimen, it was usually only possible to give cisplatin once a month.[33] In view of anxiety

**Table 17.5**  Trials ± bleomycin for germ cell cancer (for souces, see Schmoll[23])

|  | All | | 'Good risk' | | 'Poor risk' | |
|---|---|---|---|---|---|---|
|  | No. of cases | Progression free (%) | No. of cases | Progression free (%) | No. of cases | Progression free (%) |
| BEP (× 3) | ND | — | 83 | 84 | ND | — |
| vs |  |  |  |  |  |  |
| EP (× 3) | ND | — | 83 | 69 | ND | — |
| BVP | ND | — | 110 | 84 | ND | — |
| vs |  |  |  |  |  |  |
| VP | ND | — | 108 | 71 | ND | — |
| BEP | ND | — | 160 | 90 | ND | — |
| vs |  |  |  |  |  |  |
| EP | ND | — | 153 | 84 | ND | — |
| VAB-6 | ND | — | 81 | 85 | ND | — |
| vs |  |  |  |  |  |  |
| EP | ND | — | 81 | 83 | ND | — |

BEP: bleomycin, etoposide, cisplatin; EP: etoposide, cisplatin; BVP: bleomycin, vinblastine, platinum; VP: vinblastine, cisplatin; VAB: vinblastine, actinomycin D, bleomycin.
ND: not done.

about the Einhorn group's continued reporting of bleomycin-related deaths, the Memorial group then compared etoposide and cisplatin with VAB-6, and etoposide and cisplatin (EP) proved equal but less toxic.[34] Despite two subsequent trials (Table 17.5) demonstrating the importance of bleomycin in both the BVP and BEP regimens,[35] as VAB-6 was never compared with BEP, the group compounded the error further by comparing etoposide/cisplatin 3-weekly, with etoposide and carboplatin 4-weekly. This added to another of the shortcomings of the VAB-6 regimen in which the platinum was also usually given monthly. The carboplatin arm clearly did worse (Table 17.6) and the poor response of good-risk patients to carboplatin has now been confirmed by other,[36,37] though not all,[38,39] studies of carboplatin (Table 17.6). The most significant exception was a historically controlled non-randomized study by the Memorial group[37] which suggested that the bleomycin, carboplatin and etoposide regimen in poor-risk patients was at least as good as VAB-6. Furthermore, this group has salvaged cisplatin failures using carboplatin at a much higher dosage with bone marrow support, as have several other authors.[23] In addition, recent reports have demonstrated that the initial Phase 1 study of carboplatin had underestimated by nearly 50% the safe dose that could be given to elderly women with ovarian cancer without the need for haematological support.[40] As there were no

**Table 17.6**   Trials comparing cisplatin vs carboplatin for germ cell cancer (for sources, see Schmoll[23])

| | All | | 'Good risk' | | 'Poor risk' | |
|---|---|---|---|---|---|---|
| | No. of cases | Progression free (%) | No. of cases | Progression free (%) | No. of cases | Progression free (%) |
| EP | ND | — | 134 | 87 | ND | — |
| vs | | | | | | |
| EC | ND | — | 131 | 76 | ND | — |
| BEP | ND | — | 93 | 90 | ND | — |
| vs | | | | | | |
| CEB | ND | — | 88 | 80 | ND | — |
| EBCi (3 day) | 35 | 86 | 29 | 97 | 6 | 33 |
| vs | | | | | | |
| EBCa (3 day) | 26 | 73 | 21 | 81 | 5 | 40 |
| VAB-6[a] (1979–82) | ND | — | ND | — | 29 | 28 |
| VAB-6/EP[a] (1982–5) | ND | — | ND | — | 39 | 34 |
| EBC[a] (1985–8) | ND | — | ND | — | 39 | 44 |

[a]Non-randomized historical comparison.
EP: etoposide, cisplatin; EC: etoposide, carboplatin; BEP: bleomycin, etoposide, cisplatin; CEB: carboplatin, etoposide, cisplatin; EBCi: etoposide, bleomycin, cisplatin; EBCa: etoposide, bleomycin, carboplatin; VAB: vinblastine, actinomycin D, bleomycin. ND: not done.

relapses in twenty patients treated at greater than AUC-5 (5 × area under curve, i.e. glomerular filtration rate + 25) in the original germ cell cancer Phase 1/2 study by Childs *et al.*[41] and the dose–response curve appeared to be very steep (Table 17.7), these observations suggest that there is a case for further dose-escalation studies of carboplatin — particularly given the increasing evidence that the latter drug has a better late toxicity profile than cisplatin.[36]

**Table 17.7**    Relapse and AUC optimizator of carboplatin dose for germ cell cancer (adapted from Childs *et al.*[41] p. 291)

| AUC | No. of cases | Relapse rate (%) |
|---|---|---|
| <4 | 8 | 50 |
| 4–4.5 | 20 | 10 |
| 4.6–5.0 | 73 | 4 |
| >5.0 | 20 | 0 |

AUC: area under the curve.

The third school of germ cell chemotherapy was developed in the UK at Charing Cross Hospital by Newlands *et al.*[9] This group combined cisplatin into a methotrexate-containing combination developed locally for treating choriocarcinoma in women, but also including the Samuels continuous-infusion bleomycin. This regimen used some of the subsequently established erroneous principles of the VAB regimens by aiming to maximize the number of drugs in the regimen by alternating platinum, vincristine (oncovin), methotrexate and bleomycin (POMB) with actinomycin D, cyclophosphamide and etoposide (ACE). However, in contrast to the VAB regimen there remains a continued interest in the POMB regimen because, in addition to achieving somewhat better results in the high-hCG-positive patients, it is also the only combination to produce long-term cure of brain metastases without the need for concomitant radiation.[42] In addition, one study has suggested that POMB/ACE-treated patients may have a lower incidence of second germ cell cancers in the contralateral testis than occurs after the BVP/BEP regimens.[43] These two later observations might be attributed to the known ability of methotrexate to cross the blood–brain and testis barrier. This property is the basis of methotrexate's continued use in preventing cranial and testicular relapses in leukaemia. One other difference between the VAB-6 and POMB regimens was that the interval between first and second doses of cisplatin was 12–14 days compared with 28 days in the VAB-6 and 21 days in the BVP/BEP regimens. Given that, in the early studies using BVP, delay beyond 21 days was a deleterious risk factor for durable response,[44,45] it is clear that the shorter interval in the POMB regimen could be significantly advantageous.

The fourth school of germ cell cancer chemotherapy developed from Buffalo (Roswell Park) through the work of Merrin and colleagues who used weekly treatments with bleomycin, vincristine and cisplatin, 100 mg/m$^2$ (BOP).[46] Much of the data from this work is uninterpretable as the publications chiefly emphasized the surgical abilities of the hospital in undertaking major abdominal and chest surgery during a single anaesthetic to remove non-viable remnants after the chemotherapy had been completed. Most of these reports were published before issues of dose intensity had been more fully worked out. However, the idea was redeveloped by Wettlaufer et al.[47] who reported impressive results in poor-risk patients so that the Roswell Park regimen was later adopted by several authors for their so-called hybrid regimens used in poor-risk patients. High-intensity platinum/etoposide (HIPE),[48] BOP/VIP[49] and BOP/BEP,[50] have been most extensively studied, though none have proven any better than the results achieved in the small series reported by Wettlaufer using BOP alone (Table 17.8).[47]

**Table 17.8** Accelerated cisplatin ($q \leq 14$ days) as first-line treatment for 'poor risk' germ cell cancer

|  | No. of cases | Progression free (%) |
| --- | --- | --- |
| BOP | 29 | 83 |
| BOP/VIP | 91 | 66 |
| BOP/BEP | 61 | 71 |
| POMB | 22 | 56 |

BOP: bleomycin, vincristine, cisplatin; VIP: etoposide, ifosfamide, cisplatin; BEP: bleomycin, etoposide, cisplatin; POMB: platinum, vincristine, methotrexate, bleomycin.

Further support for the view that it may be the 7–10-day repeated BOP part of the hybrid regimens that is important in achieving this success comes from a study using BOP as a salvage regimen for patients who have failed a conventional 21-day BEP regimen (Table 17.9). The salvage rate is higher than that achieved by the standard VIP salvage regimen in the USA

**Table 17.9** Salvage regimens for germ cell tumours

|  | No. of cases | Continuous NEM (%) | Reference |
| --- | --- | --- | --- |
| EP/BEP salvage of BVP | 30 | 37 | Williams et al.[51] |
| VIP salvage of BVP/BEP | 48 | 15 | Loehrer et al.[20] |
| BOP salvage of BEP | 46 | 39 | Oliver (in preparation) |
| Autologous BMT salvage of BEP/VIP failure | 181 | 23 | Schmoll[33] |
| ABMT/PBSCT salvage of BEP/BOP failure | 12 | 58 | Oliver (in preparation) |

NEM: no evidence of malignancy; EP: etoposide, cisplatin; BEP: bleomycin, etoposide, cisplatin; BVP: bleomycin, vinblastine, platinum; VIP: etoposide, ifosfamide, cisplatin; BOP: bleomycin, vincristine, cisplatin; BMT: bone marrow transplant; ABMT: autologous bone marrow transplant; PBSCT: peripheral blood stem cell transplant.

(etoposide, ifosfamide, cisplatin)[44] and, even more interestingly, though subject to serious reservations because they are based on extremely small numbers, these studies also suggest that use of highly intensive chemotherapy with bone marrow or peripheral blood stem cell transplant  (PBSCT), in very high-risk patients previously treated with conventional chemotherapy and with BOP as second-line treatment, may have better third-line salvage rates than those failing VIP. To date, seven of twelve patients (58%) have been salvaged for more than 1 year compared with 23% reported in a review of 181 patients reported by Schmoll.[23]

## Grade 1 germ cell cancer (seminoma) chemotherapy studies

Most of the chemotherapy studies undertaken in seminoma have used the same combinations as used for non-seminoma (Table 17.10). This was, in part, due to early reports indicating no difference in response rates between seminoma and non-seminoma.[52] In recent years, as fewer and fewer patients have been treated in relapse after failed radiotherapy, it is becoming increasingly apparent that the results are actually better than those achieved in non-seminoma even using regimens containing etoposide and cisplatin without bleomycin.[53] However, in multivariate analysis with correction for other prognostic factors such as volume and tumour marker levels, the importance of histological subgroup as a prognostic factor is not statistically significant.

Despite these excellent results, there have been a few centres who have explored single-agent platinum in the treatment of seminoma. This is despite the knowledge since the 1960s that the single-agent response rates for seminoma and non-seminoma are different[54,55] as are, of course, the radiation response rates.[56] The anecdotal report of Samuels *et al.* (who observed four complete responses in five patients receiving weekly cisplatin and then switched to cyclophosphamide/cisplatin[57]) was the first to question whether BVP/BEP regimens should be routine for seminoma patients. The subsequent definitive publication[58] observed eight of eight durable complete responses (CRs) after single-agent treatment, suggesting that the initial Samuels failure could have been the result of a residual mass which did not progress. Though confirmed by one other study of cisplatin,[10,59]

**Table 17.10**    Response of advanced metastatic seminoma to radiation and chemotherapy (modified from Schmoll[23])

|  | No. of cases | Progression free (%) |
|---|---|---|
| Radiation  Stage 2 < 5 cm | 162 | 92 |
| Stage 2 ≥ 5 cm | 113 | 73 |
| BVP | 109 | 73 |
| BEP/EP | 46 | 96 |
| Single cisplatin | 24 | 83 |
| Single agent carboplatin | 112 | 75 |

BVP: bleomycin, vinblastine, platinum; BEP: bleomycin, etoposide, cisplatin; EP: etoposide, cisplatin.

subsequent studies with carboplatin have at first sight not been as encouraging.[10,60,61] However, the preliminary results from dosage escalation and correction for body surface area (Table 17.11) suggest that the poorer results may reflect under-dosage due to lack of appreciation of the true upper safe dosage, now known to be nearly double that used previously.[40] Clearly more data are required from studies of this rare group of patients. Perhaps the greatest encouragement justifying further pursuit of these ideas is that use of the accelerated weekly BOP regimen of Wettlaufer as salvage cured five out of five carboplatin failures.[47]

In summary, it may be concluded that BEP has established itself as the world standard for first-line treatment in both seminoma and non-seminoma. There remains dispute about the safety of single-agent platinum in seminoma and whether an accelerated dose-intensification regimen with weekly BOP is superior to VIP in the salvage setting. In addition, because BOP does less damage to the bone marrow if it fails as second line, subsequent third-line high dose treatment with stem cell protection could be more successful than after VIP failure. At present, the more intense neuro- and oto-toxicity of the BOP regimen and the more intense nausea, emesis and myelosuppression of VIP preclude their consideration as primary treatment for patients with good-prognosis metastatic disease. However, with increasing international consensus on characteristics for defining poor-prognosis patients, particularly those with less than 45% durable cure,[62] an important priority for the future will be to develop a protocol to further investigate these issues of dose intensity in the first-line setting.

There is, however, one cloud which is emerging to threaten the pre-eminence of BEP, particularly from the point of view of its suitability for use in studies of early Stage 1 and 2 germ cell cancer. This relates to the incidence of late toxicity. There have now been six studies which have reported an excess of leukaemia in patients receiving BEP compared to the number expected, and also to those observed after BVP treatment

**Table 17.11** Impact of AUC and AUC corrected to 1.8 m² surface area on relapse of metastatic seminoma after carboplatin single agent

|  | AUC uncorrected | No. of cases | Progression-free survival (%) | |
|---|---|---|---|---|
|  | ≥7.0 | 8 | 88 | P = 0.31 |
|  | <7.0 | 10 | 60 | |
|  | AUC corrected 1.8 m² |  |  | |
| All cases | ≥6.5 | 10 | 90 | P = 0.12 |
|  | <6.5 | 8 | 50 | |
| Stage 2c, 2d and 3 | ≥6.5 | 9 | 89 | P = 0.023 |
|  | <6.5 | 5 | 20 | |

AUC: area under curve.

(Table 17.12).[63] Though most of the cases have occurred in patients receiving higher than average doses, there have been a number of cases even after the routine dose used for good-risk patients. Some investigators have not observed etoposide-related leukaemia, most notably the Norwegian group (S Fossa, personal communication) which has a large proportion of its patients living in rural areas and possibly exposed to less pollution. Although worrying, the absolute incidence of leukaemia is relatively modest, particularly with the lower doses now known to cure the overwhelming majority of good-risk patients. However, it is the knowledge that many agents associated with a leukaemia risk within 5 years of exposure also have an associated increased risk of a second solid cancer — which can manifest up to 15 or 20 years after exposure — that is putting a dampener on absolute confidence in the use of the BEP regimen for early stages of disease. There are already anecdotal reports of cases of solid cancer in BEP-treated patients,[64] including one case in a patient who received BEP as adjuvant for Stage 1 disease,[65] providing a strong justification for prolonged careful follow-up of these cases.

The second late toxicity issue after BEP, which is as yet unresolved, is the issue of hypertensive heart disease that has now been reported at least anecdotally.[66] As most men cured of testicular cancer by BEP are under the age of 40 at the time of treatment, they need to be followed for a further 25 or more years before they reach the age for peak incidence of hypertensive heart disease. Already there are two early indications giving cause for concern in patients treated with BEP/BVP regimens. The first group of reports demonstrate evidence of excessively high incidence of elevated blood pressure and cholesterol level[67–70] and, in one randomized trial comparing BEP with bleomycin–etoposide–carboplatin,[70] an excess of hypertension and renal damage was clearly established as present only in the cisplatin arm, together with evidence of increased high-tone hearing loss.

The second worrying development, from the point of view of late cardiac disease, is the weight gain commonly seen after orchidectomy and demonstrated, in two studies, to be associated with increased levels of cholesterol.[67,68] These observations represent a strong justification for

**Table 17.12**   Etoposide and secondary leukaemias in testicular germ cell cancer

| No. of patients | No. AML (%) | Cumulative etoposide dose (mg/m²) for those developing AML | Reference[a] |
|---|---|---|---|
| 212 | 5 (2.4) | All > 2000 | Pedersen-Bjergaard, 1991 |
| 340 | 2 (0.6) | 1300 and 2000 | Bajorin, 1993 |
| 538 | 2 (0.37) | Both <2000 | Nichols, 1993 |
| 221 | 1[b] (0.45) | 2000 | Bokemeyer, 1993 |
| 679 | 6 (0.88) | 720, 750, 900, 3000 and 5000 | Boshoff, 1994 |
| Total 1990 | 16 (0.8) | | |

[a]For references, see Boshoff *et al.*[43]
[b]One patient developed acute lymphoblastic leukaemia.
AML: acute myeloid leukaemia.

attempting to follow up large cohorts of patients in order to establish late risks. Until this is done, the use of BEP for treating early disease should, in my view, still be confined to the clinical trial setting.

An attempt to develop alternative strategies is now being explored in the UK by an adjuvant BOP study for poor-risk Stage 1 non-seminoma patients. As the study gives two courses of BOP at a longer than normal interval than in any of the previous BOP studies, and adds two additional courses of vincristine–bleomycin, it is possible that the treatment may prove to be no better than BEP, which has a 4% recurrence rate. As the BOP regimen would still leave the patient exposed to the risk of cisplatin renal damage and later hypertensive heart disease, an alternative route for developing a safe adjuvant regimen might be to develop a carboplatin-containing version of the methotrexate-based POMB regimen, i.e. COMB. As well as reducing tumours in the contralateral testis,[43] bone marrow growth factors could be used to enable a shorter interval between treatments with carboplatin at a dose increased to the higher levels now used in ovarian cancer studies: an approach which might eliminate the 4% incidence of relapse seen after BEP. This is the current strategy now being developed in my unit, though before doing such studies it will be necessary to establish the safety of these regimens in patients with poor-risk disease.

# Assessment of comparative effectiveness and late events after radiation or surgery for early-Stage 1 and 2 non-seminoma

From the time of the earliest reports up to the modern chemotherapy era dating from the mid-1970s, there has been a continuing dispute over the relative merits of radiation versus surgical retroperitoneal lymph node dissection for non-seminoma. When analysed retrospectively, taking account of decade of diagnosis, there is no obvious difference in the effectiveness of treatment (Table 17.1), with both modalities showing substantial improvement over the 30 years that they represented the primary treatment modality. At least a part of this improvement reflected only a stage shift from improved methods for detecting metastases and staging patients.[1] If anything, these results would favour the use of adjuvant radiotherapy, as staging was purely clinical and apparent Stage 1 cases would have included 30% or more defined as Stage 2 in pathologically staged surgical studies — which would have also excluded patients with inoperable Stage 2 disease from their reports.

Despite this possible advantage, radiotherapists were the first to discontinue this modality, as early results suggested that previously irradiated patients might have more serious side-effects from chemotherapy, including treatment-related mortality, and a lower cure rate,[44,45] though this lessened with improved understanding and experience of using the drugs. By the time this was recognized, the excellent results of surveillance had been reported,[7] and the seriously increased risk of late second non-germ-cell cancers was becoming apparent, particularly in patients receiving the higher dose radiotherapy regimens for non-seminoma (Table 17.13).[71] These observations rapidly led to loss of interest in the prophylactic use of radiotherapy for non-seminoma.

**Table 17.13**   Dose and development of stomach cancer on 10–15-year follow-up of 5-year survivors after radiation for germ cell cancer[71]

|  | Number treated | Observed/expected in 5-year survivors | Relative risk |
|---|---|---|---|
| Seminoma (≤ 0.3 Gy) | 874 | 4/1.3 | 3.2 |
| Non-seminoma (0.4–0.5 Gy) | 992 | 5/0.2 | 26.3 |

For the decade that radiation oncologists were actively exploring surveillance after orchidectomy for Stage 1 disease, surgeons continued with node surgery, but developed sacral plexus sympathetic nerve sparing approaches. This substantially reduced (but did not eliminate) the risk of loss of ejaculation,[72] the most distressing complication of surgery in patients who turned out to have pathological Stage 1 disease, though the operation proved less effective for patients with Stage 2 who needed wider excision margins. With more recent data demonstrating that sperm counts after chemotherapy are possibly better than those after surgery, radiotherapy or surveillance (Table 17.14), fertility issues can no longer be used to support a surgical view of choice of treatment modality.

Despite this decade of surgical progress, surgery cannot be justified in early (Stage 1) disease as the results of surveillance are equally good. In the final analysis, taking 100 clinical Stage 1 patients undergoing surgery, the need for chemotherapy is reduced only from 30% to 20% because of the 12% relapse in the 70% who have pathological Stage 1 and the 30% relapse rate in the 30% of clinical Stage 1 patients who turn out to be pathological Stage 2. Furthermore, there have been no publications on the late events after radical lymph node surgery, the most significant of which is the need for operation for adhesions. This occurred in two of the nineteen patients in the postchemotherapy series reported from the London Hospital series, published in 1984, and followed for more than 10 years.[45]

**Table 17.14**   Germ cell cancer patients median FSH levels and change in sperm count 3 years after different management policies (Fossa *et al.*[73])

|  | FSH | Change in sperm count compared to pretreatment (%) |
|---|---|---|
| Surveillance | 7.7 | +69 |
| RLND[a] | 7.0 | + 23 |
| Chemotherapy | 8.6 | +113 |
| Radiotherapy | 8.6 | +33 |

FSH: follicle-stimulating hormone; RLND: radical lymph node dissection.

A final factor which may provide justification for adjuvant chemotherapy over surveillance is the report that tumours in the contralateral testis are more frequent after surgery than radiotherapy, and even lower after chemotherapy, albeit in the dosages used to treat metastatic disease.[75]

It is concluded that there is no longer any justification for routine use of either prophylactic radiation therapy or lymph node dissection in clinical Stage 1 non-seminoma cases. For clinical Stage 2 there remains a small area of doubt as the results from primary chemotherapy series are marginally worse than after surgery,[5] though it is unclear how much this reflects selection, with bulky cases not being included in the surgery series, or failure of chemotherapists to recognize that surgery may have an important role after chemotherapy in patients with borderline residual abnormalities.

# Surveillance vs adjuvant chemotherapy for Stage 1 non-seminoma

Data from several large-scale studies have clearly established the safety of postorchidectomy surveillance[4,7,74] compared with surgery, but have not yet quantified the psychological problems these patients face. So far, within the limits of instruments that are available to test for such problems, there is no apparent evidence of any difference between Stage 1 patients on regular surveillance and metastatic patients treated primarily by chemotherapy.[76] There is, however, some evidence at the anecdotal level that there may be a number of risks. Young patients with testicular tumours are at a very mobile time of their life, and with relapse occurring as late as 4 years after orchidectomy there are types of patients for whom such an approach is not appropriate, particularly if they are at risk of becoming lost to follow-up and later might present with an advanced, less curable stage at relapse. Increasing confidence that the acute toxicity of chemotherapy is manageable with modern antiemetics and the possibility that, like surgically treated patients, those on surveillance might have a higher incidence of tumours in the contralateral testis than radiation- or chemotherapy-treated patients[77] led to attempts to identify patients at high risk of relapse, and treating them with short-course adjuvant chemotherapy.[30]

Freedman *et al.*[77] were the first to establish a scheme for predicting relapse risk with a pathological scoring system using vascular and/or lymphatic invasion, absence of yolk sac, and presence of anaplastic areas as risk factors. This was verified in a subsequently reported prospective study.[7] Patients with three or more risk factors from this four-point scoring system had a greater than 50% risk of relapse. Use of two courses of adjuvant BEP has now been demonstrated in several series, totalling more than 100 patients, to reduce the relapse rate to 4%. Though encouraging, the overall relapse rate for Stage 1 cases falls only from 26% to 13% because of the small numbers selected for treatment (Table 17.15). With more liberal selection of patients with two or more risk factors, a reduction to an overall relapse rate of 6% has been noted — the first time that an adjuvant approach has produced better results than surgery. The recent concern arising from the risk of leukaemia in patients receiving etoposide,[63] and the

**Table 17.15**   Prognostic factors and relapse Stage 1, G2/G3 (non-seminoma) germ cell cancer on surveillance or adjuvant chemotherapy (modified from Freedman et al.[77])

| | Risk factor score (%) | | | Total |
|---|---|---|---|---|
| | 0/1 | 2 | 3 | |
| Proportion of patients | 38 | 38 | 24 | N = 233 |
| Proportion of relapse | 13 | 34 | 53 | N = 61 |
| Relapse risk, 2 years | 9 | 25 | 58 | 26%[a] |
| Relapse after BEP × 2 for patients with three risk factors | 9 | 25 | 4 | 13%[a] |
| Relapse after BEP × 2 for patients with two and three risk factors | 9 | 4 | | 6%[a] |

[a]Relapse risk for total group.
BEP: bleomycin, etoposide, cisplatin.

one anecdote of a solid cancer in an adjuvant-treated patient,[64] has put these studies on hold while a less toxic chemotherapy option is developed. The hypertension and subclinical renal and ototoxicity observed in the comparative trial of EBCi (3 day) vs EBCa (3 day), mentioned in a previous section, implies that the current British proposal by the Medical Research Council (MRC) to examine BOP will not prove to be a major gain, particularly as the decision to give two courses of cisplatin at a 2-week interval will result in the potential gain in possible reduction of the residual 4% relapse rate from short-term dose intensity being likely to be lost.

# Therapeutic options for Stage 1 and 2 seminoma

Since Maier *et al.* reported an 8% incidence of metastases at lymphadenectomy,[78] there has been no serious consideration that retroperitoneal node surgery might have a worthwhile role in early-stage seminoma. The reason for this is the high radiation-induced cure rate that has been routinely achieved since the late 1960s, when cure first reached over 90%. With the most recent overview of 2376 cases reporting 95% continuous progression-free survival and 98% cure,[8] there is at first sight little justification for considering alternative options. However, there is a well-documented increased risk of late gastrointestinal toxicity, particularly in patients with a previous history of abdominal surgery or ulcers,[79] and also an increased risk of secondary cancer, both within[80] and outside the direct field of treatment,[81] possibly reflecting the long-term degree of subtle change in T-cell immune response induced by radiotherapy.[82] This excess mortality only became apparent in patients followed up for more than 10 years,[83] and in the London Hospital series of 131 patients followed up to 3 years after treatment actuarial survival at 20 years was only 50% compared with the 75% observed in the normal population.[84]

Only half the deaths were due to secondary malignancy; excess cardiac deaths also occurred and may have been due to radiation-induced delayed arteritis of renal arteries, producing an increased incidence of hypertension. Clearly, there is room for improvement, though these extremely late toxicities may only relate to patients treated before the advent of modern linear accelerator techniques with chemotherapy (CT) planning and modern antihypertensive drugs. Equally, new treatment schedules introduced since the beginning of 1990 (using either a para-aortic strip,[85] or accelerated treatment with 20 Gy in ten fractions[86] instead of 30 Gy in fifteen fractions[87]) cannot have been adequately followed for 30 years, and might go some way to reducing the previously observed excess morbidity. However, there is clear evidence from studies measuring primary relapse-free survival that chemotherapy, even a single dose of carboplatin alone,[9] is at least as good and possibly marginally better than radiation (one relapse in 106 treated, compared with four in seventy-nine contemporary patients receiving radiotherapy).

There is a need for more widespread evaluation of this alternative option which seems to be better tolerated than radiation. With carboplatin only in widespread clinical use for the last 10 years, it is premature to conclude that there might be no late toxicity of the kind seen with radiotherapy between 15 and 30 years after treatment. Equally, with occasional late relapses of seminoma after radiation or surveillance out to 5 or more years, one could not conclude that the current results are definitive until a sizeable cohort has been followed for 10 years. However, despite these provisos, with the longest follow-up now 116 months, median follow-up for two courses being 7 years, and single-course patients all now followed for more than 2 years, the one relapse in 106 cases compares favourably with the fourteen of 499 (3%) in the latest MRC radiotherapy trial begun in 1990.[88] The issue now is how to accumulate adequate cases to resolve the question of late events, including the possibility of whether there might be a beneficial reduction in incidence of contralateral secondary germ cell testicular cancers from use of adjuvant carboplatin.

For Stage 2 seminoma, radiation has long been known to be a better option than for non-seminoma, though it is increasingly clear that there is less justification for its use as a substitute for chemotherapy (Table 17.10). For bulky Stage 2 seminoma it is already clear that chemotherapy is better. For small volume disease, a much smaller number of patients has been treated, though with 14% relapse in radiation-treated patients with low bulk (< 5 cm by computed tomography criteria) Stage 2 disease,[89] compared with none of four in the London Hospital series treated with what was an inadequate dose of carboplatin for bulky disease (Table 17.11), one suspects that there is little to be gained from continued use of radiation. However, until there are more late follow-up and toxicity data these issues, which involve the concept of altering treatment in patients with a high cure rate for a theoretical gain in terms of reduced late toxicity, cannot attract much support unless they are self-financing.

# Surveillance in Stage 1 seminoma

With more than 300 patients having now been entered into surveillance studies worldwide,[9,88–90] relapse has been documented in 20% at 4 years. Though the overall death rate obtained from these studies is even lower than after prophylactic radiotherapy, the pattern of relapse is slow and often difficult to prove.[59] Most relapses occur in the para-aortic area, occasionally in association with malignant retroperitoneal fibrosis, though relapse with signs of paraplegia is a well-recognized but rare event. This has occurred at 6 years in one of my sixty-seven patients on surveillance for more than 5 years.

Although such occurrences make it doubtful that surveillance is a safe option in a routine service setting, more detailed late follow-up of all Stage 1 patients around the world who have been entered on surveillance will clearly be important, not least to clarify whether late malignancies and vascular events 15–30 years after radiotherapy are true late effects of the treatment or perhaps a reflection of innate susceptibility in patients who develop Stage 1 seminoma.

# Management of the primary tumour

Currently, the standard diagnostic procedure for more than 95% of patients with germ cell cancer is radical orchidectomy, tracing the spermatic cord through the inguinal canal and dividing it at the internal inguinal ring. Between one-third and one-half of patients experience a variable degree of postoperative anaesthesia, due to trauma to the ileoinguinal nerve, which lasts 6–24 months. Ten per cent have a mild wound infection which delays the start of treatment, though one patient with very advanced disease, treated early in my personal series, developed late inguinal wound infection during nadir leucopenic sepsis that was complicated by ascending ileo-vena caval venous thrombosis, terminating in death with a Budd–Chiari syndrome from renal and hepatic vein thrombosis.[91] One per cent develop a persistent inguinal discomfort of such intensity that nerve blocks may be required or contemplated. A final little-documented but genuine occurrence in about one-third of patients is the development of phantom amputation symptoms in the groin, which only occur at the moment of ejaculation.

Given this catalogue of mostly minor discomforts it is surprising that, with now more than 15 years experience of curative cisplatin-based chemotherapy, there has been virtually no thought given to the possibility that there might be any option other than orchidectomy for management of the primary tumour. Despite there being at least three case reports of the use of partial orchidectomy in patients with a tumour in a solitary testis (one of whom subsequently fathered two children), many such patients are still pressured into undergoing orchidectomy for tumours in a solitary testis on the erroneous grounds that monthly testosterone replacement injections provide more than adequate replacement. Furthermore, after unilateral orchidectomy for testis cancer, more than two-thirds of patients with a tumour in one of their two testicles will have some evidence of hypogonadism (elevated follicle-stimulating hormone and/or sperm count of less than $20 \times 10^6$/ml) and about one in ten will require hormone replacement.[92] There are very few published data on the effects of chemotherapy on primary tumours, except in the minority of patients who were so ill that they underwent chemotherapy based on biopsy of metastases. Two initial reports[93,94] suggested that there might be a blood–testis barrier as there was marginally higher complete response in metastases than in the primary (Table 17.16), though in an analysis of our own somewhat larger series[95] this was not so clear-cut. In this series of thirty-two patients, fifteen did not undergo orchidectomy, having achieved a complete response to chemotherapy. One subsequently developed a second tumour of different histological type at 12 years. As the limited data available on semen cytology in patients with germ cell malignancy demonstrate malignant cells in about 50% of cases,[96] there might be a case for neoadjuvant chemotherapy before orchidectomy in such positive patients, allowing those whose testes normalized with non-surgical treatment to elect either to undergo postchemo-orchidectomy to confirm response or to keep the organ after careful consideration and signed informed consent.

**Table 17.16**　Clinical/pathological response of primary and metastases to systemic chemotherapy

| Reference | No. of cases | CR primary (%) | CR metastases (%) |
|---|---|---|---|
| Greist *et al.*[93] | 20 | 85 | 90 |
| Chong *et al.*[94] | 16 | 75 | 81 |
| Oliver *et al.*[95] | 31 | 81 | 82 |
| Total | 67 | 81 | 84 |

CR: complete response.

## Conclusions

As shown in Fig. 17.1, the results of germ cell cancer treatment have continued to improve even over the last 5 years. This has been, in part, due to the continued improvement in results of chemotherapy, first with the increased dose intensity BOP regimen, and subsequently by high dose chemotherapy with stem cell rescue, though equally important has been the increasingly early diagnosis due to increased public awareness of the disease.[95] This increased margin of safety is most dramatically demonstrated by seminoma studies from the Royal Marsden Hospital, London, reporting successful salvage of five out of five carboplatin failures using accelerated BOP.[50] Given the better understanding of the dose–response relationship of carboplatin, despite recently reported higher relapse rates with carboplatin

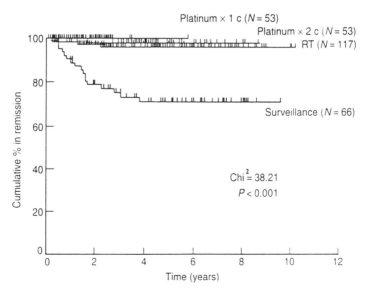

**Fig. 17.1**　Anglian Germ Cell Tumour Group study, Stage 1 seminoma (1 May 1983 to 4 March 1994). Relapse-free survival by type of treatment.

than with cisplatin, clearly further trials using this drug are justified. It might, for example, be combined in future regimens with methotrexate and vincristine plus granulocyte colony stimulating factor to enable increased dose intensity and possible increased penetration of the blood–brain and blood–testis barriers. Increasing recognition of the late vascular-, renal- and ototoxicity from cisplatin combinations, as well as the risk of leukaemia and possibly other solid cancers after etoposide treatment, is delaying widespread acceptance of BEP-type chemotherapy for good-prognosis patients. This provides additional justification for further trials of carboplatin in combination, despite the worse disease-free survival recently observed in carboplatin trials in patients with good-prognosis non-seminoma.

For Stage 1 seminoma, the simplicity of single-course carboplatin as adjuvant therapy is compelling (Fig. 17.2), but prudence is required until 5- and 10-year data are more substantial and a low cost follow-up technique has been developed, to avoid the disappointment of discovering

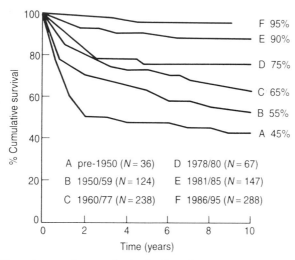

**Fig. 17.2** The change in survival of all patients of the Royal London Hospital with testis tumour (1950–95).

that delayed toxicity might have led to a 25% reduction in life expectancy after 20 years follow-up, as has been seen in recent follow-up of radiotherapy patients treated at the Royal London Hospital.

From the point of view of new approaches in early-stage cases, the observation that increasingly early diagnosis is reducing the size of tumours is important and may have valuable implications. It offers potential for lessening the degree of germinal epithelium loss by use of presurgical neoadjuvant chemotherapy.

This could in turn, enable organ conservation as a feasible and possibly routine part of the treatment of testicular cancer and would be of particular relevance in patients developing the tumour in a solitary testis.

# References

1. Blandy JP, Oliver RTD, Hope-Stone HF. A British approach to the management of patients with testicular tumours. In: JP Donohue, ed, *International Perspectives in Urology*. Baltimore: Williams & Wilkins, 1983; 207–23.
2. Donohue JP, Thornhill JA, Foster RS, *et al*. Primary retroperitoneal lymph node dissection in a clinical stage. A non-seminomatous germ cell testis cancer. Review of the Indiana University experience 1965–1989. *Br J Urol* 1993; **71**, 326–35.
3. Einhorn LH. Testicular cancer as a model for curable neoplasm: the Richard and Hinda Rosenthal Foundation Award Lecture. *Cancer Res* 1981; **41**, 3275–80.
4. Oliver RTD, Freedman L, Parkinson C, *et al*. Medical options in the management of stages 1 and 2 (N0–N3 M0) testicular germ cell tumours. *Urol Clin North Am* 1987; **14**, 721–8.
5. Horwich A, Norman A, Fisher C, *et al*. Primary chemotherapy for stage II non-seminomatous germ cell tumours of the testis. *J Urol* 1994; **151**, 72–8.
6. Logothetis CJ, Swanson DA, Dexeus F. Primary chemotherapy for clinical stage II non-seminomatous germ cell tumours of the testis: a follow-up of 50 patients. *J Clin Oncol* 1987; **5**, 906–11.
7. Read G, Stenning SP, Cullen MH, *et al*. MRC prospective study of surveillance for stage I testicular teratoma. *Clin Oncol* 1992; **10**, 1762–8.
8. Oliver RTD. A comparison of the biology and prognosis of seminoma and non-seminoma. In: A Horwich, ed, *Testicular Cancer – Investigation and Management*. London: Chapman & Hall Medical, 1991; 51–67.
9. Oliver RTD, Edmonds P, Ong JYH, *et al*. Pilot studies of 2 & 1 course carboplatin as adjuvant for stage I seminoma: should it be tested in a randomised trial against radiotherapy? *Int J Radiat Oncol Biol Phys* 1994; **29**, 3–8.
10. Oliver RTD, Love S, Ong J. Alternatives to radiotherapy in management of seminoma. *Br J Urol* 1990; **65**, 61–7.
11. Oliver RTD, Leahy M, Ong J. Should germ cell tumours of the testis be graded? *Eur J Cancer* 1995 (in press).
12. Skakkbaek NE. Possible carcinoma-in-situ of the testis. *Lancet* 1972; **ii**, 516–17.
13. Giwercman A, von der Maase H, Skakkebaek NE. Epidemiological and clinical aspects of carcinoma in situ of the testis. *Eur Urol* 1993; **23**, 104–14.
14. Chevassu M. Tumeurs du testicule. These de Paris No 193. *G Steinheil* 1906.
15. Grigor KM, Skakkebaek NE. Pathogenesis and cell biology of germ cell neoplasia: general discussion. *Eur Urol* 1993; **23**, 46–53.
16. Pugh RCB. Testicular tumours. In: RCB Pugh, ed, *Pathology of the Testis*. Oxford: Blackwell Scientific, 1976; 139–59.
17. Mostofi FK, Sobin LH. Histological typing of testis tumours. International histological classification of tumours. No 16. Geneva: World Health Organization, 1991.
18. Oliver RTD. Grading germ cell tumours as a means to resolve the last twenty years. Transatlantic conflict over testis tumour classification. In: WG Jones, ed, *Germ Cell Tumours III*. Oxford: Pergamon, 1993; 163–4.
19. Azzopardi JG, Mostofi FK, Theiss EA. Lesions of testes observed in certain patients with widespread choriocarcinoma and related tumours. The significance and genesis of hematoxylin-staining bodies in the human testis. *Am J Pathol* 1961; **38**, 207–25.
20. Higby DJ, Wallace HJ, Albert DJ, *et al*. Diaminodichloroplatinum: a phase I study showing responses in testicular and other tumors. *Cancer* 1974; **33**, 1219–55.
21. Mackenzie AR. Chemotherapy of metastatic testis cancer — results in 154 patients. *Cancer* 1966; **19**, 1369–76.

22. Samuels ML, Lanzotti VJ, Holoye PY. Combination chemotherapy in germinal cell tumors. *Cancer Treat Rev* 1976; **3**, 185–204.
23. Schmoll HJ. Biology and treatment of testicular cancer. In: Amgen/Hoffman–La Roche consultant series: *The Role of Haematological Growth Factors*. Cheshire: Gardiner/Caldwell Communications Ltd, 1994; 5–66.
24. Einhorn LH, Donohue JP. Cis-diaminodichloroplatinum, vinblastine, and bleomycin combination chemotherapy in disseminated testicular cancer. *Ann Intern Med* 1977; **87**, 293.
25. Williams SD, Birch R, Einhorn LH, *et al.* Treatment of disseminated germ-cell tumours with cisplatin, bleomycin, and either vinblastine or etoposide. *N Engl J Med* 1987; **316**, 1435–40.
26. Peckham MJ, Horwich A, Blackmore C. Etoposide and cisplatin with or without bleomycin as first line chemotherapy in patients with small volume metastases of testicular nonseminoma. *Cancer Treat Rep* 1985; **69**, 483–8.
27. Loehrer PJ, Einhorn LH, Williams SD. VP-16 plus ifosfamide plus cisplatin as salvage therapy in refractory germ cell cancer. *J Clin Oncol* 1986; **4**, 528–36.
28. Loehrer PJ, Einhorn LH, Elson P, *et al.* Phase III study of cisplatin plus etoposide with either bleomycin or ifosfamide in advanced stage germ cell tumors: an intergroup trial. *Proc ASCO* 1993; **12**, 261 (Abstract 831).
29. Newlands ES, Begent RHJ, Rustin GJS, *et al.* Further advances in the management of malignant teratoma of the testis and other sites. *Lancet* 1983; **i**, 948–51.
30. Oliver RTD, Dhaliwal HS, Hope-Stone HF, *et al.* Short course etoposide, bleomycin and cisplatin in the treatment of metastatic germ cell tumours. Appraisal of its potential as adjuvant chemotherapy for stage 1 testis tumours. *Br J Urol* 1988; **61**, 53–8.
31. Wittes RE, Yagoda A, Silvay O. Chemotherapy of germ cell tumors of the testis. 1: induction of remission with vinblastine, actinomycin D and bleomycin. *Cancer* 1976; **37**, 637–45.
32. Vugrin D, Willet F, Whitmore JR, *et al.* Vinblastine, actinomycin D, bleomycin, cyclophosphamide and cisplatinum combination chemotherapy in metastatic testis cancer — a 1 year program. *J Urol* 1982; **128**, 1205–8.
33. Bosl GJ, Gluckman R, Geller NL, *et al.* VAB-6 :an effective chemotherapy regimen for patients with germ cell tumours. *J Clin Oncol* 1986; **4**, 1493–9.
34. Loehrer PJ, Elson P, Johnson DH, *et al.* A randomised trial of cisplatin plus etoposide with or without bleomycin in favorable prognosis disseminated germ cell tumours. *Proc ASCO* 1991; **10**, 169 (Abstract 540).
35. Levi JA, Raghavan D, Harvey V, *et al.* The importance of bleomycin in combination chemotherapy for good prognosis germ cell carcinoma. *J Clin Oncol* 1993; **11**, 1300–5.
36. Bajorin DF, Sarosdy MF, Pfister DG, *et al.* Randomized trial of etoposide and cisplatin versus etoposide and carboplatin in patients with good-risk germ cell tumors: a multi-institutional study. *J Clin Oncol* 1993; **11**, 598–606.
37. Horwich A, Sleijfer D. Carboplatin-based chemotherapy in good prognosis metastatic non-seminoma of the testis (NSGCT): an interim report of an MRC/EORTC randomised trial. *Eur J Cancer, Proc ECCO 7* 1993; **29A**, 1350 (Abstract).
38. Motzer RJ, Cooper K, Geller NL, *et al.* Carboplatin, etoposide and bleomycin for patients with poor-risk germ cell tumours. *Cancer* 1990; **65**, 2465–70.
39. Wilkinson TJ, Colls BM, Schluter PJ. Increased incidence of germ cell testicular cancer in New Zealand Maoris. *Br J Cancer* 1992; **65**, 769–71.
40. Jodrell DI, Egorin MJ, Canetta RM. Relationships between carboplatin exposure and tumour response and toxicity in patients with ovarian cancer. *J Clin Oncol* 1992; **10**, 520–8.
41. Childs WJ, Nicholls EJ, Horwich A. The optimisation of carboplatin dose in

carboplatin, etoposide and bleomycin combination chemotherapy for good prognosis metastatic non-seminomatous germ cell tumours of the testis. *Ann Oncol* 1992; **3**, 291–6.

42. Crawford SM, Newlands ES, Begent RHJ, *et al.* The effect of intensity of administered treatment on the outcome of germ cell tumours treated with POMB/ACE chemotherapy. *Br J Cancer* 1989; **59**, 243–6.
43. Boshoff CH, Rustin G, Begent R, *et al.* Treatment of good risk stage II non-seminomatous testis cancer. *Lancet* 1994; **334**, 1085–6.
44. Birch R, Loehrer P, Williams S. The effect of delay of therapy on response to cisplatin chemotherapy in disseminated germ cell tumours. *Proc ASCO* 1986; **5**, 105 (Abstract).
45. Oliver RTD, Blandy JP, Hendry WF, *et al.* Evaluation of radiotherapy and/or surgicopathological staging after chemotherapy in the management of metastatic germ cell tumours. *Br J Urol* 1984; **55**, 764–8.
46. Merrin C, Beckley S, Takita H. Multimodal treatment of advanced testicular tumour with radical reductive surgery and multisequential chemotherapy with cis platinum, bleomycin, vinblastine, vincristine and actinomycin D. *J Urol* 1978; **120**, 73–4.
47. Wettlaufer JN, Feiner AS, Robinson WA. Vincristine, cisplatin and bleomycin with surgery in the management of advanced metastatic non-seminomatous testis tumours. *Cancer* 1984; **53**, 203–9.
48. Murray N, Coppin C, Swenerton K. Weekly high intensity cisplatin etoposide (HIPE) for far advanced germ cell cancers. *Proc ASCO* 1987; **6**, A394.
49. Lewis CR, Fossa SD, Mead G, *et al.* BOP/VIP — a new platinum-intensive chemotherapy regimen for poor prognosis germ cell tumours. *Ann Oncol* 1991; **2**, 203–11.
50. Horwich A, Brada M, Nicholls J, *et al.* Intensive induction chemotherapy for poor risk non-seminomatous germ cell tumours. *Eur J Cancer Clin Oncol* 1989; **25**, 177–84.
51. Williams SD, Einhorn LH, Greco FA, *et al.* VP-16-213 salvage therapy for refractory germinal neoplasms. *Cancer* 1980; **46**, 2154–8.
52. Oliver R, Edmonds P, Raja M, *et al.* BOP q7 as salvage therapy for germ cell cancer. *Ann Oncol* (submitted).
53. Mendenhall WL, Williams SD, Einhorn LH, *et al.* Disseminated seminoma — re-evaluation of treatment protocols. *J Urol* 1981; **126**, 493–5.
54. Motzer RJ, Bosl GJ, Geller NL. Advanced seminoma: the role of chemotherapy and adjunctive surgery. *Ann Intern Med* 1988; **108**, 513–18.
55. Whitmore WF, Smith WF, Yagoda A. Chemotherapy of seminoma. In: E Grundmann, ed, *Recent Results in Cancer Research*. Berlin: Springer-Verlag, 1977; 244–9.
56. Friedman M. Supervoltage roentgen therapy at Walter Reed General Hospital. *Surg Clin North Am* 1944; **24**, 1424–32.
57. Samuels M, Logothetis C, Trindade A. Sequential weekly pulse-dose cisplatinum for far-advanced seminoma. *Proc ASCO* 1980; **21**, C–415 (Abstract).
58. Logothetis CJ, Samuels ML, Ogden SL. Cyclophosphamide and sequential cisplatin for advanced seminoma: long term follow up of 52 patients. *J Urol* 1987; **138**, 789–94.
59. Oliver RTD. Limitations to the use of surveillance as an option in the management of stage I seminoma. *Int J Androl* 1987; **10**, 263–8.
60. Horwich A, Dearnaley D, A'Hern R, *et al.* The activity of single-agent carboplatin in advanced seminoma. *Eur J Cancer* 1992; **28A**, 1307–10.
61. Schmoll HJ, Harstrick A, Bokemeyer C, *et al.* Single-agent carboplatinum for advanced seminoma — a phase-II study. *Cancer* 1993; **72**, 237–43.
62. Mead GM, Stenning SP, Cullen MH, *et al.* The Second Medical Research Study of prognostic factors in nonseminomatous germ cell tumours. *Clin Oncol*

1992; **10**, 85–94.
63. Boshoff CB, Begent RHJ, Oliver RTD, *et al.* Secondary tumours following etoposide containing therapy for germ cell cancer. *Ann Oncol* 1995; **6**, 35–40.
64. Oliver RTD, Ong JYH, Raja MA, *et al.* Secondary pre-leukaemia and etoposide. *Lancet* 1991; **338**, 1269–70.
65. Hoeltl W, Pont J, Kosak D, *et al.* Treatment decision for stage I seminomatous germ cell tumours based on the risk factor 'vascular invasion'. *Br J Urol* 1992; **69**, 83–7.
66. Bissett D, Kaye SB. Myocardial infarction after chemotherapy for testicular teratoma. *Ann Oncol* 1993; **4**, 432.
67. Hansen SW, Groth S, Dangaard, *et al.* Long terms effects on renal function and blood pressure of treatment with cisplatin, vinblastine and bleomycin in patients with germ cell cancer. *J Clin Oncol* 1988; **6**, 1728–31.
68. Gietema JA, Devries EGE, Sleijfer DT. Increased incidence of cardiovascular risk factors in cured testicular cancer patients. *J Clin Oncol* 1992; **10**, 1652.
69. Raghavan D, Cox K, Childs A, *et al.* Hypercholesterolemia after chemotherapy for testis cancer. *J Clin Oncol* 1992; **10**, 1386–9.
70. Edmonds PM, Ong JHY, Raja M, *et al.* Anglian germ cell cancer group randomised phase 2 study of cisplatin and carboplatin in combination for metastatic teratoma. *Eur J Cancer* 1995 (submitted).
71. van Leeuwen FE, Stiggelbout AM, Dusebout AW. Second cancer risk following testicular cancer: follow-up of 1909 patients. *J Clin Oncol* 1993; **11**, 415–24.
72. Foster RS, Bennett R, Bihrle R, *et al.* A preliminary report: postoperative fertility assessment in nerve-sparing RPLND patients. *Eur Urol* 1993; **23**, 165–8.
73. Fossa SD, Aabyholm T, Vespestad S, *et al.* Semen quality after treatment for testicular cancer. *Eur Urol* 1993; 172–6.
74. Oliver RTD, Hope-Stone HF, Blandy JP. Justification of the use of surveillance in the management of stage 1 germ cell tumours of the testis. *Br J Urol* 1983; **55**, 760–3.
75. Osterlind A, Berthelsen JG, Abildgaard N. Risk of bilateral testicular germ cell cancer in Denmark; 1960–1984. *J Natl Cancer Inst* 1991; **83**, 1391–5.
76. Moynihan CM. Testicular cancer: the psychosocial problems of patients and their relatives. *Cancer Surv* 1987; **6**, 477–510.
77. Freedman LS, Parkinson MC, Jones WG, *et al.* Histopathology in the prediction of relapse of patients with stage 1 testicular teratoma treated by orchidectomy alone. On behalf of MRC Testicular Tumour Subgroup (Urological Working Party). *Lancet* 1987; **ii**, 294–8.
78. Maier JG, Sulak MH, Mettemeyer BT. Seminoma of the testis: analysis of treatment success and failure. *Am J Roentgenol* 1968; **102**, 596–602.
79. Hamilton C, Horwich A, Easton D, *et al.* Radiotherapy for Stage I seminoma testis: results of treatment and complications. *Radiother Oncol* 1986; **6**, 115–20.
80. van Leeuwen FE, Stiggelbout AM, Vandenbeltdusebout AW, *et al.* Second tumors after radiation treatment of testicular germ-cell tumors. *J Clin Oncol* 1993; **11**, 2286–7.
81. Hay JH, Duncan W, Kerr GR. Subsequent malignancies in patients irradiated for testicular tumours. *Br J Radiol* 1984; **57**, 597–602.
82. DeRuysscher D, Waer M, Vandeputte M, *et al.* Changes of lymphocyte subsets after local irradiation for early stage breast cancer and seminoma testis: long term increase of activated (HLA-DR+) T cells and decrease of 'naive' (CD45R) T lymphocytes. *Eur J Cancer* 1992; **28a**, 1729–34.
83. Horwich A, Bell J. Mortality and cancer incidence following radiotherapy for seminoma of the testis. *Radiother Oncol* 1994; **30**, 193–8.
84. Edmonds P, Chakraborti P, Oliver R, *et al.* Risk of a second non testis malignancy following radiotherapy for stage I seminoma. *Eur J Cancer* 1995 (submitted).

85. Fossa S, Horwich A, Stenning S. Optimum field size in the adjuvant treatment of stage 1 seminoma. *UICC XVI International Cancer Congress* 1994; OPGU2-06 (Abstract).

86. Read G, Johnston RJ. Short duration radiotherapy in stage 1 seminoma of the testis: preliminary results. *Clin Oncol* 1993; **5**, 364–6.

87. Gospodarowicz MK. The Princess Margaret Hospital experience of radiotherapy in the management of stage I and II seminoma 1981–1991. In: WG Jones, ed, *Germ Cell Tumours III*, Advances in Bioscience Vol 91. Oxford: Elsevier Science, 1994; 177–85.

88. Duchesne GM, Horwich A, Dearnaley DP. Orchidectomy alone for stage I seminoma of the testis. *Cancer* 1990; **65**, 1115–18.

89. Thomas GM, Sturgeon JF, Alison R. A study of post-orchidectomy surveillance in Stage I testicular seminoma. *J Urol* 1988; **142**, 313.

90. Maase HVD, Specht L, Jacobsen GK. Surveillance following orchidectomy for stage I seminoma of the testis. *Eur J Cancer* 1993; **29**, 1931–4.

91. Highman WJ, Oliver RTD. Diagnosis of metastases from germ cell tumours of the testis by fine needle aspiration biopsy cytology. *J Clin Pathol* 1987; **40**, 1324–33.

92. Oliver RTD. Atrophy, hormones, genes and viruses in aetiological germ cell tumours. *Cancer Surv* 1990; **9**, 263–8.

93. Greist A, Einhorn L, Williams S, *et al.* Pathologic findings at orchidectomy following chemotherapy for disseminated testicular cancer. *J Clin Oncol* 1984; **2**, 1025–7.

94. Chong C, Logothetis CJ, Voneschenbach A, *et al.* Orchidectomy in advanced germ cell cancer following intensive chemotherapy — a comparison of systemic to testicular response. *J Urol* 1986; **136**, 1221–3.

95. Oliver RTD, Ong J, Blandy J, Altman D. Testis conservation studies in germ cell cancer justified by improved primary chemotherapy response and reduced delay 1978–1994. *Lancet* 1995(submitted).

96. Brackenbury ET, Hargreave TB, Howard GCW, *et al.* Seminal fluid analysis and fine-needle aspiration cytology in the diagnosis of carcinoma in situ of the testis. *Eur Urol* 1993; **23**, 123–8.

# 18 Intraoperative radiotherapy — the Kyoto University experience

*Mitsuyuki Abe, Yuta Shibamoto and Yasumasa Nishimura*

## Introduction

Intraoperative radiotherapy (IORT) is a treatment modality in which resectable lesions are removed by surgery and unresectable remnants are sterilized by irradiation during operation. In IORT, normal organs can be shifted from the field, thereby allowing a sterilizing dose to be safely given to surgically exposed tumours or cells which are hard to eliminate by surgical operation alone. In this way the inherent problems of both radiotherapy and surgery can be solved simultaneously by IORT.[1,2]

IORT can be used either as a single treatment or as a boost to external beam radiotherapy (EBRT). The combined treatment of IORT and EBRT is generally used when the primary tumour cannot be removed by surgery or the site to be irradiated cannot be covered sufficiently by a single IORT field.

## Gastric cancer

The rationales of IORT for gastric cancer are:

1. most of the published data concerning the incidence and patterns of failure after initial treatment of gastric cancer suggest that local lymph node metastasis occurred as the only failure site in about 50% of the recurring patients;[3]
2. many patients would therefore benefit from more effective control of local disease by IORT;
3. the survival figure may thereby be improved.

## Techniques

To perform IORT, it is most convenient if all surgical procedures can be performed in a dedicated IORT room or if an operating theatre is situated adjacent to the radiation suite. Otherwise, a patient is transferred from an operating theatre to a radiation unit after the major surgical procedure.

At first, a gastrectomy is performed and as much tumour tissue as possible is extirpated. This is because large tumours require higher radiation doses than smaller ones in order to produce the same degree of regression. The abdomen is then temporarily closed and draped in a sterile fashion. The patient is covered with sterile sheets and transported to the radiation unit under general anaesthesia through non-sterile areas.

In preparing the radiation unit for IORT, no special room sterilization is necessary but two ultraviolet lamps are left turned on during the night. In the radiation unit, the abdomen is reopened and a treatment cone is inserted over the unresectable tumours or sites suspected of containing residual tumour cells before the gastroenterostomy is performed, because, at this stage, the site to be irradiated can be adequately exposed and the organs to be protected pulled aside. The treatment cone and the operation wound are covered by a sterilized sheet. During irradiation, vital signs, including electrocardiogram, pulse, and respiration of the patient are monitored using a television and a multichannel oscilloscope in the control room. After irradiation, the cone is removed from the abdomen and the gastroenterostomy is performed. The abdomen is then closed by standard techniques.

## Selection of electron energy and dose measurement

The energy is selected so that whole lesions are included within the 90% depth dose distribution volume. The dose is measured at the reference depth described in the ICRU (International Commission on Radiation Units) Report 35,[4] that is, at 1.0 cm depth from the tissue surface when the electron energies used are less than 10 MeV, and at 2.0 cm depth when they are between 10 MeV and 20 MeV.

## Radiation field

When IORT is applied to patients after curative surgery, the radiation field is positioned toward the high-risk lymph node groups along the common hepatic, the left gastric, and the splenic arteries, and around the coeliac axis. When the posterior wall of the stomach is grossly adherent to the pancreas, this part is also encompassed by the radiation field.

A pentagonally shaped treatment cone should be used so that it fits the costal arch. It is recommended that a variety of sizes and shapes of the pentagonal treatment cones be prepared so that they adequately fit the costal arch and encompass various situations of the tumour. The field is clearly illuminated by an electric lamp fixed to a telescope attached to the treatment cone. The cone is inserted into the abdomen at an inclination of about 15° so that the coeliac axis is sufficiently covered.

## Radiation dose

A single dose of 28 Gy is optimal for clinically undetectable lesions, and a single dose of 30–35 Gy (increasing with the residual tumour volume) may be potentially curative for patients who have received non-curative surgery because of an incomplete excision of metastatic lesions. IORT is not indicated for patients whose primary tumour was not resectable by gastrectomy. This is because a large primary tumour cannot be eliminated in one exposure within the tolerance limit of the normal structures suppporting or surrounding the tumour.[5] From our clinical experience, the maximum tumour size which can be eliminated by an IORT dose of 35 Gy is approximately 3 cm in diameter.

## Results

Gastric cancer patients treated at the Kyoto University are classified according to the 'General rules for gastric cancer' study in Japan.[6] The rules concerning serosal invasion and lymph node metastasis are briefly summarized below. Capital letters are used to describe gross findings and small letters are used to describe histological findings. Therefore, 'Stage' is used when the stage is classified according to the gross findings and 'stage' is used when it is classified according to the histological findings.

1. Histological classification of serosal invasion: s(–) = negative serosal invasion; s(+) = positive serosal invasion.
2. Histological classification of lymph node metastasis: n0 = no lymph node metastasis; n1 = metastasis to lymph nodes of group 1; n2 = metastasis to lymph nodes of group 2; n3 = metastasis to lymph nodes of group 3; n4 = metastasis to lymph nodes located beyond group 3. Groups 1–3 indicate the anatomical positions of the lymph nodes which are defined by the general rules.[6]

Table 18.1 demonstrates the survival rates of patients treated by operation alone and those treated by IORT at the Kyoto University Hospital from 1974 to 1984. Patients were treated by operation alone or IORT, depending on the day they were admitted to the hospital. Thus, patients who were admitted on Tuesday received an operation alone and those who were

**Table 18.1**  Five-year survival rates of patients with gastric cancer treated by operation alone or IORT according to the stages classified by the gross findings

| Tumour Stage (based on gross findings) | Operation alone | | IORT | |
|---|---|---|---|---|
| | No. of patients | 5-year survival rate (%) | No. of patients | 5-year survival rate (%) |
| I | 43 | 93 | 24 | 87 |
| II | 11 | 62 | 20 | 84 |
| III | 38 | 37 | 30 | 62 |
| IV | 18 | 0 | 27 | 15 |

admitted on Friday received IORT. Except for a few cases, chemotherapy was not used in either group of patients. Staging for the patients was performed according to the gross findings (Table 18.1).

As indicated in the table, IORT does not improve the prognosis in patients with Stage 1 disease. However, it was demonstrated that the IORT procedure improved survivals of patients with Stages II, III and IV disease. In those with Stage IV, IORT was selectively applied to patients who had direct invasion of the pancreas but had no evidence of distant metastasis, and in whom the primary tumour was removed by gastrectomy. These criteria of patient selection were also applied to patients who underwent operation alone. No patients with Stage IV who received operation alone survived for more than 2 years while those who received IORT showed a 15% 5-year survival rate.

Stage grouping based upon the histological findings were then performed in both groups and the survival rates were analysed. Histological staging was performed for ninety-four IORT patients and for 127 operation-alone patients.

Table 18.2 shows the survival rates of the operation alone and IORT groups according to the stages which were classified histologically. The IORT procedure improved survivals of patients with stages II, III and IV disease by nearly 10–20%, though this difference was not statistically significant.

**Table 18.2**   Five-year survival rates of gastric cancer patients treated by operation alone or IORT according to the stages classified by the histological findings

| Tumour stage (based on histological findings) | Operation alone | | IORT | |
|---|---|---|---|---|
| | No. of patients | 5-year survival rate (%) | No. of patients | 5-year survival rate (%) |
| I | 48 | 100 | 27 | 96 |
| II | 21 | 66 | 18 | 78 |
| III | 44 | 51 | 33 | 60 |
| IV | 14 | 14 | 16 | 33 |

The discrepancy of the survival rates analysed according to the gross and histological findings in the IORT and the operation-alone groups is caused by the fact that:

1. the number of patients enrolled in the two studies was different; and
2. the stages of some patients previously classified by the gross findings were subjected to change as a result of the classification based upon the histological findings.

Table 18.3 shows the 5-year survival rates of patients treated by operation alone or IORT according to the presence or absence of serosal invasion and the grade of the lymph node metastasis, which were examined histologically. In patients with no serosal invasion (s(−)), no differences in the

**Table 18.3** Five-year survival rates of patients with gastric cancer treated by operation alone or IORT according to the presence or absence of serosal invasion and the grade of the lymph node metastasis

| Serosal invasion (s)/ lymph node metastasis (n) | Operation alone | | IORT | |
|---|---|---|---|---|
| | No. of patients | 5-year survival rate (%) | No. of patients | 5-year survival rate (%) |
| s(−) | 109 | 87 | 32 | 94 |
| s(+) | 62 | 51 | 25 | 60 |
| n0 | 83 | 97 | 29 | 100 |
| n1(+) | 47 | 67 | 14 | 64 |
| n2(+) + n3(+) | 41 | 32 | 14 | 51 |

survival rates were observed between the operation alone and the IORT groups. However, in patients with serosal invasion (s(+)), the survival rate of the IORT group is about 10% better than the operation-alone group. With regard to lymph node metastasis, the IORT procedure did not afford any benefit if lymph node metastasis was limited within n1 groups, but was able to improve the survival of patients with n2 and n3 lymph node metastasis by nearly 19%.

## Complications

In IORT for gastric cancer, the critical organ to which exposure cannot be avoided is the pancreas. In general, a temporary increase in serum amylase and blood sugar occurs after IORT, but these return to preirradiation levels within a week.[7] Neither significant late complications nor deviation from the usual postoperative course is observed. There have been no instances of delayed wound healing.

Special attention should be paid in order to avoid including the small intestine within the radiation field during IORT.

## Indications

The indications for IORT in gastric cancer are summarized as follows:

1. there must be no metastasis to the peritoneum or the liver;
2. the primary tumour must be surgically removed;
3. all unresectable tumours must be encompassed by a single radiation field with an adequate margin;
4. IORT affords no benefit if the lymph node metastases are limited within the n1 group or serosal invasion is not found, but has potential to improve the survival of patients with serosal invasion, n2(+) or n3(+), or Stages II–IV; and
5. IORT is not indicated if the tumour size exceeds 3 cm in diameter, because the tumour can barely be eliminated by an IORT dose of 35 Gy, which is presumably the maximum safe level of radiation dose in gastric cancer treatment.

The IORT schema for gastric cancer, and the IORT field, are shown in Fig. 18.1.

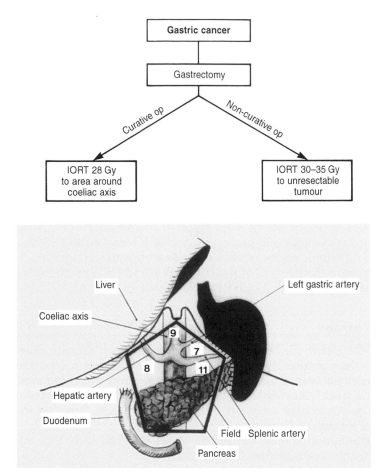

**Fig. 18.1**   IORT schema for gastric cancer and field gastric cancer with invasion of the pancreas. The field covers lymph node groups which most frequently contain metastasis and are hard to eliminate by surgery. ⑦, Lymph nodes along the left gastric artery; ⑧, lymph nodes along the common hepatic artery; ⑨, lymph nodes around the coeliac axis; and ⑪, lymph nodes along the splenic artery.

# Pancreatic cancer

In pancreatic cancer, more than 80% of patients have advanced, surgically incurable disease at the time of diagnosis. Since the tumour typically invades the surrounding soft tissues and adjacent blood vessels in most cases, surgical resection cannot prevent the possibility of local recurrence. Permanent control of this disease has only rarely been achieved with either external beam radiotherapy (EBRT) or with surgical operation as a single-treatment modality. It is therefore apparent that other treatment approaches should be considered to overcome the limitation of conventional treatments.

## Techniques

In the treatment of pancreatic cancer, IORT plus EBRT is better than IORT alone, especially when a curative operation cannot be performed. The reasons are as follows: first, a bulky tumour cannot be eliminated by a single IORT dose unless unsafe levels of radiation are delivered; second, a higher dose of radiation can be given to these tumours by EBRT plus IORT with less damage to the surrounding normal structures; and third, the risk of marginal recurrence may be decreased by using EBRT.

In all patients it is recommended that a routine gastroenterostomy and/or choledochoenterostomy or cholecystoenterostomy by-pass procedure be performed, if feasible, in order to avoid prepyloric or duodenal ulcers, obstruction, or jaundice, secondary to irradiation.

## Radiation field and dose

In the case of cancer of the head of the pancreas, great care must be taken to ensure that the duodenum is not exposed to intraoperative irradiation, but that the EBRT field covers the entire duodenal loop. This is done because cancer of the pancreatic head can invade the medial wall of the duodenum, and its entire circumference is thus at risk. Even if the small intestine is invaded by the tumour, this part should not be included in an IORT field but covered by EBRT fields in order to avoid duodenal ulcers.

External beam irradiation is given using three portals from the anterior, left and right directions. The CT simulator which we have developed is especially useful for precise definition of the radiation field for EBRT.[8,9]

When a patient has been diagnosed as inoperable, an IORT dose of 25–30 Gy is given to the tumour, followed by EBRT with 45–55 Gy over 5–7 weeks, through three portals which are positioned so that the invaded and high-risk areas around the tumour are sufficiently covered.

An IORT dose of 20–25 Gy is given to the residual tumour site if the resection was non-curative, with 15–20 Gy given to the tumour bed if the resection was curative. In both situations, this is followed by EBRT with 45–55 Gy, given in the same fashion as in an inoperable case.

## Results

Table 18.4 shows the clinical results of a non-randomized multi-institutional study which was performed in Japan between 1980 and 1985. The IORT dose ranged from 25 to 40 Gy, according to the tumour size, when it was given as a single modality. In combined therapy of EBRT and IORT, the IORT dose was 10–25 Gy, whereas the EBRT dose was 35–50 Gy, given in 1.6–1.8 Gy fractions. EBRT was given through three portals from the anterior, left and right directions. For patients treated by operation alone, the operation consisted of a by-pass procedure or various modes of tumour

**Table 18.4**  Median survival times of patients with locally advanced pancreatic cancer treated by operation, IORT, operation + EBRT, or IORT + EBRT (non-randomized, multi-institutional study)

| Treatment modality | Dose | No. of patients | Median survival time (months) |
|---|---|---|---|
| Operation | | 41 | 5.5 |
| IORT | 25–40 Gy | 49 | 5.5 |
| Op + EBRT | 40–60 Gy/6–8 weeks | 34 | 9.0 |
| IORT + EBRT | (10–25 Gy) + (35–50 Gy/5–7 weeks) | 20 | 12.0 |

resection, including pancreaticoduodenectomy, distal pancreatectomy, or partial resection of the tumour.

The median survival times for patients treated by operation + EBRT and IORT + EBRT were 9 and 12 months, respectively, while the median survival of patients treated by IORT without EBRT, or operation alone, was 5.5 months. Pain relief was obtained in about 80% of patients. About 10% of patients with cancers of the pancreatic head who received an IORT dose of more than 25 Gy developed a duodenal ulcer.

Table 18.5 shows the clinical results of patients with locally advanced pancreatic cancer treated by various treatment modalities at Kyoto University between March 1983 and December 1992. This was not a randomized clinical trial but patients' characteristics were balanced among the different treatment modalities.

IORT without EBRT was employed during the early period of our IORT study but thereafter the combination of IORT and EBRT was offered, in

**Table 18.5**  Median survival times of patients with locally advanced pancreatic cancer treated by operation, IORT, operation + EBRT, or IORT + EBRT (non-randomized, Kyoto University study)

| Operation mode | Additional treatment modality | No. of patients | Median survival time (months) |
|---|---|---|---|
| Curative resection | None | 43 | 10.5 |
| | IORT | 3 | 8.5 |
| | EBRT | 18 | 14.0 |
| | IORT + EBRT | 21 | 10.0 |
| Non-curative resection | None | 25 | 7.0 |
| | IORT | 2 | Unevaluable because too few patients |
| | EBRT | 11 | 12 |
| | IORT + EBRT | 6 | 15.5 |
| Non-resection | None | 39 | 3 |
| | IORT | 3 | 5 |
| | EBRT | 15 | 7.5 |
| | IORT + EBRT | 14 | 9 |

an attempt to give a higher radiation dose to the tumour with less damage to the surrounding normal structures, and to decrease the risk of marginal recurrence by using EBRT.

As IORT can be performed only once a week at Kyoto University Hospital, IORT with or without EBRT was used only for patients who were eventually admitted to the hospital on a Friday. Therefore, the bias of patient selection can be minimized and the number of patients treated by IORT is considerably less than that of patients treated by operation alone.

No prolongation in the median survival time due to IORT or IORT + EBRT was found in patients who received curative resection. However, in patients who underwent non-curative resection or did not have a surgical resection at all, the longest median survival time was obtained when the patients were treated by IORT combined with EBRT.

## Indications

In the treatment of pancreatic cancer, IORT combined with EBRT seems to be the most promising treatment modality, not only for patients with unresectable tumours but also for patients who have undergone tumour resection, because complete control of the tumour can only rarely be achieved, even after what is believed to be a curative operation.

The IORT schema for locally advanced pancreatic cancer is shown in Fig. 18.2.

# Brain tumours

The treatment of recurrent malignant brain tumours presents many difficulties, especially when they have recurred after a full course of EBRT. Surgical debulking is the primary treatment modality, if indicated, but is rarely curative. A second course of EBRT is often hazardous since little recovery of previous irradiation damage can be expected in normal brain tissue. In these cases, IORT may be considered to be the treatment of choice.

## Techniques and radiation dose

IORT should be given after removal of as much tumour tissue as possible. The treatment cone is placed directly onto the residual tumour or tumour bed. When IORT is applied to patients with brain tumours which have recurred after a full course of EBRT, an IORT dose of 20–30 Gy is given to the residual tumour or tumour bed after gross resection of the tumour, depending upon the histology and the tumour size. In the case of previously untreated brain tumours, it is recommended that IORT be used in combination with EBRT, especially in the case of infiltrative tumours such as glioblastoma or anaplastic astrocytoma. In these cases, an IORT dose of 15–25 Gy is given to the tumour area, in combination with EBRT to a dose of 50–65 Gy over 5–7 weeks through an extended field.

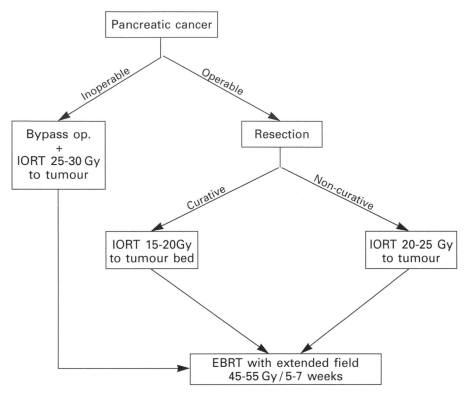

**Fig. 18.2**    IORT schema for pancreatic cancer.

## Results

Figure 18.3 shows the survival curves of patients with recurrent brain tumours treated by IORT with 25–30 Gy at Kyoto University. The histological diagnosis was glioblastoma in five patients, anaplastic oligodendroglioma in five, anaplastic astrocytoma in four, anaplastic ependymoma in two, and ependymoma in one. The seventeen patients had received EBRT (17–65 Gy; mean 53 Gy) at 4–112 months (median 39 months) before IORT. They were divided into two groups; that is, nine patients with infiltrative tumours (glioblastoma and anaplastic astrocytoma) and eight patients with less infiltrative tumours (ependymoma, anaplastic ependymoma, and anaplastic oligodendroglioma). The median survival time was 51 months for patients with less infiltrative tumours and 12 months for those with infiltrative tumours.

In order to evaluate the effectiveness of IORT, the survival time after IORT was compared with the interval from the previous operation to time of retreatment by IORT. The median interval between the previous operation and IORT was 39 months for patients with less infiltrative tumours and 15 months for those with infiltrative tumours. The post-IORT survival time was longer than the interval between the previous operation and IORT in six of the eight patients with less infiltrative tumours, but this was so in

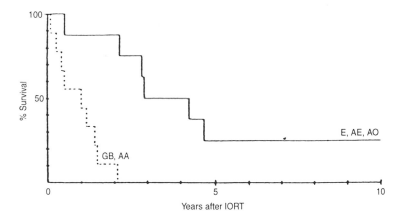

**Fig.18.3** Survival curves after IORT for recurrent brain tumours. _____, Ependymoma (E), anaplastic ependymoma (AE), and anaplastic oligoden-droglioma (AO) (*N* = 8); ...., glioblastoma (GB), and anaplastic astrocytoma

only two of the nine patients with infiltrative tumours. One patient with anaplastic ependymoma which recurred after EBRT with 50 Gy, and another with ependymoma which recurred after EBRT with 49 Gy, are currently alive with no evidence of disease at 134 and 88 months after gross resection followed by IORT, respectively.

In twelve cases, the cause of death was local tumour progression. Two patients died of spinal dissemination although local control was achieved, and one died of brain necrosis.

## Complications

Histologically proven brain necrosis occurred in the tissue volume treated by IORT in three patients, and was fatal in one of them. In eleven other patients who survived for 1 year or longer, brain necrosis did not develop. Transient postoperative meningitis occurred in three patients and this may have been related to an IORT procedure.

## Indications for treatment

IORT appears to be an effective treatment modality in selected patients, with brain tumours which have recurred after EBRT, especially in malignant but less extensive tumours which are located in peripheral (accessible) sites, preferably in the non-dominant area of the brain.

Glioblastoma is highly radioresistant and remains a very difficult tumour to treat. For selected patients with this disease, IORT plus EBRT seems to be the treatment of choice because higher radiation doses can be given by combining IORT with EBRT than by using EBRT alone. Matsutani[10] used a combination of EBRT, extensive tumour removal and IORT for primary glioblastoma which was located in relatively superficial sites of the brain, and reported a 2-year survival rate of 60%. This result seems to be encouraging.

# Osteosarcoma of the limb

Radiosensitivity of the large majority of primary bone tumours (apart from Ewing's) is very low; therefore, radiotherapy has not traditionally played an important role in treatment of these cancers. However, in IORT, a large dose can be given directly to the tumour, thereby offering the potential for long-term survival without amputation of the affected limb.

## Techniques

At first, the overlying skin is widely opened and the tumour site exposed sufficiently. Major blood vessels and nerves are detached from the bone and muscles to exclude them from the IORT field. If the major peripheral nerves are irradiated with a single dose of 25 Gy or more, severe neuralgia and/or paralysis can occur 6–24 months later.

## Radiation field and dose

With the aid of bone scintigraphy and computed tomography, potential areas of microscopic involvement are included in the treatment field with a safety margin of 5 cm from the affected bone marrow.

A single dose of 50–60 Gy is given to the exposed target area by parallel opposing portals. It is important to give systemic chemotherapy including doxorubicin and cisplatin, both before and after IORT, in order to avoid distant metastases. When a patient has developed a bone fracture, an internal prosthesis is inserted so that the affected limb is preserved.

## Results

Figure 18.4 shows the survival figures of thirty-two patients with osteosarcoma of the limb treated by IORT at Kyoto University. The patients received an IORT dose of 50 Gy or 60 Gy and systemic chemotherapy in combination with IORT. The 10-year survival rate was 46% for all patients but it has been improved to 60% for twenty-two patients treated after 1982 who received intensive chemotherapy including doxorubicin and cisplatin, before and after IORT. IORT has not yielded better survival than amputation but has improved the quality of life of these patients by contributing to the likelihood of successful preservation of the affected limb.

## Complications

The major problem of this method is fracture of the irradiated bone, which occurred in about 50% of the patients. The fracture is treated with a prothesis or by intramedullary nailing. The IORT schema for osteosarcoma is illustrated in Fig. 18.5.

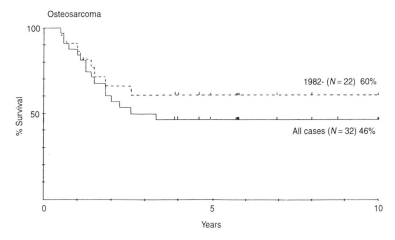

**Fig. 18.4**   Survival figures of patients with osteosarcoma treated by IORT.

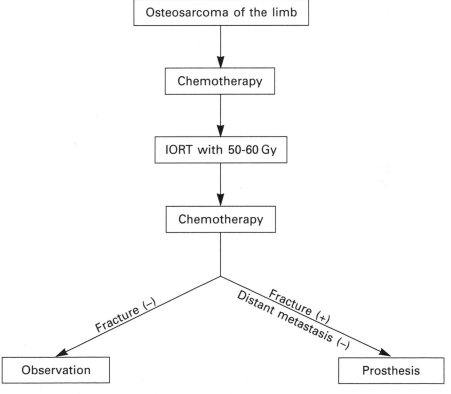

**Fig. 18.5**   IORT schema for osteosarcoma.

# Prostatic cancer

Prostatectomy has been reserved for a minority of patients, because most patients have inoperable disease at the time of diagnosis. For this group EBRT has played a major role.[11] It has been demonstrated, however, that prostatic irradiation of 65–72 Gy, with or without pelvic irradiation of 45–50 Gy, produces an overall complication rate of 24%,[12] with an approximately 10% incidence of rectovesical injuries[13] — the most common problem with EBRT. IORT using electron beams with a sharp and rapid fall-off in depth dose offers a particular advantage in the treatment of localized prostatic cancer because exposure to the bladder and the rectum can thereby be minimized.

## Techniques

The patient is placed in the exaggerated lithotomy position and an inverted U-shaped incision is made in the perineum. Dissection is continued upwards to achieve direct exposure of the prostatic tumour and separate the posterior surface of the tumour from the rectum. A Young's retractor is then passed via the urethra into the bladder. By pulling the handle of the retractor strongly towards the patient's head, the prostatic tumour can be pushed towards the perineum because the pubis acts as a fulcrum. The tumour is then positioned within a sterile treatment cone which is inserted through the perineal incision (Fig. 18.6).

## Radiation field and dose

If the tumour is larger than 4 cm in diameter, it cannot easily be covered, with a safety margin, by using a treatment cone. In such cases, EBRT should be given before IORT in an attempt to reduce the tumour size so that an IORT field can cover the tumour sufficiently. IORT is given through a perineal incision without tumour resection, using electron energies of 10–14 MeV and treatment cones of 4–5 cm in diameter.

When IORT is used for patients without pelvic lymph node metastases, a single dose of 33–35 Gy (depending upon the tumour volume) appears to be a cancericidal dose. However, for patients with suspected pelvic lymph node metastases, it is recommended that an IORT dose of 25 Gy be given in combination with an EBRT dose of 50 Gy to the whole pelvis, including the prostatic tumour.

## Results

Figure 18.7 shows the overall survival in twenty-three patients with prostatic cancer treated by IORT, with or without EBRT. Twenty-two patients had adenocarcinoma and one had transitional cell carcinoma. Twelve patients had Stage C disease, four had Stage B2, three had Stage D1, two had Stage B1 and one each had Stages A2 and D2.

In eight patients, a single IORT dose of 28–35 Gy was given, while the remaining fifteen patients received an IORT dose of 20 Gy or 25 Gy in

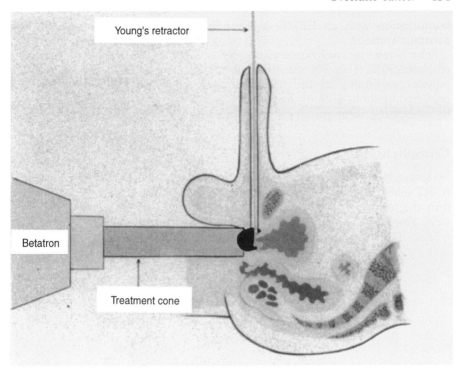

**Fig. 18.6** IORT for prostatic cancer. The tumour is pushed towards the perineum by a Young's retractor and a treatment cone inserted directly upon the tumour through the perineal incision.

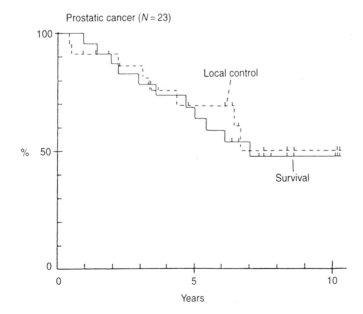

**Fig. 18.7** Survival figures of prostatic cancer patients treated by IORT.

combination with an EBRT dose of 50 Gy to the pelvis, including the prostatic tumour.

The 5-year survival rate was nearly 70% but by 10 years had decreased to about 50%. This was mainly attributed to an insufficient dose and inadequate positioning of the treatment cone, because marginal recurrence occurred in about 40% of the patients. A better prognosis might be expected by addressing these problems more effectively.

## Complications

Haematuria was observed in most patients after IORT, due not only to the IORT itself, but also to the manipulation of the Young's retractor inserted into the urethra. All patients recovered and no rectovesical complications were observed.

The IORT schema for prostatic cancer is shown in Fig. 18.8.

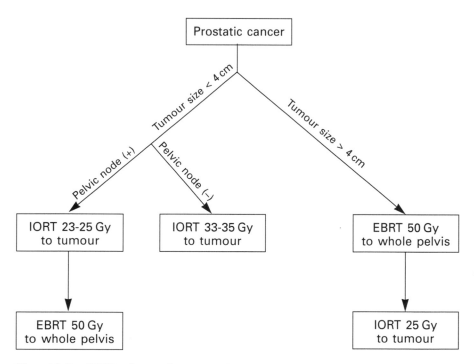

**Fig. 18.8**  IORT schema for prostatic cancer.

# Conclusions

In cancer treatment, radiotherapy has not previously played a major role in the management of tumours which are radioresistant or located near critically radiosensitive structures. On the other hand, complete elimination is difficult to attain with a surgical procedure if the tumour invades the major blood vessels. In addition, the possibility always exists that microscopic lesions remain in the tumour bed, even after what is believed to be a curative operation. We have developed intraoperative radiotherapy to overcome these limitations of radiotherapy and surgery.

Recently, great interest has been paid to the use of protons, heavy ions or pions in radiotherapy, mainly because of their excellent dose localization. However, the complexity and cost of the necessary equipment seriously limits their widespread use. Intraoperative radiotherapy will therefore continue to play an important role in the treatment of locally advanced radioresistant cancer, in which a benefit in terms of local control can translate into improvement in long-term survival.

# References

1. Abe M, Takahashi M, Yabumoto E, *et al.* Techniques, indications and results of intraoperative radiotherapy of advanced cancers. *Radiology* 1975; **116**, 693–702.
2. Abe M, Takahashi M. Intraoperative radiotherapy; the Japanese experience. *Int J Radiat Oncol Biol Phys* 1981; 7, 863–8.
3. Gunderson LL, Sosin H. Adenocarcinoma of the stomach — areas of failure in a reoperation series (second or symptomatic looks). Clinicopathologic correlation and implications for adjuvant therapy. *Int J Radiat Oncol Biol Phys* 1982; **8**, 1–11.
4. Radiation dosimetry: electrons with initial energies between 1 and 50 MeV. In: ICRU Report No. 35. Washington, DC: International Commission on Radiation Units and Measurements, 1984.
5. Abe M, Yabumoto E, Takahashi M, *et al.* Intraoperative radiotherapy of gastric cancer. *Cancer* 1974; **34**, 2034–41.
6. Japanese Research Society for Gastric Cancer. The general rules for gastric cancer in surgery and pathology. *Jap J Surg* 1981; **11**, 127–39.
7. Abe M. Intraoperative radiation therapy for gastric cancer. In: RR Dobelbower Jr, M Abe, eds, *Intraoperative Radiation Therapy*. Boca Raton, FL: CRC Press, 1989; 165–79.
8. Nishidai T, Nagata Y, Takahashi M, *et al.* CT simulator: a new 3-D planning and simulating system for radiotherapy: Part 1. Description of system. *Int J Radiat Oncol Biol Phys* 1990; **18**, 499–504.
9. Nagata Y, Nishidai T, Abe M, *et al.* CT simulator: a new 3-D planning and simulating system for radiotherapy: Part 2. Clinical application. *Int J Radiat Oncol Biol Phys* 1990; **18**, 505–13.
10. Matsutani M. Intraoperative radiation therapy for malignant brain tumors. In: RR Dobelbower Jr, M Abe, eds, *Intraoperative Radiation Therapy*. Boca Raton, FL: CRC Press, 1989; 137–58.
11. Bagshaw MA, Kaplan HS, Sagerman RH. Linear accelerator supervoltage radiotherapy. VII. Carcinoma of the prostate. *Radiology* 1965; **85**, 121–9.
12. Kurup P, Kramer TS, Lee MS, *et al.* External beam irradiation of prostatic cancer. *Cancer* 1984; **53**, 37–43.
13. Pilepich MV, Krall J, George FW, *et al.* Treatment-related morbidity in phase III RTOG studies of extended field irradiation for carcinoma of the prostate. *Int J Radiat Oncol Biol Phys* 1984; **10**, 1861–7.

# 19 Hyperthermia in the treatment of cancer: current techniques and future prospects

*Clare C Vernon*

## Introduction

All cancer treatments aim to exploit the differences between normal and malignant cells and hyperthermia is no exception. The first use of heat in cancer therapy dates back to around 3000 BC when the Edwin Smith papyrus describes the use of a 'fire drill' in a patient with breast cancer. A more validated account of tumour regression following whole body hyperthermia can be seen in W Busch's report of a sarcoma of the neck which regressed after an erysipelas-induced fever in 1866.[1] However, it was not until the 1960s that a systematic investigation of the anticancer effects of hyperthermia began, both by a variety of experimental and clinical studies and also the analysis of a vast literature of anecdotal reports. This confirmed that hyperthermia did have an antitumour effect. Techniques for heating tumours and raising temperature *in situ* were improved and the overall interest and effort in this field increased dramatically — with the result that the last few years have seen great advances.

Thermal therapy has been used in the past as cautery for superficial tumours and more recently as laser therapy, but neither of these methods delivers controllable heat. Hyperthermia as used today in the clinical setting refers to the heating of localized tumours to a temperature of 42–45°C, or whole body heating to 40–42°C. There is now a firm biological rationale for using heat in this range of temperatures, seeking to exploit weaknesses of the tumour compared with the normal tissues, and attempting to combine heat with irradiation or chemotherapy in such a way that these modalities become more cytotoxic than they would be alone.

# Rationale for the clinical use of heat

## Response of cells and tissues to hyperthermia

Temperatures of around 41°C or greater can be lethal to mammalian cells. Many tissues, especially those that are slowly dividing (or even postmitotic), respond to hyperthermia far more quickly than to ionizing radiation.[2]

### Molecular damage

With ionizing radiation the principal target is the DNA, causing cells to die when they attempt to divide. Despite the publication of numerous observations of heat-induced alterations,[3] no consensus concerning the molecular mechanisms of cell kill has emerged. Most commonly postulated mechanisms involve damage to three major cellular structures:

1. *Plasma membrane* — including receptor and transport proteins. Evidence for this is supported by the observation that membrane-active agents, e.g. local anaesthetics and aliphatic alcohols, act synergistically with heat, and cell kill by these agents alone is strikingly similar to the action of heat itself. Membrane injury causes cells to die and lyse rapidly, i.e. sooner than after equally lethal doses of ionizing radiation.
2. *Cytoskeleton* — stress fibres and spindle microtubules are rapidly disorganized, and the structure and function of mitochondria, lysosomes and protein synthesis apparatus are altered by the application of heat.
3. *Nucleus* — the nucleolus is particularly heat sensitive with the production of heat-induced specific proteins (heat-shock proteins). These are not specific to hyperthermia and can occur in a variety of stressful situations, and indeed are better named as shock proteins, rather than heat-shock proteins.

Thus, a model for heat-induced cell kill has been suggested with the disruption of critical plasma membrane structures, collapse of the cytoskeleton, absorption of protein, disruption of nuclear function and damage to critical nuclear structures. The resulting cell survival curves can be analysed by either the target-theory equation or the linear-quadratic equation, and the former is the basis for the current concept of thermal dose (to be discussed later).

### Physiology

The biological rationale[4] for combining hyperthermia and irradiation in the treatment of cancer rests in two biological mechanisms: radiosensitization and direct hyperthermic cytotoxicity. It can be hypothesized that hypoxic cells in the centre of a tumour are relatively radioresistant, but thermosensitive, whereas well-vascularized peripheral portions of the tumour are more sensitive to irradiation.

The vasculature and blood supply in tumours are generally different and inferior to that of normal tissues[5] which leads to areas of abnormal perfusion within the tumour and vascular (capillary) occlusion. This has a number of consequences and will be important for a variety of anticancer techniques.[6]

1. Some tumours, or regions within tumours, will have poorer dissipation of heat than normal tissues, and may thus become hotter than normal tissues in a localized treatment field.
2. Deficiencies in tumour vasculature result in the development of cells which are:
   (a) hypoxic — reduced $Po_2$ will not affect hyperthermia, but will reduce the effectiveness of radiotherapy and can increase the sensitivity to certain drugs (bioreductive compounds);
   (b) at low pH and/or nutrient-deficient — reduced rate of removal of waste products, in particular lactate, will lead to reduced pH which will alter the effectiveness of certain drugs, increase tissue sensitivity to hyperthermia and decrease the development of thermotolerance.
3. Cells in the DNA synthetic phase of the cell cycle are particularly sensitive to heat but relatively resistant to X-rays, so that a combined treatment with hyperthermia and radiotherapy might be advantageous in some circumstances.
4. Combining heat with chemotherapeutic drugs may enhance the therapeutic effect either by increasing drug uptake or by enhancing sensitivity to the drugs.
5. It has been suggested that neoplastic cells may be intrinsically more heat sensitive than the normal cells at risk.

There is, therefore, considerable therapeutic potential for manipulation of blood flow. Vasoactive agents can potentially be used in hyperthermal treatments, and of particular importance to hyperthermia are compounds which selectively reduce flow in tumours, e.g. hydralazine which acts on smooth muscle, thereby increasing flow to normal tissues and 'stealing' blood from the tumour. Administration of hydralazine has been shown to decrease blood flow and increase sensitivity to hyperthermia in transplanted tumours.[7]

Clearly, a greater knowledge of the effects of modifiers of blood flow could result in the design of treatment methods which take advantage of differences in the vasculature between tumours and normal tissues.[8] Several of the tools necessary for human studies of tumour blood flow and metabolism, i.e. positron emission tomography (PET) or magnetic resonance spectroscopy (MRS), are now becoming available.[9]

## Pathology

Superficially there may be acute oedema, focal haemorrhage, cellular infiltration and even necrosis, and this may be compared to a thermal burn produced by any other means. If there is no necrosis at the acute stage, then long-term effects are unlikely, and satisfactory healing will occur. However, if damage has been acutely severe, late-stage necrosis and fibrosis may occur. Clinically, hyperthermia is usually combined with radiation, which also produces similar effects, so it is difficult to separate the two components. When used correctly with radiation, hyperthermia should not increase normal skin or deep tissue reaction, in either the short or the long term.

# Thermotolerance

Survival curves after heat treatment are similar in shape to those following irradiation, the curves becoming less steep with decreasing temperatures.[10] Like conventional radiation therapy, clinical hyperthermia is usually given as several fractions. Knowledge of the biological response to fractionated hyperthermia is therefore important in rational design of treatment. A major consideration is the induction of thermotolerance, i.e. resistance to subsequent heating.[11]

Two types of thermotolerance have been identified: first, that which develops during prolonged heating below a critical temperature (about 42°C), and, second, that which develops between individual hyperthermia fractions. Small differences in tissue temperature are very likely to occur in clinical treatments, and may therefore lead to marked variations in biological responses. Below 42.5°C, and as the heating time increases, the curves flatten out, resulting in a resistant tail. This transition is thought to result from the induction of thermotolerance, i.e. resistance to subsequent heating, which is known to be reduced or abolished by low pH.

This can have a substantial effect, altering the cell survival curve by a factor of fifteen. The effect is transient, the time course depending on the particular cell type or tissue. Almost all cells and tissues show this type of thermotolerance, with no consistent indications that thermotolerance is lower in tumours than in normal tissues, despite the regions of lower pH.

Both the extent of the maximum thermotolerance and its timing have been shown both *in vitro* and *in vivo* to be related to the effectiveness of the first treatment. Thus, the greater the effectiveness of the first (or primary) heat dose, the greater is the extent of thermotolerance and the longer it takes before the maximum is reached.

A model of thermotolerance has been proposed, with three separate phases: first, *induction* or 'trigger', which can occur at any temperature; second, a *development* phase, which can only occur at temperatures below about 42°C, and, finally, *decay*. The molecular basis for thermotolerance is not well understood, but there are numerous reports that hyperthermia results in the synthesis of a specific set of proteins (heat-stress or heat-shock proteins) and there is evidence to suggest that these proteins represent a protective mechanism produced by the cell. Thermotolerance appears to be related to one such protein with molecular weight 65 000–70 000. By assaying these proteins it would be possible to watch the decay of thermotolerance and estimate the best and most effective time to give the second dose of hyperthermia. At the present time, it is best to avoid the problem of thermotolerance in the clinical situation by giving hyperthermia on a weekly basis, which allows most of the thermotolerance to decay.

Although the maximum differential might be achieved by heating at relatively low temperatures for long time periods, this may not be very practical in the clinical setting, but recent clinical results indicate its effectiveness.[12]

# Interaction between heat and ionizing radiation

The improvement in tumour kill[13] seen with the combination of radiation and hyperthermia over radiation alone can result from two independent mechanisms:

1. direct heat-induced injury, in addition to damage caused by radiation, and working at a complementary time in the cell cycle to give an improved kill for hypoxic, nutritionally deprived cells at a low pH; and
2. sensitization of the radiation effect by mild heat treatments (which alone cause no measurable effect), by reducing the capacity of the cell to repair sublethal and potentially lethal cell damage. This would appear as a reduction in the size of the shoulder of the cell survival curve, i.e. reduction in $D_0$.

For the latter effect, hyperthermia should be given after the radiation. It has been suggested that the potentiation of this component of irradiation damage by hyperthermia may last longer for tumours than for normal tissues. Hyperthermia is likely to be most effective in poorly perfused regions, which is where radiotherapy and chemotherapy are least effective. Thus, a therapeutic gain might be obtained by combined treatment.

The effect of heat in enhancing radiation response can be expressed as a thermal enhancement ratio (TER), defined as the dose of radiation required to cause a given response in the absence of hyperthermia, divided by the radiation dose required to cause the same response in combination with hyperthermia. The TER increases with the magnitude of the heat treatment. It becomes greater than 1 for heat treatments of approximately 41°C for 60 min or equivalent, up to maximum TER values of 3 or 4, beyond which the hyperthermia begins to cause direct thermal injury. The greatest TER is obtained when the two modalities are used simultaneously, utilizing both direct injury and radiosensitization effects of the hyperthermia. However, this applies for both the tumour and the normal tissue — thus, there is no therapeutic gain with simultaneous treatments (unless the tumour alone is heated). As the separation between the two modalities is increased to 2–4 hrs, data indicate that the radiation sensitization is reduced to zero, with no enhancement of the normal-tissue reaction, whilst retaining an increased response rate. With this type of sequential treatment regimen, the two treatment modalities act independently and the heat damage to tumours is greater than that to normal tissues, for the reasons given earlier.

Used in this way, the optimal dose of radiation can be given without increasing the side-effects. This is important as there is no advantage in using hyperthermia with irradiation if the same result could be obtained by merely using a higher dose of radiotherapy. An even greater therapeutic gain will be seen if the tumour is heated preferentially (as in interstitial therapy), due to abnormal tumour vasculature which will decrease cooling and alter the microenvironment.

# Thermal dose

The concept of thermal dose is a difficult one and, unlike radiotherapy, the response does not depend only on the energy delivered, but also on many other factors, including intrinsic tissue sensitivity, duration of heating, rate of heating and cooling, pH and nutrient levels, and cell cycle distribution.

Sapareto and Dewey[14] proposed that 43°C should be used as a reference temperature and that all treatment be described as equivalent minutes of heating at 43°. This has become known as the thermal isoeffect dose (TID). Despite problems, the TID has been used clinically and results can be compared with this measurement. The Dewey formula is a method of calculating this and provides a practical and reasonable method of comparing hyperthermal treatments under conditions likely to be met in practice. In practice, there is integration of the equation over the whole treatment time.

## *Dewey formula*

$$\frac{t_2}{t_1} = R^{(T_1 - T_2)} \tag{19.1}$$

where $t_1$ and $t_2$ are the heating times at temperatures $T_1$ and $T_2$ to produce equal biological effects and $R$ is a constant.

However, the formula does not apply for large variations in temperature resulting in a significant effect of step-down sensitization, nor does it account for absolute differences in sensitivity between tissues or address the problem of varying sensitivity throughout a course of fractionated heat treatments. Clearly, these effects have the potential to invalidate the above equation. However, the range of times and temperatures seen clinically are not great and the formula has been shown to hold true experimentally over the ranges commonly seen; the use of this isoeffect relationship should therefore be seen as an interim solution to the problem.

Tumour response is most likely to correlate with the minimum tumour TID[15] and complications relate better to the maximum normal-tissue temperature recorded. TIDs are not usually added from individual treatments in a treatment course to give a total for that course.

# Hyperthermia physics

Throughout the whole history of clinical applications of hyperthermia, the technical difficulties of applying heat to the body and measuring the temperature have been major factors limiting progress. Hyperthermia may be achieved by the use of microwaves, radiofrequency or ultrasound technology and is usually classified as local (deep or superficial), regional or whole body. Interstitial or intracavity hyperthermia can also be used. From the biological point of view, all methods of heat delivery produce the same result but the different uses relate to size, depth and position of the tumour, as well as different side-effects and technical problems. In regional and local hyperthermia, techniques are designed to achieve temperatures in the range 42–45°C and sometimes higher, whereas whole body hyperthermia aims for temperatures of 41–42°C.

The penetration of electromagnetically induced hyperthermia fields depends on several factors, including tissue water content, type of applicator and, especially important, the frequency of the radiation. High frequencies have poor penetration, but good localization. For deeper heating, lower frequencies must be used but, because of the longer wavelengths, a substantial loss of definition occurs and the hyperthermia becomes more regional than local. However, the relationship between field attenuation and wavelength for ultrasound gives rise to a greater potential for local heating of tumours at intermediate depth (3–5 cm) and in deep-seated (5–15 cm) sites. The short wavelength of ultrasound at the frequencies in question (in the order of 1 mm) permits highly collimated beams to be produced from transducers with dimensions of a few centimetres.

In view of the variety of tumour sizes, shapes, perfusions and locations encountered, several types of hyperthermia system have been developed. Guidelines have been formulated by the Radiation Therapy Oncology Group (RTOG)[16] and the European Society for Hyperthermic Oncology (ESHO)[17] for their use.

## Superficial hyperthermia

Electromagnetic heating is divided into radiofrequency (approximately 8–30 MHz) and microwaves (approximately 50–3000 MHz). The depth of penetration is inversely proportional to its wavelength and applicators in the range of 300–915 MHz are used. Phantom work will define the 50% specific absorbed ratio (SAR) for each applicator but implanted thermometry is always required because of the effect of blood flow on the temperature distribution. Limited field volumes mean that, to treat large areas, mechanical scanning or multiple applicators are required. Applicators require coupling water bags for cooling the skin, and, for large areas, weight and access may be a problem. Curved microwave systems are now available for chest walls or limbs. Protection from stray microwaves is needed when treating near the eye, as it is possible to induce cataracts. Microwave applicators operating at frequencies greater than about 100 MHz are usually either open-ended waveguides or microstrip antennae.[18] The latter have the advantage of being both light and small, and readily assembled into arrays, with easier conformation to body shape.

Heating of superficial sites by radiofrequency applicators in the range 8–30 MHz is normally based on either electric or magnetic devices. In the former, electrodes placed in contact with the body produce E fields perpendicular to tissue boundaries (capacitance coupling). With this technique, its low relative permittivity leads to excess heating in fat, which can be a serious limitation. Magnetic heating via coils (inductive coupling) does not have this disadvantage because the E field is normally parallel to the tissue boundaries, but this technique does suffer from the field being highly non-uniform.

Ultrasound has been used less than electromagnetic methods despite the potential advantages offered by this technique. These include the production of well-defined beams and the ability to focus energy deep into the body. However, the disadvantages of using ultrasound relate to the significant differences in acoustic impedance between soft tissue and gas or bone, leading to poor transmission across these interfaces, with considerable reflection. This contributed to pain experienced in the early days of ultrasound heating, which was often clinically limiting. More recently, multitransducer systems which offer spatial control of energy deposition have become commercially available and scanned focused ultrasound (see below) at 1–4 MHz has been used to achieve good hyperthermia treatments of recurrent tumours covering extensive areas on the chest wall. Local pain is still the most commonly reported side-effect of ultrasound-induced hyperthermia. A summary of clinical experiences of ultrasound-induced local hyperthermia is given by Hynynen.[19]

## Deep body hyperthermia

Because of localization difficulties, progress for deep body hyperthermia has been slow and cautious. The simplest method is a radiofrequency capacitive one which involves placing the patient between two large area electrodes, with an oscillating voltage. The temperatures reached with this system are limited by the fact that fat can absorb up to ten times as much heat energy as muscle. Radiofrequency can also be used in an inductive mode with magnetic coils surrounding the patient.

Annular arrays of multiple microwave applicators will produce useful hyperthermia in deep-seated tumours, and more patients have been treated using this method.[20] Better temperatures are achieved but the treatment is not always well tolerated by the patient, with both local and systemic discomfort as potential side-effects. Whilst these systems appear attractively simple at first sight, disadvantages of the method include excessive power deposition in subcutaneous fat (the orientation of the electric field is predominantly perpendicular to adipose tissue boundaries) and the lack of control over the distribution of absorbed power within the tissues.

This can be avoided if the electric field produced by the applicator is predominantly parallel to the skin. The approach most frequently adopted is to produce a field orientated in this way, and aligned along the patient's longitudinal axis from one or more radiative sources. In this way, significant power deposition deep within the patient may be achieved. Devices using this principle include annular arrays of aperture sources or dipoles and the so-called transverse electrical mode (TEM) applicator.

An early demonstration of the potential of ultrasound to heat deeply located tumours was the work of Fessenden *et al.*[21] who used a 350 kHz system with six convergent but unfocused beams. Better results are seen with focused ultrasound beams, and these may be produced by single sources using curved radiators, lenses or reflectors or from multiple sources by electronic means. Since the focal volume associated with such systems is inherently small compared with tumour volumes, mechanical scanning of the small focal volume around a predetermined trajectory within the target volume is required.[22] These scanned focused ultrasound systems have shown that bulky tumours in the breast and other superficial sites can be heated quite well, as can some tumours in the pelvic region when an adequate acoustic window is available.

An alternative method of applying heat regionally, especially to a body extremity, is to isolate major vessels and perfuse with extracorporeally heated blood. In regional hyperthermia, large volumes of the trunk or whole limbs are heated and this is usually combined with chemotherapy.

## Whole body heating

Non-invasive methods rely on external applied heat that is then absorbed and transported by blood throughout the body, and techniques include the use of hot air, hot water or wax directly on the skin or within bags or suits. Infrared or electromagnetic radiation can also be used. More invasive techniques include extracorporeal circulation or peritoneal irrigation. The main problem has been that the maximum temperature obtainable by these systems is limited by the tolerance of the heart, lungs, liver and brain, and intensive patient monitoring systems are required. Patients need heavy sedation and often general anaesthesia for temperatures greater than 41.5°C. They all require measurement of core temperature with oesophageal and rectal thermometers, and careful fluid replacement. Cardiovascular stress is a major problem with pulse rate and cardiac output frequently doubling, and therefore pulmonary catheterization may be required to monitor right pulmonary atrial pressure, pulmonary capillary wedge pressure and cardiac output.

Techniques for whole body hyperthermia have been reviewed by van der Zee *et al.*[23]

## Interstitial hyperthermia

Local hyperthermia may also be induced using devices implanted into tissue or inserted into body cavities. The difficulties in non-invasive heating have led to substantial interest in the use of invasive methods wherever clinically appropriate. Interstitial hyperthermia systems, e.g. radiofrequency (RF) or microwave antennae, and hot sources are compatible with brachytherapy methods.

The simplest method is to apply a fairly low-frequency current (200 KHz–1 MHz) to at least two planes of implanted needles, normally as used for interstitial radiotherapy. The electrodes must be insulated at the entry and exit points in order to avoid excessive heating in these regions, and it is important that they be parallel to avoid serious temperature non-uniformities. The use of coaxial microwave antennae (300–2450 MHz) has some advantages and disadvantages relative to the RF technique. A single antenna can provide useful heating to a radial distance of about 1 cm, but the effective field length is dictated by the frequency used. Flexible plastic catheters are now being introduced to improve patient comfort, especially for use with the microwave system.

The third method is hot source technique(s), which differ from the electromagnetic methods outlined above in that energy transfer from the sources is dependent entirely upon heat transfer mechanisms within the tissues. Examples include ferromagnetic seeds, tubes carrying hot water and electrically heated implants. Ferromagnetic seeds consist of thin cylinders or wires of ferromagnetic material, which when subjected to a radiofrequency magnetic field (typically 100–200 kHz) will heat to a known temperature or Curie point (40–50°C). The seeds are therefore self-regulating with automatic temperature control, and can theoretically be combined with a radioactive source such as iodine-125. Very careful planning and anatomical placement is required for their use to avoid excessive hot and cold spots within the tumour.

Detailed descriptions of interstitial hyperthermia techniques are to be found in Seegenschmiedt and Sauer.[24]

## Measurement of temperature

Because of the non-homogeneity of temperatures that may occur across the tumour, three-dimensional temperature monitoring needs to be performed routinely during the full treatment period. Temperatures measured at a single point during treatment are not representative of the temperature distributions throughout the tumour and correlate poorly with response. In clinical practice, most temperature determinations involve the use of invasive methods, e.g. implanted thermo-couples, thermistors or various devices which are not perturbed by the electromagnetic fields, such as optical methods.[25]

Thermocouples are inexpensive, easy to construct, can be made multijunctional and small (diameter approximately 0.63 mm with outer insulating sheath), but they do interfere with microwave and ultrasound fields. Thermistors which are semiconductors have high sensitivity, but also suffer from many of the above problems. Fibre-optic probes are non-perturbing in microwave fields but are expensive. Temperature accuracy better than 0.5°C and spatial resolution better than 1 cm are both feasible and essential, to ensure minimal risk of injury to normal tissues.[26] It is not possible to obtain uniform temperatures through heated volumes, because of both technical limitations and also variations in blood flow.

Non-invasive methods are urgently needed and several possible techniques are being studied. X-ray tomography can be used since the computed tomography (CT) number depends on density, and hence on temperature. Magnetic resonance imaging (MRI) can also give temperature information since the spin lattice relaxation time $T_1$ is temperature dependent. Unfortunately, both of these methods are likely to be prohibitively expensive. Microwave radiometry can give information to depths of about 3 cm, and various techniques are now being developed to improve the spatial resolution in the hope that this method may eventually prove to be clinically useful.

Most operators aim to keep the temperatures below 41°C for normal tissue. The number of temperature probes required will depend upon the tumour size and complexity; the larger the tumour, the greater the number of probes needed. Temperature probes should be placed superficially and at depth, in addition to the area expected to be at the lowest temperature and at the normal-tissue/tumour-tissue junction. Additional sensors should be placed to monitor any areas of normal tissue or tumour at risk for overheating, e.g. skin folds, scar or necrotic regions. The passage of inserted probes should be eased with local anaesthetic. Once temperature measurements have been obtained, the next problem is to relate them in a meaningful way to response, a situation for which the TID can be used.

## Thermal modelling

In most cases, the transport of heat within tissues is dominated by blood flow. The presence of large vessels and the heterogeneous nature of perfusion are the usual causes of the variations in temperature observed during hyperthermic treatments. Thermal modelling is used in order to try and predict temperature distributions from only a few measurements, and also for prediction and optimization of temperature distributions, and to assess the performance of different heating techniques.

Many studies employ a formulation known as the bioheat transfer equation. Although this can provide a useful description of the temperature field, it is important to realize that this approach is not intended to model effects related to individual vessels and the mass flow of blood. An alternative continuum approach has been to account for perfusion in terms of 'an effective thermal conductivity'; the validity of this, too, when used alone, is questionable. The problem which remains to be solved in thermal modelling is to determine the transition between continuum models and a description which takes into account individual vessels. It is likely that this will occur at the level of vessels with diameters in the range 0.5–2 mm. So far, most models are only in two dimensions, but more powerful methods leading to three-dimensional models will probably become available soon. Further details of thermal modelling have been discussed by Lagendijk[27] and Roemer.[28]

# Clinical aspects

The concept of a thermal dose has yet to be fully agreed on internationally — this would add greatly to the comparability of studies. Response to hyperthermal treatment does not appear to be strongly related to histological type or grade,[29] unlike radiotherapy and chemotherapy. Specific concerns for the use of hyperthermia as an adjunct to irradiation include details of the radiation dose and fractionation, as well as the radiation and hyperthermia scheduling.

## Prognostic factors

### Tumour volume and depth

Theoretically, larger tumours ought to be more responsive to hyperthermia as they have a relatively greater percentage of poorly perfused and hypoxic cells, and a low pH that will result in a high sensitivity to hyperthermia. Clinically, there is an inverse correlation of tumour volume and depth with response, and the calculated minimum thermal dose tends to decrease with increasing volume while the maximum and mean temperatures increase. Technically, larger volumes are more difficult to heat; in a study of patients with head and neck cancer, Valdagni et al.[30] treated N3 metastatic neck nodes and observed complete responses (CRs) in 75% with nodes <6 cm, but in only 36% with larger nodes (see Table 19.1[13,15,31-36]). However, although large volumes do respond more poorly than small volumes to the combined therapy, the adverse effect of a large volume is even greater for irradiation alone — 9% versus 69% CR.[15] It would appear that tumour size is less important for the combined modality treatments than it is for irradiation alone.

### Tumour temperature

Single-point temperature measurements are not representative of temperature distributions throughout a tumour and correlate poorly with response. The minimum temperature in a tumour is the most important variable overall in predicting CR. The duration of CR also correlates with the average measured minimum tumour temperature for all treatments in a course, and is inversely correlated with the percentage of measured intratumoral temperatures less than 41°C. Significant prognostic thermal parameters have been noted (see Table 19.2[15,32,37-41]).

### Number and timing of hyperthermia treatments

Most workers (see Table 19.3[15,30,31,42-45]) have found that one hyperthermia treatment per week is as effective as multiple treatments — this due to thermotolerance which must be allowed to decay. There is also mounting evidence that a small number of good treatments are as effective as a larger number (e.g. two vs four)[41] (see Table 19.3[15,30,31,42-45]).

Theoretically, hyperthermia will be most effective immediately after irradiation and if tumours can be selectively heated (as in interstitial hyperthermia), simultaneous or immediate treatment will produce the greatest cell kill (see Table 19.4[42,46,47]). Overgaard and Overgaard demonstrated with melanomas[46] that the timing of the radiation and hyperthermia is vitally important and that simultaneous treatments increase both normal-tissue reaction (measured by incidence of moist desquamation) and tumour response (measured by incidence of complete regression). Delaying hyperthermia until 2–4 hrs after the irradiation reduces normal-tissue reaction greater than that of tumour, while not affecting the complete response rates, compared with immediate treatment. Thus, sequential treatments with time intervals of more than 2–4 hrs increase therapeutic gain.

Recently, interesting results have been achieved with continuous low temperature hyperthermia and interstitial hyperthermia.[12]

### Radiation dose and fractionation

Valdagni *et al.*[43] reported no CRs with doses of 10–29 Gy, a 50% CR rate with 30–39 Gy and a 67% CR rate with doses of 44–49 Gy.

### Toxicities

Certain direct effects due to subacute toxicities have been attributed to hyperthermia, including superficial burns or blisters which are usually asymptomatic and heal within 2–5 days, deeper burns which require longer

**Table 19.1**  Prognostic significance of tumour size in trials of radiation therapy and hyperthermia

| Reference (year) | No. of evaluable patients (sites) | Response criteria | Tumour size | XRT + HT (%) | XRT alone (%) |
|---|---|---|---|---|---|
| Dewhirst and Sim[13,15] (1984, 1986)[a] | 227 | CR (of ≥ 1 month duration) | < 1.8 cm³<br>1.8–8.4 cm³<br>> 8.4 cm³ | 76<br>54<br>48 | 60<br>60<br>15 |
| Hiraoka et al.[31] (1984) | 36 (40) | CR (at time of maximum response) | < 4 cm<br>4–10 cm<br>> 10 cm | 100<br>55<br>0 | ND<br>ND<br>ND |
| Luk et al.[32] (1984) | 133 | CR (initial) | ≤ 3 cm<br>> 3 cm | 61<br>44 | ND<br>ND |
| Dewhirst et al.[33] (1985) | 43[b] | CR | < 2 cm³<br>2–10 cm³<br>> 10 cm³ | 86<br>86<br>57 | 50<br>0<br>13 |
| Perez et al.[34,35] (1986, 1991) | 48 (XRT + HT)<br>116 (XRT alone) | Local control (in field) | 1–3 cm<br>> 3 cm | 79<br>65 | 48<br>28 |
| Kapp et al.[36] (1987) | 18 (38) | Local control (in field) | < 5 cm³<br>> 5 cm³ | 81<br>25 | ND<br>ND |

CR: complete response; XRT: radiation therapy; HT: hyperthermia treatment; ND: not done.
[a] Spontaneous tumours in large animals.
[b] Malignant melanomas only.

**Table 19.2** Significant prognostic thermal parameters correlating with complete response

| Thermal parameters | Reference (year) | No. of evaluable sites |
|---|---|---|
| 1. Minimum tumour temperature | Dewhirst and Sim[15] (1984)<br>Oleson et al.[37] (1984)<br>Kapp et al.[38] (1985)<br>van der Zee et al.[39] (1986) | 117<br>144<br>31<br>112 |
| 2. Minimum equivalent time at 43° C | van der Zee et al.[39] (1986) | 112 |
| 3. Lowest averaged tumour temperature | Luk et al.[32] (1984) | 33 |
| 4. Average tumour temperature | Kapp et al.[38] (1985) | 31 |
| 5. Number of satisfactory heat sessions | Sapozink et al.[40] (1986)<br>Dunlop et al.[41] (1986) | 112<br>116 |

**Table 19.3** Influence of number of hyperthermia treatments on outcome in trials of radiation therapy (XRT) and adjuvant hyperthermia (HT)

| Reference (year) | No. of evaluable patients (sites) | Treatments (per week) | Outcome parameters | Actual no. of HT treatments | CR (%) |
|---|---|---|---|---|---|
| Arcangeli et al.[42] (1984) | 25 | 1 or 2 | CR at end of TX | 5<br>10 | 64 NS<br>78 |
| Dewhirst and Sim[15] (1984)[a] | 116 | 1 | CR at 1 month; duration of CR | 1<br>2<br>3<br>4 | 67 NS<br>79<br>45<br>58 |
| Hiraoka et al.[31] (1984) | 36 (40) | 2 | CR (1–8 months) | 2–7<br>8–12 | 50 NS<br>53 |
| Valdagni et al.[30] (1988) | 27 | 2 or 3 | CR at 3 months | <6<br>6<br>>6 | 67 NS<br>37<br>70 |
| Alexander et al.[44] (1987) | 44 (48) | 1 vs 2 | CR | 4<br>8 | 42 NS<br>21 |
| Kapp et al.[45] (1986) | 43 (126) | 1 vs 2 | CR at 3 weeks | 2<br>6 | 65 NS<br>73 |

NS: no statistically significant difference in CR rate.
[a] Spontaneous tumours in large animals.

**Table 19.4** Sequencing of hyperthermia (HT) and irradiation (XRT) in clinical trials

| Reference (year) | No. of evaluable patients (sites) | Treatments per week (Total no.) | Dose per fraction (Gy) | No. RTs per week (Total no.) | Timing of HT and XRT | Tumour response | Skin reaction | TGF[a] |
|---|---|---|---|---|---|---|---|---|
| | | | | | | CR (%) | MD (%) | |
| Arcangeli et al.[42] (1984) | 25 | 2 (8) | 5 | 2 (8) | RT/HT (S) | 77 | 64 | 1.14 |
| | | | | | RT, 4 hr delay HT | 67 | 46 | 1.38 |
| | 15 | 2 (5) | 6 | 2 (5) | RT/HT (S) (skin cooled) | 87 | 33 | 2.08 |
| | 26 | 3.7 | 1.52–2 | 3 (36) | RT/HT (S) | 73 | 42 | 1.57 |
| | | | | | | TCD$_{50}$ (Gy) | ED$_{50}$ (Gy) | |
| Overgaard and Overgaard[46] (1987) | 28 (65) | 2 (3) | 5–10 | 2 (3) | RT/HT (S) | 6 | 6.5 | 1.0 |
| | | | | | RT, 3–4 hr delay then HT | 6.9 | 8.5 | 1.3 |
| | | | | | RT alone | 8.8 | 8.5 | 1.0 |
| | | | | | | CR (%) | | |
| Kim et al.[47] (1984) | 48 | 2 (10) | 4 | 2 (10) | RT/HT (S) | 57 | No diff. | NA |
| | | | | | RT/HT (S) | 63 | No diff. | NA |
| | | | | | RT alone | 30 | — | — |
| | 49 | 1 (6) | 6.6 | 2 (10) | RT/HT (S) | 75 | Increased | NA |
| | | | | | RT/HT (S) | 72 | Increased | — |
| | | | | | RT alone | 59 | — | — |

CR: complete response; TCD$_{50}$: dose per fraction for 50% CR; ED$_{50}$: dose per fraction for 50% rate of severe erythema; NA: not available; S: simultaneous XRT and HT; MD: moist desquamation; TGF: therapeutic gain factor.
[a] Malignant melanoma.

periods to heal but are relatively uncommon, and ulceration developing in treated tumours and on normal tissue. This latter can persist for weeks but is usually asymptomatic. However, significant normal-tissue damage should occur to a lesser degree following the combined treatments than for irradiation alone, if hyperthermia is used correctly (i.e. with a time gap of 2–4 hrs). Acute toxicities do appear to be indicative of long-term toxicity and are relatively uncommon.

Overall, the majority of patients have not experienced excessive skin reactions from the combination therapy, beyond what might have been expected from the radiation alone. This has also been confirmed in late skin reaction studies where a minimal increase in fibrosis or induration is generally noted, particularly when high doses of irradiation have been used (Table 19.5[48]).

These studies would therefore suggest that attempts should be made to use the minimum number of hyperthermia treatments, to use active skin cooling (where the skin is not directly involved with tumour) and to restrict the maximal temperature allowed. Most workers attempt to keep the skin temperature below 41°C.

In general, hyperthermia treatment appears to be well tolerated and in a study of 100 patients conducted at the Hammersmith Hospital, London, less than 5% found either the insertion of temperature probes, or the heat itself, very unpleasant.[49] For the heating of more deeply seated tumours, however, there is a greater risk of damage. For systems using focused beams at depth, localization is difficult and visceral damage is a possibility.

**Table 19.5**  Persistent and/or late complications of radiation plus hyperthermia in sixty-five patients with ≤ 24 months follow-up

| Tumour | No. of patients | No. of fields with induration and fibrosis | No. of fields with ulceration |
|---|---|---|---|
| Breast | 15 | 31 | 3 |
| Melanoma | 2 | 2 | 1 |
| Sarcoma | 1 | 0 | 0 |
| SCC (head and neck) | 2 | 2 | 0 |
| Lymphoma | 2 | 3 | 0 |

SCC: squamous cell carcinoma.
Source: Ben-Josef and Kapp, *Int J Hyperthermia* 1992; **8**, 733–47.[48]

## Clinical results

Over 40 000 human tumours have now been treated with hyperthermia. Although the majority of these have been superficial or palliative in intent, an increasing number of studies are now being conducted that address the more important issues of hyperthermia as part of radical treatment.

## Hyperthermia alone

Hyperthermia alone has a response rate of approximately 50% with a CR rate of 10–15%, which is usually of short duration. It has been recommended as suitable treatment in certain situations, where it can be remarkably effective to control bleeding or provide pain relief.

Hyperthermia can stimulate the immune system and part of the response may be due to this ability. Melanomas in a part of the body distant to that undergoing hyperthermia have sometimes been seen to resolve. Hyperthermia alone has also been used intraoperatively for the treatment of biliary and brain tumours, but neither has been extensively investigated. Some benign diseases such as benign prostatic hypertrophy,[50] psoriasis, sinusitis and acute lung injury may also benefit from hyperthermia. Other non-malignant diseases such as menorrhagia[51] and cardiac arrhythmias can also be treated with ablative heat.

## Results from hyperthermia and radiation

Many non-randomized studies in patients with both superficial and deep-seated tumours have been performed; most have used microwave-induced heat with invasive thermometry. Commonly, temperatures of 42–44°C have been used, over 30–60 mins, following a wide variety of radiotherapy schedules, generally once or twice weekly.

### Superficial

Tumours less than 3 cm from the surface have provided the greatest experience with human tumour response to hyperthermia. Recent technical developments have produced microwave applicators and arrays of microwave and ultrasound applicators that offer many advantages: increasingly broader field size, segmental control of applicator power for greater temperature homogeneity, improved power of delivery to areas of limited access, the ability to avoid sensitive adjacent normal tissues, greater conformity to curved treatment surfaces and improved patient comfort during treatment.

Superficial malignancies which include skin nodules, melanomas, head and neck tumours and chest wall recurrences have been extensively studied. In some studies, patients have acted as their own controls, if they have had more than one lesion. A recent analysis of more than 1100 patients showed remarkably consistent results, with a CR rate of 35% for radiotherapy alone and a CR rate of 65% for the combined hyperthermia- and radiotherapy-treated patients (unpublished data from the author and Dr SB Field). The addition of hyperthermia also appeared to increase the number and speed of responses and reduce the rate of relapse, whilst not significantly increasing the toxicity.

However, a definitive Phase III trial is clearly essential to prove the effectiveness of hyperthermia and to allow it to take its correct place along with other cancer therapies. Clinical studies of hyperthermia are proceeding more rapidly in Europe than in the USA or Japan, despite more extensive government support. A concerted effort was initiated by the European Community in 1989 to cooperate aspects of multicentre clinical trials with very high standards of quality assurance, and is now being completed.

The ESHO melanoma Phase III trial has shown a positive result for hyperthermia: complete response rates of 28% for radiotherapy alone versus 46% for radiation plus hyperthermia ($P = 0.008$) at 2 years.[52] In this trial, radiation dose was also found to be extremely important, with a 56% control rate for 27 Gy in three fractions versus a 25% control rate for 24 Gy in three fractions ($P = 0.002$). The hyperthermia significantly improved the therapeutic effect of the radiation both for CR and for response duration, without significantly increasing the acute or late radiation reactions.

A second randomized trial has been undertaken by the combined Medical Research Council/European Society for Hyperthermic Oncology/Princess Margaret Hospital, Toronto (MRC/ESHO/PMH) group in patients with locally advanced or recurrent disease, closing recruitment in 1993 with over 300 patients.[53] Most of these had already failed radiation, hormone and chemotherapy treatment. Although the different groups used different radiation and hyperthermia schedules, the overall results for all groups was highly significant with a 40% CR rate for radiation alone compared with 60% for the addition of hyperthermia to radiation. Again, the addition of hyperthermia resulted in longer duration of CR rates with no increase in side-effects.

A number of tumour sites merit particular mention. Although locally advanced breast tumours may be difficult to heat because of their size, encouraging results have been seen.[54,55] In 1990, a small randomized study of head and neck primaries by Datta *et al.*[56] demonstrated significantly improved local control which translated into an improved survival. Preoperative hyperthermia and radiotherapy have been used in the former USSR[57] for advanced melanomas, colorectal cancer and Stage II and III breast cancer. All showed significant improvement in the local control rate, with improvement in survival in the melanoma and colorectal studies.

### Deep-seated tumours

The heating of deep-seated tumours is technically more difficult and limiting side-effects have included systemic heating, pain at bone interfaces when focused ultrasound is used, and preferential fat heating with capacitance-heating techniques. The placement of catheters for temperature measurement can be a problem and is usually performed under CT control. Most studies so far reported in this group have been on patients who have had prior treatment, whose life expectancy is short and in whom the aim is essentially palliation. To achieve local control in such tumours as cervical, bladder and rectal cancers could, however, lead to improved survival.

A number of studies involving the annual array system have been conducted and the limiting side-effects have mainly been due to systemic heating, which is difficult to prevent. Nonetheless, Sapozink *et al.*[40] studied twenty-three patients with advanced abdominal and pelvic tumours, and achieved response rates of 54% and 83%. Petrovich *et al.*[58] summarized the results of 353 patients treated with regional hyperthermia for a variety of abdominopelvic tumours, and observed a 10% CR and 17% PR (partial response) rate. Treatment tolerance was good in the majority of patients, but significant pain occurred in 35%. Few studies have been performed using focused ultrasound but early results indicate that it, too, may be a promising modality.[22]

In both Europe and India, Phase III studies have now commenced, particularly studying pelvic tumours. A small, randomized study by Datta *et al.*[59] for advanced cervical cancers has shown positive results. Early preliminary results from the Dutch Cancer Group (Amsterdam/Rotterdam and Utrecht)[60] have suggested improved complete response rates (58% for the combined treatments versus 37% for radiotherapy alone), which might possibly convert into a survival advantage. Here, over 180 patients with locally advanced and inoperable bladder, cervical and rectal tumours have been randomized. For the former tumours, these results are highly significant, but not as yet for rectal tumours, though these comprise a relatively small proportion of the total.

*Interstitial hyperthermia*

If hyperthermia can be strictly limited to the tumour, then simultaneous heat and irradiation gives the highest response rate, and offers the greatest theoretical advantage for interstitial treatments. Like interstitial radiotherapy, interstitial hyperthermia offers a method for providing uniform heating to small volumes below the skin surface. Tumours that have been studied include brain, breast, cervical and head and neck cancers, using radiofrequency, microwaves, hot water sources and ferromagnetic seed methods. Most Phase I–II studies have reported CR rates in the order of 55–65% for recurrent or persistent tumours. The largest series comes from the former USSR (Muratkhodzhaev *et al.*[61]) where more than 300 patients with oesophageal cancers were treated with interstitial hyperthermia, and showed both improved local control and increased survival.

*Intracavity hyperthermia*

Transrectal[62] or transurethral hyperthermia for benign prostatic hypertrophy[50] is increasingly popular, and symptomatic relief is reported in the order of 65–70%. Intracavity heating has been attempted for rectal tumours[63] with a survival at 5 years of 73.7% for 40 Gy plus heat, 58.8% for 40 Gy alone and 42.9% for 30 Gy plus heat (122 patients).

## Results for hyperthermia and chemotherapy ± irradiation

The thermal interactions[63,64] of most chemotherapeutic drugs are complex and far from being fully understood. The reasons for the increased effect seen with certain drugs in combination with hyperthermia are complex, but may be due to altered drug pharmacokinetics such as increased solubility, e.g. nitrosoureas and alkylating agents; altered plasma protein binding, e.g. cisplatinum; and activation of enzymatic processes, e.g. anthracyclines and antimetabolites. Increased drug uptake can be achieved by intra-arterial infusion, which has been attempted for limb and liver tumours, by using degradable starch microspheres to temporarily trap drugs within the circulation or by introducing liposomes containing drugs which can be triggered to release their contents at a particular temperature. There is also evidence that part of the benefit may be due to DNA effects manifesting either as increased damage or as decreased repair.

Certain drugs combine[65,66] usefully with hyperthermia and will show an additive effect. These include both the vincas and antimetabolites (methotrexate and 5-fluorouracil) (see Table 19.6). However, this does not appear to be true thermal enhancement; it does occur with the alkylating agents and the antitumour antibiotics with resultant supra-additive lethality, though the degree of effect varies between the different members of the group. In most situations, thermal enhancement will increase with temperature. Doxorubicin, bleomycin, cisplatinum and BCNU (carmustine) are all inhibited below temperatures of 37°C, probably explaining why scalp cooling reduces doxorubicin-induced alopecia. These agents all exhibit supra-additive lethality above their threshold temperatures, which increases with increasing temperature. Mitomycin C also shows marked thermal enhancement at temperatures above 42°C, and it is around this temperature that most of the group have their thesholds. Time sequencing of the hyperthermia also affects these agents — the two treatments must be given simultaneously to achieve maximum cytotoxic effect. Prolonged heating, as in whole body hyperthermia, can lead to inactivation of the drugs.

Only a few reports are available for DTIC (dacarbazine), procarbazine and podophyllotoxin — the first two do appear to have some thermal enhancement properties, the latter is only additive with heat. Not all drugs are enhanced by heat, and for some, e.g. AMSA (amsacrine) and Ara-C (cytarabine), cell killing is inhibited by heat. Some radiosensitizer drugs, e.g. misonidazole and 5-thio-D-glucose, also show increased toxicity to hypoxic cells at hyperthermic temperatures. Other drugs, e.g. ethanol, amphotericin B and cysteamine, are cytotoxic only at elevated temperatures.

Both interferon,[67] when used for melanomas and sarcomas, and *Corynebacterium parvum* show non-specific thermal enhancement of their immunostimulation.[68]

It should be remembered that although, in most cases, thermal enhancement is beneficial, it is also possible to enhance drug toxicity.[69] Most groups have found that simultaneous exposure of tumours to drugs and heat is the most effective approach and most efforts have been made, in the clinical situation, with whole body or regional hyperthermia, and to a lesser extent in local hyperthermia after failure of full dose radiotherapy.

**Table 19.6**   Chemotherapeutic drugs and hyperthermia

| Supra-additive | Additive effect | Less than addictive effect |
| --- | --- | --- |
| Mustine | Vincas | Amsacrine |
| Thiotepa | Methotrexate | Cytarabine |
| Cyclophosphamide | 5-Fluorouracil | |
| Melphalan | | |
| Mitomycin C | | |
| Nitrosoureas | | |
| Cisplatinum | | |
| Anthracyclines | | |
| Bleomycin | | |
| Misonidazole | | |
| Interferon | | |
| Lonidamine | | |
| Tumour necrosis factor | | |

Theoretically, regional perfusion allows blood to be used as the vehicle to transport and distribute both heat and drugs, as well as allowing biochemical analysis of the effects of hyperthermia. Body extremities can be heated by isolating major arteries and veins; this closed circuit system is then perfused with extracorporeally heated blood and drugs. Suitable sites include melanomas and sarcomas of the limbs, as well as primary and metastatic tumours of the liver and other organs. A variety of Phase II studies have shown significant advantages in both disease-free and actuarial survivals for patients treated in this way. The first randomized trial was completed by Ghussen *et al.*[70] in 1988, assessing these treatments in over 100 patients with Stage I–III malignant melanomas. Half received conventional surgery only and the other half hyperthermic limb perfusion together with melphalan. This study was terminated early, since long-term results revealed twenty-six recurrences in the conventional arm and only six in the combined-treatment arm. Hyperthermic infusion has also been attempted with metastatic liver tumours and advanced bladder tumours — the former with disappointing results,[71] and the latter, which also included treament by irradiation, with more 'promising' results.[72]

In a non-randomized study, treatment by regional hyperthermia for limb sarcomas (using etoposide and ifosfamide[73]) has shown an overall response rate of 37% with six out of thirty-eight CRs and four PRs for pretreated locally advanced tumours. Similar results were also obtained by the same group for pelvic tumours. Hyperthermic perfusion for hepatic colorectal metastases with 5-fluorouracil showed an improvement in survival, and for advanced bladder tumours also suggested promising results,[74] with eleven out of twenty-four patients achieving a CR.

Nature's hyperthermia, fever, is one of the body's defences against infections and no doubt involves stimulation of the immune system. It is likewise probable that whole body hyperthermia has a similar effect. Whole body hyperthermia has been used for the treatment of disseminated disease, either alone or in combination with chemotherapeutic agents. However, most of the studies so far performed are complicated by a large number of variables, including the type and stages of diseases studied, the specific drugs and the dosages used, and the degree and duration of heat employed.

Most studies have concentrated on tumours which are likely to be resistant to more conventional therapies, such as unresectable tumours of the gastrointestinal tract, e.g. pancreas, stomach and oesophagus, and lung tumours other than small-cell. In addition, tumours have also been studied which have failed standard therapy and have disseminated, e.g. lymphomas, sarcomas, leukaemia and breast cancer. Although most of these studies have reported a low CR rate (less than 10%), many have reported substantial regressions (approximately 30%), especially with regard to pain relief. This in itself may be considered remarkable, bearing in mind that most of these patients had advanced disease, thought untreatable in most cases. Promising Phase II studies were completed by Bull *et al.*[75] who treated seventeen patients with resistant sarcomas by whole body hyperthermia and BCNU (two PR, four objective responses), and Engelhardt[76] who treated fifteen patients with small cell lung cancer with whole body hyperthermia and doxorubicin, cyclophosphamide and vincristine (CR + PR fifteen of twenty-two patients in the hyperthermic arm; CR + PR eight of twenty-two for the normothermic arm).

When normal-tissue tolerance has been reached for radiotherapy, a number of studies have suggested that the combination of hyperthermia and chemotherapy might be useful, despite the fact that the vascular damage caused by the irradiation may limit the concentration of the drug reaching the tissues. Chemotherapy (doxorubicin or bleomycin) and hyperthermia have also been usefully combined for the treatment of head and neck nodes. Arcangeli *et al.*[77] found an improved response (by comparison with chemotherapy alone) in patients with advanced neck nodes (95% vs 45%). Kohno *et al.*[78] noted improved responses in patients with advanced vaginal or vulval carcinomas when hyperthermia was combined with mitomycin C and bleomycin.

### Trimodality trials

A prospective randomized trial was reported by Sugimachi *et al.*[79] in fifty-three patients treated with trimodality therapy using bleomycin given pre-operatively for carcinoma of the oesophagus, and a significant difference was found in those receiving hyperthermia. Herman *et al.*[80] reported on a group of twenty-four patients treated by hyperthermia, radiation and cis-platinum who showed a 25–67% CR (depending on the dose of cisplatinum used).

More recently, Zamboglou *et al.*[81] presented the results of a randomized trial using hyperthermia and simultaneous radiochemotherapy using mitoxantrone followed by salvage surgery in sixty-five patients with locally advanced breast cancer. Thirty-five patients (54%) who had received the trimodality treatment showed a pathologically confirmed complete response, compared with six out of forty (15%) who received radiotherapy and chemotherapy alone.

# The future

The challenge remains for physicists and engineers to develop better heating systems and non-invasive thermometry. Hyperthermia applicators are being designed to provide increasingly generous field sizes, segmental control of applicator power, output for greater temperature homogeneity, improved power delivery to areas of limited access, increased ability to avoid sensitive adjacent normal tissues, greater conformity to curved surfaces, and improved patient comfort during treatment. The ability to heat larger volumes of tumour to therapeutic temperatures will widen the scope of hyperthermia, and multiapplicator curved microwave systems are currently under investigation. Non-invasive means of thermometry such as microwave or ultrasound radiometry, applied potential tomography and MRI are among the many hopes for the future, but at present their clinical application seems likely to remain many years in the future.

The vast majority of studies so far carried out show an advantage for hyperthermia and radiation over radiation alone, and conclusive randomized Phase III studies are now appearing in press with significantly positive results. Most randomized trials will need to be multi-institutional to recruit sufficient numbers of patients quickly and it is vital that strict quality assurance guidelines are adhered to.

Although modern megavoltage radiotherapy has significantly improved the cure rate from that of conventional teletherapy at normal temperature, there is still an unacceptable rate of failure of local control. Viable cells in the residual tumour at the primary site will lead to the development of metastases and ultimately death. Probably one-third of all cancer deaths follow failure of local control in the primary tumour,[82] and if local control were improved it is probable that cure rates would be increased. Hyperthermia clearly seems to be one method of improving this, and, furthermore, the importance of local control of cancer has a critical impact on quality of life. The greatest advantage for hyperthermia at the present time appears to be in combination with radiation for the treatment of cancers where local control remains a major obstacle. These include breast, head and neck, rectal, bladder and cervical tumours. For deep-seated malignancies, technical difficulties are still considerable, but the scanned focused ultrasound system is certainly one promising way forward. It is important that studies also continue with metastatic lesions, but here the aim will be palliation, and any conclusions regarding the interaction of the two treatment modalities will be of chiefly academic rather than practical interest.

Phase III studies for whole body hyperthermia in combination with chemotherapy, rather than radiation, are also planned for the future. Tumours with a high growth fraction, e.g. small cell lung carcinomas, or perhaps some of the high-grade non-Hodgkin's lymphoma group would be suitable. Other potential uses for whole body hyperthermia include the treatment of disseminated disease (alone or with chemotherapy) or as an adjuvant with chemotherapy for micrometastatic disease. Immunotherapy or vasodilators might also be usefully combined in such studies. In the USA, Phase III trials are now ongoing for interstitial hyperthermia treatment of brain tumours.

It is possible that one day we might gain more insight into thermotolerance by investigating its relationship to heat-shock proteins. Rapid assay of heat-shock proteins might then give clues as to when to treat to get the best results. Alterations of the cellular environment by the use of vasodilators to selectively reduce tumour perfusion, or infusions of glucose to alter pH, also represent another way forward. Positron emission tomography and magnetic resonance spectroscopy are now available for studying this in humans.

There is no doubt that the availability of hyperthermia offers a significant and worthwhile improvement for selected patients and that it holds great promise as a cancer treatment in certain tumours[83] as an adjunct to both irradiation and chemotherapy, although regrettably it is time-consuming and needs a dedicated team to perform the procedure efficiently and safely. Ideally, hyperthermia units should be placed in regional referral centres to maximize their efficiency and to perform cost-effectively as part of an integrated multimodal approach to cancer treatment.

# References

1. Busch W. Verhandlungen ärtlicher Gesellschaften. *Berl Klin Wochenschr* 1986; 3, 245–6.
2. Leeper DB. Molecular and cellular mechanisms of hyperthermia alone or combined with other modalities. In: J Overgaard, ed, *Hyperthermic Oncology* 1984, Vol 2. London: Taylor & Francis, 1985; 9–40.
3. Roti-Roti JL, Wilson CF. The effects of alcohols, procaine and hyperthermia on the protein content of nuclei and chromatin. *Int J Radiat Oncol Biol Phys 1984*; **46**, 35–43.
4. Field SB. Studies relevant to a means of quantifying the effects of hyperthermia. *Int J Hyperthermia* 1987; **3**, 291–6.
5. Reinhold HS, Endrich B. Tumour microcirculation as a target for hyperthermia. *Int J Hyperthermia* 1986; **2**, 11–137.
6. Vaupel P, Kallinowski F. Physiological effects of hyperthermia. *Recent Results Cancer Res* 1987; **104**, 71–109.
7. Horsmann MR, Christiansen KL, Overgaard J. Hydralazine induced enhancement of hyperthermic damage in a C3H mammary carcinoma in vivo. *Int J Hyperthermia* 1989; **5**, 123–36.
8. Jirtle RL. Chemical modifications of tumour blood flow. *Int J Hyperthermia* 1988; **4**, 355.
9. Wilson C, Vernon CC, Lammertsma AA, *et al.* Vascular changes in tumours following hyperthermia, monitored using PET. Abstract presented at the 11th Conference of ESHO, Latina, 1990. *Strahlenther Onkol* 1990; 538.
10. Field SB. Clinical implications of thermotolerance. In: J Overgaard, ed, *Hyperthermic Oncology 1984*, Vol 2. London: Taylor & Francis, 1985; 235–44.
11. Li GC, Mivechi NF. Thermotolerance in mammalian systems: a review. In: LJ Anghilieri, J Robert, eds, *Hyperthermia in Cancer Treatment*, Vol 1, Boca Raton, FL: CRC Press, 1986; 59–77.
12. Armour EP, McEachern D, Wang Z, *et al.* Sensitivity of human cells to mild hyperthermia. *Cancer Res* 1993; **53**, 12.
13. Dewhirst MW, Sim DA. Estimation of therapeutic gain in clinical trials involving hyperthermia and radiotherapy. *Int J Hyperthermia* 1986; **2**, 165–78.
14. Sapareto SA, Dewey WC. Thermal dose determination in cancer therapy. *Int J Radiat Oncol Biol Phys* 1984; **10**, 787–800.
15. Dewhirst WC, Sim DA. The utility of thermal dose as a predictor of tumour and normal tissue responses in combined radiation and hyperthermia. *Cancer Res* 1984; **44** (Suppl), 4772s–80s.
16. Sapozink MD, Corry PM, Kapp DS, *et al.* RTOG quality assurance guidelines for clinical trials using hyperthermia for deep-seated malignancy. *Int J Radiat Oncol Biol Phys* 1991; **20**, 1109–15.
17. Hand JW, Lagendijk JJW, Bach Andersen J, *et al.* Quality assurance guidelines for ESHO protocols. *Int J Hyperthermia* 1989; **5**, 421–8.
18. Hand JW, James J (eds). *Physical Techniques in Clinical Hyperthermia*. Letchworth: Research Studies Press, 1986.
19. Hynynen K. Biophysics and technology of ultrasound hyperthermia. In: M Gauterie, ed, *Methods of External Hyperthermic Heating*. Berlin, Heidelberg, New York: Springer, 1990; 61–115.
20. Howard GCW, Sathiaseelen V, King GA, *et al.* Regional hyperthermia for extensive pelvic tumours using annular based array applicator: a feasibility study. *Br J Radiol* 1986; **59**, 1195–201.
21. Fessenden P, Lee ER, Anderson TL, *et al.* Experience with a multitransducer ultrasound system for localized hyperthermia of deep tissues. *IEEE Trans Biomed Eng* 1984; **31**, 126–35.
22. Hand JW, Vernon CC, Prior MV. Early experience of a commercial scanned

focused ultrasound hyperthermia system. *Int J Hyperthermia* 1992; **8**, 587–607.

23. van der Zee J, van Rhoon GC, Faithfull NS, *et al.* Clinical hyperthermic practice: whole-body hyperthermia. In: SB Field, JW Hand, eds, *An Introduction to the Practical Aspects of Clinical Hyperthermia*. London: Taylor & Francis, 1990; 185–212.

24. Seegenschmiedt MH, Sauer R (eds). *Interstitial and Intracavitary Thermoradiotherapy*. Berlin, Heidelberg, New York: Springer, 1993.

25. Cetas TC. Thermometry. In: SB Field, JW Hand, eds, *An Introduction to the Practical Aspects of Clinical Hyperthermia*. London: Taylor & Francis, 1990; 423–77.

26. Samulski TV, Fessenden P. Thermometry in therapeutic hyperthermia. In: M Gautherie, ed, *Methods of Hyperthermia Control*. Berlin, Heidelberg, New York: Springer, 1990; 1–34.

27. Lagendijk JW. Thermal models: principles and implementation. In: SB Field, JW Hand, eds, *An Introduction to the Practical Aspects of Clinical Hyperthermia*. London: Taylor & Francis, 1990; 478–512.

28. Roemer RB. Thermal dosimetry. In: P Gautherie, ed, *Thermal Dosimetry and Treatment Planning*. Berlin, Heidelberg, New York: Springer, 1990; 119–214.

29. Myerson RJ, Perez CA, Emani B, *et al.* Tumour control in long term survivors following superficial hyperthermia. *Int J Radiat Oncol Biol Phys* 1990; **5**, 1123–9.

30. Valdagni R, Amichetti M, Pani G. Radical radiation alone versus radical radiation plus microwave hyperthermia for N3 (TNM–UICC) neck nodes: a prospective randomized clinical trial. *Int J Radiat Oncol Biol Phys* 1988; **15**, 13–24.

31. Hiraoka M, Jo S, Takashashi M, *et al.* Clinical results of radiofrequency hyperthermia combined with radiation in the treatment of radioresistant cancer. *Cancer* 1984; **54**, 2898–904.

32. Luk KH, Pajak TF, Perez CA, *et al.* Prognostic factors for tumour response after hyperthermia and radiation. In: J Overgaard, ed, *Hyperthermic Oncology 1984*, Vol 1. London: Taylor & Francis, 1984; 353–6.

33. Dewhirst MC, Sim DA, Forsyth K, *et al.* Local tumor control and distant metastases in primary canine malignant melanomas treated with hyperthermia and/or radiotherapy. *Int J Hyperthermia* 1985; **1**, 219–34.

34. Perez CA, Kuske RR, Emami B, *et al.* Irradiation alone or combined with hyperthermia in the treatment of recurrent carcinoma of the breast in the chest wall: a non randomized comparison. *Int J Hyperthermia* 1986; **2**, 179–87.

35. Perez CA, Pajak T, Emami B, *et al.* Randomised Phase II study comparing irradiation alone or combined with hyperthermia in the superficial measurable tumours. Final report by the Radiation Therapy Oncology Group. *Am J Clin Oncol* 1991; **2**, 133–41.

36. Kapp DS, Samulski TV, Fessenden P, *et al.* Prognostic significance of tumour volume on response following local-regional hyperthermia (HT) and radiation therapy (XRT). Abstract presented at the Thirty-fifth Annual Meeting of the Radiation Research Society, Atlanta, GA, 21–26 February 1987; 17.

37. Oleson JR, Sim DA, Manning MR. Analysis of prognostic variables in hyperthermia treatments of 161 patients. *Int J Radiat Oncol Biol Phys* 1984; **10**, 2231–9.

38. Kapp DS, Samulski TV, Meyer JL, *et al.* Metastatic breast cancer with chest wall recurrences in previously irradiated areas: management with low–moderate dose irradiation therapy and hyperthermia. *Abstracts of Papers for the 33rd Annual Meeting of the Radiation Research Society* 1985; 29.

39. van der Zee J, van Putten WJL, van den Berg AP, *et al.* Retrospective analysis of the response of tumours in patients treated with a combination of radiotherapy and hyperthermia. *Int J Hyperthermia* 1986; **2**, 337–49.

40. Sapozink MD, Gibbs FA, Egger MJ, *et al.* Regional hyperthermia for clinically

advanced deep-seated pelvic malignancy. *Am J Clin Oncol* 1986; **9**, 162–9.

41. Dunlop PRC, Hand JW, Dickinson RJ, *et al.* An assessment of local hyperthermia in clinical practice. *Int J Hyperthermia* 1986; **2**, 39–50.
42. Arcangeli G, Nervi D, Cividalli A, *et al.* Problems of sequence and fractionation in the clinical application of combined heat and irradiation. *Cancer Res* 1984; **44** (Suppl), 48575–635.
43. Valdagni R, Liu FF, Kapp DS. Important prognostic factors influencing outcome of combined radiation and hyperthermia. *Int J Radiat Oncol Biol Phys* 1988; **15**, 959–72.
44. Alexander GA, Moylan DJ, Waterman FM, *et al.* A randomized trial of 1 vs 2 adjuvant hyperthermia treatments in patients with superficial metastases. Paper presented at the 7th Annual Meeting of the North American Hyperthermia Group, Atlanta, GA, 21–26 February 1987.
45. Kapp DS, Bagshaw MA, Meyer JL, *et al.* Hyperthermia as an adjuvant to radiation in the treatment of superficial metastases: a randomised trial of 2 vs 6 heat treatments. *Proceedings of the 34th Annual Meeting of the Radiation Research Society*, Las Vegas, NV, 1986; Abstract Bf-4.
46. Overgaard J, Overgaard M. Hyperthermia as an adjuvant to radiotherapy in the treatment of malignant melanoma. *Int J Hyperthermia* 1987; **3**, 483–502.
47. Kim JH, Hahn SA, Ahmed SA, *et al.* Clinical study of the sequence of combined hyperthermia and radiation therapy of malignant melanomas. In: J Overgaard, ed, *Hyperthermic Oncology*, Vol 1. London: Taylor & Francis, 1984; 387–90.
48. Ben-Yosef R, Kapp DS. Persistent and/or late complications of combined radiation and hyperthermia. *Int J Hyperthermia* 1992; **8**, 733–47.
49. Vernon CC, Field SF, Robinson Y. Do patients find hyperthermia treatments acceptable? *Abstract 12th ESHO Meeting* 1992; 446.
50. Sapozink MD, Astrahan M, Boyd S. Treatment of benign prostatic hyperplasia with transurethral hyperthermia. In: *Thirty-seventh Annual Meeting of the Radiation Research Society*, Seattle, Washington, DC, 1989; Abstract Ad-9.
51. Prior MV, Phipps JH, Roberts T, *et al.* Treatment of menorrhagia by radiofrequency heating. *Int J Hyperthermia* 1991; **7**, 213–20.
52. Overgaard J. Results of the ESHO (3–85) Phase III, a study for metastatic melanoma. *Hyperthermia Clin Oncol* 1993; **41** (Abstract).
53. Vernon CC, van der Zee J, Lui F-F. Hyperthermia as an additive to radiation vs radiation alone for the treatment of breast carcinoma — results of a collaborative Phase III trial. *Int J Radiat Oncol Biol Phys* (in press).
54. Hofman P, Knol RGF, Lagendijk JJW, *et al.* Thermoradiotherapy of primary breast carcinoma. *Int J Hyperthermia* 1989; **5**, 1–11.
55. Scott R, Gillespie B, Perez CA, *et al.* Hyperthermia in combination with definitive radiation therapy. Results of Phase II/II RTOG study 1988. *Int J Radiat Oncol Biol Phys* 1988; **3**, 711–16.
56. Datta NR, Bose AK, Kapoor HK, *et al.* Head and neck cancers: results of thermoradiotherapy versus radiotherapy. *Int J Hyperthermia* 1990; **6**, 479–86.
57. Savchenko NE, Zhakov IG, Fradkin SZ, *et al.* The use of hyperthermia in oncology. *Med Radiol* 1987; **32**, 19–24 (in Russian).
58. Petrovich Z, Langholtz B, Gibbs FA Jr. Regional hyperthermia for advanced tumours. A clinical study of 353 patients. *Int J Radiat Oncol Biol Phys* 1989; **16**, 601–7.
59. Datta NR, Bose AK, Kapoor HK. Thermoradiotherapy in the management of carcinoma cervix (IIIB): a controlled clinical study. *Indian Medical Gazette* 1987; **121**, 68–71.
60. van der Zee J. Hyperthermia combined with radiotherapy in deep seated tumours. *Abstracts of the Hyperthermia in Clinical Oncology Meeting*. Munich: BSD Medical Corp, 1993, 5.

61. Muratkhodzhaev NK, Svetitsky PV, Kochegarov AA, *et al.* Hyperthermia in therapy of cancer patients. *Med Radiol* 1987; **32**, 30–6 (in Russian).
62. Stawarz B, Smiegielski S, Petrovich Z. A comparison of transurethral and transrectal microwave hyperthermia in poor surgical risk benign prostatic hyperplasia patients. *J Urol* 1991; **146**, 353–7.
63. Qing-Shan Y, Rui-Zhi W, Guang-Qi S, *et al.* Combination preoperative radiation and endocavitary hyperthermia for rectal cancer: long-term results of 44 patients. *Int J Hyperthermia* 1993; **9**, 19–24.
64. Dahl O. Interaction of hyperthermia and chemotherapy. *Recent Results Cancer Res* 1988; **107**, 157–69.
65. Dahl O, Mella O. Hyperthermia and chemotherapeutic agents. In: SB Field, JW Hand, eds, *An Introduction to the Practical Aspects of Clinical Hyperthermia.* London: Taylor & Francis, 1990; 108–42.
66. Herman TS, Teicher BA, Jochelsen M, *et al.* Rationale for use of local hyperthermia with radiation therapy and selected anticancer drugs in locally advanced human malignancies. *Int J Hyperthermia* 1988; **4**, 143–58.
67. Lienard D, Ewalenko P, Delmotte J-J, *et al.* High-dose recombinant tumor necrosis factor alpha in combination with interferon gamma and melphalan in isolation perfusion in the limbs for melanoma and sarcoma. *J Clin Oncol* 1992; **10**, 52–60.
68. Urano M, Yamashita T, Suit HD, *et al.* Enhancement of thermal response of normal and malignant tissues by *Corynebacterium parvum*. *Cancer Res* 1984; **44**, 2341–7.
69. Wondergem J, Bulger RE, Strebel FR, *et al.* Effect of cisdiaminedichloroplatinum (II) combined with whole body hyperthermia on renal injury. *Cancer Res* 1988; **48**, 440–6.
70. Ghussen F, Kruger I, Groth W, *et al.* The role of regional hyperthermic cytostatic perfusion in the treatment of extremity melanoma. *Cancer* 1988; **61**, 654–9.
71. Aigner KR, Walther H, Helling HJ, *et al.* Pre Isolierte Leber Perfusion. *Beitr Oncol* 1985; **21**, 43–83.
72. Kubota Y, Shuin T, Miura T, *et al.* Treatment of bladder cancer with a combination of hyperthermia, radiation and bleomycin. *Cancer* 1984; **53**, 199–202.
73. Issels RD, Prenninger SW, Nagele A, *et al.* Ifosfamide plus etoposide combined with regional hyperthermia in patients with locally advanced sarcomas: a Phase II study. *J Clin Oncol* 1990; **8**, 1818–29.
74. Zhang Z, *et al.* The effect of hyperthermia–chemotherapy on bladder carcinoma: experimental and clinical studies. Abstracts of the satellite meeting of the International Congress on Hyperthermic Oncology, Beijing, China, September 1988.
75. Bull JMC, Cronau LH, Mansfield-Newman B, *et al.* Chemotherapy resistant sarcoma treated with whole body hyperthermia (WBH) combined with 1-3-bis(2-chloroethyl)-1-nitrosourea (BCNU). *Int J Hyperthermia* 1992; **8**, 297–304.
76. Engelhardt R. Summary of recent clinical experience in whole-body hyperthermia combined with chemotherapy. *Recent Results Cancer Res* 1988; **107**.
77. Arcangeli G, Cividalli A, Mauro F, *et al.* Enhanced effectiveness of Adriamycin and bleomycin combined with local hyperthermia in neck node metastases from head and neck cancer. *Tumori* 1979; **65**, 481–6.
78. Kohno F, Kaneshige E, Fugiwara K, *et al.* Thermochemotherapy for gynecological malignancies. In: J Overgaard, ed, *Hyperthermic Oncology*, Vol 1. London, Philadelphia: Taylor & Francis, 1984; 753–6.
79. Sugimachi H, Kitamura K, Baba K, *et al.* Hyperthermia combined with chemotherapy and irradiation for patients with carcinoma of the oesophagus — a prospective randomized trial. *Int J Hyperthermia* 1992; **8**, 289–95.

80.  Herman TS, Teichere BA, Chan V, *et al*. Effect of heat on the cytotoxicity and interaction with DNA of a series of platinum complexes. *Int J Radiat Oncol Biol Phys* 1989; **16(2)**, 443–9.
81.  Zamboglou N, Kolotas Ch, Audretsch W, *et al*. Hyperthermia and simultaneous radio-chemotherapy with mitoxantrone followed by salvage-surgery in local advanced breast cancer. *Abstracts of the Hyperthermia in Clinical Oncology Meeting*. Munich: BSD Medical Corp, 1993; 6.
82.  Suit HD. Potential for improving survival rates for cancer patients by improving efficiency of treatment of primary lesion. *Cancer* 1982; **50**, 1227–34.
83.  Kapp DS. Site and disease selection for hyperthermic clinical trials. *Int J Hyperthermia* 1986; **2**, 139–56.

# Further reading

The following is recommended as a 'standard textbook':
Field SB, Hand JW (eds). *An Introduction to the Practical Aspects of Clinical Hyperthermia*. London: Taylor & Francis, 1990.

# Index